Hepatic Fibrosis: Mechanisms and Therapies

Hepatic Fibrosis: Mechanisms and Therapies

Editor: Zendaya Watts

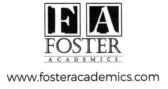

www.fosteracademics.com

www.fosteracademics.com

Cataloging-in-Publication Data

Hepatic fibrosis : mechanisms and therapies / edited by Zendaya Watts.
    p. cm.
Includes bibliographical references and index.
ISBN 978-1-64646-550-7
1. Liver--Fibrosis. 2. Liver--Fibrosis--Treatment. 3. Liver--Diseases.
4. Liver--Diseases--Treatment. I. Watts, Zendaya.
RC848.F53 H46 2023
616.362--dc23

Foster Academics,
118-35 Queens Blvd., Suite 400,
Forest Hills, NY 11375, USA

ISBN 978-1-64646-550-7 (Hardback)

Contents

Preface

Hepatic fibrosis is characterized by the scarring, overgrowth and hardening of different tissues of the liver and is caused by an excess buildup of extracellular matrix components such as collagen. It is the result of repeated wound-healing response of the liver to repeated injuries. It can be caused due to chronic liver diseases such as cystic fibrosis (CF), hepatitis B and hepatitis C. Cystic fibrosis refers to a type of inherited disease characterized by the accumulation of thick and sticky mucus that can harm many organs of the body. CF may lead to hepatic fibrosis, by causing mucus build up and blockage of the bile ducts in the liver. Scar tissues from fibrosis cannot repair themselves and also block the flow of blood within the liver, which leads to gradual death of even the healthy liver cells. This process leads to the creation of even more scar tissues. This book will help new researchers by foregrounding their knowledge on the mechanisms and therapies of hepatic fibrosis. It will serve as a valuable source of reference for graduate and postgraduate students.

The information shared in this book is based on empirical researches made by veterans in this field of study. The elaborative information provided in this book will help the readers further their scope of knowledge leading to advancements in this field.

Finally, I would like to thank my fellow researchers who gave constructive feedback and my family members who supported me at every step of my research.

Editor

New Drugs for Hepatic Fibrosis

Liang Shan[1,2,3,4], Fengling Wang[1], Dandan Zhai[1], Xiangyun Meng[1], Jianjun Liu[1*†] and Xiongwen Lv[2,3,4*†]

[1]Department of Pharmacy, The Second People's Hospital of Hefei, Hefei Hospital Affiliated to Anhui Medical University, Hefei, China, [2]Anhui Province Key Laboratory of Major Autoimmune Diseases, Anhui Medical University, Hefei, China, [3]Inflammation and Immune Mediated Diseases Laboratory of Anhui Province, Hefei, China, [4]The Key Laboratory of Major Autoimmune Diseases, Hefei, China

*Correspondence:
Jianjun Liu
Jianjun_liu2020@163.com
Xiongwen Lv
xiongwen_lv2019@163.com

The morbidity and mortality of hepatic fibrosis caused by various etiologies are high worldwide, and the trend is increasing annually. At present, there is no effective method to cure hepatic fibrosis except liver transplantation, and its serious complications threaten the health of patients and cause serious medical burdens. Additionally, there is no specific drug for the treatment of hepatic fibrosis, and many drugs with anti-hepatic fibrosis effects are in the research and development stage. Recently, remarkable progress has been made in the research and development of anti-hepatic fibrosis drugs targeting different targets. We searched websites such as PubMed, ScienceDirect, and Home-ClinicalTrials. gov and found approximately 120 drugs with anti-fibrosis properties, some of which are in phase II or III clinical trials. Additionally, although these drugs are effective against hepatic fibrosis in animal models, most clinical trials have shown poor results, mainly because animal models do not capture the complexity of human hepatic fibrosis. Besides, the effect of natural products on hepatic fibrosis has not been widely recognized at home and abroad. Furthermore, drugs targeting a single anti-hepatic fibrosis target are prone to adverse reactions. Therefore, currently, the treatment of hepatic fibrosis requires a combination of drugs that target multiple targets. Ten new drugs with potential for development against hepatic fibrosis were selected and highlighted in this mini-review, which provides a reference for clinical drug use.

Keywords: anti-hepatic fibrosis drug, hepatic fibrosis, HSCs, inflammation, oxidative stress

INTRODUCTION

Hepatic fibrosis is one of the most important manifestations of chronic liver injury (Roehlen et al., 2020). At present, the mechanism of its occurrence has not yet been clarified and there is a lack of effective treatment drugs (Gilgenkrantz et al., 2021). Hepatic fibrosis is a necessary process for most chronic liver diseases to develop into cirrhosis. Hepatic fibrosis is a pathological process of abnormal deposition of extracellular matrix (ECM) in liver tissue caused by a persistent injury-repair response, which further leads to abnormal changes in liver structure and function (Boyer-Diaz et al., 2021). The activation of hepatic stellate cells (HSCs) is the central link in the occurrence of hepatic fibrosis, and the inflammatory response to liver cell injury plays a key role in the development of fibrosis (Chen et al., 2021).

Hepatic fibrosis is caused by a variety of etiological factors, including alcoholism, viral hepatitis, autoimmune hepatitis, non-alcoholic steatohepatitis (NASH), primary biliary cirrhosis, and primary bile duct cirrhosis (intrinsic and extrinsic factors). Hepatic fibrosis is an inflammation disorder, and cytotoxicity, liver damage, and excessive accumulation of fat can cause the liver inflammatory

TABLE 1 | List of drugs currently being evaluated in phase II and phase III clinical trials.

Drug(s)	Mechanism	Research Unit	Research State	Trial Identification
Belapectin	Gal-3	Galectin Therapeutics	II	NCT02421094
Cenicriviroc	CCR2/5	Takeda	III	NCT03028740
Elafibranor	PPAR-α/δ	Genfit	III	NCT02704403
Emricasan	Pan-caspase	Conatus Pharmaceutical	IIb	NCT02686762
Liraglutide	GLP-1	Novo Nordisk	III	NCT02654665
Obeticholic acid	FXR	Intercept	III	NCT02548351
Pentoxifylline	TNF-α	US Pharm Holdings	II	NCT02283710
Pirfenidone	PDE	Marnac	II	NCT02161952
Simtuzumab	LOXL2	Gilead	II	NCT01707472
Sorafenib	VEGFR-2/PDGF-β	Bayer	III	NCT01849588

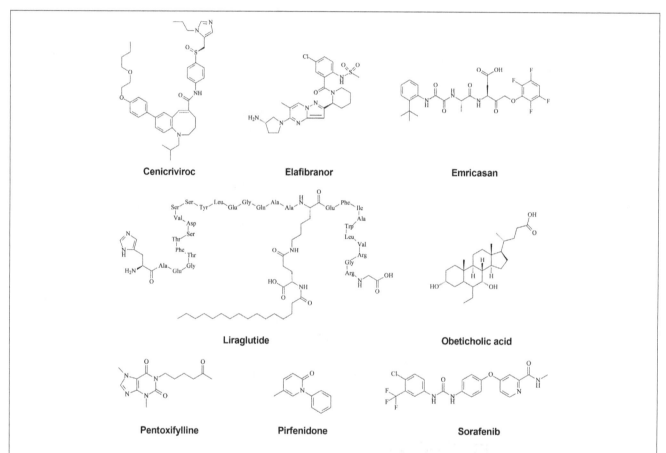

FIGURE 1 | Structural formula of new drugs with anti-hepatic fibrosis effects. (1) Cenicriviroc is a dual antagonist of CCR2/5, which also inhibits both HIV-1 and HIV-2, and displays potent anti-hepatic fibrosis activity. (2) Elafibranor is a double agonist of PPARα/δ, and both animal experiments and clinical trials have found that it has anti-hepatic fibrosis activity. (3) Emricasan is an irreversible pan-caspase inhibitor, which is currently in a phase 2 clinical trial to test its efficacy in treating liver injury and fibrosis, although its clinical trial results are controversial. (4) Liraglutide is a GLP-1 receptor agonist used clinically to treat type 2 diabetes, which functions by ameliorating the progression of NAFLD in patients with T2DM. (5) Obeticholic acid is a potent, selective, and orally active FXR agonist; FXR has been shown to reduce inflammatory mediator expression in HSCs via the induction of PPARγ, suggesting that FXR is an ideal target for the treatment of hepatic fibrosis. (6) Pentoxifylline is an orally active non-selective PDE inhibitor, with anti-inflammatory and anti-proliferation effects. PDE has a strong anti-fibrosis effect but needs more in-depth research. (7) Pirfenidone has broad-spectrum anti-fibrosis effects and is the first drug to demonstrate some efficacy for IPF, which was approved by the FDA in 2008. The mechanism of action of Pirfenidone may be related to the reduction of TGF-β-induced signal transduction pathways. (8) Sorafenib is a multikinase inhibitor of Raf-1, B-Raf, and VEGFR-2, an inhibitor of tyrosine protein kinases that targets the Raf/Mek/Erk pathway. Animal experiments have shown that Sorafenib has anti-fibrosis effects, and the mechanism may be related to inhibiting the TGF-β1/Smad3 pathway.

response. Inflammatory cytokines released by inflammatory cells promote the activation of HSCs, which leads to an increase in ECM release and ultimately causes hepatic fibrosis. Intrinsic factors encompass genetic alterations of cellular pathways leading to the activation of inflammatory pathways such as nuclear factor kappa-light-chain-enhancer of activated B cells

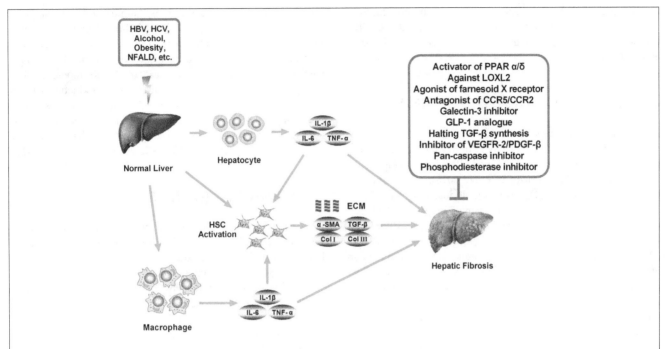

FIGURE 2 | Main targets of new drugs against hepatic fibrosis. Hepatic fibrosis can be induced by various factors, including HBV, HCV, alcohol, obesity, and NFALD, all of which can stimulate the normal liver to induce an inflammatory response. Various cells in the liver, mainly hepatocytes, macrophages, and HSCs, secrete inflammatory cytokines (mainly IL-1β, IL-6, and TNF-α) after receiving stimulation. A large number of inflammatory cytokines continuously stimulate HSCs, inducing activation, proliferation, and the secretion of many fibrosis cytokines, including α-SMA, TGF-β, collagen-I, and Collagen-III, which are important components of the ECM. The chronic accumulation of ECM eventually leads to hepatic fibrosis. Inhibiting the activation and proliferation of HSCs and reducing the accumulation of ECM are the most important methods to reverse hepatic fibrosis. Numerous recent studies have found many targets for inhibiting the process of hepatic fibrosis, which has led to the development of novel therapeutic drugs, mainly activators of PPAR α/δ, agonists of FXR, antagonists of CCR2/5, Galectin-3 inhibitor, GLP-1 analog, inhibitors of VEGFR-2/PDGF-β, LOXL2 inhibitor, Pan-caspase inhibitor, a Phosphodiesterase inhibitor, and TGF-β signaling inhibitors.

(NF-κB), among others. Extrinsic components include inflammatory pathways activated by the liver microenvironment, such as chemokines, cytokines, and adhesion molecules. Although 120 drugs are currently being evaluated for treating hepatic fibrosis, none have yet been approved by the United States Food and Drug Administration (FDA) to treat the disease (Roehlen et al., 2020; Gilgenkrantz et al., 2021). However, many phases II and III clinical trials are ongoing, and a new chapter for treating hepatic fibrosis is expected in the near future (**Table 1**) (**Figure 1**). The main reason for the failure of the 120 drugs is that most are in the stage of animal experiments or clinical trials, with different shortcomings and a lack of adequate data on evidence-based medicine.

BELAPECTIN (GALACTOARABINO-RHAMNOGALACTURONATE, GR-MD-02)

Belapectin is a galectin-3 antagonist developed by Galectin (Rotman and Sanyal, 2017; Neuschwander-Tetri, 2020). Early preclinical studies have shown that Belapectin is a candidate drug for anti-fibrosis research and can reverse the degree of hepatic fibrosis in steatohepatitis mice and prevent collagen deposition

before the occurrence of fibrotic cells (**Figures 2, 3**) (Rotman and Sanyal, 2017; Iacobini et al., 2011). Elevated galactosin-3 levels are associated with NASH and induce hepatic fibrosis in mice (Iacobini et al., 2011; Harrison et al., 2016). Belapectin, an inhibitor of galactosin-3, can alleviate hepatic fibrosis and portal hypertension in rats and was shown to be safe and well-tolerated in a phase I trial (NCT01899859) (Harrison et al., 2016). Galectin is currently in a phase III trial to evaluate Belapectin for the prevention and treatment of nonalcoholic fatty liver disease (NAFLD), portal hypertension, fibrosis, psoriasis, liver function decline, and other diseases (Chalasani et al., 2020).

Belapectin single and three weekly repeated at 2, 4, and 8 mg/kg demonstrated no meaningful clinical differences in treatment-emergent adverse events, vital signs, electrocardiographic findings, or laboratory tests. Pharmacokinetic parameters showed a dose-dependent relationship, with evidence of drug accumulation following 8 mg/kg (Harrison et al., 2016). Results of a 52-weeks phase IIb trial suggest that Belapectin is an effective anti-fibrotic drug for compensatory NASH cirrhosis (NCT02462967) (Chalasani et al., 2020). Because the treatment can take many years, there is an urgent need for effective drug candidates with good safety and tolerability (NCT02421094) (Harrison et al., 2018b). Overall, the clinical success of Belapectin indicates a promising path for the continued clinical development of Belapectin in compensatory NASH cirrhosis, which could make it the first anti-fibrosis drug candidate to win approval from NASH regulators (Chalasani et al., 2018).

CENICRIVIROC (TAK-652, TBR-652)

Cenicriviroc is a chemokine receptor 2/5 (CCR2/5) antagonist that acts differently from previous anti-HIV1 drugs and holds great promise in the field of anti-AIDS drugs (**Figure 1**) (Friedman et al., 2016; Friedman et al., 2018). The formula of Cenicriviroc is $C_{41}H_{52}N_4O_4S$, with a molecular weight of 696.94. Studies have found that monocyte chemokine protein-1 (MCP-1), chemokine C-C motif chemokine 2 (CCL2), and regulated upon activation, normal T cells expressed and secreted (RAN-TES) can promote the aggregation of monocytes/macrophages in blood to liver inflammatory sites through CCR2/5, as well as produce various cytokines, such as transforming growth factor-β (TGF-β), tumor necrosis factor-α (TNF-α), interleukin-1β (IL-1β), and IL-6, to further activate HSCs and generate ECM, which leads to the formation of hepatic fibrosis (NCT02217475) (Friedman et al., 2016; Lefebvre et al., 2016a; Lefebvre et al., 2016b). Additionally, CCR2 and CCR5 are highly expressed in activated HSCs, which directly or indirectly mediate various biological functions of HSCs after binding with its ligand and participate in the formation of hepatic fibrosis (NCT02217475) (Lefebvre et al., 2016a; Lefebvre et al., 2016b). Therefore, CCR2 and CCR5 have become important targets for anti-fibrosis therapy (**Figures 2, 3**).

Cenicriviroc is a novel oral drug developed in collaboration between Takeda and Tobira Therapeutics. The plasma half-life of Cenicriviroc is 30–40 h, and it can be administered once a day (NCT02217475) (Lefebvre et al., 2016a; Friedman et al., 2016). Cenicriviroc has shown good safety, providing new ideas and methods for the clinical prevention and treatment of hepatic fibrosis (Lefebvre et al., 2016a; Friedman et al., 2016). Animal experiments have shown that Cenicriviroc significantly alleviates thioacetamide (TAA)-induced hepatic fibrosis in rats, mainly by inhibiting HSC synthesis of collagen I, thereby inhibiting collagen deposition in the liver and reducing liver tissue inflammation (Lefebvre et al., 2016b; Kruger et al., 2018). Therefore, Cenicriviroc may represent an effective drug against hepatic fibrosis.

Clinical studies have found that Cenicriviroc has excellent pharmacokinetic properties in the human body and is well tolerated without causing dose-limiting adverse reactions (Friedman et al., 2016; Friedman et al., 2018). Cenicriviroc is also well absorbed and slowly eliminated (Anstee et al., 2020; Reimer et al., 2020). Additionally, the majority of adverse reactions were mild (grade 1 or 2) and dose-independent, with gastrointestinal disturbances (63%) and systemic adverse reactions (37%) being the most common. Grade 3 adverse events (abscesses) were reported by one subject in each of the placebo and 75 mg (qd) groups, but they were not considered to be related to the product. There were no grade 4 adverse reactions, severe adverse reactions, death, or withdrawal from

the study due to adverse reactions (Sumida and Yoneda, 2018; Sumida et al., 2019). A phase II trial showed that Cenicriviroc rapidly blocks CCR2 and CCR5 (Sumida and Yoneda, 2018; Sumida et al., 2019), and it has been shown that 150 mg Cenicriviroc can be used to treat mild and moderate liver injury, with good tolerance. The pharmacokinetic data of Cenicriviroc is relatively complete and it represents a promising drug for treating hepatic fibrosis (Lefebvre et al., 2016a). Cenicriviroc is currently in a phase III trial (NCT03028740) (Sumida and Yoneda, 2018; Pedrosa et al., 2020).

ELAFIBRANOR (GFT505)

Elafibranor is a double agonist of peroxisome proliferator-activated receptors α/δ (PPARα/δ) developed by Genfit, France; its molecular formula is $C_{22}H_{24}O_4S$, and its molecular weight is 384.489 (Boeckmans et al., 2019; Cheng et al., 2019). The chemical structure is shown in **Figure 1**. Elafibranor alleviates NASH symptoms through various mechanisms, including increased fatty acid oxidation, improved lipid profile, increased insulin sensitivity, and anti-inflammatory and anti-fibrosis effects (**Figures 2, 3**) (Alukal and Thuluvath, 2019; Ratziu et al., 2019).

Animal experiments have shown that Elafibranor administration can effectively reduce hepatic steatosis, inflammation, fibrosis, and the level of liver dysfunction biomarkers, as well as inhibit the expression of pro-inflammatory and pro-fibrosis genes; it is effective in both the prevention and treatment of hepatic fibrosis (Schuppan et al., 2018; Baandrup Kristiansen et al., 2019; Roth et al., 2019). Elafibranor treatment protects against hepatic steatosis and inflammatory progression (Ratziu et al., 2016; Baandrup Kristiansen et al., 2019), and has shown preventive and therapeutic effects on CCl₄-induced hepatic fibrosis in rats (Schuppan et al., 2018). In pharmacokinetic studies conducted in rats, Elafibranor and its metabolites were rapidly excreted into bile and underwent extensive enterohepatic circulation (Schuppan et al., 2018). High concentrations of Elafibranor and/or its metabolites were detected in the liver and intestines, with little distribution in other tissues (Schuppan et al., 2018; Roth et al., 2019).

No toxicity or carcinogenesis of Elafibranor was found in long-term animal toxicity tests (Roth et al., 2019; Gore et al., 2020). From 2011 to 2015, Genfit completed a series of phase I clinical trials of Elafibranor, which were found to be both safe and well-tolerated. The safety of Elafibranor is generally good in many clinical trials, and no serious adverse events have occurred to date (Boeckmans et al., 2019; Cheng et al., 2019; Alukal et al., 2016). In completed phase II clinical trials, Elafibranor has shown a certain therapeutic efficacy and good safety and tolerability (Ratziu et al., 2016; Alukal and Thuluvath, 2019). Fast-track approval was granted by the FDA in February 2014, and a phase III clinical trial began in March 2016 (Ratziu et al., 2016; Alukal and Thuluvath, 2019). In January 2018, Genfit announced that the FDA had approved Elafibranor for the pediatric study program and would begin a clinical trial for the treatment of pediatric NASH. Elafibranor is currently in phase III of the clinical trial,

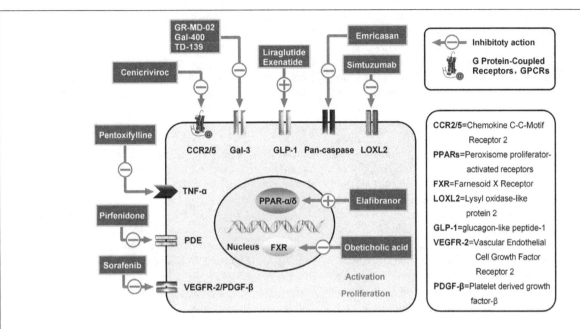

FIGURE 3 | Potential candidates for hepatic fibrosis and their mechanisms of action. Inhibiting the activation and proliferation of HSCs is an important method for the prevention and treatment of hepatic fibrosis. Various representative drugs have emerged for different targets. (1) PPARs are members of the nuclear receptor superfamily, and the PPAR agonist Elafibranor can inhibit liver fibrosis through direct anti-inflammatory effects and indirect improvement of the oxidative stress state. (2) Additionally, a representative FXR receptor agonist, Obeticholic acid, has been shown to reduce liver inflammation and promote ECM degradation to alleviate hepatic fibrosis. (3) Simtuzumab is a monoclonal antibody currently being developed by Gilead for NASH, cirrhosis, and advanced hepatic fibrosis blocking of LOXL2. LOXL2 is a protease that modifies the ECM by promoting the cross-linking of collagen fibers and is believed to play an important role in tumor progression and fibrosis. (4) Emricasan is an irreversible pan-caspase inhibitor, which can reduce the activity of caspases to improve the inflammatory environment and inhibit HSC activation. (5) The GLP-1R agonist Liraglutide can inhibit the formation of ECM and reduce the liver inflammatory response and fibrosis process. (6) Belapectin is a galectin-3 antagonist, which can alleviate hepatic fibrosis and portal hypertension in rats and was found to be safe and well-tolerated in a phase I trial. (7) The CCR2/5 antagonist Cenicriviroc can improve hepatic fibrosis by inhibiting liver inflammation. Cenicriviroc is not only effective for early hepatic fibrosis but also feasible for maintenance treatment in patients with advanced fibrosis. (8) Pentoxifylline is a non-specific PDE inhibitor, which can increase intracellular cAMP concentration and plays an anti-hepatic fibrosis role by inhibiting TNF-α production. (9) Attenuating TGF-β-induced signal transduction pathways can inhibit hepatic fibrosis, such as via Pirfenidone (10) Sorafenib can inhibit VEGFR-2 and PDGF-β to alleviate hepatic fibrosis.

and subgroup analyses of results support its potential efficacy in patients with severe NASH (Boeckmans et al., 2019; Cheng et al., 2019). Currently, there is no approved effective drug for NASH (Alukal and Thuluvath, 2019; Boeckmans et al., 2019). Of nearly 200 candidates in development worldwide, Elafibranor is one of the most highly anticipated drugs for NASH to hit the market.

In a 52-weeks phase II study in patients with NASH without cirrhosis, 276 patients were randomly assigned to receive Elafibranor at either 80 mg or 120 mg daily or a placebo. Even though the trial was not designed with antifibrotic goals, it is worth noting that among the patients who responded to 120 mg Elafibranor (n = 17), there was a reduction in fibrosis ($p < 0.001$) compared to non-responders to the same regimen. However, at present, there are limited pharmacokinetic data on this drug in the human body, which needs further study (Ratziu et al., 2016). On 11 May 2020, Genfit announced that in its phase III trial of Elafibranor in the treatment of NASH, the drug failed to significantly improve patients' NASH histological symptoms, and in some cases, exacerbated hepatic fibrosis compared to placebo (Guaraldi et al., 2020; Shen and Lu, 2021). A total of 1070 patients with NASH were randomized (2:1) to receive Elafibranor 120 mg/day or a placebo (Guaraldi et al., 2020; Shen and Lu, 2021). After 72 weeks, 19.2% and 14.7% of

patients treated with Elafibranor and placebo had improved NASH histology without worsening hepatic fibrosis, respectively, 24.5% and 22.4% of patients with at least a grade of fibrosis improvement, however, these results were not statistically significant. The safety of Elafibranor was consistent with the results of previous studies (Guaraldi et al., 2020; Shen and Lu, 2021) in that no adverse effects, such as increased fluid retention and heart failure, were mediated by PPARγ (Guaraldi et al., 2020; Shen and Lu, 2021).

EMRICASAN (IDN-6556, PF-03491390)

Emricasan is a pioneering and irreversible pan-caspase inhibitor that is orally administered (**Figure 1**) (Garcia-Tsao et al., 2019; Barreyro et al., 2015). The formula of Emricasan is $C_{26}H_{27}F_4N_3O_7$, and its molecular weight is 569.50. Emricasan can be retained in the liver for a long time and can reduce the activity of caspases, which mediate inflammation, cell death, and apoptosis (Garcia-Tsao et al., 2019; Barreyro et al., 2015; Gracia-Sancho et al., 2019). By reducing the activity of these enzymes, Emricasan may block the development of liver disease (Gracia-Sancho et al., 2019; Shiffman et al., 2019). Emricasan, developed by Conatus, has been shown in preclinical studies to reduce apoptosis, improve the inflammatory environment and inhibit HSC activation (**Figures 2, 3**) (Barreyro et al., 2015; Gracia-Sancho et al., 2019; Shiffman et al., 2019).

Emricasan reduced liver damage in NASH but had no significant effect on metabolic disorders (Frenette et al., 2019; Harrison et al., 2020). Emricasan was previously demonstrated to inhibit some of the liver enzymes which lead to liver inflammation and fibrosis (Frenette et al., 2019; Harrison et al., 2020). In a mouse model of NASH, treatment with Emricasan attenuated hepatic fibrosis and the activation of HSCs (Barreyro et al., 2015; Gracia-Sancho et al., 2019). Emricasan is currently in a phase II clinical trial to test its efficacy in treating liver injury and fibrosis through chronic HCV infection (Frenette et al., 2019). In two previous trials, Emricasan was both well-tolerated and safe, and the results were consistent with those of 19 previous clinical studies (Frenette et al., 2019; Shiffman et al., 2019). Emricasan treatment was safe and well-tolerated, with adverse events, severe events, abnormal experimental results, vital signs, cancers, and infections occurring at similarly low rates in the Emricasan treatment group and placebo groups (Frenette et al., 2019; Shiffman et al., 2019; Harrison et al., 2020). The most common adverse reactions in the Emricasan group were headache (16%), nausea (14%), and fatigue (9%) (Frenette et al., 2019; Shiffman et al., 2019; Harrison et al., 2020). Results from a multicenter phase b clinical trial suggest that Emricasan improves liver function in patients with severe cirrhosis (NCT02686762) (Garcia-Tsao et al., 2020). Moreover, a 28-days randomized clinical trial of Emricasan assessed the efficacy, safety, and tolerability of Emricasan in subjects with NAFLD, in which the subjects were randomized to Emricasan 25 mg twice daily or a matching placebo. The results showed that Emricasan decreased ALT and biomarkers in subjects with NAFLD and raised AST after 28 days (NCT02077374). Emricassan has a high first-pass metabolism, but the current pharmacokinetic data are mainly from animal experiments, with a lack of complete human experimental data (Garcia-Tsao et al., 2019).

LIRAGLUTIDE (VICTOZA)

Liraglutide is a Glucagon-Like Peptide (GLP-1) analog developed by Novo Nordisk to decrease blood sugar in patients with type 2 diabetes mellitus (T2DM) (**Figure 1**) (Kahal et al., 2014; Zoubek et al., 2017). The formula of Liraglutide is $C_{172}H_{265}N_{43}O_{51}$, and its molecular weight is 3751.26. GLP-1 can increase insulin release, decrease glucagon secretion, reduce hepatic steatosis, and improve hepatic fibrosis (Fagone et al., 2016; Briand et al., 2020). GLP-1R agonists can reduce liver cell apoptosis and endoplasmic reticulum stress through various mechanisms. Previuous studies of mechanisms have been proposed, including an increase in cyclic adenosine monophosphate (cAMP) production, activation of an AMP-activated protein kinase (AMPK)-dependent pathway in hepatocytes increasing fatty acid oxidation and decrease in lipogenesis, and/or an increase in hepatic insulin signaling and sensitivity with GLP-

1 and subsequent improvement of the hepatic glucose metabolism. Additionally, Liraglutide has been found to reduce fatty acid accumulation, in mice fed a high-fat diet by enhancing autophagy and reducing endoplasmic reticulum stress-related apoptosis. Furthermore, the GLP-1R agonist can reduce liver cell apoptosis and endoplasmic reticulum stress by inhibiting activation of the NACHT, LRR and PYD domains-containing protein 3 (NALP3) inflammasome and NF-κB signaling pathway. Besides, Liraglutide can promote liver glucose and lipid metabolism, and inhibit the secretion of inflammatory cytokines, which may explain its ability to alleviate the process of hepatic fibrosis (Kahal et al., 2014; Zoubek et al., 2017; Fagone et al., 2016). Studies have also shown that Liraglutide can inhibit the formation of ECM, reduce the liver inflammatory response and fibrosis process, and slow and improve the progression of NAFLD in patients with T2DM (**Figures 2, 3**) (Kahal et al., 2014; Fagone et al., 2016; Zoubek et al., 2017).

The results of animal experiments showed that Liraglutide could significantly reduce collagen fibers in NAFLD models (Fagone et al., 2016; Choi et al., 2019; Briand et al., 2020). Moreover, Liraglutide significantly reduced levels of inflammatory factors, such as IL-6 and TNF-α, and liver fibrosis factors in the NAFLD model group (Fagone et al., 2016; Choi et al., 2019; Briand et al., 2020). Liraglutide may play an important role in NAFLD by activating the SIRT1/AMPK pathway, regulating key regulatory molecules of lipid synthesis and metabolism, and inhibiting the *de novo* synthesis of fatty acids (Kahal et al., 2014). Early intervention with Liraglutide can reduce blood glucose, inhibit fat synthesis, reduce insulin resistance, inflammation, fibrosis, and oxidative stress damage, thereby alleviating NAFLD, which may be related to the activation of SIRT1/AMPK and its downstream genes (Kahal et al., 2014). These results indicate that Liraglutide may represent a potential drug for the treatment of NAFLD, with SIRT1 as a potential therapeutic target.

Recently, in addition to its good hypoglycemic effect, Liraglutide has also been shown to inhibit myocardial fibrosis, renal fibrosis, and hepatic fibrosis (Kahal et al., 2014). Current studies suggest that inflammation is the core cause of hepatic fibrosis, which is mainly associated with NF-κB activation, and initiation of the NF-κB signaling pathway (Gilgenkrantz et al., 2021). Therefore, inhibiting NF-κB mitigates various inflammatory liver diseases, including hepatic fibrosis. Liraglutide may play anti-inflammatory and anti-fibrosis roles by inhibiting the activation of NF-κB and reducing the production of superoxide (Fagone et al., 2016). Liraglutide can also reduce the degree of tissue collagen deposition and improve tissue fibrosis (Armstrong and Newsome, 2015; Choi et al., 2019; Briand et al., 2020), and may play an anti-fibrosis role by regulating some important links in the fibrotic process (Armstrong et al., 2015; Armstrong et al., 2016; Gaborit et al., 2016; Choi et al., 2019). The data from genetic toxicity studies show that Liraglutide is not toxic in the human body (Armstrong et al., 2015; Armstrong et al., 2016; Gaborit et al., 2016). Results of a phase II multicentered trial showed improvement in NASH and no further increase in hepatic fibrosis in 39% of participants in the treatment group compared to only 9% in the placebo group (NCT02654665). Pharmacokinetic studies have shown that about 99% of Liraglutide binds to albumin in the body, allowing it to escape glomerular filtration and extend its duration of action (Alruwaili et al., 2021). It is expected to be one of the candidate drugs for the treatment of hepatic fibrosis in the future.

OBETICHOLIC ACID (INT-747, 6-ECDCA, 6A-ETHYLCHENODEOXYCHOLIC ACID)

Farnesoid X Receptor (FXR) is a member of the nuclear receptor superfamily and is classified as NR1H4 (**Figure 1**) (Eslam et al., 2019; Anfuso et al., 2020). FXR is mainly expressed in the enterohepatic system, FXRα1/2 and FXRα3/4 are expressed in the liver, while FXRα3/4 is mainly expressed in the intestine. FXR is widely involved in the pathophysiological processes of many diseases in the enterohepatic system (Armstrong et al., 2015; Gawrieh et al., 2019). Activated FXR plays a protective role in various chronic liver diseases (Brunt et al., 2019; Eaton et al., 2020), and FXR agonists include Obecholic Acid, GW4064, WAY-362450, PR20606, GS9674, and LJN452, which are a batch of synthetic or semi-synthetic FXR agonists. Among them, GW4064 and Obecholic Acid are widely used. The formula of Obecholic Acid is $C_{26}H_{44}O_4$, and its molecular weight is 420.63. GW4064 is a synthetic nonsteroidal FXR agonist (**Figures 2, 3**).

FXR has been found to be associated with hepatic fibrosis, cirrhosis, and portal hypertension (Younossi et al., 2019; Hindson, 2020; Siddiqui et al., 2020). The activation of HSCs is a key factor in the development of hepatic fibrosis, and it has been previously reported that FXR activation mitigates hepatic inflammation. One mechanism by which FXR reduces inflammatory mediator expression in HSCs is via the induction of PPARγ. Additionally, FXR activation represses gluconeogenesis, TG synthesis, and VLDL export via SHP, a primary FXR-responsive gene, which contributes to regulating FXR target genes. FXR modulates many genes by regulating SHP. Besides, regulation of the MMP/TIMP balance is essential for the transition of the physiological ECM into pathological ECM. The FXR agonist Obecholic Acid has been shown to induce MMP2-9 activity and a dose-dependent reduction of collagen. Therefore, FXR inhibits HSC activation by activating the PPARγ and SHP-TIMP pathways. Additionally, FXR improves portal hypertension by increasing eNOs activity and reducing vascular remodeling (Anfuso et al., 2020). These findings, together with the regulation of metabolic and inflammatory functions, strongly suggest that FXR is an ideal target for the treatment of hepatic fibrosis, cirrhosis, and portal hypertension (Brunt et al., 2019; Gawrieh et al., 2019; Younossi et al., 2019). Studies have shown that the FXR agonist Obecholic Acid can reduce liver inflammation and fibrosis in TAA-induced toxic cirrhosis, and even reverse hepatic fibrosis (Anfuso et al., 2020). FXR inhibits the negative regulator NF-κB by up-regulating IκBα, resulting in reduced expression of pro-fibrotic cytokines and related markers of hepatocyte transformation, thereby weakening the effect of inflammatory cytokines (Younossi et al., 2019).

Hepatic fibrosis is caused by persistent liver injury and is characterized by inflammation, activation of HSCs, accumulation of ECM, and destruction of the liver structure. HSCs proliferate and transform into myofibroblasts, which deposit collagen I and fibronectin in the ECM and eventually produce fibrogenic cytokines (Brunt et al., 2019; Eslam et al., 2019; Anfuso et al., 2020). FXR prevents the activation of HSCs through FXR-PPARγ or FXR-SHP-TIMP pathways. In animal models of hepatic fibrosis induced by TAA, bile duct ligation (BDL), and CCl₄, Obecholic Acid significantly reduced the expression of hepatic fibrosis genes and proteins, as well as the area of hepatic fibrosis parenchymal tissue (Eslam et al., 2019; Anfuso et al., 2020). The FXR agonist Obecholic Acid has also been shown to increase the interaction between FXR and Smad3 and alleviate CCl₄-induced liver injury and fibrosis. Studies have shown that FXR gene knockout mice can increase liver inflammation and fibrosis, suggesting that the loss of FXR function is more likely to induce liver inflammation and fibrosis. Clinical trials also showed that Obecholic Acid significantly improves hepatic fibrosis, ballooning degeneration, steatosis, and lobular infiltration (Brunt et al., 2019; Younossi et al., 2019). In addition to Obecholic Acid, other FXR agonists such as PX-102, Way-362450, and EDP-305 have been shown to have protective effects against diet-induced fibrosis such as MCD (Anfuso et al., 2020). Taken together, these preclinical studies support the anti-fibrosis effects of FXR agonists.

The FXR agonist obecholangitis was approved by the FDA on 27 May 2016, for treating primary biliary cholangitis (PBC) in adults (Eaton et al., 2020). Results from two phase II clinical trials showed that Obecholic Acid significantly improved the disease activity scores in patients with NAFLD, as well as steatosis, lobular inflammation, ballooning degeneration, and hepatic fibrosis (Younossi et al., 2019; Anfuso et al., 2020). The results of a phase II clinical trial (NCT00501592) showed that Obeticholic Acid significantly improved insulin sensitivity in patients with T2DM complicated with NAFLD, significantly improved hepatic fibrosis, and liver enzymology indexes ($p < 0.05$). Additionally, there were no adverse reactions during the trial, and both safety and tolerability were good. However, elevated serum alkaline phosphatase and total cholesterol concentrations in patients during the study should be seriously considered.

Recently, a phase III clinical trial of Obecholic Acid in the treatment of NASH with fibrosis has been completed (Younossi et al., 2019; Hindson, 2020). In the trial, 18% of patients who received 10 mg Obecholic Acid and 23% who received 25 mg Obecholic Acid showed improvement in hepatic fibrosis. Another double-blind placebo-controlled trial investigating the efficacy and safety of Obecholic Acid in the treatment of type 2 diabetes complicated by NAFLD also demonstrated a significant reduction in hepatic fibrosis markers in patients taking 25 mg Obecholic Acid (Younossi et al., 2019; Hindson, 2020). These clinical studies demonstrate that the FXR agonist Obecholic Acid is promising for the treatment of hepatic fibrosis. Recently, some scholars have suggested that specific micro RNA is also a target gene of FXR, which can regulate the process of hepatic fibrosis. After mice and human HSCs were treated with the FXR agonist GW4064, miR-

29a levels increased, ECM accumulation decreased, and hepatic fibrosis was alleviated. Additionally, the level of FXR in liver tissue of patients with severe hepatic fibrosis was decreased and the level of miR-199a-3p was increased, while the expression of miR-199a-3p was inhibited after activation of FXR, which further inhibited the proliferation of HSCs and alleviated hepatic fibrosis.

Since Obecholic Acid was marketed in May 2016, 19 deaths have been confirmed, of which 8 have provided the cause of death information and seven patients with moderate to severe liver dysfunction may have been caused by the use of the drug beyond the recommended dose (Younossi et al., 2019). The FDA recommends that physicians determine a patient's baseline liver function before administering Obecholic Acid and strictly adhere to the approved dosing regimen (Younossi et al., 2019; Siddiqui et al., 2020). The most common adverse reactions shown in clinical trials were severe pruritus, which resulted in discontinued treatment in some patients at higher doses. Some patients also experienced fatigue, abdominal pain and discomfort, arthralgia, constipation, elevated blood sugar, elevated blood lipids, dizziness, and dysarthria, which may be caused by cerebral ischemia. The observed increase in LDL and decrease in HDL suggest that this drug may lead to the occurrence of cardiovascular and cerebrovascular events (Eslam et al., 2019; Younossi et al., 2019; Siddiqui et al., 2020). However, these adverse reactions can be effectively alleviated after dose control and medication regimen adjustment. Obecholic Acid is subject to enterohepatic circulation, and the pharmacokinetic parameters of the active metabolites show that food may increase its absorption (Wang et al., 2021).

PENTOXIFYLLINE

Pentoxifylline, a derivative of Methylxanthine, is a non-specific phosphodiesterase inhibitor developed by Pharm Holdings, with various pharmacological characteristics, mainly used in cerebrovascular diseases (**Figure 1**) (Oberti et al., 1997; Desmoulière et al., 1999; Chooklin and Perejaslov, 2003). The formula of Methylxanthine is $C_{13}H_{18}N_4O_3$, and its molecular weight is 278.31. Recent studies have found that Pentoxifylline also has a strong anti-fibrosis effect, which can effectively inhibit hepatic fibrosis, kidney fibrosis, and skin scar formation (Peterson, 1993; Pinzani et al., 1996; Verma-Gandhu et al., 2007). Pentoxobromine is a first-line drug for the treatment of AH, which has anti-inflammatory, anti-hepatic fibrosis, and immunological regulation effects (Louvet et al., 2008; Ali et al., 2018). However, the specific mechanism of Pentoxifylline is still unclear (**Figures 2, 3**).

The Hedgehog signaling pathway plays an important role in cell differentiation and proliferation during embryonic development. Recent studies have found that the hedgehog signaling pathway is involved in the repair of liver injury and the occurrence of hepatic fibrosis (Solhi et al., 2022). Furthermore, Pentoxifylline may block the activation of HSCs by inhibiting the hedgehog signaling pathway and inhibit the occurrence of hepatic fibrosis in Schistosoma, and is therefore expected to be an effective drug for the prevention and treatment

of Schistosoma in clinical practice. Additionally, PPAR-α and NF-κB P65 have been studied in many fields and are closely related to AH due to their anti-inflammatory, anti-oxidation, and anti-hepatic fibrosis effects, and regulation of fat metabolism (Ali et al., 2018). Current studies have found that Pentoxifylline can treat AH in rats, and its mechanism may be related to the upregulation of PPAR-α expression and downregulation of NF-κB P65 expression (Satapathy et al., 2007; Ali et al., 2018).

Through non-selective inhibition of phosphodiesterase, Pentoxifylline reduces intracellular cAMP hydrolysis to 5-AMP and increases intracellular cAMP concentrations, inducing corresponding changes in cells and inhibition of the calcium ion influx (Pinzani et al., 1996). Pentoxifylline improves hemorheology in many complementary ways, including reducing blood and plasma viscosity, reducing plasma fibrinogen, and promoting fibrinolysis. Additionally, Pentoxifylline improves blood permeability in tissues by enhancing the plasticity of erythrocytes and reducing neutrophil activation. Pentoxifylline has a protective effect on the liver by improving liver hemorheology and has anti-inflammatory and anti-fibrosis effects (Zein et al., 2012; Park et al., 2014). As an anti-inflammatory and anti-fibrosis drug, Pentoxifylline can inhibit the production of TNF-α, a pro-inflammatory cytokine, at 400 mg/day, 3 times per day for 28 days, which can effectively delay the disease progression in patients with severe alcoholic liver disease. Additionally, the anti-fibrosis and anti-inflammatory effects of Pentoxifylline have certain protective effects on the liver. The mechanism of action of Pentoxifylline is completely different from that of other commonly used liver protective drugs, so a combination of Pentoxifylline can produce complementary effects (Lebrec et al., 2010; Zein et al., 2012; Park et al., 2014).

As a non-specific phosphodiesterase inhibitor, Pentoxifylline has anti-inflammatory and anti-fibrosis effects, improves hepatic hemorheology, inhibits hyperplasia, and has certain effects on the prevention and treatment of cirrhosis and reduces mortality of liver disease (Ali et al., 2018). Existing clinical evidence shows that Pentoxifylline combined with corticosteroids can reduce the risk of death in severe alcoholic hepatitis (Louvet et al., 2008). Pentoxifylline can improve the histological characteristics of NAFLD/NASH, prevent hepatic steatosis, and improve liver function in patients with non-dyslipidemia NAFLD (Satapathy et al., 2007; Zein et al., 2012). Furthermore, Pentoxifylline can improve the survival rate of patients with HRS and is expected to be a therapeutic drug for HRS. Pentoxifylline hit the market earlier, and its efficacy, toxicity, and pharmacokinetic data are relatively complete. Previous studies have found that Pentoxifylline can be rapidly and widely absorbed from the gastrointestinal tract of animals and humans and rapidly metabolized systemically (Ward and Clissold, 1987).

PIRFENIDONE

Pirfenidone, chemically known as 5-Methyl-N-phenyl-2-1H-pyridone, is a new kind of pyridinone compound with a broad spectrum of anti-fibrosis effects, which can prevent and reverse the formation of fibrosis and scars (**Figure 1**) (Grizzi, 2009; Di Sario et al., 2002). The formula of Pirfenidone is $C_{12}H_{11}NO$, and its molecular weight is 185.22. Pirfenidone, marketed by Shionogi in 2008 and approved by the FDA, is the first drug to demonstrate some efficacy for idiopathic pulmonary fibrosis (IPF) in a repeated, randomized, placebo-controlled phase III clinical trial (Armendáriz-Borunda et al., 2006; Verma et al., 2017; Sandoval-Rodriguez et al., 2020). Moreover, it also has a good effect on fibrosis diseases, such as renal interstitial fibrosis and hepatic fibrosis. However, its mechanism of action for treating IPF is still unclear (Benesic et al., 2019; Zhang et al., 2019). Current studies have shown that Pirfenidone can reduce the proliferation of lung fibroblasts and their differentiation into myofibroblasts by attenuating TGF-β-induced signal transduction pathways (Smad3, P38, and Akt), decreasing the expression of recombinant Heat Shock Protein 47 (HSP47) induced by TGF-β, reducing the expression of α-SMA and collagen I (**Figures 2**, **3**) (Di Sario et al., 2002; Benesic et al., 2019; Sandoval-Rodriguez et al., 2020).

Pirfenidone can inhibit the proliferation of hepatocytes and promote hepatocyte apoptosis by inhibiting the Wnt/β-Catenin signaling pathway, which is an effective oral small-molecule drug for the treatment of fibrosis. Many studies have found that Pirfenidone has important anti-inflammatory and anti-fibrosis effects *in vivo* and *in vitro* (Di Sario et al., 2002; Grizzi, 2009; Benesic et al., 2019). Pirfenidone can regulate TGF-β and TNF-α and inhibit fibroblast proliferation and collagen synthesis (García et al., 2002; Salah et al., 2019; Ullah et al., 2019). Moreover, Pirfenidone can significantly alleviate hepatic fibrosis induced by CCl_4 in mice; this effect is closely related to the mechanism of reducing expression levels of PI3K and PKB in the mouse liver (Grizzi, 2009; Benesic et al., 2019). These results suggest that Pirfenidone is a potential therapeutic agent for hepatic fibrosis.

Of the 978 adverse events reported, 17% were nausea and vomiting, 16% were diarrhea, 10% were fatigue, 9% were loss of appetite, 6% were dyspepsia, 6% were rash (n = 59), 5% were headache, and 10% were others (Maher et al., 2020). The incidence of other adverse events was lower than 5%; the most common was acute respiratory failure (2 cases), indicating that the disease is progressive (Maher et al., 2020). Overall, these data suggest that long-term oral administration of Pirfenidone does not increase the risk of ADRs, which is consistent with the known safety characteristics of Pirfenidone. Pirfenidone is a small synthetic molecule with high oral bioavailability, which is primarily metabolized via the liver, although the specific mode of metabolism remains unknown. Currently, the pharmacokinetic data obtained are from trials with small sample sizes, and large-scale clinical trial data are still needed (Cho and Kopp, 2010).

SIMTUZUMAB (GS-6624, INN, SIM)

Simtuzumab is a monoclonal antibody that targets blocking Lysyl Oxidase Like Protein-2 (LOXL2) (Harrison et al., 2018a; Fickert, 2019). LOXL2 is a protease that modifies the ECM by promoting cross-linking of collagen fibers, is believed to play an important role in tumor progression and fibrosis, with the potential to inhibit tumor progression and reverse fibrosis (**Figures 2**, **3**) (Muir et al., 2019; Sanyal et al., 2019).

It has been reported that LOXL2 can promote the occurrence of liver cell fibrosis by catalyzing collagen cross-linking (Meissner et al., 2016; Raghu et al., 2017). Researchers have investigated the safety and efficacy of Simtuzumab in patients with advanced fibrosis caused by NASH (Meissner et al., 2016; Sanyal et al., 2019). In a double-blind study of 219 patients with bridging fibrosis caused by NASH, the patients were randomly assigned (in a 1:1:1 ratio) to a subcutaneous injection of Simtuzumab (75 or 125 mg) or placebo each week for 240 weeks. The experiment was stopped after week 96, and the results showed that liver collagen levels were significantly reduced in all three groups of patients with bridging fibrosis, including those who were given a placebo (Sanyal et al., 2019).

Gilead designed five phase II trials for Simtuzumab to investigate the potential of Simtuzumab in the treatment of pancreatic cancer, colorectal cancer, myeloid fibrosis, IPF, and hepatic fibrosis (Harrison et al., 2018a; Fickert, 2019). To date, two phase II trials of Simtuzumab have failed in pancreatic cancer and colorectal cancer, the remaining three remain to be observed. The latter two indications (pulmonary fibrosis and hepaitc fibrosis) may be the best bet for Simtuzumab. Gilead is currently investigating the efficacy of Simtuzumab for treating IPF (Fickert, 2019; Muir et al., 2019; Sanyal et al., 2019).

A multicenter phase II trial evaluated the efficacy and safety of Selonsertib (a selective inhibitor of ASK1) or in combination with Simtuzumab in patients with NASH and stage 2 or 3 hepatic fibrosis (Harrison et al., 2018b). A total of 72 patients were randomized to open treatment for 24 weeks. Patients were treated with 6 mg or 18 mg Selonsertib orally once daily along with or without a weekly injection of 125 mg Simtuzumab, or with Simtuzumab alone. The results showed that hepatic fibrosis improved in 20% of patients treated with Simtuzumab alone after 24 weeks of treatment. The improvement of hepatic fibrosis was related to decreased liver hardness, reduced collagen content and inflammation of liver lobules, as well as an improvement in serum biomarkers of apoptosis and necrosis (Harrison et al., 2018a). There were no significant differences in side effects among the three treatment groups. At present, no pharmacodynamic and pharmacokinetic assays are available to assess whether LOXL2 is indeed effectively inhibited in the human liver, and further studies are needed (Fickert, 2019).

SORAFENIB (BAY43-9006, NEXAVAR)

Sorafenib is a small molecule compound whose chemical name is 4-[4-({[4-chloro-3-(trifluoromethyl) phenyl] carbamoyl} amino) phenoxy]-Nmethylpyridine-2-carboxamide (**Figure 1**) (Thabut et al., 2011; Liu et al., 2018), the formula is $C_{21}H_{16}ClF_3N_4O_3$, and the molecular weight is 464.82. Sorafenib is an oral multiple kinase inhibitor and a novel multi-molecular target chemotherapy drug. Sorafenib mainly functions by inhibiting tumor cell proliferation, inhibiting angiogenesis, and promoting tumor cell apoptosis (Chen et al., 2014; Deng et al., 2013). Clinically, Sorafenib is mostly used for the treatment of advanced malignant tumors, particularly liver cancer (Lin et al., 2016; Faivre et al., 2020).

Sorafenib can prolong the survival of patients with advanced HCC by 3 months on average, but due to congenital or acquired resistance of patients, it is usually not longer than 6 months before Sorafenib resistance occurs (**Figures 2, 3**) (Faivre et al., 2020).

Hepatic fibrosis, as an important feature of the pathogenesis of chronic liver diseases, has always been one of the important topics in the field of liver disease research and treatment (Ma et al., 2017; Sung et al., 2018). The causes of hepatic fibrosis are complex, TGF-β is the most important known factor promoting hepatic fibrosis (Deng et al., 2013; Ma et al., 2017; Faivre et al., 2020). Hepatic parenchymal cells secrete TGF-β during injury and inflammation, stimulate and activate HSCs, induce epithelial-mesenchymal transition (EMT) of hepatic parenchymal cells, then form activated myofibroblasts and increase the synthesis of ECM such as collagen, thus promoting the occurrence of fibrosis disease (Deng et al., 2013; Lin et al., 2016; Sung et al., 2018). Therefore, therapeutic strategies targeting TGF-β signaling provide the possibility for the eventual prevention and treatment of hepatic fibrosis.

The effective treatment of hepatic fibrosis is an urgent problem to be solved. Studies have shown that combined treatment with Sorafenib and Fluvastatin can reduce collagen deposition and protein expression of α-SMA, down-regulate the content of hyaluronic acid (HA), and the expression of mesenchymal markers in rats with hepatic fibrosis induced by diethylnitrosamine (DEN). Our results suggest that combination therapy can inhibit the progression of hepatic fibrosis by inhibiting the TGF-β1/Smad3 pathway. As such, Sorafenib and fluvastatin may be a potential treatment for hepatic fibrosis. The present study found that Sorafenib can significantly inhibit the TGF-β signal, thereby inhibiting TGF-β-mediated EMT and apoptosis of hepatic parenchymal cells (Thabut et al., 2011; Ma et al., 2017). By establishing a mouse model of hepatic fibrosis induced by CCl$_4$, researchers found that feeding Sorafenib to model mice effectively reduced EMT and apoptosis in liver parenchymal cells, and improved and repaired hepatic fibrosis symptoms in mice (Ma et al., 2017; Sung et al., 2018). This work provides a new mechanism for Sorafenib to improve hepatic fibrosis, as well as a theoretical and experimental basis for whether the drug can be finally applied in the clinical treatment of organ fibrosis. Although Sorafenib is a potential therapeutic agent for hepatic fibrosis, it has side effects such as hand-foot syndrome, diarrhea, and hypertension due to oral administration and its non-specific uptake by normal tissues. In addition, the poor water solubility of Sorafenib decreases the efficiency of its absorption by the gastrointestinal tract, leading to poor pharmacokinetics. Future preparation formulation studies of the drug should address these issues (Lin et al., 2016).

CONCLUSION AND FUTURE DIRECTIONS

It should be noted that the development of drugs specific to hepatic fibrosis is still in its infancy. Additionally, most drugs are in phase of animal experiments or clinical trials and have various disadvantages, including lack of chronic toxicity, pharmacokinetic studies, and adequate evidence-based medicine. The occurrence and development of hepatic fibrosis is a complex process with many factors and steps. Single drugs often cause obvious adverse reactions due to large doses, single drug targets, and other factors, prices of them are often expensive. Therefore, drug combination has shown advantages of improving efficacy and reducing toxicity in clinical studies, and multi-target anti-hepatic fibrosis drugs are an important direction of future drug R&D.

Commonly used anti-hepatic fibrosis drugs include immunosuppressants, glucocorticoids, and non-specific anti-inflammatory drugs, but these drugs have more adverse reactions and poor efficacy. Moreover, due to individual differences, some patients may have adverse reactions. We found the central event in fibrogenesis appears to be the activation of HSCs, which is a complex process, leading to multiple potential targets for therapeutic interventions. Targeting only one of these targets is difficult to play an anti-hepatic fibrosis effect immediately. With the development of molecular biology, molecular targeted therapy has broad clinical application prospects beyond conventional drug therapy. Additionally, traditional Chinese medicine has unique therapeutic advantages. Therefore, the combined application of different drugs for treating hepatic fibrosis is the direction of future clinical research. Most drugs for hepatic fibrosis are still in the experimental stage. With further research on its formation mechanism and the development of new drugs, hepatic fibrosis may eventually be reversed.

AUTHOR CONTRIBUTIONS

Writing of the manuscript: LS, FW, and DZ; developing the idea for the article and critically revising it: XM and JL; supervision: XL. All of the authors have read and approved the final version of the manuscript.

ACKNOWLEDGMENTS

We thank LetPub (www.letpub.com) for its linguistic assistance during the preparation of this manuscript.

REFERENCES

Ali, F. E. M., Bakr, A. G., Abo-Youssef, A. M., Azouz, A. A., and Hemeida, R. A. M. (2018). Targeting Keap-1/Nrf-2 Pathway and Cytoglobin as a Potential Protective Mechanism of Diosmin and Pentoxifylline against Cholestatic Liver Cirrhosis. *Life Sci.* 207, 50–60. doi:10.1016/j.lfs.2018.05.048

Alruwaili, H., Dehestani, B., and Le Roux, C. W. (2021). Clinical Impact of Liraglutide as a Treatment of Obesity. *Clin. Pharmacol.* 13, 53–60. doi:10.2147/CPAA.S276085

Alukal, J. J., and Thuluvath, P. J. (2019). Reversal of NASH Fibrosis with Pharmacotherapy. *Hepatol. Int.* 13 (5), 534–545. doi:10.1007/s12072-019-09970-3

Anfuso, B., Tiribelli, C., Adorini, L., and Rosso, N. (2020). Obeticholic Acid and INT-767 Modulate Collagen Deposition in a NASH *In Vitro* Model. *Sci. Rep.* 10 (1), 1699. doi:10.1038/s41598-020-58562-x

Anstee, Q. M., Neuschwander-Tetri, B. A., Wong, V. W., Abdelmalek, M. F., Younossi, Z. M., Yuan, J., et al. (2020). Cenicriviroc for the Treatment of Liver Fibrosis in Adults with Nonalcoholic Steatohepatitis: AURORA Phase 3 Study Design. *Contemp. Clin. Trials* 89, 105922. doi:10.1016/j.cct.2019.105922

Armendariz-Borunda, J., Islas-Carbajal, M. C., Meza-Garcia, E., Rincon, A. R., Lucano, S., Sandoval, A. S., et al. (2006). A Pilot Study in Patients with Established Advanced Liver Fibrosis Using Pirfenidone. *Gut* 55 (11), 1663–1665. doi:10.1136/gut.2006.107136

Armstrong, M. J., Gaunt, P., Aithal, G. P., Barton, D., Hull, D., Parker, R., et al. (2016). Liraglutide Safety and Efficacy in Patients with Non-alcoholic Steatohepatitis (LEAN): a Multicentre, Double-Blind, Randomised, Placebo-Controlled Phase 2 Study. *Lancet* 387 (10019), 679–690. doi:10.1016/S0140-6736(15)00803-X

Armstrong, M. J., and Newsome, P. N. (2015). Trials of Obeticholic Acid for Non-alcoholic Steatohepatitis. *Lancet* 386 (9988), 28. doi:10.1016/S0140-6736(15)61199-0

Armstrong, M. J., Gaunt, P., Aithal, G. P., Parker, R., Barton, D., Hull, D., et al. (2015). G01 : Liraglutide Is Effective in the Histological Clearance of Non-alcoholic Steatohepatitis in a Multicentre, Doubleblinded, Randomised, Placebo-Controlled Phase II Trial. *J. Hepatology* 62, S187. doi:10.1136/gutjnl-2015-309861.16 10.1016/S0168-8278(15)30002-7

Baandrup Kristiansen, M. N., Veidal, S. S., Christoffersen, C., Feigh, M., Vrang, N., Roth, J. D., et al. (2019). Validity of Biopsy-Based Drug Effects in a Diet-Induced Obese Mouse Model of Biopsy-Confirmed NASH. *BMC Gastroenterol.* 19 (1), 228. doi:10.1186/s12876-019-1149-z

Barreyro, F. J., Holod, S., Finocchietto, P. V., Camino, A. M., Aquino, J. B., Avagnina, A., et al. (2015). The Pan-Caspase Inhibitor Emricasan (IDN-6556) Decreases Liver Injury and Fibrosis in a Murine Model of Non-alcoholic Steatohepatitis. *Liver Int.* 35 (3), 953–966. doi:10.1111/liv.12570

Benesic, A., Jalal, K., and Gerbes, A. L. (2019). Acute Liver Failure during Pirfenidone Treatment Triggered by Co-medication with Esomeprazole. *Hepatology* 70 (5), 1869–1871. doi:10.1002/hep.30684

Boeckmans, J., Natale, A., Rombaut, M., Buyl, K., Rogiers, V., De Kock, J., et al. (2019). Anti-NASH Drug Development Hitches a Lift on PPAR Agonism. *Cells* 9 (1), 37. doi:10.3390/cells9010037

Boyer-Diaz, Z., Aristu-Zabalza, P., Andrés-Rozas, M., Robert, C., Ortega-Ribera, M., Fernández-Iglesias, A., et al. (2021). Pan-PPAR Agonist Lanifibranor Improves Portal Hypertension and Hepatic Fibrosis in Experimental Advanced Chronic Liver Disease. *J. Hepatol.* 74 (5), 1188–1199. doi:10.1016/j.jhep.2020.11.045

Briand, F., Duparc, T., Heymes, C., Bonada, L., and Sulpice, T. (2020). A 3-week Nonalcoholic Steatohepatitis Mouse Model Allows the Rapid Evaluation of Liraglutide and Elafibranor Benefits on NASH. *Metabolism* 104, 154113. doi:10.1016/j.metabol.2019.12.059

Brunt, E. M., Kleiner, D. E., Wilson, L. A., Sanyal, A. J., and Neuschwander-Tetri, B. A. (2019). Improvements in Histologic Features and Diagnosis Associated with Improvement in Fibrosis in Nonalcoholic Steatohepatitis: Results from the Nonalcoholic Steatohepatitis Clinical Research Network Treatment Trials. *Hepatology* 70 (2), 522–531. doi:10.1002/hep.30418

Chalasani, N., Abdelmalek, M. F., Garcia-Tsao, G., Vuppalanchi, R., Alkhouri, N., Rinella, M., et al. (2020). Effects of Belapectin, an Inhibitor of Galectin-3, in Patients with Nonalcoholic Steatohepatitis with Cirrhosis and Portal Hypertension. *Gastroenterology* 158 (5), 1334–1345. e5. doi:10.1053/j.gastro.2019.11.296

Chalasani, N., Garcia-Tsao, G., Goodman, Z., Lawitz, E., and Harrison, S. (2018). A Multicenter, Randomized, Double-Blind, Plb-Controlled Trial of Galectin-3 Inhibitor (Gr-md-02) in Patients with Nash Cirrhosis and Portal Hypertension. *J. Hepatol.* 68 (1), S100–S101. doi:10.1016/S0168-8278(18)30420-3

Chen, H., Cai, J., Wang, J., Qiu, Y., Jiang, C., Wang, Y., et al. (2021). Targeting Nestin+ Hepatic Stellate Cells Ameliorates Liver Fibrosis by Facilitating TβRI Degradation. *J. Hepatol.* 74 (5), 1176–1187. doi:10.1016/j.jhep.2020.11.016

Chen, Y., Huang, Y., Reiberger, T., Duyverman, A. M., Huang, P., Samuel, R., et al. (2014). Differential Effects of Sorafenib on Liver versus Tumor Fibrosis

Mediated by Stromal-Derived Factor 1 Alpha/C-X-C Receptor Type 4 axis and Myeloid Differentiation Antigen-Positive Myeloid Cell Infiltration in Mice. *Hepatology* 59 (4), 1435–1447. doi:10.1002/hep.26790

Cheng, H. S., Tan, W. R., Low, Z. S., Marvalim, C., Lee, J., and Tan, N. S. (2019). Exploration and Development of PPAR Modulators in Health and Disease: An Update of Clinical Evidence. *Int. J. Mol. Sci.* 20 (20), 5055. doi:10.3390/ijms20205055

Cho, M. E., and Kopp, J. B. (2010). Pirfenidone: an Anti-fibrotic Therapy for Progressive Kidney Disease. *Expert Opin. Investig. Drugs* 19 (2), 275–283. doi:10.1517/13543780903501539

Choi, Y. J., Song, J., Johnson, J., Hellerstein, M., and Mcwherter, C. (2019). Fri-329-comparison of Seladelpar and Combinations with Liraglutide or Selonsertib for Improvement of Fibrosis and NASH in a Diet-Induced and Biopsy-Confirmed Mouse Model of Nash. *J. Hepatol.* 70 (1), e541. doi:10.1016/S0618-8278(19)31070-9

Chooklin, S. N., and Perejaslov, A. A. (2003). Mechanism of Pentoxifylline Action on Liver Fibrosis. *J. Hepatol.* 38 (S2), 75. doi:10.1016/S0168-8278(03)80311-2

Deng, Y. R., Ma, H. D., Tsuneyama, K., Yang, W., Wang, Y. H., Lu, F. T., et al. (2013). STAT3-mediated Attenuation of CCl4-Induced Mouse Liver Fibrosis by the Protein Kinase Inhibitor Sorafenib. *J. Autoimmun.* 46, 25–34. doi:10.1016/j.jaut.2013.07.008

Desmoulière, A., Xu, G., Costa, A. M., Yousef, I. M., Gabbiani, G., and Tuchweber, B. (1999). Effect of Pentoxifylline on Early Proliferation and Phenotypic Modulation of Fibrogenic Cells in Two Rat Models of Liver Fibrosis and on Cultured Hepatic Stellate Cells. *J. Hepatol.* 30 (4), 621–631. doi:10.1016/s0168-8278(99)80192-5

Di Sario, A., Bendia, E., Svegliati Baroni, G., Ridolfi, F., Casini, A., Ceni, E., et al. (2002). Effect of Pirfenidone on Rat Hepatic Stellate Cell Proliferation and Collagen Production. *J. Hepatol.* 37 (5), 584–591. doi:10.1016/s0168-8278(02)00245-3

Eaton, J. E., Vuppalanchi, R., Reddy, R., Sathapathy, S., Ali, B., and Kamath, P. S. (2020). Liver Injury in Patients with Cholestatic Liver Disease Treated with Obeticholic Acid. *Hepatology* 71 (4), 1511–1514. doi:10.1002/hep.31017

Eslam, M., Alvani, R., and Shiha, G. (2019). Obeticholic Acid: towards First Approval for NASH. *Lancet* 394 (10215), 2131–2133. doi:10.1016/S0140-6736(19)32963-0

Fagone, P., Mangano, K., Pesce, A., Portale, T. R., Puleo, S., and Nicoletti, F. (2016). Emerging Therapeutic Targets for the Treatment of Hepatic Fibrosis. *Drug Discov. Today* 21 (2), 369–375. doi:10.1016/j.drudis.2015.10.015

Faivre, S., Rimassa, L., and Finn, R. S. (2020). Molecular Therapies for HCC: Looking outside the Box. *J. Hepatol.* 72 (2), 342–352. doi:10.1016/j.jhep.2019.09.010

Fickert, P. (2019). Is This the Last Requiem for Simtuzumab. *Hepatology* 69 (2), 476–479. doi:10.1002/hep.30309

Frenette, C. T., Morelli, G., Shiffman, M. L., Frederick, R. T., Rubin, R. A., Fallon, M. B., et al. (2019). Emricasan Improves Liver Function in Patients with Cirrhosis and High Model for End-Stage Liver Disease Scores Compared with Placebo. *Clin. Gastroenterol. Hepatol.* 17 (4), 774–783. e4. doi:10.1016/j.cgh.2018.06.012

Friedman, S. L., Ratziu, V., Harrison, S. A., Abdelmalek, M. F., Aithal, G. P., Caballeria, J., et al. (2018). A Randomized, Placebo-Controlled Trial of Cenicriviroc for Treatment of Nonalcoholic Steatohepatitis with Fibrosis. *Hepatology* 67 (5), 1754–1767. doi:10.1002/hep.29477

Friedman, S., Sanyal, A., Goodman, Z., Lefebvre, E., Gottwald, M., Fischer, L., et al. (2016). Efficacy and Safety Study of Cenicriviroc for the Treatment of Non-alcoholic Steatohepatitis in Adult Subjects with Liver Fibrosis: CENTAUR Phase 2b Study Design. *Contemp. Clin. Trials* 47, 356–365. doi:10.1016/j.cct.2016.02.012

Gaborit, B., Darmon, P., Ancel, P., and Dutour, A. (2016). Liraglutide for Patients with Non-alcoholic Steatohepatitis. *Lancet* 387 (10036), 2378–2379. doi:10.1016/S0140-6736(16)30734-6

García, L., Hernández, I., Sandoval, A., Salazar, A., Garcia, J., Vera, J., et al. (2002). Pirfenidone Effectively Reverses Experimental Liver Fibrosis. *J. Hepatol.* 37 (6), 797–805. doi:10.1016/s0168-8278(02)00272-6

Garcia-Tsao, G., Bosch, J., Kayali, Z., Harrison, S. A., Abdelmalek, M. F., Lawitz, E., et al. (2020). Randomized Placebo-Controlled Trial of Emricasan for Non-alcoholic Steatohepatitis-Related Cirrhosis with Severe Portal Hypertension. *J. Hepatol.* 72 (5), 885–895. doi:10.1016/j.jhep.2019.12.010

Garcia-Tsao, G., Fuchs, M., Shiffman, M., Borg, B. B., Pyrsopoulos, N., Shetty, K., et al. (2019). Emricasan (IDN-6556) Lowers Portal Pressure in Patients with Compensated Cirrhosis and Severe Portal Hypertension. *Hepatology* 69 (2), 717–728. doi:10.1002/hep.30199

Gawrieh, S., Guo, X., Tan, J., Lauzon, M., Taylor, K. D., Loomba, R., et al. (2019). A Pilot Genome-wide Analysis Study Identifies Loci Associated with Response to Obeticholic Acid in Patients with NASH. *Hepatol. Commun.* 3 (12), 1571–1584. doi:10.1002/hep4.1439

Gilgenkrantz, H., Mallat, A., Moreau, R., and Lotersztajn, S. (2021). Targeting Cell-Intrinsic Metabolism for Antifibrotic Therapy. *J. Hepatol.* 74 (6), 1442–1454. doi:10.1016/j.jhep.2021.02.012

Gore, E., Bigaeva, E., Oldenburger, A., Jansen, Y., Schuppan, D., Boersema, M., et al. (20202019). Investigating Fibrosis and Inflammation in an *Ex Vivo* NASH Murine Model. *Am. J. Physiol. Gastrointest. Liver Physiol.* 318 (2), G336–G351. doi:10.1152/ajpgi.0020910.1152/ajpgi.00209.2019

Gracia-Sancho, J., Manicardi, N., Ortega-Ribera, M., Maeso-Díaz, R., Guixé-Muntet, S., Fernández-Iglesias, A., et al. (2019). Emricasan Ameliorates Portal Hypertension and Liver Fibrosis in Cirrhotic Rats through a Hepatocyte-Mediated Paracrine Mechanism. *Hepatol. Commun.* 3 (7), 987–1000. doi:10.1002/hep4.1360

Grizzi, F. (2009). Pirfenidone: a Potential Therapeutic Option in the Treatment of Liver Fibrosis. *Clin. Exp. Pharmacol. P* 36 (10), 961–962. doi:10.1111/j.1440-1681.2009.05262.x

Guaraldi, G., Maurice, J. B., Marzolini, C., Monteith, K., Milic, J., Tsochatzis, E., et al. (2020). New Drugs for NASH and HIV Infection: Great Expectations for a Great Need. *Hepatology* 71 (5), 1831–1844. doi:10.1002/hep.31177

Harrison, S. A., Abdelmalek, M. F., Caldwell, S., Shiffman, M. L., Diehl, A. M., Ghalib, R., et al. (2018a). Simtuzumab Is Ineffective for Patients with Bridging Fibrosis or Compensated Cirrhosis Caused by Nonalcoholic Steatohepatitis. *Gastroenterology* 155 (4), 1140–1153. doi:10.1053/j.gastro.2018.07.006

Harrison, S. A., Dennis, A., Fiore, M. M., Kelly, M. D., Kelly, C. J., Paredes, A. H., et al. (2018b). Utility and Variability of Three Non-invasive Liver Fibrosis Imaging Modalities to Evaluate Efficacy of GR-MD-02 in Subjects with NASH and Bridging Fibrosis during a Phase-2 Randomized Clinical Trial. *PloS one* 13 (9), e0203054. doi:10.1371/journal.pone.0203054

Harrison, S. A., Goodman, Z., Jabbar, A., Vemulapalli, R., Younes, Z. H., Freilich, B., et al. (2020). A Randomized, Placebo-Controlled Trial of Emricasan in Patients with NASH and F1-F3 Fibrosis. *J. Hepatol.* 72 (5), 816–827. doi:10.1016/j.jhep.2019.11.024

Harrison, S. A., Marri, S. R., Chalasani, N., Kohli, R., Aronstein, W., Thompson, G. A., et al. (2016). Randomised Clinical Study: GR-MD-02, a Galectin-3 Inhibitor, vs. Placebo in Patients Having Non-alcoholic Steatohepatitis with Advanced Fibrosis. *Aliment. Pharm. Ther.* 44 (11-12), 1183–1198. doi:10.1111/apt.13816

Hindson, J. (2020). Obeticholic Acid for the Treatment of NASH. *Nat. Rev. Gastroenterol. Hepatol.* 17 (2), 66. doi:10.1038/s41575-020-0264-1

Iacobini, C., Menini, S., Ricci, C., Blasetti Fantauzzi, C., Scipioni, A., Salvi, L., et al. (2011). Galectin-3 Ablation Protects Mice from Diet-Induced NASH: a Major Scavenging Role for Galectin-3 in Liver. *J. Hepatol.* 54 (5), 975–983. doi:10.1016/j.jhep.2010.09.020

Kahal, H., Abouda, G., Rigby, A. S., Coady, A. M., Kilpatrick, E. S., and Atkin, S. L. (2014). Glucagon-like Peptide-1 Analogue, Liraglutide, Improves Liver Fibrosis Markers in Obese Women with Polycystic Ovary Syndrome and Nonalcoholic Fatty Liver Disease. *Clin. Endocrinol.* 81 (4), 523–528. doi:10.1111/cen.12369

Kruger, A. J., Fuchs, B. C., Masia, R., Holmes, J. A., Salloum, S., Sojoodi, M., et al. (2018). Prolonged Cenicriviroc Therapy Reduces Hepatic Fibrosis Despite Steatohepatitis in a Diet-Induced Mouse Model of Nonalcoholic Steatohepatitis. *Hepatol. Commun.* 2 (5), 529–545. doi:10.1002/hep4.1160

Lebrec, D., Thabut, D., Oberti, F., Perarnau, J. M., Condat, B., Barraud, H., et al. (2010). Pentoxifylline Does Not Decrease Short-Term Mortality but Does Reduce Complications in Patients with Advanced Cirrhosis. *Gastroenterology* 138 (5), 1755–1762. doi:10.1053/j.gastro.2010.01.040

Lefebvre, E., Gottwald, M., Lasseter, K., Chang, W., Willett, M., Smith, P. F., et al. (2016a). Pharmacokinetics, Safety, and CCR2/CCR5 Antagonist Activity of Cenicriviroc in Participants with Mild or Moderate Hepatic Impairment. *Clin. Transl. Sci.* 9 (3), 139–148. doi:10.1111/cts.12397

Lefebvre, E., Moyle, G., Reshef, R., Richman, L. P., Thompson, M., Hong, F., et al. (2016b). Antifibrotic Effects of the Dual CCR2/CCR5 Antagonist Cenicriviroc in Animal Models of Liver and Kidney Fibrosis. *PloS one* 11 (6), e0158156. doi:10.1371/journal.pone.0158156

Lin, T., Gao, D. Y., Liu, Y. C., Sung, Y. C., Wan, D., Liu, J. Y., et al. (2016). Development and Characterization of Sorafenib-Loaded PLGA Nanoparticles for the Systemic Treatment of Liver Fibrosis. *J. Control Release* 221, 62–70. doi:10.1016/j.jconrel.2015.11.003

Liu, C. H., Chern, G. J., Hsu, F. F., Huang, K. W., Sung, Y. C., Huang, H. C., et al. (2018). A Multifunctional Nanocarrier for Efficient TRAIL-Based Gene Therapy against Hepatocellular Carcinoma with Desmoplasia in Mice. *Hepatology* 67 (3), 899–913. doi:10.1002/hep.29513

Louvet, A., Diaz, E., Dharancy, S., Coevoet, H., Texier, F., Thévenot, T., et al. (2008). Early Switch to Pentoxifylline in Patients with Severe Alcoholic Hepatitis Is Inefficient in Non-responders to Corticosteroids. *J. Hepatol.* 48 (3), 465–470. doi:10.1016/j.jhep.2007.10.010

Ma, R., Chen, J., Liang, Y., Lin, S., Zhu, L., Liang, X., et al. (2017). Sorafenib: A Potential Therapeutic Drug for Hepatic Fibrosis and its Outcomes. *Biomed. Pharmacother.* 88, 459–468. doi:10.1016/j.biopha.2017.01.107

Maher, T. M., Corte, T. J., Fischer, A., Kreuter, M., Lederer, D. J., Molina-Molina, M., et al. (2020). Pirfenidone in Patients with Unclassifiable Progressive Fibrosing Interstitial Lung Disease: a Double-Blind, Randomised, Placebo-Controlled, Phase 2 Trial. *Lancet Respir. Med.* 8 (2), 147–157. doi:10.1016/S2213-2600(19)30341-8

Meissner, E. G., McLaughlin, M., Matthews, L., Gharib, A. M., Wood, B. J., Levy, E., et al. (2016). Simtuzumab Treatment of Advanced Liver Fibrosis in HIV and HCV-Infected Adults: Results of a 6-month Open-Label Safety Trial. *Liver Int.* 36 (12), 1783–1792. doi:10.1111/liv.13177

Muir, A. J., Levy, C., Janssen, H., Montano-Loza, A. J., Shiffman, M. L., Caldwell, S., et al. (2019). Simtuzumab for Primary Sclerosing Cholangitis: Phase 2 Study Results with Insights on the Natural History of the Disease. *Hepatology* 69 (2), 684–698. doi:10.1002/hep.30237

Neuschwander-Tetri, B. A. (2020). Therapeutic Landscape for NAFLD in 2020. *Gastroenterology* 158 (7), 1984–1998. e3. doi:10.1053/j.gastro.2020.01.051

Oberti, F., Pilette, C., Rifflet, H., Maïga, M. Y., Moreau, A., Gallois, Y., et al. (1997). Effects of Simvastatin, Pentoxifylline and Spironolactone on Hepatic Fibrosis and Portal Hypertension in Rats with Bile Duct Ligation. *J. Hepatol.* 26 (6), 1363–1371. doi:10.1016/s0168-8278(97)80473-4

Park, S. H., Kim, D. J., Kim, Y. S., Yim, H. J., Tak, W. Y., Lee, H. J., et al. (2014). Pentoxifylline vs. Corticosteroid to Treat Severe Alcoholic Hepatitis: a Randomised, Non-inferiority, Open Trial. *J. Hepatol.* 61 (4), 792–798. doi:10.1016/j.jhep.2014.05.014

Pedrosa, M., Seyedkazemi, S., Francque, S., Sanyal, A., Rinella, M., Charlton, M., et al. (2020). A Randomized, Double-Blind, Multicenter, Phase 2b Study to Evaluate the Safety and Efficacy of a Combination of Tropifexor and Cenicriviroc in Patients with Nonalcoholic Steatohepatitis and Liver Fibrosis: Study Design of the TANDEM Trial. *Contemp. Clin. Trials* 88, 105889. doi:10.1016/j.cct.2019.105889

Peterson, T. C. (1993). Pentoxifylline Prevents Fibrosis in an Animal Model and Inhibits Platelet-Derived Growth Factor-Driven Proliferation of Fibroblasts. *Hepatology* 17 (3), 486–493. doi:10.1016/0270-9139(93)90062-r

Pinzani, M., Marra, F., Caligiuri, A., DeFranco, R., Gentilini, A., Failli, P., et al. (1996). Inhibition by Pentoxifylline of Extracellular Signal-Regulated Kinase Activation by Platelet-Derived Growth Factor in Hepatic Stellate Cells. *Br. J. Pharmacol.* 119 (6), 1117–1124. doi:10.1111/j.1476-5381.1996.tb16012.x

Raghu, G., Brown, K. K., Collard, H. R., Cottin, V., Gibson, K. F., Kaner, R. J., et al. (2017). Efficacy of Simtuzumab versus Placebo in Patients with Idiopathic Pulmonary Fibrosis: a Randomised, Double-Blind, Controlled, Phase 2 Trial. *Lancet Respir. Med.* 5 (1), 22–32. doi:10.1016/S2213-2600(16)30421-0

Ratziu, V., Harrison, S. A., Francque, S., Bedossa, P., Lehert, P., Serfaty, L., et al. (2016). Elafibranor, an Agonist of the Peroxisome Proliferator-Activated Receptor-α and -δ, Induces Resolution of Nonalcoholic Steatohepatitis without Fibrosis Worsening. *Gastroenterology* 150 (5), 1147–1159. e5. doi:10.1053/j.gastro.2016.01.038

Reimer, K. C., Wree, A., Roderburg, C., and Tacke, F. (2020). New Drugs for NAFLD: Lessons from Basic Models to the Clinic. *Hepatol. Int.* 14 (1), 8–23. doi:10.1007/s12072-019-10001-4

Roehlen, N., Crouchet, E., and Baumert, T. F. (2020). Liver Fibrosis: Mechanistic Concepts and Therapeutic Perspectives. *Cells* 9 (4), 875. doi:10.3390/cells9040875

Roth, J. D., Veidal, S. S., Fensholdt, L., Rigbolt, K., Papazyan, R., Nielsen, J. C., et al. (2019). Combined Obeticholic Acid and Elafibranor Treatment Promotes Additive Liver Histological Improvements in a Diet-Induced Ob/ob Mouse Model of Biopsy-Confirmed NASH. *Sci. Rep.* 9 (1), 9046. doi:10.1038/s41598-019-45178-z

Rotman, Y., and Sanyal, A. J. (2017). Current and Upcoming Pharmacotherapy for Non-alcoholic Fatty Liver Disease. *Gut* 66 (1), 180–190. doi: doi:10.1136/gutjnl-2016-312431

Salah, M. M., Ashour, A. A., Abdelghany, T. M., Abdel-Aziz, A. H., and Salama, S. A. (2019). Pirfenidone Alleviates Concanavalin A-Induced Liver Fibrosis in Mice. *Life Sci.* 239, 116982. doi:10.1016/j.lfs.2019.116982

Sandoval-Rodriguez, A., Monroy-Ramirez, H. C., Meza-Rios, A., Garcia-Bañuelos, J., Vera-Cruz, J., Gutiérrez-Cuevas, J., et al. (2020). Pirfenidone Is an Agonistic Ligand for PPARα and Improves NASH by Activation of SIRT1/LKB1/pAMPK. *Hepatol. Commun.* 4 (3), 434–449. doi:10.1002/hep4.1474

Sanyal, A. J., Harrison, S. A., Ratziu, V., Abdelmalek, M. F., Diehl, A. M., Caldwell, S., et al. (2019). The Natural History of Advanced Fibrosis Due to Nonalcoholic Steatohepatitis: Data from the Simtuzumab Trials. *Hepatology* 70 (6), 1913–1927. doi:10.1002/hep.30664

Satapathy, S. K., Sakhuja, P., Malhotra, V., Sharma, B. C., and Sarin, S. K. (2007). Beneficial Effects of Pentoxifylline on Hepatic Steatosis, Fibrosis and Necroinflammation in Patients with Non-alcoholic Steatohepatitis. *J. Gastroenterol. Hepatol.* 22 (5), 634–638. doi:10.1111/j.1440-1746.2006.04756.x

Schuppan, D., Ashfaq-Khan, M., Yang, A. T., and Kim, Y. O. (2018). Liver Fibrosis: Direct Antifibrotic Agents and Targeted Therapies. *Matrix Biol.* 68-69, 435–451. doi:10.1016/j.matbio.2018.04.006

Shen, B., and Lu, L. G. (2021). Efficacy and Safety of Drugs for Nonalcoholic Steatohepatitis. *J. Dig. Dis.* 22 (2), 72–82. doi:10.1111/1751-2980.12967

Shiffman, M., Freilich, B., Vuppalanchi, R., Watt, K., Chan, J. L., Spada, A., et al. (2019). Randomised Clinical Trial: Emricasan versus Placebo Significantly Decreases ALT and Caspase 3/7 Activation in Subjects with Non-alcoholic Fatty Liver Disease. *Aliment. Pharm. Ther.* 49 (1), 64–73. doi:10.1111/apt10.1111/apt.15030

Siddiqui, M. S., Van Natta, M. L., Connelly, M. A., Vuppalanchi, R., Neuschwander-Tetri, B. A., Tonascia, J., et al. (2020). Impact of Obeticholic Acid on the Lipoprotein Profile in Patients with Non-alcoholic Steatohepatitis. *J. Hepatol.* 72 (1), 25–33. doi:10.1016/j.jhep.2019.10.006

Solhi, R., Lotfi, A. S., Lotfinia, M., Farzaneh, Z., Piryaei, A., Najimi, M., et al. (2022). Hepatic Stellate Cell Activation by TGFβ Induces Hedgehog Signaling and Endoplasmic Reticulum Stress Simultaneously. *Toxicol Vitro* 80, 105315. doi:10.1016/j.tiv.2022.105315

Sumida, Y., Okanoue, T., and Nakajima, A. (2019). Phase 3 Drug Pipelines in the Treatment of Non-alcoholic Steatohepatitis. *Hepatol. Res.* 49 (11), 1256–1262. doi:10.1111/hepr.13425

Sumida, Y., and Yoneda, M. (2018). Current and Future Pharmacological Therapies for NAFLD/NASH. *J. Gastroenterol.* 53 (3), 362–376. doi:10.1007/s00535-017-1415-1

Sung, Y. C., Liu, Y. C., Chao, P. H., Chang, C. C., Jin, P. R., Lin, T. T., et al. (2018). Combined Delivery of Sorafenib and a MEK Inhibitor Using CXCR4-Targeted Nanoparticles Reduces Hepatic Fibrosis and Prevents Tumor Development. *Theranostics* 8 (4), 894–905. doi:10.7150/thno.21168

Thabut, D., Routray, C., Lomberk, G., Shergill, U., Glaser, K., Huebert, R., et al. (2011). Complementary Vascular and Matrix Regulatory Pathways Underlie the Beneficial Mechanism of Action of Sorafenib in Liver Fibrosis. *Hepatology* 54 (2), 573–585. doi:10.1002/hep.24427

Ullah, A., Wang, K., Wu, P., Oupicky, D., and Sun, M. (2019). CXCR4-targeted Liposomal Mediated Co-delivery of Pirfenidone and AMD3100 for the Treatment of TGFβ-Induced HSC-T6 Cells Activation. *Int. J. Nanomedicine* 14, 2927–2944. doi:10.2147/IJN.S171280

Verma, N., Kumar, P., Mitra, S., Taneja, S., Dhooria, S., Das, A., et al. (2017). Drug Idiosyncrasy Due to Pirfenidone Presenting as Acute Liver Failure: Case Report and Mini-Review of the Literature. *Hepatol. Commun.* 2 (2), 142–147. doi:10.1002/hep4.1133

Verma-Gandhu, M., Peterson, M. R., and Peterson, T. C. (2007). Effect of Fetuin, a TGFbeta Antagonist and Pentoxifylline, a Cytokine Antagonist on Hepatic Stellate Cell Function and Fibrotic Parameters in Fibrosis. *Eur. J. Pharmacol.* 572 (2-3), 220–227. doi:10.1016/j.ejphar.2007.06.039

Wang, M. N., Yu, H. T., Li, Y. Q., Zeng, Y., Yang, S., Yang, G. P., et al. (2021). Bioequivalence and Pharmacokinetic Profiles of Generic and Branded Obeticholic Acid in Healthy Chinese Subjects under Fasting and Fed Conditions. *Drug Des. Devel Ther.* 15, 185–193. doi:10.2147/DDDT10.2147/DDDT.S289016

Ward, A., and Clissold, S. P. (1987). Pentoxifylline. A Review of its Pharmacodynamic and Pharmacokinetic Properties, and its Therapeutic Efficacy. *Drugs* 34 (1), 50–97. doi:10.2165/00003495-198734010-00003

Younossi, Z. M., Ratziu, V., Loomba, R., Rinella, M., Anstee, Q. M., Goodman, Z., et al. (2019). Obeticholic Acid for the Treatment of Non-alcoholic Steatohepatitis: Interim Analysis from a Multicentre, Randomised, Placebo-Controlled Phase 3 Trial. *Lancet* 394 (10215), 2184–2196. doi:10.1016/S0140-6736(19)33041-7

Zein, C. O., Lopez, R., Fu, X., Kirwan, J. P., Yerian, L. M., McCullough, A. J., et al. (2012). Pentoxifylline Decreases Oxidized Lipid Products in Nonalcoholic Steatohepatitis: New Evidence on the Potential Therapeutic Mechanism. *Hepatology* 56 (4), 1291–1299. doi:10.1002/hep.25778

Zhang, Y., Jones, K. D., Achtar-Zadeh, N., Green, G., Kukreja, J., Xu, B., et al. (2019). Histopathological and Molecular Analysis of Idiopathic Pulmonary Fibrosis Lungs from Patients Treated with Pirfenidone or Nintedanib. *Histopathology* 74 (2), 341–349. doi:10.1111/his.13745

Zoubek, M. E., Trautwein, C., and Strnad, P. (2017). Reversal of Liver Fibrosis: From Fiction to Reality. *Best. Pract. Res. Clin. Gastroenterol.* 31 (2), 129–141. doi:10.1016/j.bpg.2017.04.005

2

Curdione and Schisandrin C Synergistically Reverse Hepatic Fibrosis via Modulating the TGF-β Pathway and Inhibiting Oxidative Stress

Wenzhang Dai[1,2†], Qin Qin[1†], Zhiyong Li[1†], Li Lin[1], Ruisheng Li[1], Zhie Fang[1], Yanzhong Han[1], Wenqing Mu[1], Lutong Ren[1], Tingting Liu[1], Xiaoyan Zhan[1,3*], Xiaohe Xiao[1,2,3*] and Zhaofang Bai[1,3*]

[1] Senior Department of Hepatology, The Fifth Medical Center of Chinese PLA General Hospital, Beijing, China, [2] School of Pharmacy, Hunan University of Chinese Medicine, Changsha, China, [3] China Military Institute of Chinese Materia, The Fifth Medical Centre, Chinese PLA General Hospital, Beijing, China

*Correspondence:
Xiaoyan Zhan
xyzhan123@163.com
Xiaohe Xiao
pharmacy_302@126.com
Zhaofang Bai
baizf2008@hotmail.com

†These authors have contributed equally to this work and share first authorship

Hepatic fibrosis is the final pathway of several chronic liver diseases, which is characterized by the accumulation of extracellular matrix due to chronic hepatocyte damage. Activation of hepatic stellate cells and oxidative stress (OS) play an important role in mediating liver damage and initiating hepatic fibrosis. Hence, hepatic fibrosis can be reversed by inhibiting multiple channels such as oxidative stress, liver cell damage, or activation of hepatic stellate cells. Liuwei Wuling Tablets is a traditional Chinese medicine formula with the effect of anti- hepatic fibrosis, but the composition and mechanism of reversing hepatic fibrosis are still unclear. Our study demonstrated that one of the main active components of the Chinese medicine Schisandra chinensis, schisandrin C (Sin C), significantly inhibited oxidative stress and prevented hepatocyte injury. Meanwhile one of the main active components of the Chinese medicine Curdione inhibited hepatic stellate cell activation by targeting the TGF-β1/Smads signaling pathway. The further *in vivo* experiments showed that Sin C, Curdione and the combination of both have the effect of reversing liver fibrosis in mice, and the combined effect of inhibiting hepatic fibrosis is superior to treatment with Sin C or Curdione alone. Our study provides a potential candidate for multi-molecular or multi-pathway combination therapies for the treatment of hepatic fibrosis and demonstrates that combined pharmacotherapy holds great promise in the prevention and treatment of hepatic fibrosis.

Keywords: schisandrin C, Curdione, hepatic fibrosis, oxidative stress, TGF-β1/Smads signaling pathway

Abbreviations: ALT, alanine aminotransferase; APAP, acetaminophen; AST, aspartate aminotransferase; BJRG, Biejia Ruangan tablets; CCK-8, cell counting kit-8; CFDA, Chinese State Food and Drug Administration; DBIL, direct bilirubin; ECM, extracellular matrix; ELISA, enzyme-linked immunosorbent assay; FZHY, Fuzheng Huayu capsules; GSH, glutathione; HSC, hepatic stellate cells; Hyp, hydroxyprolinein; LCA, lithocholic acid; LWWL, Liuwei Wuling tablets; MDA, malondialdehyde; NAC, nacetylcysteine; NF-κB, nuclear factor kappa-B; OS, oxidative stress; PXR, pregnane X receptor; ROS, reactive oxygen species; SinC, Schisandrin C; TBIL, total bilirubin; TCM, traditional Chinese medicine; TGF-β1, transforming growth factor-β1.

INTRODUCTION

Hepatic fibrosis is a compensatory pathological process in which abnormal proliferation of connective tissue in the liver occurs when the liver is injured by various chronic inflammations, which leads to excessive deposition of extracellular matrix (ECM) (Sánchez-Valle et al., 2012). It is the common pathological basis of a variety of chronic liver diseases, including chronic viral hepatitis, alcoholic steatohepatitis, non-alcoholic steatohepatitis and drug-induced liver injury (Cordero-Espinoza and Huch, 2018). It will gradually develop into liver cirrhosis and even hepatocellular carcinoma if without timely intervention (Huang et al., 2017; Cordero-Espinoza and Huch, 2018; Pan et al., 2020). Therefore, reversal of hepatic fibrosis is significant for the prevention and the treatment of cirrhosis and liver diseases. Thus far, several potential chemotherapeutic and biological agents have been developed for the intervention of hepatic fibrosis. However, there remains a lack of effective anti-hepatic fibrosis drugs in the clinic (Fagone et al., 2016; Schuppan et al., 2018).

The activation of hepatic stellate cells (HSC) is a central part of hepatic fibrosis. After hepatocytes are invaded by various inflammatory factors, cytokines such as transforming growth factor-β1 (TGF-β1) secreted by hepatocytes, immune cells, and platelets stimulate the sustained proliferation and chemotaxis of HSC (Elpek, 2014; Kumar et al., 2017; Xu et al., 2020). TGF-β/Smad is the main signal transduction pathway of liver fibrosis (Xu et al., 2016). TGF-β1 plays a key role in the process of HSC activation and proliferation. It promotes the up-regulation of pathway related proteins α-SMA and Smad3 by regulating the Smads signaling pathway, and secretes a large amount of ECM, leading to the development of fibrosis (Nagase et al., 2006; Wu et al., 2016; Mu et al., 2018). Multiple small molecules targeting TGF-β1 have been found to have the potential to prevent and treat hepatic fibrosis (Fagone et al., 2016). Some studies have demonstrated that small molecule combination or combined pharmacotherapy is a potential strategy for the prevention and treatment of hepatic fibrosis, which has been successfully used to treat hepatic fibrosis in animal models (Yang et al., 2012; Sung et al., 2018). The occurrence of oxidative stress has been detected in almost all clinical and experimental settings of chronic liver disease, and oxidative stress plays an important role in generating liver injury and initiating hepatic fibrosis by producing mitochondrial reactive oxygen species (ROS) (Parola and Robino, 2001; Sánchez-Valle et al., 2012). Reactive oxygen species-mediated hepatic fibrosis is due to the excessive production of ROS in the liver, which leads to peroxidative damage of hepatocytes (Gandhi, 2012; Islam et al., 2017; Sun et al., 2018). In addition, there is evidence show that some antioxidants have a therapeutic effect on hepatic fibrosis or cirrhosis (Guimarães et al., 2006).

In recent years, Traditional Chinese Medicine (TCM) formulations have shown unique advantages in anti-hepatic fibrosis. For example, Fuzheng Huayu Capsules (FZHY), Biejia Ruangan Tablets (BJRG), and other TCM compound preparations have been approved to treat hepatic fibrosis in the clinic by China Food and Drug Administration (Guo et al., 2004;

Zhang and Schuppan, 2014). Besides, studies have confirmed that the active compound polyphenol rosmarinic acid combined with baicalin in the herbal prescription Yang-Gan-Wan has the effect of treating hepatic fibrosis (Yang et al., 2012). Liuweiwuling tablets (LWWL) is a TCM formula approved by the Chinese State Food and Drug Administration (CFDA) to reduce transaminase levels caused by liver disease with chronic hepatitis B. And which is composed of six herbs, namely Schisandra, Ligustrum lucidum, Forsythia, Zedoary Turmeric, Perennial Sow Thistle, and Ganoderma lucidum spores (Liu et al., 2018a,b; Ai et al., 2021). Our previous studies have found that LWWL can inhibit the activation of HSC by regulating nuclear factor kappa-B (NF-κB) and TGF-β/Smad signaling pathways, and exert its protective effect on hepatic fibrosis induced by carbon tetrachloride (CCl₄) and bile duct ligation (BDL) in rats (Liu et al., 2018b; Sun et al., 2018). In addition, the bioactive lignan can inhibit the proliferation of HSC-T6 cells, and the monomeric component schisandrin B (Sin B) has been shown block HSC activation by inhibiting TGF-β/Smad signaling pathway and reduce hepatic fibrosis progress in rats (Huang et al., 2011; Chen et al., 2013, 2017).

Schisandrin C (Sin C), one of the lignans of Schisandra chinensis, has been proven to resist cholestatic liver injury caused by lithocholic acid (LCA) in mice by stimulating pregnane X receptor (PXR) and to affect the antioxidant enzyme activity in rat liver microsomes to exert antioxidant effects (Lu and Liu, 1991; Fan et al., 2019). In recent years, it has been found that Sin C may be the main active substance of LWWL against hepatic fibrosis *in vivo* (Liu et al., 2018a,b). Curdione is a sesquiterpenoid component isolated from Curcuma zedoaria (Berg.) Rosc, which has the potential to inhibit the proliferation of hepatic fibroblasts. Curdione has been reported to improve pulmonary fibrosis by inhibiting the activation of the TGF-β pathway, but experimental studies of this component against hepatic fibrosis have not been reported in the literature (Park et al., 2005; Liu et al., 2020). In this study, we proved that the combination of Curdione and Sin C synergistically reverse hepatic fibrosis via modulating the TGF-β pathway and inhibiting oxidative stress, suggesting regulating multiple signal transduction pathways to combined pharmacotherapy is a valid strategy for the treatment of hepatic. And the combination of Curdione and Sin C may be used as a potential therapeutic drug for the hepatic fibrosis.

EXPERIMENTAL

Mice

SPF class C57BL/6 mice (Male) were purchased from Beijing SPF Biotechnology Co., Ltd. All mice were used at approximately weighting 18–20 g. The animals were housed at Fifth Medical Centre, Chinese PLA General Hospital for 1 week prior to the initiation of this study. All animal care and experimental procedures in this study were performed in accordance with the guidelines for care and use of laboratory animals of Fifth Medical Centre, Chinese PLA General Hospital. This study was reviewed and approved by the animal ethics committee of the Fifth Medical Centre, Chinese PLA General Hospital (Beijing, China).

Reagents and Chemicals

Schisandrin A, Schisandrin B, Schisandrin C (SinC), Schisandrol B, Isocurcumenol, Curdione, Curcumenol, Specnuezhenide, Salidroside, Phillyrin, Esculetin, Apigenin, and SYBR Green Mix were purchased from MedChemExpress (NJ, United States). Anti-Collagen1 (1:500), anti-mouse-Smad2/3 (1:2,000), and anti-mouse-P-Smad3 (1:1,000) primary and horseradish peroxidase-conjugated secondary antibodies (1:5,000) were purchased from Cell Signaling Technology (Boston, United States). The mouse Collagen IV enzyme-linked immunosorbent assay (ELISA) kits and anti-human Smad3 (1:500), anti-human P-Smad3 (1:2,000) were purchased from Abcam (Cambridge, United Kingdom). Anti-human α-SMA (1:1,000) was purchased from ABclonal (Wuhan, China) and anti-GAPDH (1:5,000) was obtained from Proteintech (Chicago, United States). The kits for determining alanine aminotransferase (ALT), aspartate aminotransferase (AST) activity, total bilirubin (TBIL), and direct bilirubin (DBIL) content were obtained from Jiancheng (Nanjing, China). Malondialdehyde (MDA) and glutathione (GSH) test kits were supplied by KANGLANG (Shanghai, China). Lactate Dehydrogenase (LDH) cytotoxicity assay kit was purchased from Beyotime (Shanghai, China). Mouse tissue hydroxyproline (Hyp) levels were measured by enzyme-linked immunosorbent assay (ELISA) kits (Cloud-Clone Corp, Houston, TX, United States). MitoSOX^{TM} Red mitochondrial superoxide indicator was manufactured by Invitrogen (Carlsbad, CA, United States). Enhanced chemiluminescent reagents was purchased from Millipore (Beijing, MA, United States).

Animal Experiment Protocol

This experiment was divided into the following groups, including control group (Control), model group (MCD feed), positive drug (colchicine) group (Col, 0.2 mg/kg), Sin C administration group alone (200 mg/kg), Cur administration group alone (50 mg/kg), Sin C + Cur combined administration group (200 + 50 mg/kg). The experimental modeling lasted for 6 weeks. After the C57BL/6 mice were adaptively reared for 1 week, used MCD feed to conduct an experimental model. Except for the normal control group, the other groups were given the solvent and administered according to the above-mentioned protocol for 6 weeks.

Serum Biochemistry

Blood samples were centrifugated at 1,500 g for 15 min to separate serum. The serum ALT and AST levels, TBIL and DBIL contents were measured using commercial kits.

Enzyme-Linked Immunosorbent Assay

Mouse liver samples were homogenized with extraction buffer to extract the proteins, then each sample was normalized by the total protein concentration. Then the levels of Collagen IV and hydroxyprolinein liver were determined using the assay kits in accordance with the manufacturer's instructions. Supernatants from cell culture were assayed with MDA according to manufacturer's instructions.

Cell Culture and Treatment

LX-2 and L0-2 cells were cultured in RPMI 1640 and Dulbecco's modified eagle medium (DMEM) medium containing 10% fetal bovine serum (FBS) and 1% penicillin/streptomycin (P/S), respectively. All cells were cultured in a sterile cell culture incubator at 37°C with 5% CO_2.

CCK-8 Assay for Cell Viability

L02 and LX-2 cells were seeded overnight in 96-well plates at a density of 1.5×10^4 and 2.5×10^4 cells/well, respectively, and treated with SinC and Curdione (0–120 μM) for 24 h. Subsequently, the cell counting kit-8 (CCK-8) working solution was added to the cells according to the manufacturer's instructions and incubated at 37°C for 30 min. Measure the absorbance at 450 nm with a microplate reader (BioTek, VT, United States).

Lactate Dehydrogenase Assay

L02 cells were seeded in a 24-well plate overnight at a density of 1.5×10^4 cells/well and the cells were treated with SinC for 6 h, and exposed to APAP (20 mM) for 12 h. Then LDH release was determined using the LDH Assay according to the manufacturer's instructions.

Measurement of Cellular Reactive Oxygen Species

The L02 cells were pretreated with Schisandrin A (40 μM), Schisandrin B (40 μM), Schisandrin C (SinC) (40 μM), Schisandrol B (40 μM), Isocurcumenol (40 μM), Curdione (40 μM), Curcumenol (40 μM), Specnuezhenide (40 μM), Salidroside (40 μM), Phillyrin (40 μM), Esculetin (40 μM), Apigenin (40 μM) for 6 h and exposed to APAP (20 mM) for 12 h. Next, the ROS levels were determined according to the previous description with some modifications (Shi et al., 2020). In addition, the determination of ROS generation with different concentrations of Sin C (10, 20, and 40 μM) in the presence or absence of APAP as described in the previous step.

Cell Culture Treatments and Sample Collection

LX-2 cells were seeded in a 24-well plate at a concentration of 7.5×10^4 cells/well and placed in the incubator overnight. The cells were treated with Curdione for 1 h, and exposed to TGF-β1 (10 ng/ml) for 24 h. The supernatant was then discarded and 1 × Laemmli sample loading buffer or TRIZOL (Invitrogen) was added to lyse the cells and the samples were collected for downstream experiments.

Western Blotting

The expressions of Collagen I, P-Smad3, Smad3, and α-SMA in mice liver tissue and LX-2 cells were analyzed by Immunoblot performed as described previously (Ai et al., 2021).

Curdione and Schisandrin C Synergistically Reverse Hepatic Fibrosis via Modulating the TGF-β Pathway...

17

Real-Time Quantitative Polymerase Chain Reaction

Quantitative Polymerase Chain Reaction (Q-PCR) analysis was used to determine gene expression in LX-2 cells and mouse liver tissue from each experimental group 25. TRIZOL (Invitrogen) reagent was used to extract total RNA from mouse liver tissue and LX-2 cells, according to the supplier's instruction. RT Master Mix for qPCR was employed based on the manufacturer's instructions for the amplification of the target gene. Use the instrument to amplify each target gene following previous methods. Primer sequences are shown in **Table 1**.

Statistical Analyses

Prism 6 (GraphPad Software, CA, United States) software was used for statistical analysis, and the experimental data were presented as mean ± standard deviation (Mean ± SD). One way ANOVA followed by an unpaired Student's t-test or Dunnett's multiple comparison *post hoc* test were used, and the difference was statistically significant with $P < 0.05$.

RESULTS

Numerous Drugs Have the Ability to Inhabit Acetaminophen-Induced Oxidative Stress and TGF-β1/Smad-Mediated Activation of Hepatic Stellate Cells *in vitro*

The composition and mechanism of LWWL reversal of hepatic fibrosis are not yet clear. Persistent hepatocyte damage is the fundamental factor of fibrosis. The accumulation of ROS in cells will cause cell oxidative damage. It is also one of

the important causes of fibrosis (Islam et al., 2017). Hence, it can be achieved by inhibiting the accumulation of ROS, reduce hepatocyte damage to reverse hepatic fibrosis. To further evaluate the effect of LWWL on hepatic fibrosis, twelve active constituents in the LWWL [schisandrin A, schisandrin B, schisandrin C (Sin C), schisandrol B, isocurcumenol, curdione, curcumenol, specnuezhenide, salidroside, phillyrin, esculetin, and apigenin] were chosen for testing. Acetaminophen (APAP) is a commonly used antipyretic and analgesic drug. Excessive use can cause oxidative damage to hepatocytes (Yan et al., 2018). Acetaminophen pretreatment on L02 cells will cause the accumulation of ROS. Hence, APAP-primed L02 cells were treated with twelve drugs for 6 h. The results showed that Schisandrin A, Schisandrin B, Schisandrin C, and Esculetin could inhibit the accumulation of ROS caused by APAP as the same as nacetylcysteine (NAC). Nacetylcysteine as the precursor of GSH is the only antidote for APAP overdose, which can significantly inhibit the accumulation of ROS caused by APAP (Corcoran et al., 1985; Corcoran and Wong, 1986). Among them, SinC showed the most potent effect on inhibiting the accumulation of ROS (**Figures 1A,B**). Moreover, The TGF-β1/Smad pathway plays a key role in the hepatic fibrosis pathway (Xu et al., 2016). Hence, we used TGF-β1 stimulation to activate the TGF-β1/Smad signaling pathway, and then pretreated with twelve drugs to observe the effects of these drugs on the TGF-β1/Smad signaling pathway. The result showed that Curdione had the strongest effect (**Figure 1C**). Therefore, we next separately focused on investigating the effect of Sin C on oxidative stress, the influence of Curdione on the TGF-β1/Smad signaling pathway and the role of the combination of two components in hepatic fibrosis.

Schisandrin C Inhibits Acetaminophen-Induced Oxidative Stress *in vitro* in a Dose-Dependent Manner

The chemical structure of Sin C is shown in **Figure 2A**. we treated APAP primed L02 cells with the twelve drugs for 24 h. CCK-8 assay results showed that cell viability was not affected by Sin C or Curdione treatment compared with control cells (at a concentration of 0–120 μM) (**Figure 2B**), indicating that Sin C and Curdione had no significant toxic effects on L02 cells within the effective concentration range. And then, we examined whether Sin C suppressed hepatocyte damage in an effective concentration range (0, 10, 20, and 40 μM). At the same time, the ability of Sin C to eliminate intracellular ROS on hepatocytes was further examined by using the MitoSOX™ Mitochondrial Superoxide Red Fluorescent Probe. The results showed that Sin C treatment increased cell viability in a dose-dependent manner and inhibited the accumulation of ROS in L02 cells (**Figures 2C–G**). In addition, Sin C also inhibited the release of LDH and the production of MDA in the cell supernatant in the presence of APAP. After in the same conditions, L02 cells were treated with Sin C only, the result showed the accumulation of ROS *in vivo* was not affected (**Figure 2H**).

TABLE 1 | Primer sequences for Real–time quantitative polymerase chain reaction.

Target gene		Sequence (5′–3′)
mouse Acta2	Forward	CCCAGACATCAGGGAGTAATGG
	Reverse	TCTATCGGATACTTCAGCGTCA
mouse Collagen I	Forward	CTGGCGGTTCAGGTCCAAT
	Reverse	TTCCAGGCAATCCACGAGC
mouse GAPDH	Forward	TGGCCTTCCGTGTTCCTAC
	Reverse	GAGTTGCTGTTGAAGTCGCA
mouse Smad3	Forward	TCTCCCCGAATCCGATGTCC
	Reverse	GCTGGTTCAGCTCGTAGTAGG
mouse TGF-β1	Forward	CTTCAATACGTCAGACATTCGGG
	Reverse	GTAACGCCAGGAATTGTTGCTA
human Acta2	Forward	CAGGGCTGTTTTCCCATCCAT
	Reverse	GCCATGTTCTATCGGGTACTTC
human Collagen I	Forward	GTCGAGGGCCAAGACGAAG
	Reverse	CAGATCACGTCATCGCACAAC
human Smad3	Forward	CCATCTCCTACTACGAGCTGAA
	Reverse	CACTGCTGCATTCCTGTTGAC
human GAPDH	Forward	AGCCACATCGCTCAGACAC
	Reverse	GCCCAATACGACCAAATCC

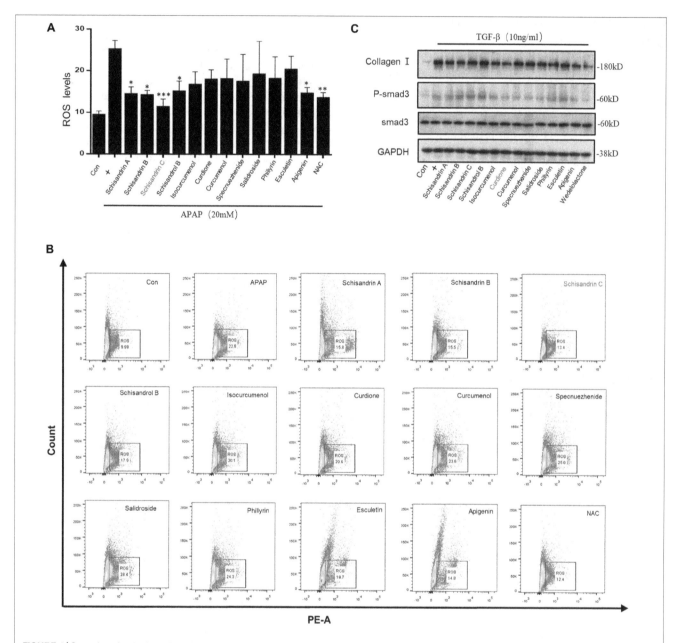

FIGURE 1 | Screening of active ingredients *in vitro* based on inhibiting oxidative stress and blocking TGF-β1/Smad-mediated hepatic stellate cells (HSC) activation. **(A,B)** The percentage of ROS positive cells were detected with MitoSox staining and analyzed by FACS. **(C)** Western blot analysis of Collagen I, Smad3, p-Smad3, GAPDH in LX-2 cells treated with twelve active ingredients (40 μM) in Liuwei Wuling tablets (LWWL) and then stimulated with TGF-β1 (10 ng/ml). Data are expressed as the mean ± SD of three independent experiments in panels **(A,B)**, $^*p < 0.05$, $^{**}p < 0.01$, and $^{***}p < 0.001$.

Curdione Prevents Hepatic Stellate Cell Activation *in vitro* Mediated by TGF-β1/Smad Signaling Pathway

The chemical structure of Curdione is shown in **Figure 3A**. The TGF-β1/Smad signaling pathway mediates the continuous synthesis of collagen in activating HSCs and plays a central role in the pathogenesis of hepatic fibrosis (Mu et al., 2018). Our results showed that cell viability was not affected by Curdione treatment for 24 h compared with control cells (at a concentration of 0–120 μM Curdione) (**Figure 3C**), indicating that Curdione

had no significant toxic effects on LX-2 cells within the effective concentration range. Based on these results, we investigated whether Curdione had an effect on inhibiting TGF-β1/Smad signaling *in vitro*. LX-2 cells were pretreated with Curdione (0, 10, 20, and 40 μM) for 1 h and then exposed to TGF-β1 (10 ng/ml) for a further 24 h. Our results showed that there was a decrease in expression and phosphorylation of Smad3 in the TGF-β1 signaling after Curdione pretreatment (**Figures 3B,D**). Curdione also down-regulated α-SMA and collagen I expression mediated by TGF-β1 in a dose-dependent manner (**Figures 3B,D**).

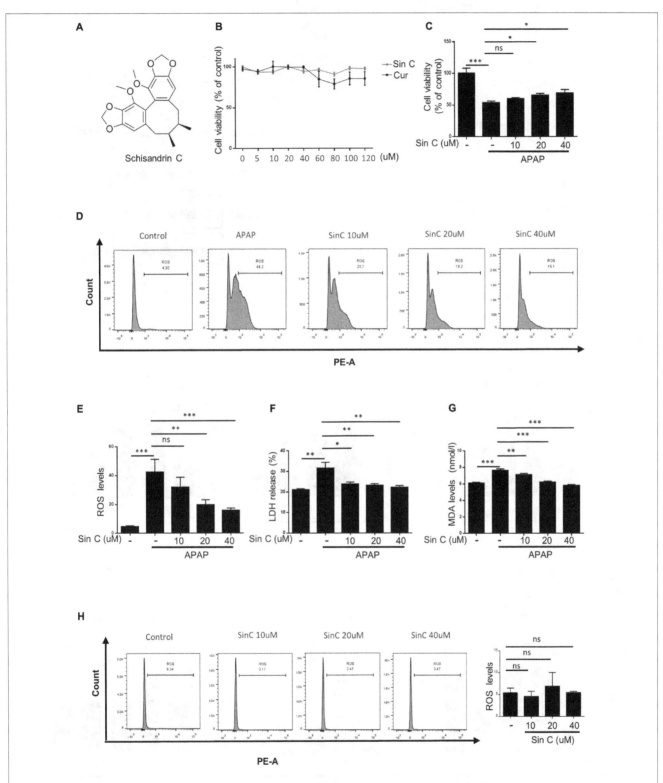

FIGURE 2 | Schisandrin (Sin C) inhibits acetaminophen (APAP)-induced oxidative stress *in vitro*. **(A)** Structure of Sin C. **(B)** The Cell viability of L02 cells treated with different concentrations of Sin C and Curdione was determined using CCK-8 kit. **(C–G)** L02 cells were pretreated with SinC (10, 20, and 40 μM) for 6 h and then exposed to APAP (20 mM) for a further 12 h. The survival rate by CCK-8 **(C)** and the release of LDH **(D)** and MDA **(E)** were detected. **(F–G)** The percentage of reactive oxygen species (ROS) positive cells were detected with MitoSox staining and analyzed by FACS. **(H)** L02 cells were treated with SinC (10, 20, and 40 μM) for 18 h without any treatment and the percentage of ROS positive cells were detected with MitoSox staining and analyzed by FACS. Data are expressed as the mean ± SD of three independent experiments, $^*p < 0.05$, $^{**}p < 0.01$, and $^{***}p < 0.001$; ns, not significant.

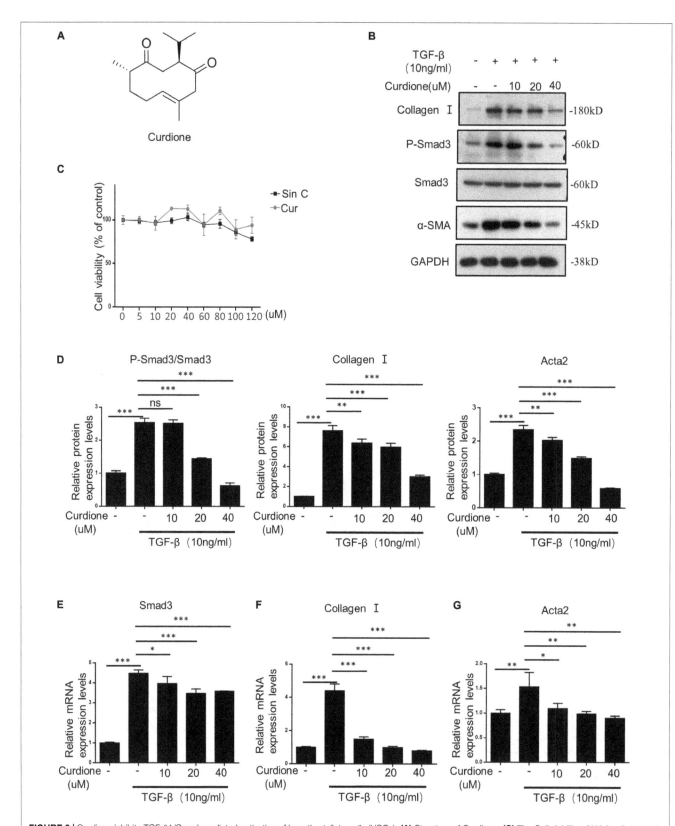

FIGURE 3 | Curdione inhibits TGF-β1/Smad-mediated activation of hepatic stellate cells (HSCs). **(A)** Structure of Curdione. **(C)** The Cell viability of LX-2 cells treated with different concentrations of SinC and Curdione was determined using CCK-8 kit. LX-2 cells treated with Curdione (10, 20, and 40 μM) and then stimulated with TGF-β1 (10 ng/ml), the protein of Collagen I, α-SMA, Smad3, p-Smad3, GAPDH were detected by Western blot analysis **(B,D)**. And quantitative PCR analysis of Collagen I, α-SMA, Smad3 mRNA levels **(E–G)**. Data are expressed as the mean ± SD of three independent experiments in panels **(C–G)**, *$p < 0.05$, **$p < 0.01$, and ***$p < 0.001$; ns, not significant.

Similarly, Curdione inhibited the mRNA levels of Smad3, α-SMA and collagen I (**Figures 3E–G**). Combining the above results, we reveal that Curdione suppresses the activation of HSCs by targeting the TGF-β1/Smad signaling pathway.

The Combination of Schisandrin C and Curdione Significantly Alleviates Hepatic Fibrosis in Mice With MCD-Induced Hepatic Fibrosis

We have demonstrated *in vitro* that Sin C had the effect of resisting oxidative stress and protecting hepatocytes, and Curdione could target and regulate the TGF-β1/Smad pathway. We further evaluated whether the Sin C and Curdione combined mediated anti-hepatic fibrosis effect is better than the effect of Sin C and Curdione alone in the MCD-induced hepatic fibrosis mouse model. The MCD diet was used to induce hepatic fibrosis and the mice were randomly divided into six groups, except for the control group, all the other groups were fed with MCD fodder. Compared with control group, model group mice showed the histopathological changes of HE and Masson confirmed hepatocytes injury and hepatic fibrosis. Curdione, Sin C, and their combined treatment groups showed good effects in preventing hepatic fibrosis. Moreover, the coordinate repression of Curdione and Sin C on hepatic fibrosis was significantly superior than Curdione or Sin C alone (**Figures 4A,B**). Hyproxyproline is a unique amino acid component of collagen in the body. Together with Collagen IV, it serves as an important indicator of collagen metabolism in the body (Attallah et al., 2007; Mak and Mei, 2017). Consistent with the results of liver histopathological evaluation, the combination therapy of Curdione and Sin C also reduced the content of hydroxyproline and Collagen IV in liver tissue more effectively than Curdione or Sin C alone (**Figures 5E,F**). In addition, the serum levels of ALT, AST, DBIL, and TBIL in mice induced by MCD are consistent with histopathological analysis (**Figures 5A–D**).

The Combination of Schisandrin C and Curdione Reduces MCD-Induced Hepatic Fibrosis by Regulating the TGF-β1/Smad Pathway and Inhibiting Oxidative Stress

Excessive consumption of GSH is a important way to produce ROS that leads to cell oxidative damage (Wu et al., 2019). For this reason, we measured the level of GSH in liver tissue. The results showed that Curdione and Sin C alone or in combination with both increased the consumption of GSH caused by MCD to varying degrees (**Figure 6B**). α-SMA is a unique marker that activates HSC to cause hepatic fibrosis, so we detected the expression of α-SMA by immunohistochemical staining and qPCR (**Figures 6A,C**). Our immunohistochemical results showed that Curdione and Sin C treatment reduced collagen I and α-SMA expression in MCD-induced hepatic fibrosis mice (**Figure 6A**). As revealed by qPCR analysis (**Figures 6C,D**), Curdione and Sin C treatment also significantly reduced the MCD-induced increase

in collagen I and α-SMA mRNA levels. The activation and continuous activation of HSC are regulated by the TGF-β1/Smad signaling pathway mediated by TGF-β1 (Inagaki and Okazaki, 2007; Dewidar et al., 2019). Therefore, we used western blotting to detect the expression of P-Smad 3/Smad 3 in liver tissue. Compared with the control group, the protein expression level of P-Smad 3/Smad 3 in the model group was significantly increased, and the protein level decreased after the administration of Curdione, Sin C, and the combination of Curdione and Sin C (**Figure 6G**). Moreover, the combination group was significantly better than the single administration group. Q-PCR analysis of TGF-β1 and Smad 3 mRNA level is consistent with protein expression level (**Figures 6E,F**).

DISCUSSION

Our present research demonstrates that SinC, Curdione, or the combination of SinC and Curdione can reverse hepatic fibrosis *in vivo*, evidenced by the alleviation of pathological lesions and the changes in biochemical indicators. Among them, the combined effect of SinC and Curdione in inhibiting hepatic fibrosis is better than SinC or Curdione alone. In addition, SinC can inhibit the accumulation of ROS *in vitro*, improve cell survival, and reduce the release of LDH and Curdione can block the activation of HSC by acting on TGF-β1/Smad signaling pathway. Our research confirms the combination of drugs that inhibits oxidative stress *in vivo*, reduces hepatocyte damage and blocks the TGF-β1/Smad pathway to reduce ECM deposition will more effectively solve hepatic fibrosis.

Hepatic fibrosis is secondary to liver damage (Gieling et al., 2009; Aydın and Akçalı, 2018). Hepatocyte damage can further promote the activation of HSC in the liver (Aydın and Akçalı, 2018). Therefore, reversing hepatocyte damage is one of the important ways to prevent and treat hepatic fibrosis. The production of ROS in the liver is an important cause of hepatocyte damage (Lee et al., 2015). When the liver is stimulated by foreign substances such as acetaminophen and ethanol, it will cause excessive accumulation of ROS in the liver and further aggravate hepatocyte damage (McGill and Jaeschke, 2013). In addition, the further stimulate the activation of HSC can be mediated by ROS or other secretions such as superoxide anion (Cheng et al., 2019). After HSCs are activated by ROS, they further promote the excessive secretion and accumulation of ECM, leading to hepatic fibrosis. In our research, we found that SinC can reduce the accumulation of ROS, the release of LDH and MDA in cells, and protect LO2 cells from APAP damage. In MCD-induced hepatic fibrosis model mice, it plays a superior role in protecting liver and anti-oxidation. This indicates that SinC can reverse hepatic fibrosis by inhibiting oxidative stress and reduce further damage to hepatocytes.

The key to hepatic fibrosis is the activation of HSC (Bataller and Brenner, 2005), which can mediate TGF-β1/Smad signaling pathway and cause the formation of hepatic fibrosis

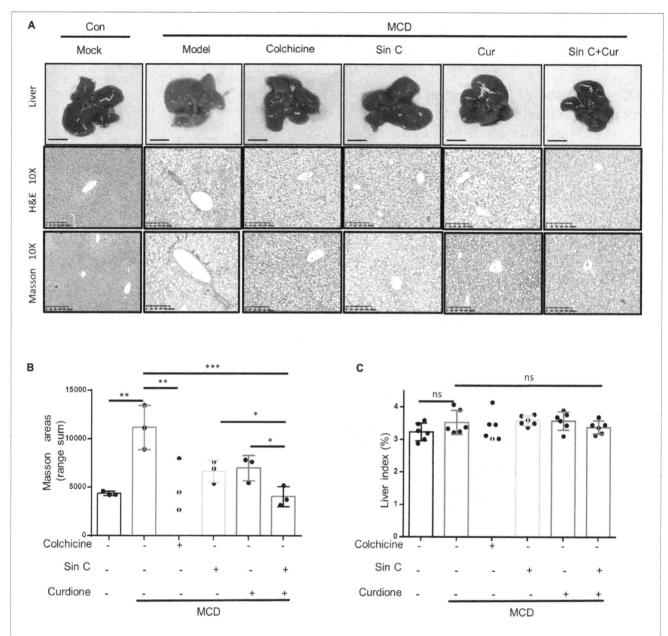

FIGURE 4 | The combination of Sin C and Curdione treatment significantly improved the histopathological changes in the liver of mice induced by MCD feed. The mice were pretreated with SinC, Curdione or combination of SinC and Curdione vehicle by gavage and fed with MCD feed for 6 weeks. Histopathological changes in the liver **(A)**, Scale bars represent 200 μm Quantitative results of Masson staining sections **(B)** and liver coefficients **(C)**. Data are expressed as the mean ± SD from three independent mice samples **(A,B)**, $^*p < 0.05$, $^{**}p < 0.01$, and $^{***}p < 0.001$; ns, not significant.

(Inagaki and Okazaki, 2007). Studies have shown that TGF-β1 siRNA significantly down-regulates the expression of TGF-β1, thereby inhibiting the activation and proliferation of HSCs, and reversing rat hepatic fibrosis (Hafez et al., 2017). The TGF-β1/Smad signaling pathway can enhance the activation of stellate cells and play an important role in the excessive accumulation of ECM components induced by TGF-β1 (Lang et al., 2011; Duan et al., 2014). Our data showed that the expression of p-Smad3 in LX-2 cells was up-regulated under the stimulation of TGF-β1, as well as the activated HSC markers

α-SMA and collagen I. In addition, the expression of TGF-β1 and p-Smad3 in the liver tissue of mice with hepatic fibrosis induced by MCD was also up-regulated. However, Curdione partially reversed the levels of p-Smad3, α-SMA, and collagen I in LX-2 cells and mouse liver tissue in response to TGF-β1 (Zhou et al., 2017). The above data indicate that Curdione can inhibit TGF-β1-induced HSC activation by modulating TGF-β1/Smad signaling.

To date, there is no internationally recognized safe, effective and liver-targeted drug that has been approved

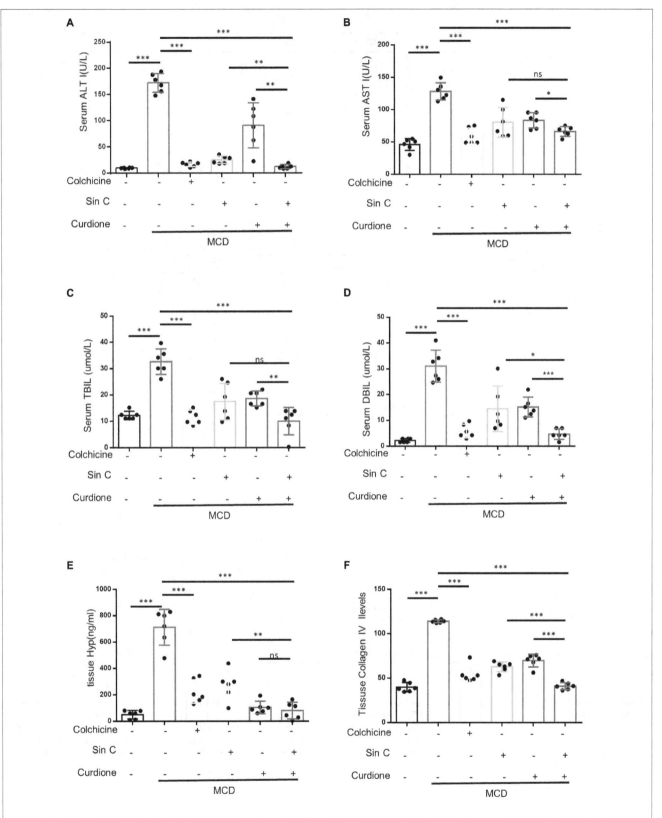

FIGURE 5 | A combination of Sin C and Curdione treatment dramatically inhibits hepatic fibrosis and injury in MCD feed fed-induced mice. Mice were treated as described in **Figure 4**. Serum level of ALT **(A)**, AST **(B)**, TBIL **(C)**, and DBIL **(D)** were detected. The amount of hydroxyproline **(E)** and Collagen IV **(F)** in liver of mice were measured using commercial ELISA kits. Data are expressed as the mean ± SD from six independent mice samples, $*p < 0.05$, $**p < 0.01$, and $***p < 0.001$; ns, not significant.

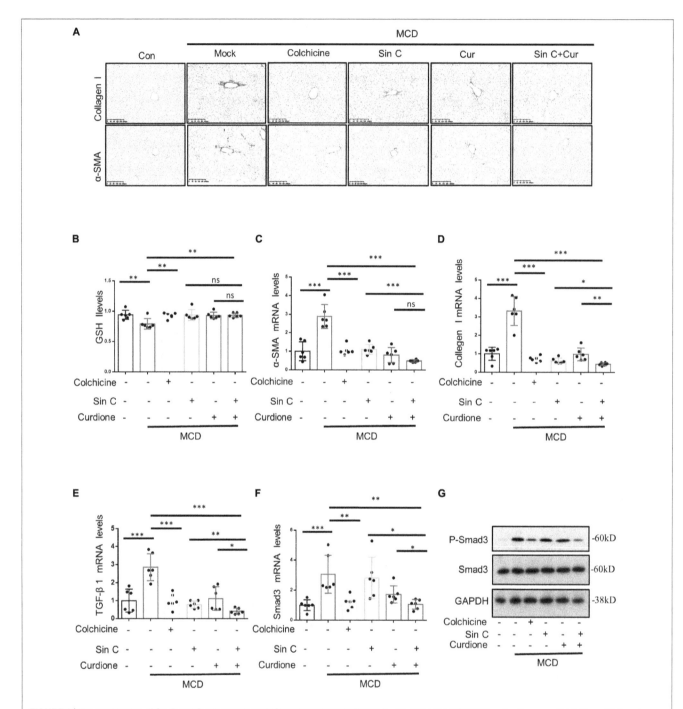

FIGURE 6 | The combination of Sin C and Curdione reduces MCD-induced hepatic fibrosis by regulating the TGF-β1/Smad pathway and inhibiting oxidative stress. Immunohistochemical staining of α-SMA and collagen I **(A)** The amount of glutathione (GSH) **(B)** in liver of mice were measured using commercial ELISA kits. Quantitative polymerase chain reaction (PCR) analysis of mRNA levels of α-SMA, Collagen I, TGF-β 1, and Smad3 **(C–F)**. Western blot analysis of p-Smad3, Smad3, and GAPDH in livers from control, MCD fed-induced hepatic fibrosis mice, MCD fed-induced hepatic fibrosis mice treated with colchicine (0.2 mg/kg), Sin C (200 mg/kg), Curdione (50 mg/kg) or combination of Curdione and Sin C **(G)**. Data are expressed as the mean ± SD from six independent mice samples **(B–F)**, $*p < 0.05$, $**p < 0.01$, and $***p < 0.001$; ns, not significant.

by the FDA for the treatment of human hepatic fibrosis (Campana and Iredale, 2017), the general treatment is to eliminate chronic stress and liver transplantation. Combination therapies that target multiple pathways or involve multiple key molecules are considered to have great promise for the treatment of hepatic fibrosis (Trautwein et al., 2015).

Hepatocyte damage and HSCs activation are important reasons for the development of hepatic fibrosis. SinC and Curdione can reverse hepatic fibrosis by inhibiting oxidative stress, protecting hepatocytes and regulating TGF-β1/Smad signal pathway to block HSC activation, respectively. More importantly, the two combined play a superior role in reversing hepatic fibrosis, and can be used as a promising candidate for the treatment of hepatic fibrosis.

REFERENCES

Ai, Y., Shi, W., Zuo, X., Sun, X., Chen, Y., Wang, Z., et al. (2021). The combination of schisandrol B and wedelolactone synergistically reverses hepatic fibrosis via modulating multiple signaling pathways in mice. *Front. Pharmacol.* 12:655531. doi: 10.3389/fphar.2021.655531

Attallah, A. M., Toson, E. A., Shiha, G. E., Omran, M. M., Abdel-Aziz, M. M., and El-Dosoky, I. (2007). Evaluation of serum procollagen aminoterminal propeptide III, laminin, and hydroxyproline as predictors of severe fibrosis in patients with chronic hepatitis C. *J. Immunoassay Immunochem.* 28, 199–211. doi: 10.1080/15321810701454649

Aydın, M. M., and Akçalı, K. C. (2018). Liver fibrosis. *Turk. J. Gastroenterol.* 29, 14–21. doi: 10.5152/tjg.2018.17330

Bataller, R., and Brenner, D. A. (2005). Liver fibrosis. *J. Clin. Invest.* 115, 209–218. doi: 10.1172/JCI24282

Campana, L., and Iredale, J. P. (2017). Regression of liver fibrosis. *Semin. Liver Dis.* 37, 1–10. doi: 10.1055/s-0036-1597816

Chen, Q., Zhang, H., Cao, Y., Li, Y., Sun, S., Zhang, J., et al. (2017). Schisandrin B attenuates CCl(4)-induced liver fibrosis in rats by regulation of Nrf2-ARE and TGF-β/Smad signaling pathways. *Drug Des. Devel. Ther.* 11, 2179–2191. doi: 10.2147/DDDT.S137507

Chen, Y. C., Liaw, C. C., Cheng, Y. B., Lin, Y. C., Chen, C. H., Huang, Y. T., et al. (2013). Anti-liver fibrotic lignans from the fruits of Schisandra arisanensis and Schisandra sphenanthera. *Bioorg. Med. Chem. Lett.* 23, 880–885. doi: 10.1016/j.bmcl.2012.11.040

Cheng, Q., Li, C., Yang, C. F., Zhong, Y. J., Wu, D., Shi, L., et al. (2019). Methyl ferulic acid attenuates liver fibrosis and hepatic stellate cell activation through the TGF-β1/Smad and NOX4/ROS pathways. *Chem. Biol. Interact.* 299, 131–139. doi: 10.1016/j.cbi.2018.12.006

Corcoran, G. B., Todd, E. L., Racz, W. J., Hughes, H., Smith, C. V., and Mitchell, J. R. (1985). Effects of N-acetylcysteine on the disposition and metabolism of acetaminophen in mice. *J. Pharmacol. Exp. Ther.* 232, 857–863.

Corcoran, G. B., and Wong, B. K. (1986). Role of glutathione in prevention of acetaminophen-induced hepatotoxicity by N-acetyl-L-cysteine in vivo: studies with N-acetyl-D-cysteine in mice. *J. Pharmacol. Exp. Ther.* 238, 54–61.

Cordero-Espinoza, L., and Huch, M. (2018). The balancing act of the liver: tissue regeneration versus fibrosis. *J. Clin. Invest.* 128, 85–96. doi: 10.1172/JCI93562

Dewidar, B., Meyer, C., Dooley, S., and Meindl-Beinker, A. N. (2019). TGF-β in hepatic stellate cell activation and liver fibrogenesis-updated 2019. *Cells* 8:1419. doi: 10.3390/cells8111419

Duan, W. J., Yu, X., Huang, X. R., Yu, J. W., and Lan, H. Y. (2014). Opposing roles for Smad2 and Smad3 in peritoneal fibrosis in vivo and in vitro. *Am. J. Pathol.* 184, 2275–2284. doi: 10.1016/j.ajpath.2014.04.014

Elpek, G. (2014). Cellular and molecular mechanisms in the pathogenesis of liver fibrosis: an update. *World J. Gastroenterol.* 20, 7260–7276. doi: 10.3748/wjg. v20.i23.7260

Fagone, P., Mangano, K., Pesce, A., Portale, T. R., Puleo, S., and Nicoletti, F. (2016). Emerging therapeutic targets for the treatment of hepatic fibrosis. *Drug Discov. Today* 21, 369–375. doi: 10.1016/j.drudis.2015.10.015

Fan, S., Liu, C., Jiang, Y., Gao, Y., Chen, Y., Fu, K., et al. (2019). Lignans from Schisandra sphenanthera protect against lithocholic acid-induced cholestasis by pregnane X receptor activation in mice. *J. Ethnopharmacol.* 245:112103. doi: 10.1016/j.jep.2019.112103

AUTHOR CONTRIBUTIONS

WD, QQ, ZL, XZ, ZB, and XX participated in research design. WD, QQ, and ZL wrote or contributed to the writing of the manuscript. WD, QQ, ZL, LL, RL, and TL conducted experiments. XZ, ZB, and XX contributed new reagents or analytic tools. YH, ZF, and LR performed data analysis. All authors contributed to the article and approved the submitted version.

Gandhi, C. R. (2012). Oxidative stress and hepatic stellate cells: a paradoxical relationship. *Trends Cell Mol. Biol.* 7, 1–10.

Gieling, R. G., Wallace, K., and Han, Y. P. (2009). Interleukin-1 participates in the progression from liver injury to fibrosis. *Am. J. Physiol. Gastrointest. Liver Physiol.* 296, G1324–G1331. doi: 10.1152/ajpgi.90564.2008

Guimarães, E. L., Franceschi, M. F., Grivicich, I., Dal-Pizzol, F., Moreira, J. C., Guaragna, R. M., et al. (2006). Relationship between oxidative stress levels and activation state on a hepatic stellate cell line. *Liver Int.* 26, 477–485. doi: 10.1111/j.1478-3231.2006.01245.x

Guo, S. G., Zhang, W., Jiang, T., Dai, M., Zhang, L. F., Meng, Y. C., et al. (2004). Influence of serum collected from rat perfused with compound Biejiaruangan drug on hepatic stellate cells. *World J. Gastroenterol.* 10, 1487–1494. doi: 10.3748/wjg.v10.i10.1487

Hafez, M. M., Hamed, S. S., El-Khadragy, M. F., Hassan, Z. K., Al Rejaie, S. S., Sayed-Ahmed, M. M., et al. (2017). Effect of ginseng extract on the TGF-β1 signaling pathway in CCl(4)-induced liver fibrosis in rats. *BMC Complement. Altern. Med.* 17:45. doi: 10.1186/s12906-016-1507-0

Huang, H. C., Lin, Y. C., Fazary, A. E., Lo, I. W., Liaw, C. C., Huang, Y. Z., et al. (2011). New and bioactive lignans from the fruits of Schisandra sphenanthera. *Food Chem.* 128, 348–357. doi: 10.1016/j.foodchem.2011.03.030

Huang, Y., Deng, X., and Liang, J. (2017). Modulation of hepatic stellate cells and reversibility of hepatic fibrosis. *Exp. Cell Res.* 352, 420–426. doi: 10.1016/j.yexcr.2017.02.038

Inagaki, Y., and Okazaki, I. (2007). Emerging insights into Transforming growth factor beta Smad signal in hepatic fibrogenesis. *Gut* 56, 284–292. doi: 10.1136/gut.2005.088690

Islam, M. A., Al Mamun, M. A., Faruk, M., Ul Islam, M. T., Rahman, M. M., Alam, M. N., et al. (2017). Astaxanthin ameliorates hepatic damage and oxidative stress in carbon tetrachloride-administered rats. *Pharmacognosy Res.* 9, S84–S91. doi: 10.4103/pr.pr_26_17

Kumar, S., Wang, J., Shanmukhappa, S. K., and Gandhi, C. R. (2017). Toll-like receptor 4-independent carbon tetrachloride-induced fibrosis and lipopolysaccharide-induced acute liver injury in mice: role of hepatic stellate cells. *Am. J. Pathol.* 187, 1356–1367. doi: 10.1016/j.ajpath.2017.01.021

Lang, Q., Liu, Q., Xu, N., Qian, K. L., Qi, J. H., Sun, Y. C., et al. (2011). The antifibrotic effects of TGF-β1 siRNA on hepatic fibrosis in rats. *Biochem. Biophys. Res. Commun.* 409, 448–453. doi: 10.1016/j.bbrc.2011.05.023

Lee, Y. A., Wallace, M. C., and Friedman, S. L. (2015). Pathobiology of liver fibrosis: a translational success story. *Gut* 64, 830–841. doi: 10.1136/gutjnl-2014-306842

Liu, H., Dong, F., Li, G., Niu, M., Zhang, C., Han, Y., et al. (2018a). Liuweiwuling tablets attenuate BDL-induced hepatic fibrosis via modulation of TGF-β/Smad and NF-κB signaling pathways. *J. Ethnopharmacol.* 210, 232–241. doi: 10.1016/j.jep.2017.08.029

Liu, H., Zhang, Z., Hu, H., Zhang, C., Niu, M., Li, R., et al. (2018b). Protective effects of Liuweiwuling tablets on carbon tetrachloride-induced hepatic fibrosis in rats. *BMC Complement. Altern. Med.* 18:212. doi: 10.1186/s12906-018-2276-8

Liu, P., Miao, K., Zhang, L., Mou, Y., Xu, Y., Xiong, W., et al. (2020). Curdione ameliorates bleomycin-induced pulmonary fibrosis by repressing TGF-β-induced fibroblast to myofibroblast differentiation. *Respir. Res.* 21:58. doi: 10.1186/s12931-020-1300-y

Lu, H., and Liu, G. T. (1991). Effect of dibenzo[a,c]cyclooctene lignans isolated from Fructus schizandrae on lipid peroxidation and anti-oxidative enzyme activity. *Chem. Biol. Interact.* 78, 77–84. doi: 10.1016/0009-2797(91)90104-F

Mak, K. M., and Mei, R. (2017). Basement membrane type IV collagen and laminin: an overview of their biology and value as fibrosis biomarkers of liver disease. *Anat. Rec.* 300, 1371–1390. doi: 10.1002/ar.23567

McGill, M. R., and Jaeschke, H. (2013). Metabolism and disposition of acetaminophen: recent advances in relation to hepatotoxicity and diagnosis. *Pharm. Res.* 30, 2174–2187. doi: 10.1007/s11095-013-1007-6

Mu, M., Zuo, S., Wu, R. M., Deng, K. S., Lu, S., Zhu, J. J., et al. (2018). Ferulic acid attenuates liver fibrosis and hepatic stellate cell activation via inhibition of TGF-β/Smad signaling pathway. *Drug Des. Devel. Ther.* 12, 4107–4115. doi: 10.2147/DDDT.S186726

Nagase, H., Visse, R., and Murphy, G. (2006). Structure and function of matrix metalloproteinases and TIMPs. *Cardiovasc. Res.* 69, 562–573. doi: 10.1016/j.cardiores.2005.12.002

Pan, X., Ma, X., Jiang, Y., Wen, J., Yang, L., Chen, D., et al. (2020). A comprehensive review of natural products against liver fibrosis: flavonoids, quinones, lignans, phenols, and acids. *Evid. Based Complement. Alternat. Med.* 2020:7171498. doi: 10.1155/2020/7171498

Park, S. D., Jung, J. H., Lee, H. W., Kwon, Y. M., Chung, K. H., Kim, M. G., et al. (2005). Zedoariae rhizoma and curcumin inhibits platelet-derived growth factor-induced proliferation of human hepatic myofibroblasts. *Int. Immunopharmacol.* 5, 555–569. doi: 10.1016/j.intimp.2004.11.003

Parola, M., and Robino, G. (2001). Oxidative stress-related molecules and liver fibrosis. *J. Hepatol.* 35, 297–306. doi: 10.1016/S0168-8278(01)00142-8

Sánchez-Valle, V., Chávez-Tapia, N. C., Uribe, M., and Méndez-Sánchez, N. (2012). Role of oxidative stress and molecular changes in liver fibrosis: a review. *Curr. Med. Chem.* 19, 4850–4860. doi: 10.2174/092986712803341520

Schuppan, D., Ashfaq-Khan, M., Yang, A. T., and Kim, Y. O. (2018). Liver fibrosis: direct antifibrotic agents and targeted therapies. *Matrix Biol.* 68-69, 435–451. doi: 10.1016/j.matbio.2018.04.006

Shi, W., Xu, G., Zhan, X., Gao, Y., Wang, Z., Fu, S., et al. (2020). Carnosol inhibits inflammasome activation by directly targeting HSP90 to treat inflammasome-mediated diseases. *Cell Death Dis.* 11:252. doi: 10.1038/s41419-020-2460-x

Sun, J., Wu, Y., Long, C., He, P., Gu, J., Yang, L., et al. (2018). Anthocyanins isolated from blueberry ameliorates CCl(4) induced liver fibrosis by modulation of oxidative stress, inflammation and stellate cell activation in mice. *Food Chem. Toxicol.* 120, 491–499. doi: 10.1016/j.fct.2018.07.048

Sung, Y. C., Liu, Y. C., Chao, P. H., Chang, C. C., Jin, P. R., Lin, T. T., et al. (2018). Combined delivery of sorafenib and a MEK inhibitor using CXCR4-targeted nanoparticles reduces hepatic fibrosis and prevents tumor development. *Theranostics* 8, 894–905. doi: 10.7150/thno.21168

Trautwein, C., Friedman, S. L., Schuppan, D., and Pinzani, M. (2015). Hepatic fibrosis: concept to treatment. *J. Hepatol.* 62, S15–S24. doi: 10.1016/j.jhep.2015.02.039

Wu, C. T., Deng, J. S., Huang, W. C., Shieh, P. C., Chung, M. I., and Huang, G. J. (2019). Salvianolic acid C against acetaminophen-induced acute liver injury by attenuating inflammation, oxidative stress, and apoptosis through inhibition of the Keap1/Nrf2/HO-1 signaling. *Oxid. Med. Cell Longev.* 2019:9056845. doi: 10.1155/2019/9056845

Wu, X., Wu, X., Ma, Y., Shao, F., Tan, Y., Tan, T., et al. (2016). CUG-binding protein 1 regulates HSC activation and liver fibrogenesis. *Nat. Commun.* 7:13498. doi: 10.1038/ncomms13498

Xu, F., Liu, C., Zhou, D., and Zhang, L. (2016). TGF-β/SMAD pathway and its regulation in hepatic fibrosis. *J. Histochem. Cytochem.* 64, 157–167. doi: 10.1369/0022155415627681

Xu, Y., Sun, X., Zhang, R., Cao, T., Cai, S. Y., Boyer, J. L., et al. (2020). A positive feedback loop of TET3 and TGF-β1 promotes liver fibrosis. *Cell Rep.* 30, 1310.e5–1318.e5. doi: 10.1016/j.celrep.2019.12.092

Yan, H., Huang, Z., Bai, Q., Sheng, Y., Hao, Z., Wang, Z., et al. (2018). Natural product andrographolide alleviated APAP-induced liver fibrosis by activating Nrf2 antioxidant pathway. *Toxicology* 396-397, 1–12. doi: 10.1016/j.tox.2018.01.007

Yang, M. D., Chiang, Y. M., Higashiyama, R., Asahina, K., Mann, D. A., Mann, J., et al. (2012). Rosmarinic acid and baicalin epigenetically derepress peroxisomal proliferator-activated receptor γ in hepatic stellate cells for their antifibrotic effect. *Hepatology* 55, 1271–1281. doi: 10.1002/hep.24792

Zhang, L., and Schuppan, D. (2014). Traditional Chinese Medicine (TCM) for fibrotic liver disease: hope and hype. *J. Hepatol.* 61, 166–168. doi: 10.1016/j.jhep.2014.03.009

Zhou, L., Dong, X., Wang, L., Shan, L., Li, T., Xu, W., et al. (2017). Casticin attenuates liver fibrosis and hepatic stellate cell activation by blocking TGF-β/Smad signaling pathway. *Oncotarget* 8, 56267–56280. doi: 10.18632/oncotarget.17453

3

Gut Microbiome Contributes to Liver Fibrosis Impact on T Cell Receptor Immune Repertoire

Qing Liang[1], Meina Zhang[1], Yudi Hu[1], Wei Zhang[2], Ping Zhu[3], Yujie Chen[1], Pengxin Xue[1], Qiyuan Li[1] and Kejia Wang[1]*

[1] National Institute for Data Science in Health and Medicine, School of Medicine, Xiamen University, Xiamen, China,
[2] Department of Pathology, The 971 Hospital of People's Liberation Army Navy, Qingdao, China, [3] Department of Gynecology and Obstetrics, The 971 Hospital of People's Liberation Army Navy, Qingdao, China

*Correspondence:
Kejia Wang
wangkejia@xmu.edu.cn

Gut microbiota (GM) modifies the intrahepatic immune microenvironment, but the underlying mechanisms remain poorly understood. Liver fibrosis-associated imprinting is predicted to be reflected in GM. This study investigated the link between GM and the intrahepatic T cell receptor (TCR) immune repertoire (IR), and whether GM modulates the intrahepatic immune microenvironment via TCR IR during liver fibrosis. We analyzed the correlation between GM and TCR IR during liver fibrogenesis. Accordingly, 16S rRNA gene sequencing (16S-seq) and bulk immune repertoire sequencing (IR-seq) were performed to characterize GM and intrahepatic TCR IR. Fecal microbial transplant (FMT) and TCRβ knockout (Tcrb^{KO}) mouse models were employed to determine the biological link between GM and TCR IR in liver fibrosis. We found that GM and intrahepatic TCR IR are highly correlated, with both showing reduced diversity and centralized distribution during liver fibrosis. The restoration of normal intestinal microbiota may reshape intrahepatic TCR IR and delay liver fibrosis. Interestingly, TCR IR ablation abrogated the impact of GM on liver fibrogenesis. Furthermore, GM modulated hepatic stellate cell (HSC) activation via TCR IR-mediated intrahepatic immune milieu. Our study demonstrates that GM, which exhibits cross-talk with the intrahepatic TCR IR, influences the intrahepatic immune microenvironment and liver fibrosis progression.

Keywords: gut microbiome, T cell receptor, immune repertoire, liver fibrosis, immune microenvironment

INTRODUCTION

The gut microbiota (GM) (comprising more than 100 trillion bacteria) represents a "footprint" of genetic and environmental factors. The GM has been implicated in the pathophysiology of many intestinal and extraintestinal diseases (Tilg et al., 2016). GM, considered a virtual organ, forms axes with various extraintestinal organs, including the brain, liver, and kidney as well as cardiovascular and endocrine systems. Characteristically, the gut-liver axis is a close anatomical, functional, and bidirectional interaction that occurs primarily through the portal circulation (Milosevic et al., 2019). Intestinal antigens (IAg) (originating either from pathogenic microorganisms or from food) that enter the portal circulation, are captured by intrahepatic antigen-presenting cells (APCs), leading to T cell receptor (TCR) recognition and hence the activation of the adaptive immune system. The interaction between the GM and intrahepatic immune microenvironment is regulated and stabilized by a complex network of factors including IAg, immune cells, and cytokines. GM dysbiosis leads to the excessive production of bacterial fragments and products [including lipopolysaccharides (LPS), peptidoglycans, and flagellin], which reach the liver through the portal system, contributing to chronic inflammation and liver fibrosis (Zhou et al., 2019). Emerging evidence suggests that the GM is altered following intestinal microbiota transplantation in patients with pre-cirrhotic liver disease and cirrhosis (Ohtani and Kawada, 2019; Bajaj and Khoruts, 2020). Liver fibrogenesis triggers an upsurge in the number of bacteria in circulation, indicating that intestinal microbiota modify the progression of liver fibrosis (Tilg et al., 2016).

The liver is structurally and functionally heterogeneous and is known to induce immune tolerance and immunity (Breous et al., 2009). In the liver, cell types such as hepatocytes, immune cells, and hepatic stellate cells (HSC) interact with each other. Recent studies have investigated the crucial role of different intrahepatic immunocyte subsets (including T cells, B cells, neutrophils, macrophages, and innate lymphoid cells) in the progression of liver inflammation and fibrosis (Koyama and Brenner, 2017; Tosello-Trampont et al., 2017; Wahid et al., 2018). An aberrant intrahepatic immune microenvironment (aberrant immune cell distribution and cytokines/chemokine secretion) induces HSC transdifferentiation from quiescent lipocytes into myofibroblast-like cells to drive fibrogenesis (Friedman, 2008; Higashi et al., 2017). Evidence from studies indicates that adaptive immune cells, especially T and B cells, can modulate inflammation and fibrosis in response to liver injury (Novobrantseva et al., 2005; Holt et al., 2006; Hammerich et al., 2014). However, the links between GM and the adaptive immune system in the pathogenic progression of liver fibrosis and whether GM modulates HSC activation in the intrahepatic immune microenvironment under the context of chronic liver injury remain largely unknown.

T cells, expressing a TCR heterodimer consisting of αβ or γδ chains, belong to the T lymphocyte subset. The complementarity-determining region 3 (CDR3) region of TCRβ plays a critical role in the major histocompatibility complex (MHC)-peptide complex recognition, which determines antigen recognition, immune activation, clonal expansion, and selection for T cells (Pannetier et al., 1993; Nikolich-Zugich et al., 2004). The CDR3 region is composed of variable (V), diversity (D), and the joining (J) domains spanning from the terminus of the V domain to the beginning of the J domain. It is thought that the hypervariable CDR3 region of TCRβ, referred to as the TCR IR, mediates endogenous or exogenous stimuli (infection and disease) and undergoes reconstitution in response to various antigens (Mikszta et al., 1999). In addition to TCR-mediated Ag recognition and pathogen clearance, our preceding work demonstrated an immunoregulatory function of TCR IR reconstitution in other immune cells in the hepatic immune microenvironment (Liang et al., 2018).

Despite all this knowledge, it remains unknown how various components of GM interact with intrahepatic TCR immune repertoire (IR). Next-generation sequencing (NSG) provides a tool for describing the features of TCR IR and the distribution of GM. In this study, we analyzed the GM profiles and TCR distribution using 16S rRNA gene sequencing (16S-seq) and bulk immune repertoire sequencing (IR-seq) to reveal the variations in GM and TCR IR during liver fibrogenesis, as well as associations between GM shift and TCR transformation. In addition, fecal microbial transplant (FMT) and TCRβ knockout (Tcrb^KO) mouse models were employed to determine the functional link between GM and TCR IR in liver fibrosis.

MATERIALS AND METHODS

Animal Models and Fecal Microbial Transplantation (FMT)

Wild-type C57BL/6 (WT) and Tcrb^KO mice were housed in pathogen-free animal rooms at the Animal Care Center of Xiamen University. All animal experiments were approved and conducted in accordance with the Guidelines of the Xiamen University Committee on Animal Care and Use (XMULAC20190061). For FMT, 8 to 12-week-old male mice were recolonized by FMT from WT mice. Mice were administered stool by oral gavage using animal feeding needles, given three times per week before CCl$_4$ injection and once per week after CCl$_4$ injection until the end point. To induce chronic liver fibrosis, mice were injected intraperitoneally with CCl$_4$ (Sigma-Aldrich, St. Louis, MO, United States) at a dose of 1 μl/g body weight mixed with olive oil three times per week for 8 weeks. Animals were sacrificed 24 h after the last injection, and samples were harvested for subsequent analyses.

DNA Extraction and 16S rRNA Sequencing

Cecal content was aseptically collected into 1.5 ml Eppendorf tubes. Microbial DNA was extracted using the HiPure stool DNA Kits (Magen, Guangzhou, China) according to the manufacturer's protocols. The 16S rRNA V3-V4 region of the ribosomal RNA gene was amplified by PCR (94°C for 2 min, followed by 30 cycles at 98°C for 10 s, 62°C for 30 s, 68°C for 30 s, and a final extension at 68°C for 5 min). Amplicons were extracted from 2% agarose gels and purified using the AxyPrep DNA Gel Extraction Kit (Axygen Biosciences, Union City, CA, United States). Purified amplicons were pooled in equimolar, paired, and sequenced on the Novaseq 6000 platform (Illumina, San Diego, CA, United States) using the 2 × 250 bp paired-end protocol.

Isolation of Intrahepatic Immunocytes and Flow Cytometry

Mouse intrahepatic immunocytes were isolated as previously described (Liang et al., 2018). The isolated immunocytes were incubated with fluorescently conjugated antibodies directed against mouse CD45 (FITC, I3/2.3, Cat#: 147709), B220

(PE, RA3-6B2, Cat#: 103207), CD3e (APC, 145-2C11, Cat#: 100312), TCRβ (FITC, clone: H57-597, Cat#: 109205), and TCRγδ (APC, clone: GL3, Cat#: 118115) from Biolegend (San Diego, CA, United States) for 20 min at 4°C in the dark. B cells (CD45$^+$ and B220$^+$), γδT cells (CD3e$^+$ and TCRγδ$^+$), and αβT cells (CD3e$^+$ and TCRβ$^+$) were obtained from intrahepatic immunocytes by flow cytometry. For cytokine detection, the selected cells were stained with antibodies against murine tumor necrosis factor α (TNF-α) and interleukin-17 (IL-17) from BD PharMingen (Mountain View, CA, United States) for 20 min at 4°C in the dark after incubation with permeabilization buffer. The stained cells were examined on a Beckman CytoFlex S (Beckman Coulter, Inc., Kraemer Boulevard Brea, CA, United States) and analyzed with the FlowJo software (version 10.0, TreeStar, Ashland, OR, United States).

Construction, Sequencing, and Data Processing for TCR IR

The RNAprep Pure Cell/Bacteria Kit (Tiangen Biotech, Beijing, China) was used to extract total RNA from intrahepatic immune cells according to the manufacturer's specifications. Then, 200 ng of total RNA was reverse-transcribed into cDNA using a Transcriptor First Strand cDNA Synthesis Kit (Roche Applied Science, Penzberg, Germany) on a C1000 Touch^{TM} Thermal Cycler (Bio-Rad Inc., Hercules, CA, United States). Two-round nested amplicon arm-PCR with specific primers was performed using 2 × SanTaq PCR Mix (Sangon Biotech, Shanghai, China) as previously described (Liang et al., 2018). Amplicons were extracted from 2% agarose gels and purified using the AxyPrep DNA Gel Extraction Kit (Axygen Biosciences, Union City, CA, United States). Purified amplicons were paired-end sequenced (PE250) on the Illumina platform according to standard protocols.

The clean data were harvested by filtering the low-quality sequences. The V, D, and J segments of the TCRβ consensus sequences were identified using the BLAST software (v2.2.25) in the international ImMunoGeneTics (IMGT) information system (IMGT)[1] by a standard algorithm. The Gini index, Shannon diversity, and CDR3 clustering were calculated using the QIIME (version 1.9.1).

Statistical Analysis

All statistical data were analyzed using the GraphPad Prism 8.0 Package (GraphPad Software, La Jolla, CA, United States). Data are presented as the mean ± standard deviation (SD). Student's t-test or the Welch t-test was used to compare values between the two groups. The means of multiple groups were compared using one-way analysis of variance (ANOVA) followed by Tukey's HSD test for mean separation. Statistical significance was accepted at $P < 0.05$. *$P < 0.05$; **$P < 0.01$; ***$P < 0.001$.

Additional methods are provided in the **Supplementary Material**.

[1]http://www.imgt.org/

RESULTS

GM Dysbiosis Occurs in Liver Fibrosis

To characterize GM variations in the context of liver fibrosis, we constructed and sequenced 16S rRNA amplicon libraries from cecal content. Mice were administered 0.9% saline (Saline group) or CCl$_4$ by intraperitoneal injection (CCl$_4$ group) three times a week for 8 weeks. This induced distinct changes in microbiota composition due to fibrogenesis compared to controls as revealed by principal component analysis (PCA) (**Figure 1A** and **Supplementary Table 1**). The operational taxonomic units (OTUs) were observed by the Bray-Curtis distance analysis (**Figure 1B** and **Supplementary Table 2**). Interestingly, liver fibrosis caused an obvious decrease in OTUs (**Figure 1C**). We further measured microbial diversity using different methodologies (rank-abundance, ACE index, Shannon and Simpson index). The results showed that the diversity of GM was significantly lower in the CCl$_4$ group than in the saline group (**Figures 1D,E**). Subsequently, we assessed the enrichment of specific bacterial communities in each group at the phylum level (**Figure 1F** and **Supplementary Figure 1A**). Bacteroidetes and Firmicutes were the most abundant in control mice, which was consistent with a previous study (Liu et al., 2016). Of note, liver fibrosis markedly increased Verrucomicrobia abundance while it decreased Bacteroidetes abundance (**Figure 1G**). To explore the potential function of GM in fibrogenesis, Phylogenetic Investigation of Communities by Reconstruction of Unobserved States (PICRUSt) was employed to predict the Kyoto Encyclopedia of Genes and Genomes (KEGG) pathways associated with components of the GM. **Supplementary Figure 1B** shows that a majority of functional biomarkers were enriched in metabolic pathways and less so in "Replication and repair," "Membrane transport," "Cell motility" as well as "Immune system" processes (**Supplementary Table 3**). Notably, liver fibrosis reinforced these pathway enrichments (**Supplementary Figure 1C** and **Supplementary Table 4**). These data suggest that liver fibrosis triggers GM dysbiosis, especially altering microbiota abundance and decreasing diversity.

Liver Fibrosis Decreases Diversity of Intrahepatic TCR IR

The changes in TCR IR in liver fibrosis were examined with bulk IR-seq. A total of 23 distinct V gene segments and 12 distinct J gene segments were identified from all samples (**Supplementary Table 5**). The most frequent V and J gene segments in the saline group were TRBV1 (37.58%) and TRBJ1-1 (15.02%). The most frequent V and J gene segments in the CCl$_4$ group were TRBV1 (40.61%) and TRBJ2-1 (17.01%) (**Supplementary Figure 2A**). Based on the usage frequency of V and J gene segments, heat maps were generated as shown in **Supplementary Figure 2B**. The usage patterns of most V and J gene segments were similar between the two groups, but significant usage differences for four V gene segments were observed, including TRBV15, TRBV17, TRBV12-2, and TRBV23

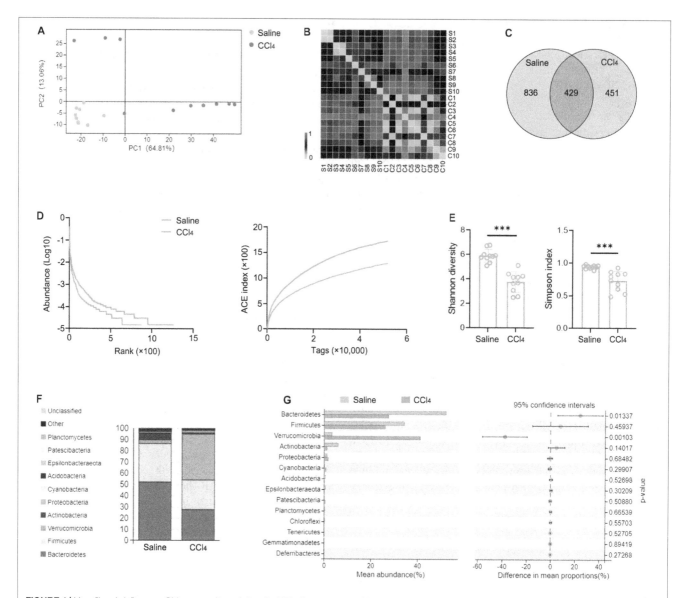

FIGURE 1 | Liver fibrosis influences GM community and diversity. WT mice were treated three times weekly with CCl₄ or 0.9% saline for 8 weeks. The 16S rRNA-seq data from cecal content were evaluated (*N* = 10). **(A,B)** Beta diversity determined by PCA **(A)** and Bray-Curtis distance **(B)**, showing closeness and distance between the two groups. **(C)** Venn analysis was performed to identify unique and common OTUs. **(D,E)** Alpha diversity determined by rank-abundance (left), ACE curve (right) **(D)**, Shannon diversity (left), and the Simpson index (right) **(E)** were used to measure the diversity of GM. **(F,G)** The composition **(F)** and abundance **(G)** of GM at the phylum taxonomic level. ***P < 0.001.

(**Supplementary Figure 2C**). We also analyzed the composition of VJ segments and VDJ segments. A total of 276 distinct VJ segments and 537 distinct VDJ segments were identified from all samples (**Supplementary Table 5**). Strikingly, multiple VJ and VDJ segments were absent in the CCl₄ group but were present in the saline group (**Figures 2A,B**). Of note, the usage of 13 VJ segments and nine VDJ segments in the CCl₄ group was significantly lower than in the saline group (**Figure 2C** and **Supplementary Figure 2D**).

CDR3 amino acid (AA) clonotypes determine the diversity of the TCR IR. Thus, we investigated the effect of fibrogenesis on the diversity of CDR3 AA clonotypes. Overall, 384,216 distinct CDR3 AA clonotypes were identified from all samples

(**Supplementary Table 6**). Although the overlap rate and length of CDR3 AA clonotypes were similar between the saline group and the CCl₄ group (**Figure 2D** and **Supplementary Figure 2E**), CDR3 AA clones and shared CDR3 AA clones were lower in the CCl₄ treatment group (**Figure 2E**). The Gini index and Shannon diversity revealed that liver fibrosis remarkably narrowed the diversity of CDR3 AA (**Figure 2F**). In addition, rank-abundance analysis demonstrated shrunken CDR3 AA richness and evenness in the CCl₄ group compared to the saline group (**Figure 2G**). Although the total CDR3 AA clonal frequencies were nearly identical in the two groups, fibrogenesis caused obvious distinct usage in high-frequency CDR3 AA clonotypes (cut-off threshold

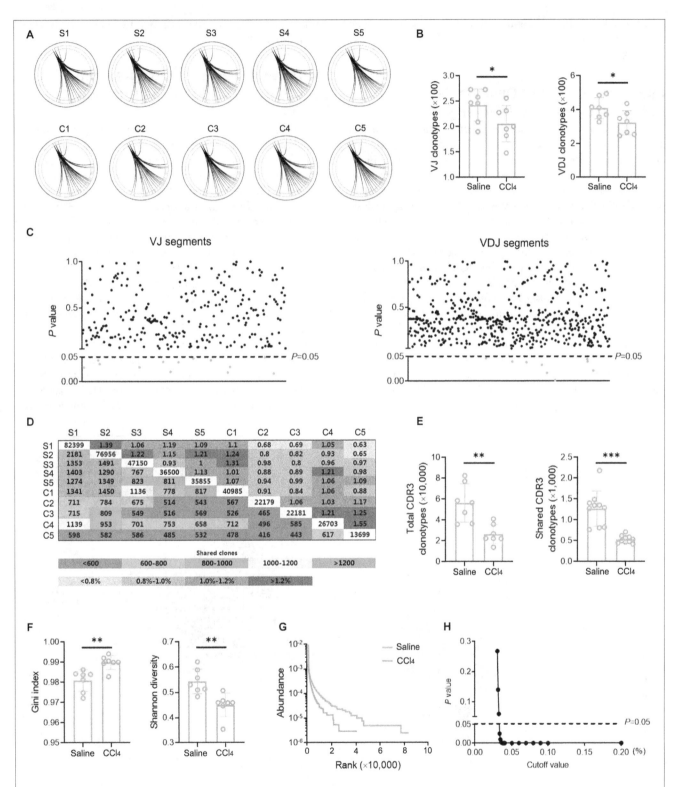

FIGURE 2 | Fibrogenesis diminishes intrahepatic TCR diversity. WT mice were treated three times weekly with CCl₄ or 0.9% saline for 8 weeks. TCR IR-seq data from intrahepatic isolated immune cells were evaluated (N = 5–7). **(A)** Circle diagram showing the composition of VJ segments. **(B)** Quantification of the composition of VJ segments (left) and VDJ segments (right). **(C)** The frequencies of VJ segments (left) and VDJ segments (right) that had significant differences (P < 0.05). Green color indicated downregulation. **(D)** Quantification (colored plots) and frequency (gray plots) of TCR CDR3 AA clones between two groups. Uncolored plots indicate the total clones per sample. **(E)** The total (left) and shared (right) CDR3 AA clones in each group. **(F)** The Gini index (left) and Shannon diversity (right) CDR3 AA clones in each group. **(G)** Rank-abundance showing CDR3 AA richness and evenness. **(H)** Comparison of clone frequencies for intrahepatic TCR CDR3 AA (dotted line indicates P = 0.05). The cut-off value depends on the clonal frequency exceeding a certain threshold. *P < 0.05; **P < 0.01; ***P < 0.001.

>0.033%, $P < 0.05$) (**Figure 2H**). These data indicate that liver fibrosis can reset intrahepatic TCR IR, thereby lowering diversity.

Intrahepatic TCR IR Diversity Is Associated With GM Diversity

The conclusion presented above indicate that liver fibrosis narrows the diversity of GM and intrahepatic TCR IR. To delineate the correction between the GM and TCR IR, a similar sequence clustering method for the CDR3 sequence was used in this work, and a total of 50 CDR3 clusters were identified (**Supplementary Table 7**). Clustering analysis revealed an aggregated expression of specific CDR3 clusters in liver fibrosis, and the expression of CDR3 clusters was spread and even in the saline group (**Figure 3A**). A similar phenomenon was observed in bacterial communities (at species level), and liver fibrosis obviously enhanced the abundance of *Akkermansia muciniphila* (*A. muciniphila*) and reduced the abundance of *Lachnospiraceae_bacterium_DW17* (**Figure 3B**, **Supplementary Figure 3**, and **Supplementary Table 8**). In addition, a significant positive association was observed between CDR3 AA clonotypes/Shannon diversity and OTU clonotypes/Shannon diversity (**Figures 3C,D**). Collectively, these data indicate that liver fibrosis induces the expression of the high-frequency CDR3 cluster and intestinal bacterial

communities and that intrahepatic TCR IR diversity is associated with GM diversity.

GM Participates in the Progression of Liver Fibrosis and Shapes Intrahepatic TCR IR

To determine whether GM can influence the progression of liver fibrosis, we performed fecal microbial transplantation (FMT). Fecal material from WT mice (FMT group) or 0.9% saline (UnFMT group) was transplanted by oral gavage three times a week. After 2 weeks, the mice were administered a CCl_4 injection three times a week for 8 weeks (**Figure 4A**). The abundance and diversity of OTUs in FMT mice and UnFMT mice were also measured (**Supplementary Table 9**). As expected, an obvious change in microbiota composition (**Figure 4B**) and an increase in microbial diversity were observed in the FMT group (**Figures 4C,D**). Of note, FMT reversed the effect of fibrogenesis on the abundance of Verrucomicrobia and Bacteroidetes (**Figures 4E,F**). Subsequently, we assessed the progression of liver fibrosis in the context of GM changes. Masson staining and Sirius red assays revealed that FMT alleviated CCl_4-induced liver fibrosis and *Collagen*-I expression (*Col1*) (**Figures 4G,H**). Consistently, a significant reduction in HSCs activation was observed in mice that received FMT compared with

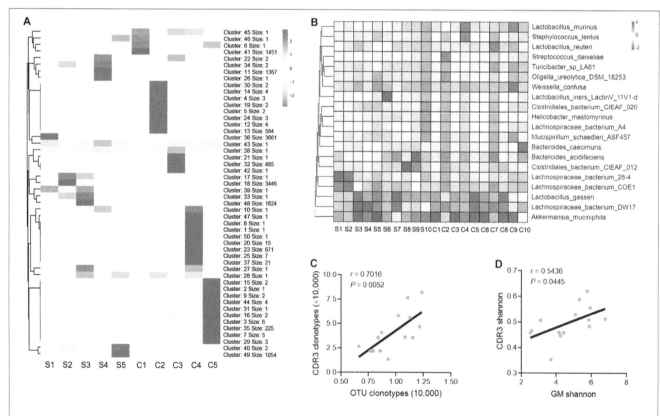

FIGURE 3 | TCR IR distribution is associated with GM distribution. **(A)** Heat maps showing the hierarchical clustering of intrahepatic TCR CDR3 AA clusters (N = 5). **(B)** Heat maps showing the abundance of GM at the species taxonomic level (N = 10). **(C,D)** A plot of CDR3 AA clonotypes versus OUT clonotypes **(C)** and CDR3 AA Shannon diversity versus OTU Shannon diversity **(D)**. Pearson's r values and the corresponding P-value are shown (N = 7).

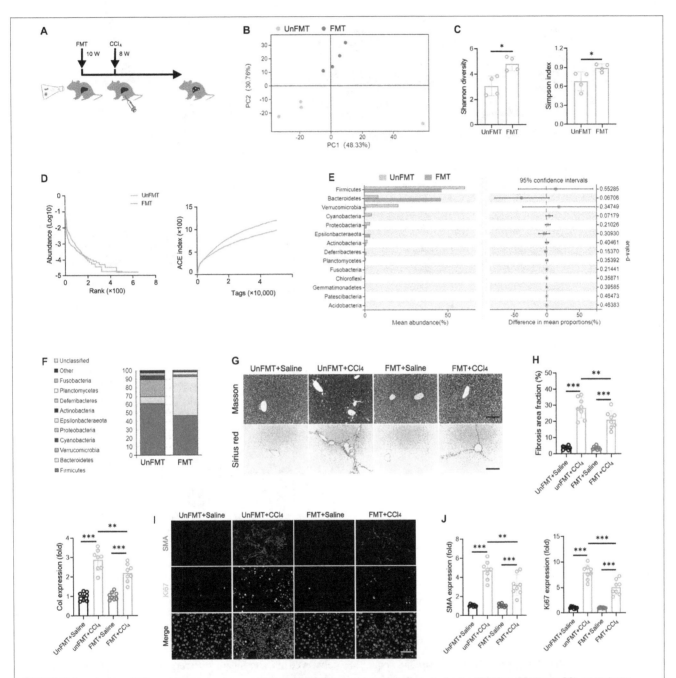

FIGURE 4 | Gut microbiota (GM) regulates the development of liver fibrosis. **(A)** Experimental procedure of extracting FMT from WT mice in CCl₄-treated mice (N = 4–8). **(B)** Beta diversity as determined by PCA, showing closeness between FMT mice and UnFMT mice. **(C,D)** Alpha diversity by Shannon diversity (left), Simpson index (right) **(C)**, rank-abundance (left), and ACE curve (right) **(D)**, showing the diversity of GM. **(E,F)** The composition **(E)** and the abundance **(F)** of GM at the phylum taxonomic level. **(G)** Representative images of Masson trichrome staining and Sirius red staining of FMT and UnFMT mice liver after CCl₄ or 0.9% saline treatment for 8 weeks. Scale bar, 100 μm. **(H)** Quantification of fibrosis area fraction (left) and *Collagen*-I expression (right) as shown in **(G)**. **(I)** Liver sections were stained for SMA (red) and Ki67 (green) to identify the proliferative HSCs. Representative images are shown. Scale bar, 100 μm. **(J)** Quantification of SMA (left) and Ki67 (right) expression as shown in **(I)**. *P < 0.05; **P < 0.01; ***P < 0.001.

saline (UnFMT) (**Figures 4I,J**). Collectively, these results suggest that FMT delays liver fibrosis progression by modulating HSC activation.

To investigate whether GM can influence intrahepatic TCR IR, we performed bulk IR-seq to assess variations in TCR IR. Interestingly, the distribution and abundance of V, J, VJ, and

VDJ segments was not significantly different between FMT mice and UnFMT mice (**Supplementary Figure 4** and **Supplementary Table 10**). However, it was noted that FMT ameliorated the inhibitory effect of fibrogenesis on CDR3 AA clonotypes (**Figures 5A,B** and **Supplementary Table 11**) and CDR3 AA diversity (as shown by the Gini index, Shannon diversity, and

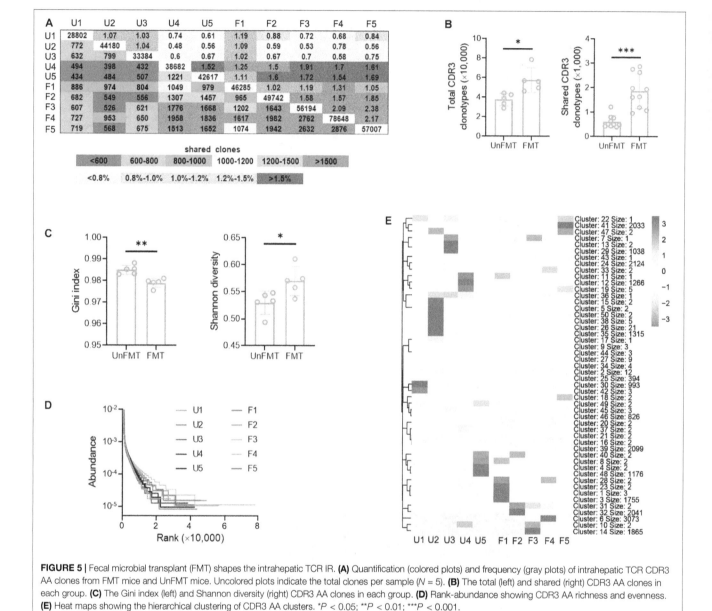

FIGURE 5 | Fecal microbial transplant (FMT) shapes the intrahepatic TCR IR. **(A)** Quantification (colored plots) and frequency (gray plots) of intrahepatic TCR CDR3 AA clones from FMT mice and UnFMT mice. Uncolored plots indicate the total clones per sample (*N* = 5). **(B)** The total (left) and shared (right) CDR3 AA clones in each group. **(C)** The Gini index (left) and Shannon diversity (right) CDR3 AA clones in each group. **(D)** Rank-abundance showing CDR3 AA richness and evenness. **(E)** Heat maps showing the hierarchical clustering of CDR3 AA clusters. *P < 0.05; **P < 0.01; ***P < 0.001.

rank-abundance analysis) (**Figures 5C,D**). A similar sequence clustering analysis performed to detect CDR3 cluster changes, revealed that liver fibrosis led to the aggregation of specific CDR3 clusters, whereas FMT led to the diffusion of CDR3 clusters (**Figure 5E** and **Supplementary Table 12**). These data demonstrate that GM can shape the intrahepatic TCR IR.

The GM/TCR IR/Immune Milieu Axis Modulates Liver Fibrosis

Thus far, we have demonstrated that GM regulates liver fibrosis and intrahepatic TCR IR. A key question yet to be answered is whether TCR IR mediates the effects of GM in liver fibrosis. To answer this question, Tcrb^{KO} mice were subjected to FMT derived from WT mice (**Figure 6A**). We

observed no significant differences in appearance, architecture, fibrogenesis, and inflammation between WT mice and Tcrb^{KO} mice (**Supplementary Figures 5A–C**). The deletion of TCRβ in the Tcrb^{KO} mice was confirmed by immunofluorescence analysis and cytometry assay (**Supplementary Figures 5D,E**). TCR IR ablation reversed the suppressive effect of FMT on liver fibrogenesis and fibrogenic gene expression (**Figures 6B,C**). Notably, SMA and Ki67 expression restored HSC activation in Tcrb^{KO} mice that received FMT (**Figures 6D,E**). These results indicate that TCR IR mediates the effects of GM on liver fibrosis.

We then co-cultured primary HSCs (isolated from fibrotic liver) with or without T cells (isolated from normal liver) to verify whether T cells alone are responsible for HSC activation. Interestingly, we found no differences in HSC

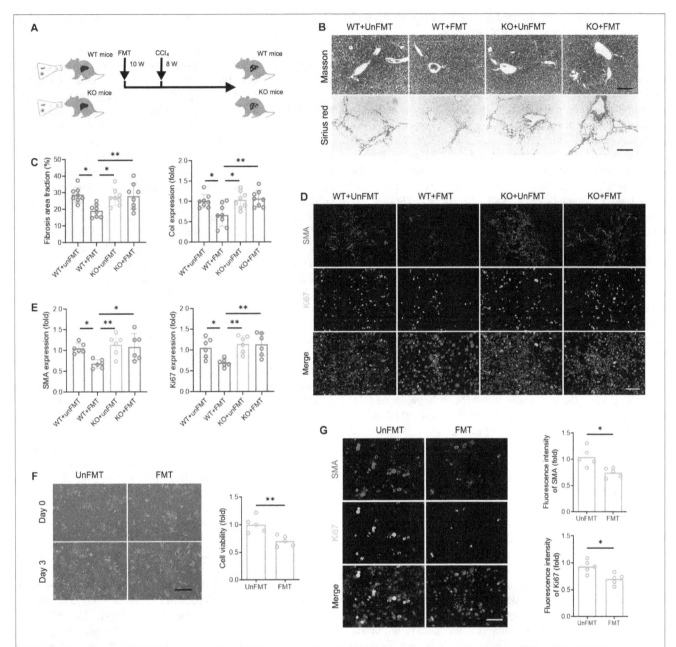

FIGURE 6 | Deficiency of TCR IR abrogates the effects of GM on liver fibrosis. **(A)** Experimental procedure of extracting FMT and CCl₄ treatment in WT mice and Tcrb^KO mice (N = 6–8). **(B)** Representative images of Masson staining and Sirius red staining of WT mouse and Tcrb^KO mouse livers after CCl₄ treatment for 8 weeks. Scale bar, 100 μm. **(C)** Quantification of fibrotic area fraction (left) and *Collagen*-I expression (right) as shown in **(B)**. **(D)** Liver sections were stained for SMA (red) and Ki67 (green) to identify the proliferative HSCs. Representative images are shown. Scale bar, 100 μm. **(E)** Quantification of SMA (left) and Ki67 (right) expression as shown in **(D)**. **(F)** Representative images showing day 0 and day 3 co-cultures of primary HSCs (isolated from 6-week CCl₄-treated liver) with intrahepatic immune cell (isolated from WT + UnFMT or WT + FMT mice liver after CCl₄ treatment for 8 weeks) (left). Scale bar, 50 μm. Cell viability was estimated using the CCK-8 assay (right) after co-culture for 3 days (N = 5). **(G)** Immunofluorescence staining for SMA (red) and Ki67 (green) performed to identify the proliferating HSCs. Representative images are shown (left). Scale bar, 50 μm. Quantification of SMA (up) and Ki67 expression (down) (N = 5). *P < 0.05; **P < 0.01.

growth and proliferation among the different treatment groups, indicating that TCR IR is not the only driver of HSC activation (**Supplementary Figure 6**). Instead, other factors contribute to this process. To explore the regulatory role of the intrahepatic immune microenvironment on HSCs, co-cultures of mouse primary HSCs with intrahepatic immune cells, isolated from the WT + UnFMT group and the

WT + FMT group, were performed for 3 days. A CCK-8 assay and Ki67 immunostaining were performed to confirm the HSC activation *in vitro*. Co-culture with intrahepatic immune cells isolated from the WT + FMT group notably inhibited HSC growth and proliferation compared with co-culture with intrahepatic immune cells isolated from the WT + UnFMT group (**Figures 6F,G**). Taken together, these results demonstrated that HSC activation is modulated by the intrahepatic immune microenvironment rather than by T cells alone.

Due to the compromised immune milieu in the fibrotic livers, we investigated whether TCRβ deficiency affects liver fibrosis by influencing the recruitment and activation of neighboring immunocyte subsets. We performed mass cytometry (CyTOF), targeting a global panel of 38 markers, and generated a detailed profile of the intrahepatic immune microenvironment (**Supplementary Figure 7A**). Characterization of the markers revealed nine distinct immunocyte subsets, including B cells, dendritic cells (DCs), macrophages, natural killer (NK) cells, neutrophils, CD4 T cells, CD8 T cells, γδ T cells, and natural killer T lymphocytes (NKT) in the liver (**Figure 7A, Supplementary Figures 7B,C, and Supplementary Table 13**). Of note, Tcrb^{KO} mice revealed abnormal B cell and γδ T cell expansion due to αβ T cell deficiency during liver fibrosis (**Figures 7B–D**). Compared with the UnFMT group, FMT gave rise to expanded CD8 T cells and shrunken B cells in WT mice liver (**Figures 7E,F and Supplementary Figures 7D,E**). Interestingly, expanded B cells with enhanced TNF-α levels (**Figures 7E–G**) and expanded γδ T cells with enhanced IL-17 levels were found in CCl$_4$-treated Tcrb^{KO} mice with or without FMT (**Figures 7H–J**). However, FMT did not affect the distribution and activation of B cells and γδ T cells during liver fibrosis in Tcrb^{KO} mice (**Figures 7E–J**), suggesting that GM can shape intrahepatic immune cells by TCR IR. Collectively, these results suggest that FMT delays liver fibrosis progression by influencing TCR IR-mediated intrahepatic immune milieu.

DISCUSSION

Liver fibrosis may interfere with gut-bacterial interactions, leading to GM dysbiosis (Tilg et al., 2016; Tripathi et al., 2018b). Our data demonstrate that liver fibrogenesis is accompanied with reduced diversity of GM and decreased abundance of Bacteroidetes, an observation that was consistent with previous studies (Chen et al., 2011; Bajaj et al., 2014). Interestingly, liver fibrosis boosted *A. muciniphila* abundance. *A. muciniphila*, considered a promising probiotic, is known to have important value in improving host metabolic functions and immune responses (Derrien et al., 2017; Plovier et al., 2017; Zhang et al., 2019). Recent studies support a protective effect of *A. muciniphila* against hepatic injury, steatosis, and neutrophil infiltration (Wu et al., 2017; Kim et al., 2020). *A. muciniphila* also protects against ethanol-induced gut leakiness, enhanced mucus thickness, and tight-junction expression (Grander et al., 2018). In our study, CCl$_4$ treatment enhanced *A. muciniphila* abundance, which may be explained as a feedback mechanism responding to hepatic injury. The breakdown of gut barrier integrity is mainly driven by gut inflammation and dysbiosis, both of which trigger bacterial translocation. Microorganisms and microorganism-derived molecules translocate to the liver through the portal system and interact with the intrahepatic immune microenvironment, causing inflammation and hepatic injury (Tripathi et al., 2018a). Although higher microbial

diversity is known to modify the immune state, the "bridge" between GM and immune function is not entirely clear.

Identifying and tracking TCR IR by NSG provides a novel strategy to investigate the dynamics and distribution of all T cell clonotypes. TCR IR therefore serves as a "footprint" of immune status (Calis and Rosenberg, 2014). Emerging studies suggest that TCR IR participates in various liver diseases (including viral hepatitis, liver regeneration, hepatocellular carcinoma, primary sclerosing cholangitis, and alcoholic liver disease) (Chen et al., 2016; Huang et al., 2016; Liaskou et al., 2016; Jiang et al., 2018). In this study, we demonstrate the resetting of intrahepatic TCR IR in response to chronic liver injury, showing an intact characteristic of V, D, J, VJ, and VDJ segment usage and the distribution of CDR3 AA clonotypes during liver fibrosis. A lower diversity of CDR3 AA clonotypes along with diminished and centralized VJ and VDJ segments were observed during fibrogenesis. This is consistent with a recent work describing that liver remodeling leads to a remarkably lower TCR IR diversity and high-frequency TCR clonotypes expression (Liang et al., 2018).

Through a "gut-microbiome-liver" axis, the intestinal microbiome controls liver and immune functions (Woodhouse et al., 2018). Indeed, liver cirrhosis can be considered a microbiota-driven disorder, and a strong link between the GM and liver cirrhosis and its complications has been demonstrated (Adolph et al., 2018). The exact mechanism by which GM regulates liver fibrogenesis remains unclear. Previous studies have examined the metabolic role of GM in the liver. In the current study, the majority of functional biomarkers of GM were enriched in the metabolic pathways in liver fibrosis. However, the immune regulatory effects of GM in the liver should not be overlooked. The liver receives stimuli from the intestines that induce intrahepatic T cells recognition due to TCR IR reconstitution. Any change, therefore, in the GM composition will modify TCR IR reconstitution, thereby reshaping the intrahepatic immune microenvironment and the development of liver disease. In this study, changes in the distribution and diversity of GM correlated with changes in TCR IR during liver fibrosis. In addition, FMT restored the intrahepatic TCR IR diversity and improved liver fibrogenesis, while TCR IR ablation reversed the impact of FMT on fibrogenesis. These results suggest that intrahepatic TCR IR mediates the biological effect of GM in the development of liver fibrosis. Interestingly, although decreasing the GM by antibiotics or blocking their receptors results in decreased inflammatory and fibrogenic signaling in the liver (Fouts et al., 2012), the GM diversity plays an indispensable role in the maintenance of liver homeostasis. Furthermore, FMT did not alter the abundance of Verrucomicrobia and Bacteroidetes indicating that the normal balance in GM communities (both dominant microorganisms and inferior microorganisms) may prevent the development of liver fibrosis.

We also elucidated the potential mechanism by which TCR IR regulates HSC activation in a fibrotic liver. An interesting observation was that co-culturing HSCs with T cells isolated from WT mouse liver did not alter HSC activation and proliferation. In contrast, co-culturing HSCs with all

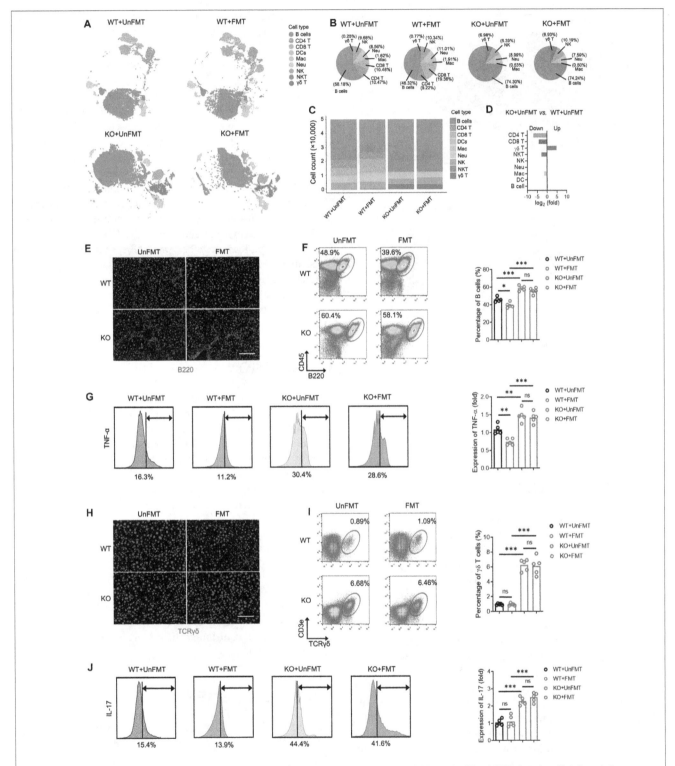

FIGURE 7 | TCR IR influences intrahepatic immune microenvironment. **(A)** *t* distributed stochastic neighbor embedding (*t*SNE) clustering of intrahepatic immune cells from WT mice that received UnFMT, WT mice that received FMT, Tcrb^KO mice that received UnFMT, and Tcrb^KO mice that received FMT after 8-week CCl₄ treatment, colored by immune cell type (*N* = 4–5). **(B,C)** The percentage **(B)** and the cell count **(C)** of each cell type. **(D)** The ratio [Tcrb^KO mice with UnFMT versus WT mice with UnFMT, log₂(fold)] of distribution of each immune cell type. **(E)** Representative immunofluorescence image of B220 staining (red) in liver sections. Scale bar, 100 μm. **(F)** Representative cytometry plots of intrahepatic B cells (CD45⁺ and B220⁺) are shown. Quantification of the percentage of B cells. **(G)** Intrahepatic B cells were gated and used to test for expression of TNF-α. **(H)** Representative immunofluorescence image of TCRγδ (red) staining in liver sections. Scale bar, 100 μm. **(I)** Representative cytometry plots of intrahepatic γδT cells (CD3e⁺ and TCRγδ⁺) are shown. Quantification of the percentage of γδT cells. **(J)** Intrahepatic γδT cells were gated and used to test for expression of IL-17. *P < 0.05; **P < 0.01; ***P < 0.001.

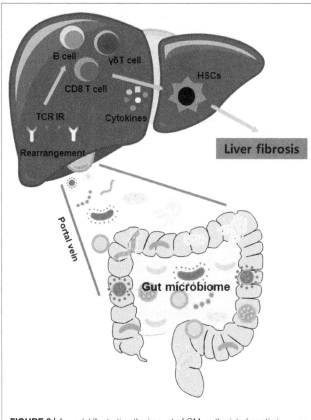

FIGURE 8 | A model illustrating the impact of GM on the intrahepatic immune microenvironment in liver fibrosis.

immune cells isolated from FMT mouse liver suppressed HSC proliferation. This is in full agreement with our earlier conclusion that hepatic functions are regulated by many factors in the intrahepatic immune microenvironment and not solely by T cells (Liang et al., 2018). Accumulating studies indicate that HSCs receive many signals from hepatic immunocytes and in turn, produce many fibrotic mediators that broadcast the signals, thereby influencing liver fibrosis progression (Higashi et al., 2017; Tsuchida and Friedman, 2017). In this work, the intrahepatic immune cell landscape during liver fibrosis was examined using CyTOF. We found that FMT diminished B cells and expanded CD8$^+$ T cells, thereby alleviating liver fibrogenesis as previously reported (Novobrantseva et al., 2005; Holt et al., 2006; Guidotti et al., 2015). Interestingly, TCR IR deficiency resulted in an aberrant intrahepatic immune microenvironment (expanded B cells with an enhanced TNF-α level, and expanded γδT cells with an enhanced IL-17 level) both in the Tcrb^{KO}+UnFMT group and the Tcrb^{KO}+FMT group during liver fibrogenesis. Indeed, B cell and γδT cell expansion

are a normal characteristic of Tcrb^{KO} mice due to αβ T cell deficiency. However, FMT did not affect the distribution and activation of B cells and γδ T cells during liver fibrosis in Tcrb^{KO} mice, suggesting that TCR IR mediates the effects of GM on intrahepatic immune cells.

Liver injury leads to increases in the production of expanded T cell subsets from extrahepatic recruitment (Liang et al., 2018). Although the nature of the crosstalk between T cells and other immune cells is still unclear, recruited T cells pass through the liver vasculature, closely interacting with resident immunocytes, including intrahepatic γδT cells, NK cells, and Kupffer cells, on which they can directly exert their immunoregulatory effects (Heymann and Tacke, 2016; Liang et al., 2018). Conventionally, T cells are regulated by environmental stimuli via TCR and TCR-dependent environmental exposures (Xiao and Cai, 2017). The TCR IR patterns together with the specific TCR signaling associated with environmental exposures, jointly regulate the intrahepatic immune microenvironment. The reconstitution of TCR IR in the fibrotic liver observed in this study, provides novel insights into the immunosurveillance and immunoregulation of TCR IR that are synergistic with other immunocytes.

CONCLUSION

We demonstrated a connection between GM, TCR IR, and the intrahepatic immune microenvironment. The dysbiosis of intestinal microbiota precipitated an unfavorable intrahepatic immune microenvironment, characterized by abnormal distribution and the activation of immune cell subsets due to TCR IR rearrangement (**Figure 8**). Thus, manipulation of GM may be an effective therapeutic opportunity to rebuild the intrahepatic immune microenvironment, hence improving liver fibrosis.

AUTHOR CONTRIBUTIONS

KW conceived and designed the study, and wrote the manuscript. QL, MZ, WZ, PZ, and YC performed the experiments. QL and YH analyzed the CyTOF data. KW and QYL analyzed the 16S rRNA-seq data. KW and PX analyzed the bulk IR-seq data. All authors contributed to the article and approved the submitted version.

ACKNOWLEDGMENTS

We thank Prof. Changchun Xiao (Xiamen University) and Prof. Guo Fu (Xiamen University) for technical support.

REFERENCES

Adolph, T. E., Grander, C., Moschen, A. R., and Tilg, H. (2018). Liver-microbiome axis in health and disease. *Trends Immunol.* 39, 712–723. doi: 10.1016/j.it.2018.05.002

Bajaj, J. S., Heuman, D. M., Hylemon, P. B., Sanyal, A. J., White, M. B., Monteith, P., et al. (2014). Altered profile of human gut microbiome is associated with cirrhosis and its complications. *J. Hepatol.* 60, 940–947. doi: 10.1016/j.jhep.2013.12.019

Bajaj, J. S., and Khoruts, A. (2020). Microbiota changes and intestinal microbiota transplantation in liver diseases and cirrhosis. *J. Hepatol.* 72, 1003–1027. doi: 10.1016/j.jhep.2020.01.017

Breous, E., Somanathan, S., Vandenberghe, L. H., and Wilson, J. M. (2009). Hepatic regulatory T cells and Kupffer cells are crucial mediators of systemic T cell tolerance to antigens targeting murine liver. *Hepatology* 50, 612–621. doi: 10.1002/hep.23043

Calis, J. J., and Rosenberg, B. R. (2014). Characterizing immune repertoires by high throughput sequencing: strategies and applications. *Trends Immunol.* 35, 581–590. doi: 10.1016/j.it.2014.09.004

Chen, Y., Xu, Y., Zhao, M., Liu, Y., Gong, M., Xie, C., et al. (2016). High-throughput T cell receptor sequencing reveals distinct repertoires between tumor and adjacent non-tumor tissues in HBV-associated HCC. *Oncoimmunology* 5:e1219010. doi: 10.1080/2162402x.2016.1219010

Chen, Y., Yang, F., Lu, H., Wang, B., Chen, Y., Lei, D., et al. (2011). Characterization of fecal microbial communities in patients with liver cirrhosis. *Hepatology* 54, 562–572. doi: 10.1002/hep.24423

Derrien, M., Belzer, C., and De Vos, W. M. (2017). *Akkermansia muciniphila* and its role in regulating host functions. *Microb. Pathog.* 106, 171–181. doi: 10.1016/j.micpath.2016.02.005

Fouts, D. E., Torralba, M., Nelson, K. E., Brenner, D. A., and Schnabl, B. (2012). Bacterial translocation and changes in the intestinal microbiome in mouse models of liver disease. *J. Hepatol.* 56, 1283–1292. doi: 10.1016/j.jhep.2012.01.019

Friedman, S. L. (2008). Mechanisms of hepatic fibrogenesis. *Gastroenterology* 134, 1655–1669. doi: 10.1053/j.gastro.2008.03.003

Grander, C., Adolph, T. E., Wieser, V., Lowe, P., Wrzosek, L., Gyongyosi, B., et al. (2018). Recovery of ethanol-induced *Akkermansia muciniphila* depletion ameliorates alcoholic liver disease. *Gut* 67, 891–901. doi: 10.1136/gutjnl-2016-313432

Guidotti, L. G., Inverso, D., Sironi, L., Di Lucia, P., Fioravanti, J., Ganzer, L., et al. (2015). Immunosurveillance of the liver by intravascular effector CD8(+) T cells. *Cell* 161, 486–500. doi: 10.1016/j.cell.2015.03.005

Hammerich, L., Bangen, J. M., Govaere, O., Zimmermann, H. W., Gassler, N., Huss, S., et al. (2014). Chemokine receptor CCR6-dependent accumulation of gammadelta T cells in injured liver restricts hepatic inflammation and fibrosis. *Hepatology* 59, 630–642. doi: 10.1002/hep.26697

Heymann, F., and Tacke, F. (2016). Immunology in the liver–from homeostasis to disease. *Nat. Rev. Gastroenterol. Hepatol.* 13, 88–110. doi: 10.1038/nrgastro.2015.200

Higashi, T., Friedman, S. L., and Hoshida, Y. (2017). Hepatic stellate cells as key target in liver fibrosis. *Adv. Drug Deliv. Rev.* 121, 27–42. doi: 10.1016/j.addr.2017.05.007

Holt, A. P., Stamataki, Z., and Adams, D. H. (2006). Attenuated liver fibrosis in the absence of B cells. *Hepatology* 43, 868–871. doi: 10.1002/hep.21155

Huang, Y., Ma, H., Wei, S., Luo, G., Sun, R., Fan, Z., et al. (2016). Analysis of the complementarity determining regions beta-chain genomic rearrangement using high-throughput sequencing in periphery cytotoxic T lymphocytes of patients with chronic hepatitis B. *Mol. Med. Rep.* 14, 762–768. doi: 10.3892/mmr.2016.5329

Jiang, Q., Liu, Y., Xu, B., Zheng, W., Xiang, X., Tang, X., et al. (2018). Analysis of T cell receptor repertoire in monozygotic twins concordant and discordant for chronic hepatitis B infection. *Biochem. Biophys. Res. Commun.* 497, 153–159. doi: 10.1016/j.bbrc.2018.02.043

Kim, S., Lee, Y., Kim, Y., Seo, Y., Lee, H., Ha, J., et al. (2020). *Akkermansia muciniphila* prevents fatty liver disease, decreases serum triglycerides, and maintains gut homeostasis. *Appl. Environ. Microbiol.* 86:e03004-19.

Koyama, Y., and Brenner, D. A. (2017). Liver inflammation and fibrosis. *J. Clin. Invest.* 127, 55–64.

Liang, Q., Liu, Z., Zhu, C., Wang, B., Liu, X., Yang, Y., et al. (2018). Intrahepatic T cell receptor beta immune repertoire is essential for liver regeneration. *Hepatology* 68, 1977–1990. doi: 10.1002/hep.30067

Liaskou, E., Klemsdal Henriksen, E. K., Holm, K., Kaveh, F., Hamm, D., Fear, J., et al. (2016). High-throughput T-cell receptor sequencing across chronic liver diseases reveals distinct disease-associated repertoires. *Hepatology* 63, 1608–1619. doi: 10.1002/hep.28116

Liu, H. X., Rocha, C. S., Dandekar, S., and Wan, Y. J. (2016). Functional analysis of the relationship between intestinal microbiota and the expression of hepatic genes and pathways during the course of liver regeneration. *J. Hepatol.* 64, 641–650. doi: 10.1016/j.jhep.2015.09.022

Mikszta, J. A., Mcheyzer-Williams, L. J., and Mcheyzer-Williams, M. G. (1999). Antigen-driven selection of TCR In vivo: related TCR alpha-chains pair with diverse TCR beta-chains. *J. Immunol.* 163, 5978–5988.

Milosevic, I., Vujovic, A., Barac, A., Djelic, M., Korac, M., Radovanovic Spurnic, A., et al. (2019). Gut-liver axis, gut microbiota, and its modulation in the management of liver diseases: a review of the literature. *Int. J. Mol. Sci.* 20:395. doi: 10.3390/ijms20020395

Nikolich-Zugich, J., Slifka, M. K., and Messaoudi, I. (2004). The many important facets of T-cell repertoire diversity. *Nat. Rev. Immunol.* 4, 123–132. doi: 10.1038/nri1292

Novobrantseva, T. I., Majeau, G. R., Amatucci, A., Kogan, S., Brenner, I., Casola, S., et al. (2005). Attenuated liver fibrosis in the absence of B cells. *J. Clin. Invest.* 115, 3072–3082. doi: 10.1172/jci24798

Ohtani, N., and Kawada, N. (2019). Role of the gut-liver axis in liver inflammation, fibrosis, and cancer: a special focus on the gut microbiota relationship. *Hepatol. Commun.* 3, 456–470. doi: 10.1002/hep4.1331

Pannetier, C., Cochet, M., Darche, S., Casrouge, A., Zoller, M., and Kourilsky, P. (1993). The sizes of the CDR3 hypervariable regions of the murine T-cell receptor beta chains vary as a function of the recombined germ-line segments. *Proc. Natl. Acad. Sci. U.S.A.* 90, 4319–4323. doi: 10.1073/pnas.90.9.4319

Plovier, H., Everard, A., Druart, C., Depommier, C., Van Hul, M., Geurts, L., et al. (2017). A purified membrane protein from *Akkermansia muciniphila* or the pasteurized bacterium improves metabolism in obese and diabetic mice. *Nat. Med.* 23, 107–113. doi: 10.1038/nm.4236

Tilg, H., Cani, P. D., and Mayer, E. A. (2016). Gut microbiome and liver diseases. *Gut* 65, 2035–2044. doi: 10.1136/gutjnl-2016-312729

Tosello-Trampont, A., Surette, F. A., Ewald, S. E., and Hahn, Y. S. (2017). Immunoregulatory role of NK cells in tissue inflammation and regeneration. *Front. Immunol.* 8:301. doi: 10.3389/fimmu.2017.00301

Tripathi, A., Debelius, J., Brenner, D. A., Karin, M., Loomba, R., Schnabl, B., et al. (2018a). Publisher correction: the gut-liver axis and the intersection with the microbiome. *Nat. Rev. Gastroenterol. Hepatol.* 15:785. doi: 10.1038/s41575-018-0031-8

Tripathi, A., Debelius, J., Brenner, D. A., Karin, M., Loomba, R., Schnabl, B., et al. (2018b). The gut-liver axis and the intersection with the microbiome. *Nat. Rev. Gastroenterol. Hepatol.* 15, 397–411.

Tsuchida, T., and Friedman, S. L. (2017). Mechanisms of hepatic stellate cell activation. *Nat. Rev. Gastroenterol. Hepatol.* 14, 397–411.

Wahid, B., Ali, A., Rafique, S., Saleem, K., Waqar, M., Wasim, M., et al. (2018). Role of altered immune cells in liver diseases: a review. *Gastroenterol. Hepatol.* 41, 377–388. doi: 10.1016/j.gastrohep.2018.01.014

Woodhouse, C. A., Patel, V. C., Singanayagam, A., and Shawcross, D. L. (2018). Review article: the gut microbiome as a therapeutic target in the pathogenesis and treatment of chronic liver disease. *Aliment. Pharmacol. Ther.* 47, 192–202. doi: 10.1111/apt.14397

Wu, W., Lv, L., Shi, D., Ye, J., Fang, D., Guo, F., et al. (2017). Protective effect of *Akkermansia muciniphila* against immune-mediated liver injury in a mouse model. *Front Microbiol* 8:1804. doi: 10.3389/fmicb.2017.01804

Xiao, X., and Cai, J. (2017). Mucosal-associated invariant T cells: new insights into antigen recognition and activation. *Front. Immunol.* 8:1540. doi: 10.3389/fimmu.2017.01540

Zhang, T., Li, Q., Cheng, L., Buch, H., and Zhang, F. (2019). *Akkermansia muciniphila* is a promising probiotic. *Microb. Biotechnol.* 12, 1109–1125. doi: 10.1111/1751-7915.13410

Zhou, R., Fan, X., and Schnabl, B. (2019). Role of the intestinal microbiome in liver fibrosis development and new treatment strategies. *Transl. Res.* 209, 22–38. doi: 10.1016/j.trsl.2019.02.005

4

The Combination of Schisandrol B and Wedelolactone Synergistically Reverses Hepatic Fibrosis *via* Modulating Multiple Signaling Pathways in Mice

Yongqiang Ai[1†], Wei Shi[1†], Xiaobin Zuo[1†], Xiaoming Sun[1†], Yuanyuan Chen[1], Zhilei Wang[1], Ruisheng Li[2], Xueai Song[3], Wenzhang Dai[1], Wenqing Mu[1], Kaixin Ding[1], Zhiyong Li[1], Qiang Li[1], Xiaohe Xiao[1,3]*, Xiaoyan Zhan[1,3]* and Zhaofang Bai[1,3]*

[1]Department of Hepatology, The Fifth Medical Centre, Chinese PLA General Hospital, Beijing, China, [2]Research Center for Clinical and Translational Medicine, The Fifth Medical Center of Chinese PLA General Hospital, Beijing, China, [3]China Military Institute of Chinese Materia, The Fifth Medical Centre, Chinese PLA General Hospital, Beijing, China

*Correspondence:
Zhaofang Bai
baizf2008@hotmail.com
Xiaoyan Zhan
xyzhan123@163.com
Xiaohe Xiao
pharmacy_302@126.com

[†]These authors have contributed equally to this work.

Hepatic fibrosis represents an important event in the progression of chronic liver injury to cirrhosis, and is characterized by excessive extracellular matrix proteins aggregation. Early fibrosis can be reversed by inhibiting hepatocyte injury, inflammation, or hepatic stellate cells activation, so the development of antifibrotic drugs is important to reduce the incidence of hepatic cirrhosis or even hepatic carcinoma. Here we demonstrate that Schisandrol B (SolB), one of the major active constituents of traditional hepato-protective Chinese medicine, Schisandra sphenanthera, significantly protects against hepatocyte injury, while Wedelolactone (WeD) suppresses the TGF-β1/Smads signaling pathway in hepatic stellate cells (HSCs) and inflammation, the combination of the two reverses hepatic fibrosis in mice and the inhibitory effect of the combination on hepatic fibrosis is superior to that of SolB or WeD treatment alone. Combined pharmacotherapy represents a promising strategy for the prevention and treatment of liver fibrosis.

Keywords: schisandrol B, wedelolactone, hepatic fibrosis, combined pharmacotherapy, TGF-β1/smads signaling pathway

INTRODUCTION

Hepatic fibrosis is caused by chronic injury and persistent excessive inflammation, which is accompanied with chronic HBV or HCV infection, alcoholic steatohepatitis, NASH, and biliary diseases (Cordero-Espinoza and Huch, 2018). Hepatic fibrosis is a key process in the development of chronic injury to cirrhosis, eventually leading to liver failure and even hepatocellular carcinoma with a worldwide mortality. Once chronic injury or persistent inflammation is resolved, hepatic fibrosis can be regressed (Bansal and Chamroonkul, 2019). Therefore, treatment of hepatic fibrosis is important for the prevention of cirrhosis and related diseases. At present, many potential therapeutic drugs including chemicals and biological drugs have been developed to prevent and treat hepatic fibrosis (Fagone et al., 2016; Schuppan et al., 2018), but there is still a lack of effective antifibrotic drugs in clinic.

Many evidences demonstrated that hepatic stellate cells (HSCs) and macrophages play the key role in driving hepatic fibrogenesis (Bataller and Brenner, 2005; Seki and Schwabe, 2015). Quiescent

HSCs can rapidly differentiate into myofibroblast with increased extracellular matrix (ECM) synthesis and deposition in response to fibrogenic stimuli, including transforming growth factor-β1 (TGF-β1) and platelet-derived growth factor (PDGF) (Liu et al., 2006; Inagaki and Okazaki, 2007), so activated HSCs are central to the pathogenesis of hepatic fibrosis. Chronic injury-mediated macrophages recruitment and activation may promote the survival of activated HSCs via Toll-like receptor 4 (TLR4)-dependent production of chemokines and pro-inflammatory cytokines, such as interleukin-1β (IL-1β) and tumor necrosis factor-α (TNF-α) (Pradere et al., 2013). If the recruited inflammatory cells are not effectively resolved, they can further exacerbate the tissue injury, thereby resulting in hepatic fibrosis (Krenkel et al., 2018). As TGF-β1 has been considered as the key cytokine in the activation of HSCs, multiple small molecules or antibodies that target TGF-β1 have potential value in prevention and treatment of hepatic fibrosis (Fagone et al., 2016). But TGF-β1 is a multifunctional cytokine with broad biological activities involving multiple biological functions, such as embryogenesis, immunity, carcinogenesis and inflammation (Wynn and Ramalingam, 2012; Wu et al., 2017), whether long-term inhibition of TGF-β1 activity is beneficial to patients with hepatic fibrosis remains to be further studied. Some studies have demonstrated that the combination of small molecules has been successfully used in the treatment of liver fibrosis in animal models (Yang et al., 2012; Sung et al., 2018), suggesting that combined pharmacotherapy will represent a promising strategy for the prevention and treatment of hepatic fibrosis.

Some Traditional Chinese Medicine (TCM) formulations have been approved by the China Food and Drug Administration and are widely used for the treatment of hepatic fibrosis, such as Biejiaruangan Compound and Fuzheng Huayu (FZHY) (Zhang and Schuppan, 2014). Besides, the herbal prescription Yang-Gan-Wan and its active compound polyphenolic rosmarinic acid combined with baicalin has also been proved to be able to treat hepatic fibrosis (Yang et al., 2012). Liuweiwuling tablets (LWWL) is a Chinese Medicine formula which is composed of six herbs: *Schisandrae chinensis fructus, Fructus Ligustri Lucidi, Forsythiae fructus, Curcumae rhizoma, Perennial sow thistle, and Ganoderma spore* and is well known for protection against liver injury in patients with chronic hepatitis B in China (Xin et al., 2009; Lei et al., 2015; Du and Jaeschke, 2016). Clinical studies have also confirmed that LWWL also has definite therapeutic effects on liver fibrosis, we also demonstrated that LWWL could attenuate hepatic fibrosis via modulation of TGF-β1 and NF-κB signaling pathways in BDL and CCL4-induced hepatic fibrosis rat models (Liu et al., 2018a; Liu et al., 2018b). Schisandrol B (SolB) is one of the main active ingredients isolated from *Schisandrae chinensis fructus*, and has been shown to have definite hepatoprotective effects in APAP and cholestasis induced liver injury models (Jiang et al., 2015; Zeng et al., 2017). Wedelolactone (WeD) is a coumarin isolated from Eclipta prostrate L, which exhibits anti-inflammatory effects (Yuan et al., 2013; Luo et al., 2018; Zhu et al., 2019), it also has anti-fibrotic effects on human hepatic stellate cell line LX-2 (Xia et al., 2013). In our study, we demonstrate that the combination of SolB and WeD synergistically reverses hepatic fibrosis via modulating multiple signaling pathways, suggesting that the combination of SolB and WeD may be developed as potential candidate for the treatment of liver fibrosis.

MATERIALS AND METHODS

Mice
Six-to-eight-week-old female C57BL/6 mice were purchased from SPF Biotechnology Co., Ltd. (Beijing, China). All animals were maintained under 12 h light/dark conditions at 22–24°C with unrestricted access to food and water for the duration of the experiment. All animal protocols in this study were performed according to the guidelines for care and use of laboratory animals and approved by the animal ethics committee of the Fifth Medical Center, Chinese PLA General Hospital (Beijing, China).

Reagents and Antibodies
Nigericin, dimethyl sulfoxide, and ultrapure lipopolysaccharide (LPS) were purchased from Sigma (Munich, Germany). SolB, WeD, and colchicine were obtained from TargetMol (Boston, MA, United States). Anti-mouse-Collagen1 (1:1000), anti-mouse-Smad2/3 (1:1000), and anti-mouse-P-Smad3 (1:1000) were purchased from Cell Signaling Technology (Boston, MA, United States). Anti-mouse-P-IκBα (1:1000), anti-mouse-IκBα (1:1000), anti-mouse -P-IKK (1:1000), anti-mouse-IKK (1:1000), anti-human Smad3 (1:1000), anti-human P-Smad3 (1:1000), and anti-human α-SMA (1:1000) were purchased from Proteintech (Chicago, IL, United States). Anti-mouse-IL-1β, anti-mouse-NLRP3 (1:2000), and anti-mouse-ASC (1:1000) were purchased from Santa Cruz Biotechnology (Beijing, China). Anti-mouse -caspase-1 p20 (1:1000), anti-mouse-caspase-1 p45 (1:1000), anti-mouse-pro-IL-1β (1:1000), and anti-GAPDH (1:2000) were purchased from Proteintech (Chicago, IL, United States).

Cell Culture
Bone marrow-derived macrophages (BMDMs) were isolated from the femoral bone marrow of 10°week-old female C57BL/6 mice and cultured in Dulbecco's modified Eagle's medium (DMEM) supplemented with 10% fetal bovine serum (FBS), 1% penicillin/streptomycin (P/S), and 50 ng/ml murine macrophage colony-stimulating factor. LX-2 and L0-2 cells were grown in RPMI 1640 medium. All cell lines were cultured under a humidified 5% (v/v) CO_2 atmosphere at 37°C.

Animal Experiments
Four-to-five-week-old female C57BL/6 mice were purchased from SPF Biotechnology Co., Ltd. (Beijing, China). All animals were maintained under 12 h light/dark conditions at 22–24°C with unrestricted access to food and water for the duration of the experiment, except during fasting tests. All animal protocols in this study were performed according to the guidelines for care and use of laboratory animals and approved by the animal ethics committee of the Fifth Medical Center, Chinese PLA General Hospital. For experiments with BDL, mice were randomly divided into six groups. From days 7 to 21 after surgery, the

sham group and the mice with successful development of the disease were divided into groups and administered drugs by gavage with a dose of 2 ml/kg once a day. The mice were divided into the following groups: sham operation group (Control), model group (BDL/CCl$_4$-induced hepatic fibrosis model group), colchicine positive group (0.2 mg/kg), WeD 20 mg/kg group, SolB 40 mg/kg group, and WeD 20 mg/kg in combination with SolB 40 mg/kg group. Eight mice were included in each group. The body weight was measured daily. The animals were euthanized in random order between 9:00 am and 11:00 am after an overnight fast. Samples of serum and liver were collected for further analysis.

Serum Biochemistry and Liver Histology

Alanine transaminase (ALT) and aspartate transaminase (AST) were analyzed using kits from Thermo Fisher Scientific (Cincinnati, OH, United States). Formalin-fixed tissue was embedded in paraffin, and sections were stained with Masson, hematoxylin and eosin (H&E), and Sirius red stains. Liver histology was blindly assessed for inflammation, necrosis, and bile duct proliferation. Hydroxyproline levels in the liver were measured as described.

Quantitative Real-Time Polymerase Chain Reaction

qPCR method was used to detect gene expression in liver tissue of mice in each group. After RNA extraction, Reverse transcription kit was used to reverse transcription RNA cDNA, and the specific operation was carried out strictly in accordance with the kit instructions. Using a qPCR instrument to amplify each gene and its GAPDH, qPCR reaction system: cDNA1µL, SYBR Green Mix 5 , 0.5 µl of upstream and downstream primers, DEPC water 3 µl. Reaction conditions 95°C 3 min, 95°C 3 s, 60°C 30 s, 95°C 15 s, 60°C 1 min, 95°C 15 s, Cycle 50 times. Each sample contains two multiple holes, gene expression levels were quantitatively analyzed by 2-ΔΔCt method.

Western Blotting

Immunoblot analysis was used to evaluate the expression of Collagen1, p-Smad3, Smad2/3, p-IκB, IκBα, IKK, p-IKK, NLRP3, Lamin B, α-SMA, caspase-1 p20, IL-1β p17, pro-IL-1β, caspase-1 p45, NLRP3, and ASC. GAPDH and Lamin B served as loading controls in cell lysates. The samples were boiled at 105°C for 15 min. The protein samples were resolved using 12 or 10% sodium dodecyl sulfate-polyacrylamide gel electrophoresis (SDS-PAGE) gels and transferred to a nitrocellulose membrane *via* a wet-transfer system. The membranes were subsequently incubated with 5% fat-free milk for 1 h at room temperature followed by incubation overnight with primary antibodies at 4°C. Blots were washed thrice with Tris-buffered saline Tween-20 (TBST) and incubated with corresponding horseradish peroxidase-conjugated secondary antibody (1:5000) for 1 h at room temperature. This step was followed by washing with TBST thrice, and the signals were analyzed using the enhanced chemiluminescent reagent (Promega, Beijing, China) detection system.

Infammasome Activation

BMDMs were seeded at 5×10^5 cells/well in 24-well plates overnight. The following day, the medium was replaced, and cells were stimulated with 50 ng/ml LPS for 4 h. The medium was then changed to opti-MEM containing WeD or SolB for 1 h. For inducing the activation of NLRP3 infammasome, cells were stimulated with nigericin (7.5 µmol/L) for 45 min.

NF-κB Signing Pathway Activation

BMDMs were seeded at 5×10^5 cells/well in 24-well plates overnight. BMDMs were treated with WeD or SolB for an hour and then stimulated with LPS (50 ng/ml) for 0, 5, 15, 30, and 60 min.

TGF-β1 in Combination With LPS Induced Hepatocyte Injury *in vitro*

We seeded BMDMs at 5×10^5 cells/well in 24-well plates overnight. The medium was then replaced with 1640 medium without FBS, then give SolB or WeD for an hour, followed by treatment with TGF-β1 (5 ng/ml) alone or in combination with LPS (50 ng/ml).

Cell Viability Assay

The cell counting kit-8 (CCK-8) assay was used to detect the viability of cells. L0-2 cells were seeded in a 96-well growth-medium plate overnight at 8.5×10^4 cells/well. The cells were then incubated at 37°C followed by individual treatments with WeD or SolB for 24 h. These cells were incubated with CCK-8 for 30 min. The optical density (O.D.) values were determined at the wavelength of 450 nm. The half-maximal inhibitory concentration (IC50) of WeD or SolB was evaluated using the software Prism 6 (GraphPad Software, San Diego, CA, United States).

APAP-Induced Hepatocyte Injury *in vitro*

To induce hepatocyte injury, L0-2 cells were seeded at 8.5×10^3 cells/well in 96-well plates overnight. The following day, the medium was replaced with DMEM containing APAP (22 mmol/L) and SolB or WeD (5, 10, 20, 40 µmol/L).

Enzyme-Linked Immunosorbent Assay

Supernatants from cell culture were assayed with mouse TNF-α and mouse IL-6 according to manufacturer's instructions (Dakewe, Beijing, China).

Lactate Dehydrogenase Assay

L0-2 cells were treated with WeD and SolB separately. The release of LDH into the culture supernatants was evaluated using the LDH cytotoxicity assay kit (Beyotime, Shanghai, China) according to the manufacturer's instructions.

Statistical Analysis

Statistical analysis was performed using the software Prism 6 (GraphPad Software, San Diego, CA, United States). All experimental data were expressed as mean ± standard error of the mean (SD). One-way ANOVA was used for multiple comparisons followed by Tukey's *post hoc* test or Dunnett's test for comparison between two groups. The differences with $p < 0.05$ were considered statistically significant.

RESULTS

SolB Significantly Inhibited Hepatocyte Injury *in vitro*

Persistent hepatocyte injury or death, as an main driver of fibrosis and liver inflammation, could initiate and perpetuate sterile inflammatory responses and HSCs activation, so hepatic fibrosis can be reversed by inhibiting hepatocyte injury or eliminating the triggering factors (Cordero-Espinoza and Huch, 2018; Bansal and Chamroonkul, 2019). *S. sphenanthera* is a traditional hepato-protective Chinese medicine, so we test the effect of the constituents of *S. sphenanthera* on APAP-induced hepatocyte injury. The data showed that several constituents could improve cell viability of LO-2 cells exposed to acetaminophen, and Schisandrol B (SolB) is the most effective constituent (**Figure 1A**). We then tested the effect of the SolB on hepatocyte survival by the CCK8 assay and the result showed that SolB were not toxic to LO-2 cells, even at concentrations up to 200 μmol/L (**Figure 1B**). We next examined whether SolB inhibited hepatocyte injury at a wide range of concentrations (0, 5,10, 20, and 40 μM). The result showed that SolB treatment dose-dependently improved cell viability and inhibited LDH release in LO-2 cells exposed to acetaminophen (**Figures 1C,D**). The protective effects of SolB on hepatocytes was further examined using Annexin V-FITC Apoptosis detection kit, the result showed that SolB treatment significantly inhibited acetaminophen-induced apoptosis of LO-2 cells (**Figure 1E**). These results indicated the protective effect of SolB against hepatocyte injury.

SolB Attenuates Hepatic Injury and Fibrosis Induced by BDL in Mice

Considering the obviously hepato-protective effect, we tested the role of SolB in mouse model of hepatic fibrosis induced by bile duct ligation (BDL) ligation. The livers of mice treated with colchicine (colchicine has been used for the treatment of liver fibrosis (Rambaldi and Gluud, 2005) and was used as a positive control in this study, 0.2 mg/kg per day) or SolB (10, 20, and 40 mg/kg per day, respectively) exhibited a remarkably lower cirrhotic appearance with varying degrees (**Figures 2A–D**). Furthermore, the histological assessment of liver sections by H&E staining, Sirius red, and Masson staining demonstrated that treatment with SolB inhibited hepatic injury and fibrosis in mice induced by BDL (**Figures 2A,B**). Consistent with the histopathology analysis, SolB treatment reversed the increase in ALT, AST, DBIL, TBIL, and TBA serum levels induced by BDL in a dose-dependent manner in mice (**Figures 2C,D**; **Supplementary Figures S1A–C**).

HSCs play a crucial role in hepatic fibrosis, which can be activated upon persistent liver injury and leads to the deposition of ECM components including collagen 1 (Shang et al., 2018).

The α-smooth muscle actin (α-SMA) is a unique marker of activated HSCs (Nouchi et al., 1991). Hence, we analyzed the expression of α-SMA by immunohistochemical staining (**Figure 2A**) and qPCR (**Figure 2E**) in all groups. The results demonstrated that SolB inhibited the expression of α-SMA in mice with hepatic fibrosis induced by BDL in a dose-dependent manner. Our results also showed that treatment with SolB reduced the number of macrophages, staining by specific marker of F4/80, in mice induced by BDL. Consequently, this observation indicated that SolB inhibited the activation of HSCs *in vivo*. Activation and survival of HSCs are regulated by transforming growth factor-beta (TGF-β) and platelet-derived growth factor (PDGF) signaling pathways (Pinzani 2002; Kikuchi et al., 2017; Dewidar et al., 2019). The expression of TGF-β and PDGF was also inhibited by SolB treatment in mice with hepatic fibrosis induced by BDL, as evidenced by qPCR (**Figures 2F,G**). BDL significantly promoted collagen I gene expression compared to that in the normal mice, while SolB treatment significantly abrogated BDL-induced upregulation of collagen I, as revealed by immunoblotting (**Figure 2H**; **Supplementary Figure S1D**) and qPCR analysis (**Supplementary Figure S1E**). More importantly, we observed that SolB inhibited both the phosphorylation of Smad3 and the expression of Smad2/3 in a dose-dependent manner (**Figure 2H**; **Supplementary Figure S1E**). We also have evaluated macrophages (by F4/80) in the liver of the BDL-induced hepatic fibrosis mice. Our results showed that treatment with SolB reduced the number of macrophages, staining by specific marker of F4/80, in mice induced by BDL (**Supplementary Figure S1F**). These results demonstrated that SolB attenuates hepatic injury and fibrosis induced by BDL in mice.

WeD Inhibits TGF-β1/Smad-Mediated Activation of HSCs *in vitro*

Combination therapy for liver fibrosis is considered to be very attractive. Targeting several vital but very different pathways to reduce chronic inflammation and ECM deposition would more effectively address liver fibrosis (Schuppan and Kim, 2013; Schuppan, 2015). So we reasoned that the combination of SolB with another compound that target HSC activation would exhibit better anti-fibrosis effect. Activated HSCs play a central role in the pathogenesis of hepatic fibrogenesis, in which a continuous synthesis of collagen is mediated by the TGF-β1/Smad signaling pathway (Lee and Friedman, 2011). We screened compounds that could inhibit TGF-β1/Smad signaling in LX-2 cells (human hepatic stellate cell line) and found that Wedelolactone (WeD) could suppress TGF-β1/Smad pathway (**Supplementary Figures S2A,B**). Next we tested whether WeD could inhibit TGF-β1/Smad signaling to suppress the activation of HSCs *in vitro*. We detected the expression and phosphorylation of Smad3 in the TGF-β1 signaling cascade. The result demonstrated a reduction in the expression of Smad3 and its phosphorylation after treatment with WeD in LX-2 cells pretreated with TGF-β1 (**Figure 3A**; **Supplementary Figure S2C**). WeD also inhibited TGF-β1-mediated induction of α-SMA (**Figures 3A,B**; **Supplementary Figure S2C**). These

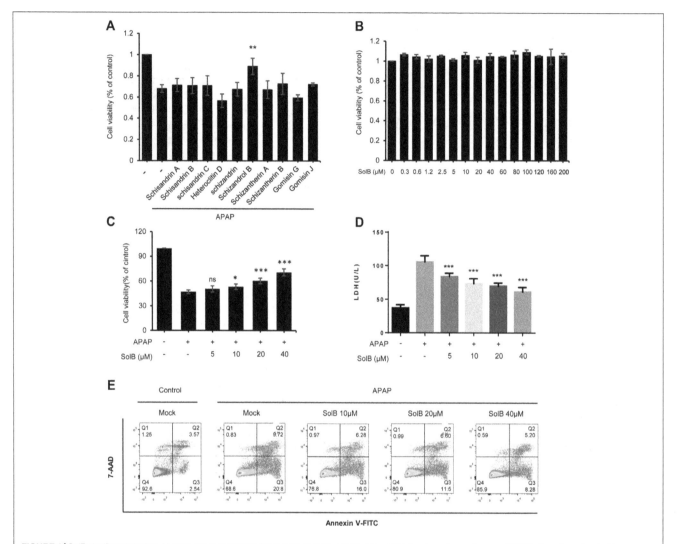

FIGURE 1 | SolB significantly inhibited hepatocyte injury *in vitro* **(A)** The effect of the constituents of *Schisandra sphenanthera* on APAP-induced hepatocyte injury **(B)** Cell viability of L02 cells treated with SolB for 24 h were detected **(C,D)** Survival rate by CCK-8 **(C)** and the release of LDH **(D)** of L02 cells treated with SolB and then exposed to APAP **(E)** Early apoptotic of L02 cells were treated with SolB and then exposed to APAP, and detected by Flow cytometry. Data are expressed as Mean ± SD from three biological replicates (*n* = 3). Statistics differences were analyzed using One-way ANOVA followed by Dunnett's test:*p < 0.05, **p < 0.01, ***p < 0.001; NS, no significance.

results demonstrated that WeD could suppress the activation of HSCs by targeting the TGF-β1/Smad signaling pathway.

WeD Blocks the Production of TNF-α and IL-1β in Macrophages

Previous studies have demonstrated that TNF-α and IL-1β produced by hepatic macrophages can promote the survival of activated HSCs (Gieling et al., 2009; Osawa et al., 2013; Pradere et al., 2013). Wedelolactone has been reported to be an inhibitor of IKK that is critical for activation of NF-κB by mediating phosphorylation and degradation of IκBα (Kobori et al., 2004), activation of NF-κB signaling leads to expression of downstream target genes including TNF-α and IL-6. Hence, we next tested whether WeD affected the

production of TNF-α and IL-6 in LPS-treated macrophages, the result showed that WeD dose-dependently inhibited the production of TNF-α and IL-6 in LPS-treated BMDMs (**Figures 3C,D**). The maturation and release of IL-1β are mediated by the inflammasome. WeD has been reported to inhibit the activation of the NLRP3 inflammasome (Wei et al., 2017; Cheng et al., 2019). We further confirmed the effect of WeD on NLRP3 inflammasme activation and release of IL-1β. Our data showed that WeD inhibited nigericin-induced caspase-1 cleavage and IL-1β production in a dose-dependent manner in LPS-primed BMDMs (**Figure 3E; Supplementary Figure S2D**), suggesting that WeD inhibited the production of IL-1β by directly blocking the activation of the NLRP3 inflammasome. Taken together, these results demonstrated that WeD can directly inhibit the production of TNF-α and IL-1β in macrophages.

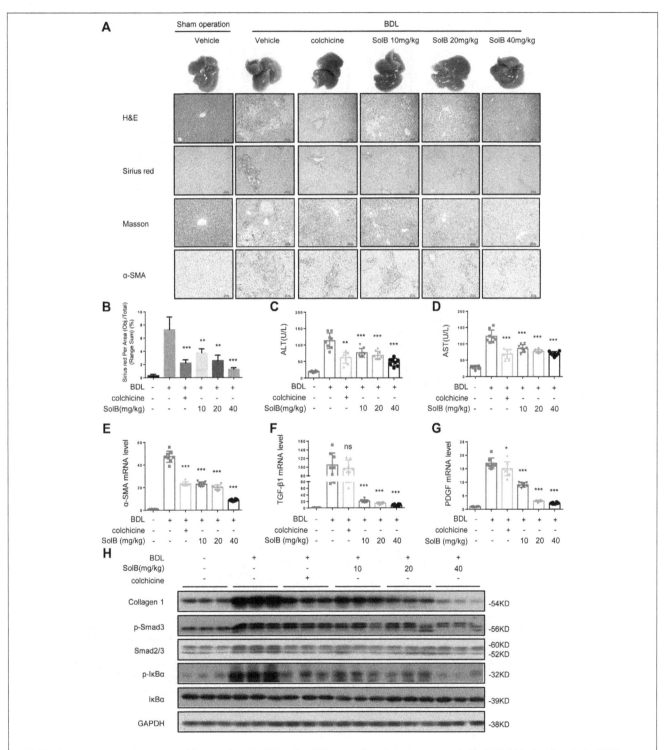

FIGURE 2 | SolB attenuates hepatic injury and fibrosis induced by BDL in mice **(A)** Images of livers from sham-operated mice (SHAM), bile duct-ligated mice (BDL), BDL-mice treated with SolB. Representative micrographs of liver H&E staining, Sirius red, Masson staining and α-SMA were shown. Scale bars represent 50 μm **(B)** Quantitative results of Sirius red staining sections **(C,D)** Serum level of ALT **(C)** and AST **(D)** of sham-operated mice (SHAM), bile duct-ligated mice (BDL) and BDL-mice treated with SolB or colchicine (0.2 mg/kg) **(E–G)** Quantitative PCR analysis of mRNA levels of α-SMA **(E)**, TGF-β1 **(F)**, and PDGF **(G)** in livers from sham-operated mice, BDL mice, BDL-mice treated with SolB **(H)** Western blot analysis of Collagen1, p-Smad3, Smad2/3, P-IκBα, IκBα, and GAPDH in livers from sham-operated mice, BDL mice, BDL-mice treated with SolB. Data are expressed as Mean ± SD (n = 8 or 3 mice). Statistics differences were analyzed using One-way ANOVA followed by Dunnett's test: $^*p < 0.05$, $^{**}p < 0.01$, $^{***}p < 0.001$. NS, no significance.

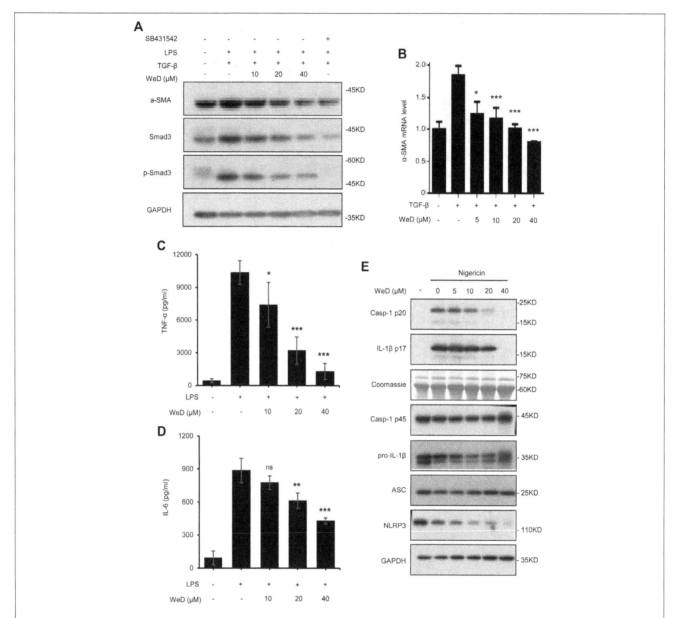

FIGURE 3 | WeD inhibits TGF-β1/Smad-mediated activation of HSCs and blocks the production of TNF-α and IL-1β in macrophages **(A)** Western blot analysis of α-SMA, Smad3, p-Smad3, GAPDH in LX-2 cells treated with WeD (10, 20, 40 μM) and then stimulated with TGF-β1 (5 ng/ml) combined with LPS (50 ng/ml) **(B)** Quantitative PCR analysis of mRNA levels of α-SMA of LX-2 cells treated with WeD and then stimulated with TGF-β1 (5 ng/ml) **(C,D)** ELISA of TNF-α **(C)** and IL-6 **(D)** in SN of BMDMs treated with WeD (10, 20, 40 μM) and then stimulated with LPS (50 ng/ml) **(E)** Western blot analysis of caspase-1 (p20) and IL-1β in SN and pro- IL-1β, caspase-1 (p45), NLRP3 and ASC in WCL of LPS-primed BMDMs treated with WeD (5, 10, 20, 40 μM) and then stimulated with nigericin. Data are expressed as Mean ± SD from three biological replicates (n = 3). Statistics differences were analyzed using One-way ANOVA followed by Dunnett's test: *p < 0.05, **p < 0.01, ***p < 0.001. NS, no significance.

WeD Attenuates Hepatic Injury and Fibrosis Induced by BDL in Mice

Considering the inhibitory effect of WeD on HSC activation and inflammation, we further tested the role of WeD in liver fibrosis in a mouse model of hepatic fibrosis induced by BDL. Our result of histological assessment of liver sections by H&E staining, Sirius red, and Masson staining showed that treated with WeD significantly alleviated hepatic injury and fibrosis in BDL-induced

mice (**Figures 4A,B**). Consistent with the histopathology analysis, WeD treatment reduced the ALT, AST, DBIL, TBIL, and TBA serum levels induced by BDL in a dose-dependent manner in mice (**Figures 4C,D**; **Supplementary Figure S3A–C**).

It has been reported that HSCs play a crucial role in hepatic fibrosis and α-SMA is a unique marker of activated HSCs (Nouchi et al., 1991; Shang et al., 2018). So we detected the expression of α-SMA by immunohistochemical staining and qPCR. Our result

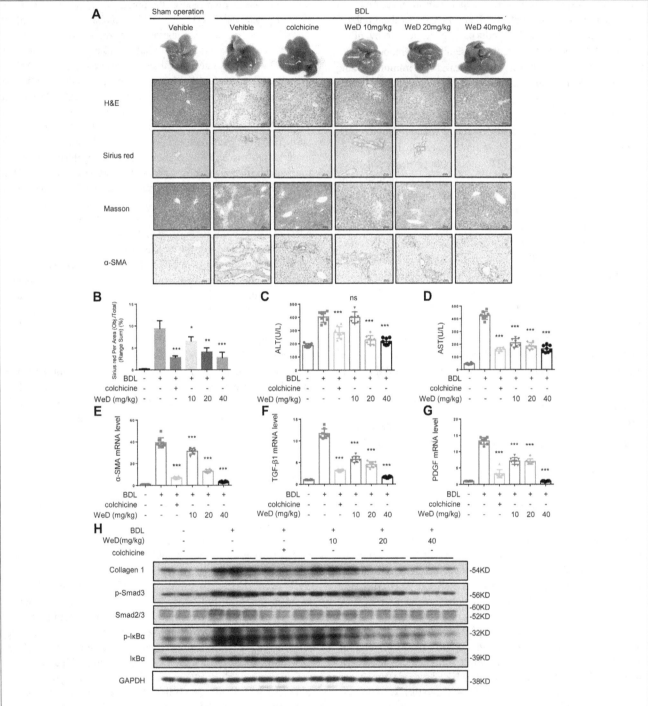

FIGURE 4 | WeD attenuates hepatic injury and fibrosis induced by BDL in mice **(A)** Images of livers from sham-operated mice (SHAM), bile duct-ligated mice (BDL), BDL-mice treated with WeD. Representative micrographs of liver H&E staining, Sirius red, Masson staining, and α-SMA were shown. Scale bars represent 50 μm **(B)** Quantitative results of Sirius red staining sections **(C,D)** Serum level of ALT **(C)** and AST **(D)** of sham-operated mice (SHAM), bile duct-ligated mice (BDL) and BDL-mice treated with WeD or colchicine (0.2 mg/kg) **(E–G)** Quantitative PCR analysis of mRNA levels of α-SMA **(E)**, TGF-β1 **(F)**, and PDGF **(G)** in livers from sham-operated mice, BDL mice, BDL-mice treated with WeD **(H)** Western blot analysis of Collagen1, p-Smad3, Smad2/3, P-IκBα, IκBα and GAPDH in livers from sham-operated mice, BDL mice, BDL-mice treated with WeD. Data are expressed as Mean ± SD (n = 8 or 3 mice). Statistics differences were analyzed using One-way ANOVA followed by Dunnett's test: *$p < 0.05$, **$p < 0.01$, ***$p < 0.001$. NS, no significance.

showed that the expression of α-SMA in mice with hepatic fibrosis induced by BDL could be reduced by WeD treatment (**Figures 4A,E**). Our results showed that treatment with WeD reduced the number of macrophages, staining by specific marker of F4/80, in mice induced by BDL. Consequently, this observation demonstrated that WeD also inhibited the activation of HSCs *in vivo*. Then we examined the expression of TGF-β and PDGF in mice. The data showed that the expression of TGF-β and PDGF was also inhibited by WeD treatment with BDL-induced hepatic fibrosis by qPCR (**Figures 4F,G**). WeD treatment also significantly reduced BDL-induced increase of collagen I, as revealed by immunoblotting (**Figure 4H; Supplementary Figure S3H**) and qPCR analysis (**Supplementary Figure S3D**). Consistent with the effect *in vitro*, WeD inhibited both the phosphorylation of Smad3 and the expression of Smad3 in a dose-dependent manner (**Figure 4H; Supplementary Figure S3H**). we have evaluated macrophages (by F4/80) in the liver of the BDL-induced hepatic fibrosis mice. Our results showed that treatment with WeD reduced the number of macrophages, staining by specific marker of F4/80, in mice induced by BDL (**Supplementary Figure S3G**). We have demonstrated that WeD dose-dependently inhibited the production of TNF-α and IL-6 in LPS-treated BMDMs and the production of IL-1β by directly blocking the activation of the NLRP3 inflammasome in BMDMs. Consistent with the effect in BMDMs, WeD treatment could inhibit the expression of IL-β and IL-6 (**Supplementary Figure S3E,F**). The results demonstrated that WeD could attenuate inflammation in liver *in vivo*. Thus, these results demonstrated that WeD attenuates hepatic injury and fibrosis induced by BDL in mice and inhibited the TGF-β/Smad-mediated activation of HSCs *in vivo*.

A Combination of SolB and WeD Significantly Inhibits Hepatic Fibrosis and Injury in Mice With CCl₄-Induced Hepatic Fibrosis

Next we examined if SolB and WeD would show protective effects in another hepatic fibrosis mouse model. We evaluated the anti-fibrosis effect of SolB and WeD in CCl4-induced hepatic fibrosis model mice, and the data showed that both SolB and WeD alleviated hepatic fibrosis induced by CCl₄ in mice, suggesting their potent anti-fibrosis effect. Next we tested whether the anti-fibrosis effect mediated by the combination of SolB and WeD was more potent in comparison with that mediated by individual treatments of SolB and WeD. Mice with CCl₄-induced hepatic fibrosis were randomly divided into five groups and received gavages with PBS (model group), colchicine (a positive control drug), 20 mg/kg WeD, 40 mg/kg SolB, or a combination of WeD (20 mg/kg) and SolB (40 mg/kg). Compared with control mice, mice with CCl₄-induced hepatic fibrosis showed serve hepatocyte damage and hepatic fibrosis, evidenced by HE, Sirius red staining, and Masson staining (**Figures 5A–C**). WeD, SolB and their combination treatment were all shown to prevent the progression of liver fibrosis in the mouse model with CCl₄-induced hepatic fibrosis. The synergistic inhibitory effect of SolB and WeD on hepatic fibrosis was significantly better than that of WeD or SolB (**Figures 5A–C**). Consistent with the results of liver histology assessment, combined treatment of WeD and SolB also more efficiently reduced the hydroxyproline content in liver tissues than WeD or SolB alone (**Figure 5E**).

To further examine the antifibrotic effect of SolB combined with WeD, the expression of α-SMA was evaluated by immunohistochemistry, results showed that CCl₄ significantly

promoted α-SMA expression in the portal area of fibrotic liver tissue, while treatment with WeD, SolB, or their combination suppressed the expression of α-SMA in fibrotic liver tissues (**Figures 5A,D**). Furthermore, the expression of α-SMA in mice co-treated with SolB and WeD was significantly lower than that in mice treated with WeD or SolB alone (**Figures 5A,D**). Moreover, compared with the individual WeD or SolB treatment, the combined treatment of WeD and SolB more effectively reduced the mRNA level of α-SMA in liver tissues of mice (**Figure 5F**). Previous studies have shown that cytoglobin, which is the fourth globin in mammals and function as a local gas sensor, is a promising new marker that discriminates between myofibroblasts derived from stellate cells and those from portal fibroblasts (Kawada, 2015; Thuy et al., 2015). Thus, we evaluated the cytoglobin by qPCR in CCl4-induced hepatic fibrosis mice, and the results showed that combination treatment of WeD and SolB significantly reduced the expression of cytoglobin induced by CCl4 in mice compared to that by treatment with WeD and SolB alone, suggesting that the combination of WeD and SolB is more effective in the treatment of liver fibrosis (**Supplementary Figure S4A**). Western blot analysis also demonstrated that combination treatment of WeD and SolB significantly decreased the expression of collagen and Smad as well as phosphorylation of IκB and Smad3 induced by CCl₄ in mice compared to that by treatment with WeD and SolB alone, suggesting that WeD combined with SolB could inhibit the activity of the TGF-β1 and NF-κB pathway more effectively than WeD or SolB alone *in vivo* (**Figure 5G; Supplementary Figure S4B**). These results indicate that the combination of WeD and SolB is more effective in the treatment of liver fibrosis owing to the regulation of several signaling pathways associated with hepatic fibrosis.

DISCUSSION

In this study, we demonstrate that SolB, WeD or the combination of SolB and WeD could reverse hepatic fibrosis *in vivo* and the inhibitory effect of combination of SolB and WeD on hepatic fibrosis is superior to that of SolB or WeD treatment alone. SolB reverses hepatic fibrosis by inhibiting hepatocyte injury, and WeD could block the production of TNF-α and IL-1β in macrophages and the activation of TGF-β1/Smad signaling pathway in activated HSCs. Our result confirms that combination pharmacotherapy targeting several vital but very different pathways to reduce chronic inflammation and ECM deposition would more effectively address liver fibrosis.

Schisandra sphenanthera is the dried ripe fruit of S. sphenanthera Rehd. et Wils, it is a traditional Chinese medicine widely used for its protective effects in liver, kidney, and heart (Panossian and Wikman, 2008). Recent studies report that Schisandra sphenanthera possesses hepatoprotective effects against viral or chemical hepatitis (Zhu et al., 2000; Teraoka et al., 2012). Hepatocyte injury, a primary inducer of hepatic fibrosis, can promote inflammation and activation of HSCs in liver, therefore, reversal of hepatocyte injury is one of the important ways to prevent and treat hepatic fibrosis (Lee et al., 2015). Our result showed that SolB is the most effective constituent of Schisandra sphenanthera to protect against APAP-induced injury in LO-2 cells, it showed obviously anti-fibrotic effect in

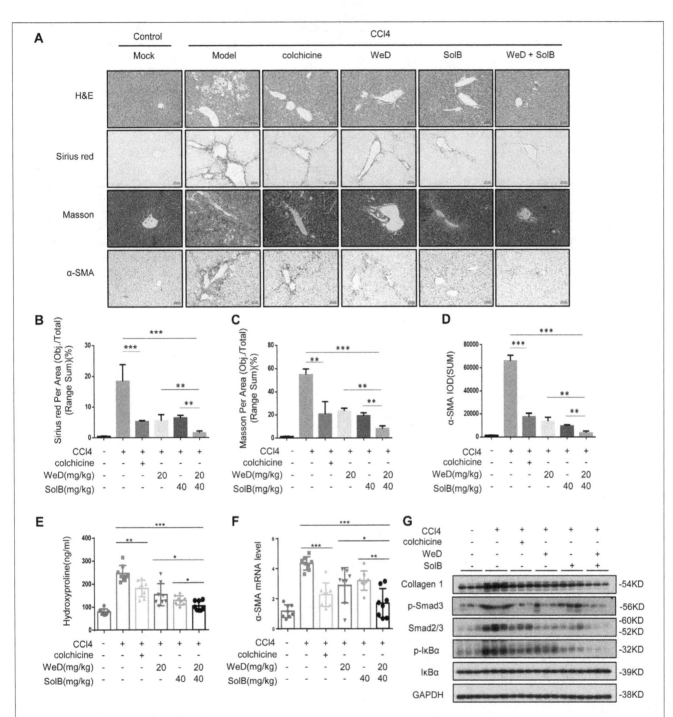

FIGURE 5 | A combination of SolB and WeD treatment dramatically inhibits hepatic fibrosis and injury in CCL4-induced hepatic fibrosis mice **(A)** Images of livers from control, CCL4-induced hepatic fibrosis mice, CCL4-induced hepatic fibrosis mice treated with colchicine (0.2 mg/kg), SolB (40 mg/kg), WeD (20 mg/kg) or combination of SolB (40 mg/kg) and WeD (20 mg/kg). Representative micrographs of liver H&E staining, Sirius red, Masson, and α-SMA staining were shown. Scale bars represent 50 μm **(B–D)** Quantitative results of Sirius red **(B)**, Masson **(C)**, and α-SMA **(D)** staining sections **(E)** Serum level of hydroxyproline of control, CCL4-induced hepatic fibrosis mice, CCL4-induced hepatic fibrosis mice treated with colchicine (0.2 mg/kg), SolB (40 mg/kg), WeD (20 mg/kg) or combination of SolB and WeD **(F)** Quantitative PCR analysis of mRNA levels of α-SMA in livers from control, CCL4-induced hepatic fibrosis mice, CCL4-induced hepatic fibrosis mice treated with colchicine (0.2 mg/kg), SolB (40 mg/kg), WeD (20 mg/kg) or combination of SolB and WeD. **(G)** Western blot analysis of Collagen1, p-Smad3, Smad2/3, p-IκBα, IκBα and GAPDH in livers from control, CCL4-induced hepatic fibrosis mice, CCL4-induced hepatic fibrosis mice treated with colchicine (0.2 mg/kg), SolB (40 mg/kg), WeD (20 mg/kg) or combination of SolB and WeD. Data are expressed as Mean ± SD (n = 8 or 3 mice). Statistics differences were analyzed using One-way ANOVA followed by Tukey's *post hoc* test: *p < 0.05, **p < 0.01, ***p < 0.001. NS, no significance.

BDL and CCl4-induced liver fibrosis model mice, indicating the potential of SolB to be used in the treatment of liver fibrosis. In addition, Many studies have shown that SolB could inhibit liver injury by regulating multiple pathways (Jiang et al., 2015; Jiang et al., 2016; Lu et al., 2016; Zeng et al., 2017), these studies may help explain the target of SolB in the prevention and treatment of liver injury and the related mechanism.

Hepatic stellate cell activation and chronic inflammation are also important contributors to the development of liver fibrosis (Bataller and Brenner, 2005; Seki and Schwabe, 2015). TGF-β plays a critical role in the activation of HSCs, inhibiting TGF-β activity is a potential and effective treatment for hepatic fibrosis (Gyorfi et al., 2018; Dewidar et al., 2019). Our data showed that Wedelolactone (WeD), a coumarin isolated from Eclipta prostrate L exhibiting hepatoprotective effect and anti-fibrotic effect on human hepatic stellate cell line LX-2 (Xia et al., 2013; Lu et al., 2016; Luo et al., 2018), inhibited TGF-β-mediated induction of Smad3 and its phosphorylation, suggesting that WeD could directly target TGF-β/Smads signaling pathway to inhibit the activation of HSCs. Recent studies also demonstrate the role of WeD in anti-inflammation, WeD is an inhibitor of IKK that is critical for activation of NF-κB (Luo et al., 2018), it has also been reported to suppress NLRP3 infammasome activation (Wei et al., 2017; Cheng et al., 2019). Our data also confirmed the inhibitory effect of WeD on production of TNF-α and IL-1β in macrophages, which are involved in the progression of fibrogenesis through promoting survival and activation of HSCs (Gieling et al., 2009; Osawa et al., 2013; Pradere et al., 2013).

Hepatocyte injury, triggered by multifarious factors, is the main driver of chronic liver inflammation and fibrosis (Luedde et al., 2014; Seki and Schwabe, 2015). Meanwhile, previous studies have demonstrated that apoptotic hepatocyte could promote the secretion of pro-inflammatory and profibrogenic cytokines from macrophages, and to directly promote HSC activation (Canbay et al., 2003; Zhan et al., 2006; Seki and Schwabe, 2015). HSCs, which is the main executors of fibrogenesis, interact with hepatocytes, hepatic macrophages, lymphocytes and endothelial cells resulting in the promotion of fibrogenesis (Bataller and Brenner, 2005; Bansal and Chamroonkul, 2019). Moreover, it has been suggested that damage-associated molecular patterns (DAMPs), which are released by dead or damaged cells, may also directly or indirectly promote fibrosis (Luedde et al., 2014; Seki and Schwabe, 2015). Elevation in ALT and AST has been

regarded as the indicators of hepatocyte injury (Luedde et al., 2014; Seki and Schwabe, 2015). In our study, we have detected the level of serum ALT and AST in CCl4/BDL-induced hepatic fibrosis mice, and the results suggested that SolB, WeD or the combination of SolB and WeD treatment reversed the increase in ALT and AST serum levels induced by CCl4 or BDL, suggesting that the treatment reduced hepatocyte injury in vivo.

Combination therapies that address two or more key molecular players and/or pathways are considered to hold much promise for treatment of liver fibrosis (Trautwein et al., 2015). Hepatocyte injury, inflammation, or hepatic stellate cells (HSCs) activation are important contributors to the development of liver fibrosis (Bataller and Brenner, 2005; Gieling et al., 2009; Seki and Schwabe, 2015). In our studies, we show that SolB inhibited hepatocyte injury, while WeD blocked HSC activation and inflammatory cytokines production in macrophage. The inhibitory effect of the combination of SolB and WeD on hepatic fibrosis is superior to that of individual SolB or WeD treatments in CCl4-induced liver fibrosis model mice, as evidenced by the histopathological assessment, quantitative analysis of fibrogenesis and anti-fibrinogenic genes or the expression of proteins such as collagen I and α-SMA. Our study indicated that combination therapy with two compounds (SolB and WeD) targeting different pathways exhibit better anti-fibrotic effect. Taken together, our data demonstrate that SolB and WED reverses the progress of liver fibrosis by targeting different cells and pathways, the inhibitory effect of the combination of the two on hepatic fibrosis is superior to that of SolB or WeD alone. Combination of SolB and WeD may be a potential candidate for the prevention and treatment of liver fibrosis.

AUTHOR CONTRIBUTIONS

ZB and XZ supervised the project. ZB and XX acquired funding for the study. ZB designed the experiment. YA performed the most of the experiments. WS performed the mechanistic studies and analyzed the data. XZu and XSu performed the BDL-induced hepatic fibrosis experiments. YC performed the experiment of the TGF β1-mediated induction of α-SMA. ZW, RL, and XSo help performed the CCL4-induced hepatic fibrosis experiment in mice. WD, WM, and KD help analyzed the data of mice experiments. ZL and QL help analyzed the immune-histochemistry data. ZB and XZh wrote and revised the manuscript.

REFERENCES

Bansal, M. B., and Chamroonkul, N. (2019). Antifibrotics in Liver Disease: Are We Getting Closer to Clinical Use? Hepatol. Int. 13, 25–39. doi:10.1007/s12072-018-9897-3

Bataller, R., and Brenner, D. A. (2005). Liver Fibrosis. J. Clin. Invest. 115, 209–218. doi:10.1172/jci24282

Canbay, A., Feldstein, A. E., Higuchi, H., Werneburg, N., Grambihler, A., Bronk, S. F., et al. (2003). Kupffer Cell Engulfment of Apoptotic Bodies Stimulates Death Ligand and Cytokine Expression. Hepatology 38, 1188–1198. doi:10.1053/jhep.2003.50472

Cheng, M., Lin, J., Li, C., Zhao, W., Yang, H., Lv, L., et al. (2019). Wedelolactone Suppresses IL-1β Maturation and Neutrophil Infiltration in Aspergillus fumigatus Keratitis. Int. Immunopharmacol. 73, 17–22. doi:10.1016/j.intimp.2019.04.050

Cordero-Espinoza, L., and Huch, M. (2018). The Balancing Act of the Liver: Tissue Regeneration versus Fibrosis. J. Clin. Invest. 128, 85–96. doi:10.1172/jci93562

Dewidar, B., Meyer, C., Dooley, S., and Meindl-Beinker, A. N. (2019). TGF-β in Hepatic Stellate Cell Activation and Liver Fibrogenesis-Updated 2019. Cells 8, 8. doi:10.3390/cells8111419

Du, K., and Jaeschke, H. (2016). Liuweiwuling Tablets Protect against Acetaminophen Hepatotoxicity: What Is the Protective Mechanism? World J. Gastroenterol. 22, 3302–3304. doi:10.3748/wjg.v22.i11.3302

Fagone, P., Mangano, K., Pesce, A., Portale, T. R., Puleo, S., and Nicoletti, F. (2016). Emerging Therapeutic Targets for the Treatment of Hepatic Fibrosis. Drug Discov. Today 21, 369–375. doi:10.1016/j.drudis.2015.10.015

Gieling, R. G., Wallace, K., and Han, Y.-P. (2009). Interleukin-1 Participates in the Progression from Liver Injury to Fibrosis. Am. J. Physiol.-Gastrointestinal Liver Physiol. 296, G1324–G1331. doi:10.1152/ajpgi.90564.2008

Györfi, A. H., Matei, A.-E., and Distler, J. H. W. (2018). Targeting TGF-β Signaling for the Treatment of Fibrosis. *Matrix Biol.* 68-69, 8–27. doi:10.1016/j.matbio.2017.12.016

Inagaki, Y., and Okazaki, I. (2007). Emerging Insights into Transforming Growth Factor Smad Signal in Hepatic Fibrogenesis. *Gut* 56, 284–292. doi:10.1136/gut.2005.088690

Jiang, Y.-m., Wang, Y., Tan, H.-S., Yu, T., Fan, X.-M., Chen, P., et al. (2016). Schisandrol B Protects against Acetaminophen-Induced Acute Hepatotoxicity in Mice via Activation of the NRF2/ARE Signaling Pathway. *Acta Pharmacol. Sin* 37, 382–389. doi:10.1038/aps.2015.120

Jiang, Y., Fan, X., Wang, Y., Chen, P., Zeng, H., Tan, H., et al. (2015). Schisandrol B Protects against Acetaminophen-Induced Hepatotoxicity by Inhibition of CYP-Mediated Bioactivation and Regulation of Liver Regeneration. *Toxicol. Sci. : official J. Soc. Toxicol.* 143, 107–115. doi:10.1093/toxsci/kfu216

Kawada, N. (2015). Cytoglobin as a Marker of Hepatic Stellate Cell-Derived Myofibroblasts. *Front. Physiol.* 6, 329. doi:10.3389/fphys.2015.00329

Kikuchi, A., Pradhan-Sundd, T., Singh, S., Nagarajan, S., Loizos, N., and Monga, S. P. (2017). Platelet-Derived Growth Factor Receptor α Contributes to Human Hepatic Stellate Cell Proliferation and Migration. *Am. J. Pathol.* 187, 2273–2287. doi:10.1016/j.ajpath.2017.06.009

Kobori, M., Yang, Z., Gong, D., Heissmeyer, V., Zhu, H., Jung, Y.-K., et al. (2004). Wedelolactone Suppresses LPS-Induced Caspase-11 Expression by Directly Inhibiting the IKK Complex. *Cell Death Differ* 11, 123–130. doi:10.1038/sj.cdd.4401325

Krenkel, O., Puengel, T., Govaere, O., Abdallah, A. T., Mossanen, J. C., Kohlhepp, M., et al. (2018). Therapeutic Inhibition of Inflammatory Monocyte Recruitment Reduces Steatohepatitis and Liver Fibrosis. *Hepatology* 67, 1270–1283. doi:10.1002/hep.29544

Lee, U. E., and Friedman, S. L. (2011). Mechanisms of Hepatic Fibrogenesis. *Best Pract. Res. Clin. Gastroenterol.* 25, 195–206. doi:10.1016/j.bpg.2011.02.005

Lee, Y. A., Wallace, M. C., and Friedman, S. L. (2015). Pathobiology of Liver Fibrosis: a Translational success story. *Gut* 64, 830–841. doi:10.1136/gutjnl-2014-306842

Lei, Y.-C., Li, W., and Luo, P. (2015). Liuweiwuling Tablets Attenuate Acetaminophen-Induced Acute Liver Injury and Promote Liver Regeneration in Mice. *World J. Gastroenterol.* 21, 8089–8095. doi:10.3748/wjg.v21.i26.8089

Liu, H., Dong, F., Li, G., Niu, M., Zhang, C., Han, Y., et al. (2018a). Liuweiwuling Tablets Attenuate BDL-Induced Hepatic Fibrosis via Modulation of TGF-β/Smad and NF-κB Signaling Pathways. *J. ethnopharmacology* 210, 232–241. doi:10.1016/j.jep.2017.08.029

Liu, H., Zhang, Z., Hu, H., Zhang, C., Niu, M., Li, R., et al. (2018b). Protective Effects of Liuweiwuling Tablets on Carbon Tetrachloride-Induced Hepatic Fibrosis in Rats. *BMC Complement. Altern. Med.* 18, 212. doi:10.1186/s12906-018-2276-8

Liu, X., Hu, H., and Yin, J. Q. (2006). Therapeutic Strategies against TGF-β Signaling Pathway in Hepatic Fibrosis. *Liver Int. : Official J. Int. Assoc. Study Liver* 26, 8–22. doi:10.1111/j.1478-3231.2005.01192.x

Lu, Y., Hu, D., Ma, S., Zhao, X., Wang, S., Wei, G., et al. (2016). Protective Effect of Wedelolactone against CCl 4 -induced Acute Liver Injury in Mice. *Int. Immunopharmacol.* 34, 44–52. doi:10.1016/j.intimp.2016.02.003

Luedde, T., Kaplowitz, N., and Schwabe, R. F. (2014). Cell Death and Cell Death Responses in Liver Disease: Mechanisms and Clinical Relevance. *Gastroenterology* 147, 765–783.e764. doi:10.1053/j.gastro.2014.07.018

Luo, Q., Ding, J., Zhu, L., Chen, F., and Xu, L. (2018). Hepatoprotective Effect of Wedelolactone against Concanavalin A-Induced Liver Injury in Mice. *Am. J. Chin. Med.* 46, 819–833. doi:10.1142/s0192415x1850043x

Nouchi, T., Tanaka, Y., Tsukada, T., Sato, C., and Marumo, F. (1991). Appearance of Alpha-Smooth-Muscle-Actin-Positive Cells in Hepatic Fibrosis. *Liver* 11, 100–105. doi:10.1111/j.1600-0676.1991.tb00499.x

Osawa, Y., Hoshi, M., Yasuda, I., Saibara, T., Moriwaki, H., and Kozawa, O. (2013). Tumor Necrosis Factor-Alpha Promotes Cholestasis-Induced Liver Fibrosis in the Mouse through Tissue Inhibitor of Metalloproteinase-1 Production in Hepatic Stellate Cells. *PLoS One* 8, e65251. doi:10.1371/journal.pone.0065251

Panossian, A., and Wikman, G. (2008). Pharmacology of Schisandra Chinensis Bail.: an Overview of Russian Research and Uses in Medicine. *J. ethnopharmacology* 118, 183–212. doi:10.1016/j.jep.2008.04.020

Pinzani, M. (2002). PDGF and Signal Transduction in Hepatic Stellate Cells. *Front. Biosci.* 7, d1720–d1726. doi:10.2741/a875

Pradere, J.-P., Kluwe, J., De Minicis, S., Jiao, J.-J., Gwak, G.-Y., Dapito, D. H., et al. (2013). Hepatic Macrophages but Not Dendritic Cells Contribute to Liver Fibrosis by Promoting the Survival of Activated Hepatic Stellate Cells in Mice. *Hepatology* 58, 1461–1473. doi:10.1002/hep.26429

Rambaldi, A., and Gluud, C. (2005). Colchicine for Alcoholic and Non-Alcoholic Liver Fibrosis and Cirrhosis. *Cochrane Database Syst. Rev.* (2), CD002148. doi:10.1002/14651858

Schuppan, D., Ashfaq-Khan, M., Yang, A. T., and Kim, Y. O. (2018). Liver Fibrosis: Direct Antifibrotic Agents and Targeted Therapies. *Matrix Biol.* 68-69, 435–451. doi:10.1016/j.matbio.2018.04.006

Schuppan, D., and Kim, Y. O. (2013). Evolving Therapies for Liver Fibrosis. *J. Clin. Invest.* 123, 1887–1901. doi:10.1172/jci66028

Schuppan, D. (2015). Liver Fibrosis: Common Mechanisms and Antifibrotic Therapies. *Clin. Res. Hepatol. Gastroenterol.* 39 (Suppl. 1), S51–S59. doi:10.1016/j.clinre.2015.05.005

Seki, E., and Schwabe, R. F. (2015). Hepatic Inflammation and Fibrosis: Functional Links and Key Pathways. *Hepatology* 61, 1066–1079. doi:10.1002/hep.27332

Shang, L., Hosseini, M., Liu, X., Kisseleva, T., and Brenner, D. A. (2018). Human Hepatic Stellate Cell Isolation and Characterization. *J. Gastroenterol.* 53, 6–17. doi:10.1007/s00535-017-1404-4

Sung, Y.-C., Liu, Y.-C., Chao, P.-H., Chang, C.-C., Jin, P.-R., Lin, T.-T., et al. (2018). Combined Delivery of Sorafenib and a MEK Inhibitor Using CXCR4-Targeted Nanoparticles Reduces Hepatic Fibrosis and Prevents Tumor Development. *Theranostics* 8, 894–905. doi:10.7150/thno.21168

Teraoka, R., Shimada, T., and Aburada, M. (2012). The Molecular Mechanisms of the Hepatoprotective Effect of Gomisin A against Oxidative Stress and Inflammatory Response in Rats with Carbon Tetrachloride-Induced Acute Liver Injury. *Biol. Pharm. Bull.* 35, 171–177. doi:10.1248/bpb.35.171

Thuy, L. T. T., Matsumoto, Y., Thuy, T. T. V., Hai, H., Suoh, M., Urahara, Y., et al. (2015). Cytoglobin Deficiency Promotes Liver Cancer Development from Hepatosteatosis through Activation of the Oxidative Stress Pathway. *Am. J. Pathol.* 185, 1045–1060. doi:10.1016/j.ajpath.2014.12.017

Trautwein, C., Friedman, S. L., Schuppan, D., and Pinzani, M. (2015). Hepatic Fibrosis: Concept to Treatment. *J. Hepatol.* 62, S15–S24. doi:10.1016/j.jhep.2015.02.039

Wei, W., Ding, M., Zhou, K., Xie, H., Zhang, M., and Zhang, C. (2017). Protective Effects of Wedelolactone on Dextran Sodium Sulfate Induced Murine Colitis Partly through Inhibiting the NLRP3 Inflammasome Activation via AMPK Signaling. *Biomed. Pharmacother.* 94, 27–36. doi:10.1016/j.biopha.2017.06.071

Wu, L., Zhang, Q., Mo, W., Feng, J., Li, S., Li, J., et al. (2017). Quercetin Prevents Hepatic Fibrosis by Inhibiting Hepatic Stellate Cell Activation and Reducing Autophagy via the TGF-β1/Smads and PI3K/Akt Pathways. *Sci. Rep.* 7 (7), 9289. doi:10.1038/s41598-017-09673-5

Wynn, T. A., and Ramalingam, T. R. (2012). Mechanisms of Fibrosis: Therapeutic Translation for Fibrotic Disease. *Nat. Med.* 18, 1028–1040. doi:10.1038/nm.2807

Xia, Y., Chen, J., Cao, Y., Xu, C., Li, R., Pan, Y., et al. (2013). Wedelolactone Exhibits Anti-fibrotic Effects on Human Hepatic Stellate Cell Line LX-2. *Eur. J. Pharmacol.* 714, 105–111. doi:10.1016/j.ejphar.2013.06.012

Xin, S. J., Han, J., and Ding, J. B. (2009). The Clinical Study of Liuweiwuling Tablet on Patients with Chronic Hepatitis B. *Chin. J. Integrated Traditional West. Med. Liver Dis.*

Yang, M. D., Chiang, Y.-M., Higashiyama, R., Asahina, K., Mann, D. A., Mann, J., et al. (2012). Rosmarinic Acid and Baicalin Epigenetically Derepress Peroxisomal Proliferator-Activated Receptor γ in Hepatic Stellate Cells for Their Antifibrotic Effect. *Hepatology* 55, 1271–1281. doi:10.1002/hep.24792

Yuan, F., Chen, J., Sun, P.-p., Guan, S., and Xu, J. (2013). Wedelolactone Inhibits LPS-Induced Pro-inflammation via NF-kappaB Pathway in RAW 264.7 Cells. *J. Biomed. Sci.* 20, 84. doi:10.1186/1423-0127-20-84

Zeng, H., Jiang, Y., Chen, P., Fan, X., Li, D., Liu, A., et al. (2017). Schisandrol B Protects against Cholestatic Liver Injury through Pregnane X Receptors. *Br. J. Pharmacol.* 174, 672–688. doi:10.1111/bph.13729

Zhan, S.-S., Jiang, J. X., Wu, J., Halsted, C., Friedman, S. L., Zern, M. A., et al. (2006). Phagocytosis of Apoptotic Bodies by Hepatic Stellate Cells Induces NADPH Oxidase and Is Associated with Liver Fibrosisin Vivo. *Hepatology* 43, 435–443. doi:10.1002/hep.21093

Zhang, L., and Schuppan, D. (2014). Traditional Chinese Medicine (TCM) for Fibrotic Liver Disease: hope and Hype. *J. Hepatol.* 61, 166–168. doi:10.1016/j.jhep.2014.03.009

Zhu, M.-M., Wang, L., Yang, D., Li, C., Pang, S.-T., Li, X.-H., et al. (2019). Wedelolactone Alleviates Doxorubicin-Induced Inflammation and Oxidative Stress Damage of Podocytes by IκK/IκB/NF-κB Pathway. *Biomed. Pharmacother.* 117, 109088. doi:10.1016/j.biopha.2019.109088

Zhu, M., Yeung, R. Y., Lin, K. F., and Li, R. C. (2000). Improvement of Phase I Drug Metabolism with Schisandra Chinensis against CCl4 Hepatotoxicity in a Rat Model. *Planta Med.* 66, 521–525. doi:10.1055/s-2000-11202

5

Pulmonary Arterial Hypertension and Consecutive Right Heart Failure Lead to Liver Fibrosis

Florian Hamberger[1†], Ekaterina Legchenko[2†], Philippe Chouvarine[2],
Young Seon Mederacke[1], Richard Taubert[1], Martin Meier[3], Danny Jonigk[4,5],
Georg Hansmann[2*‡] and Ingmar Mederacke[1*‡]

[1] Department of Gastroenterology, Hepatology and Endocrinology, Hannover Medical School, Hannover, Germany,
[2] Department of Pediatric Cardiology and Critical Care, Hannover Medical School, Hannover, Germany, [3] Laboratory Animal
Science, Small Animal Imaging Center, Hannover Medical School, Hannover, Germany, [4] Institute of Pathology, Hannover
Medical School, Hannover, Germany, [5] Member of the German Center for Lung Research (DZL), Biomedical Research in
Endstage and Obstructive Lung Disease Hannover (BREATH), Hannover, Germany

*Correspondence:
Ingmar Mederacke
mederacke.ingmar@mh-hannover.de
Georg Hansmann
georg.hansmann@gmail.com

† These authors have contributed
equally to this work and share first
authorship
‡ These authors have contributed
equally to this work and share senior
authorship

Hepatic congestion occurs in patients with right heart failure and can ultimately lead to liver fibrosis or cardiac cirrhosis. Elevated pulmonary arterial pressure is found in patients with hepatic congestion. However, whether pulmonary arterial hypertension (PAH) can be a cause of liver fibrosis is unknown. The aim of this study was to investigate whether rats in the SuHx model with severe PAH develop liver fibrosis and to explore the mechanisms of congestive hepatic fibrosis both in rats and humans. To achieve this, PAH was induced in six to eight-week old male Sprague Dawley rats by a single subcutaneous injection of the VEGFR 2 inhibitor SU5416 and subsequent hypoxia for 3 weeks, followed by a 6-week period in room air. SuHx-exposed rats developed severe PAH, right ventricular hypertrophy (RVH), and consecutive right ventricular failure. Cardiac magnetic resonance imaging (MRI) and histological analysis revealed that PAH rats developed both hepatic congestion and liver fibrosis. Gene set enrichment analysis (GSEA) of whole liver RNA sequencing data identified a hepatic stellate cell specific gene signature in PAH rats. Consistently, tissue microarray from liver of patients with histological evidence of hepatic congestion and underlying heart disease revealed similar fibrogenic gene expression patterns and signaling pathways. In conclusion, severe PAH with concomitant right heart failure leads to hepatic congestion and liver fibrosis in the SU5416/hypoxia rat PAH model. Patients with PAH should therefore be screened for unrecognized liver fibrosis.

Keywords: congestive hepatopathy, pulmonary arterial hypertension, liver fibrosis, hepatic stellate cells, hypoxia

INTRODUCTION

Liver fibrosis or cirrhosis are the long-term consequences of chronic liver injury and do not only occur as a sequelae of primary hepatic diseases such as infectious viral hepatitis or alcoholic liver disease, but can also develop secondary to heart disease (1). While *acute* right or left heart failure with low cardiac output can result in ischemic hepatitis with a rapid increase in aminotransferase levels (2), *chronic* congestive heart failure causes elevated central venous pressure, congestive hepatopathy (3, 4), and eventually liver fibrosis or cardiac cirrhosis (5). The etiology of right heart failure predisposing to hepatic congestion include tricuspid regurgitation, mitral stenosis, cardiomyopathy, constrictive pericarditis, and/or pulmonary hypertension (PH) in its precapillary, postcapillary or combined forms (cor pulmonale) (6–8). Moreover, chronic hepatic congestion after the Fontan procedure (no subpulmonary ventricle) causes liver fibrosis in almost all patients with single ventricle physiology, and up to 40% of those patients present with bridging fibrosis 10 years following Fontan procedure (9). All these conditions lead to elevated right sided filling pressure, but it is not known to what extent pulmonary vascular alterations such as PH, defined as a mean pulmonary artery pressure (mPAP) >20 mmHg (10, 11), predispose or cause hepatic congestion and liver fibrosis. A study investigating hemodynamic alterations in patients with chronic congestion observed an elevated average mPAP of 35 mmHg in patients with chronic hepatic congestion (12). Pulmonary arterial hypertension (PAH) is characterized by obliteration of small pulmonary arteries, increased pulmonary vascular resistance, and isolated precapillary PH with normal left-sided filling pressure. In contrast, one of the major causes of post-capillary PH is left heart disease with elevated left-sided filling pressure. Both HFpEF (heart failure with preserved ejection fraction) and HFrEF (heart failure with reduced ejection fraction) can cause PH (13–16), however, recent studies suggest that PH is more common in patients with HFpEF (38% in HFpEF vs. 22.6% in HFrEF) (17, 18).

Patients with progressive PH may develop right heart failure with elevated right-sided filling pressure, subsequent increase in central venous pressure and potentially congestive hepatopathy (3, 4). However, clinical evaluation for liver fibrosis or cirrhosis in patients with heart or lung disease and biventricular circulation is not routinely performed, although higher liver fibrosis scores are associated with increased risks of all-cause mortality among patients with coronary artery disease (19) or HFpEF (20).

The mechanisms underlying liver fibrosis in right, left or biventricular heart failure are incompletely understood. It has been proposed that congestive cirrhosis is a response to intrahepatic thrombosis (21) and hypercoagulation (22–25). However, there is an unmet need for a small animal model with heart failure and consecutive hepatic fibrosis or cirrhosis to study the underlying mechanisms more in detail (26, 27).

None of the published models on right ventricular (RV) pressure or volume overload studied or even demonstrated that consecutive congestive heart failure—when evident—causes substantial liver fibrosis (27–30). Toxin-induced models of RV hypertrophy or failure such as monocrotaline (27) are suboptimal since they are associated with liver toxicity (31) and myocarditis (32).

The SU5416/hypoxia (SuHx) rat model, i.e., a combination of vascular endothelial growth factor 2 (VEGFR2) blockade and chronic hypoxia, is one of the most established PAH models that can be used to induce PH and subsequent right heart failure in rats (27, 32, 33). The aim of this study was to investigate whether rats in the SuHx model with severe PAH develop liver fibrosis and to explore the mechanisms of such congestive hepatic fibrosis both in rats and humans.

MATERIALS AND METHODS

Study Design: SU5416/Hypoxia Rat PAH Model

All animal experiments were conducted under the approval of the Niedersaechsisches Landesamt für Verbraucherschutz und Lebensmittelsicherheit (LAVES; #15/2022).

Six- to eight-week-old male Sprague Dawley rats were purchased from Charles River (Germany), matched by age, and separated into three different treatment groups. The untreated control group (ConNx) was kept in room air (FiO$_2$ 0.21) for the whole duration of the experiment (9 weeks). The control/hypoxia group (ConHx) was injected once s.c. with vehicle DMSO, then exposed to chronic hypoxia (FiO$_2$ 0.1) for 3 weeks, followed by a 6-week period in room air. The SU5416/hypoxia group (SuHx) was treated with VEGFR2 inhibitor SU5416 (Sigma-Aldrich, St. Louis, MO, USA) (1x SU5416, 20 mg/kg per dose, s.c. dissolved in DMSO) and subsequently exposed to chronic hypoxia (3 weeks), followed by 6 weeks of room air (**Figure 1A**). At the end of the experiment, when severe PAH and right ventricular (RV) dysfunction were evident, echocardiography (ECHO), cardiac magnetic resonance imaging (MRI), and cardiac catheterization (closed chest) were performed as described previously (33). Subsequently, the animals were sacrificed and organs were harvested for further analysis.

Immunohistochemical Staining and Microscopy

Tissue from rat livers was collected from the median and left lateral lobes, fixed with 4% paraformaldehyde, embedded in paraffin and cut to yield 2 μm sections. Afterwards the slides were deparaffinized and rehydrated with xylene and graded ethanol. Hematoxylin and Eosin (H&E), Masson's Trichrome and Picrosirius Red stainings were done according to routine protocols. For immunohistochemistry (IHC), antigen retrieval was performed with either citrate buffer (ab93678, Abcam, Cambridge, UK) or Tris-EDTA buffer (ab93684, Abcam, Cambridge, UK), depending on the antibody used. Primary and secondary antibodies were used as follows: CD3 (1:200, ab16669, Abcam, Cambridge, UK), CD19 (1:100, MAB7489, R&D Systems, Minneapolis, MN, USA), CD68 (1:100, MCA341R, Bio-Rad, Hercules, CA, USA), Von Willebrand Factor (1:200, A0082, Agilent Dako, Santa Clara, CA, USA), Fibrin (1:250, MABS2155, Sigma-Aldrich, St. Louis, MO, USA), mouse anti-rabbit IgG-HRP (1:500, sc-2357, Santa Cruz Biotechnology, Dallas, TX, USA), goat anti-mouse IgG-HRP (1:500, sc-2005, Santa Cruz Biotechnology, Dallas, TX, USA). Antibodies were visualized using ImmPACT DAB solution (Vector Laboratories, Burlingame, CA, USA) and counterstained with hematoxylin solution. The stained tissue sections were scanned with an Aperio CS2 (Leica, Wetzlar, Germany) slide scanner and analyzed with ImageJ software (Version 1.51n).

RNA Isolation

Liver tissue collected for RNA isolation was snap frozen in liquid nitrogen and stored at −80°C. For RNA extraction, the tissue was

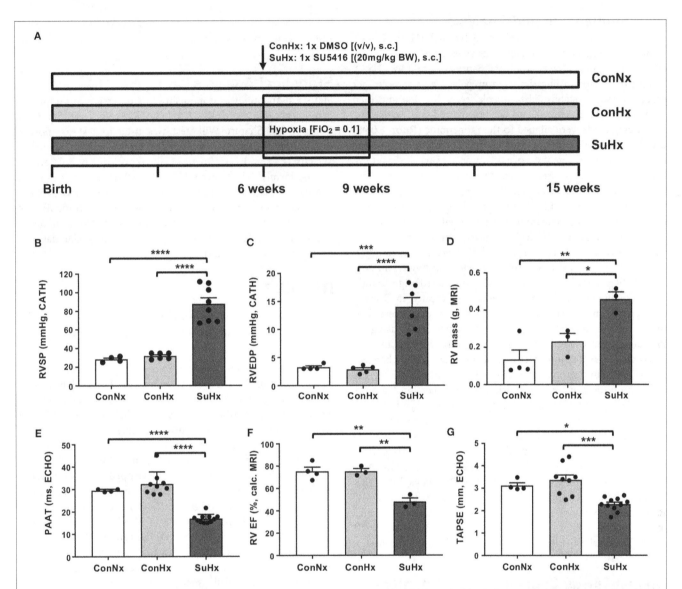

FIGURE 1 | The SU5416/hypoxia model leads to severe PAH in rats. **(A)** Experimental setup. Six- to eight-week-old male Sprague Dawley rats were purchased from Charles River and divided into three different treatment groups: (i) Normoxia (ConNx), (ii) Hypoxia (ConHx) [injected once s.c. with vehicle (DMSO), then exposed to chronic hypoxia (FiO₂ 0.1) for 3 weeks, followed by a 6-week period in room air (FiO₂ 0.21)], (iii) SU5416/hypoxia (SuHx) [injected with the VEGFR2 inhibitor SU5416 (Sigma), 20 mg/kg per dose s.c. dissolved in DMSO and subsequently exposed to chronic hypoxia (3 weeks), followed by 6 weeks of room air]. **(B–D)** Right ventricular systolic pressure (RVSP), right ventricular end diastolic pressure (RVEDP), both measured by heart catheterization, and right ventricular (RV) mass, measured by MRI of analyzed rats. **(E–G)** Pulmonary artery acceleration time (PAAT), measured by echocardiography (ECHO), right ventricular ejection fraction (RV EF), calculated from MRI data and tricuspid annular peak systolic excursion (TAPSE), measured by ECHO. Means ± SEM, ConNx $n = 13$, ConHx $n = 12$, SuHx $n = 7$, ANOVA-Bonferroni *post-hoc* test, $*p < 0.05$, $**p < 0.01$, $***p < 0.001$, $****p < 0.0001$.

submerged in TRIzol (Life Technologies, Carlsbad, CA, USA), subjected to a tissue grinder and was further processed according to the TRIzol manufacturer's protocol.

Reverse Transcription and Quantitative PCR

Reverse transcription was performed with the High-Capacity cDNA Reverse Transcription Kit (Applied Biosystems, Waltham, MA, USA) and qPCR was run on an ABI 7300 Real-Time PCR System (Applied Biosystems, Waltham, MA,

USA) using qPCR Master Mix Plus (Eurogentec, Seraing, Belgium) and TaqMan Probes (ThermoFisher Scientific, Waltham, MA, USA). The following primers were used: *Acta2* (Mm01546133_m1), *Col1a1* (Mm00801666_g1), *Timp1* (Mm00441818_m1), *TNFa* (Mm00443258_m1), *Desmin* (Mm00802455_m1), *vWF* (Rn01492158_m1), *CD4* (Rn00562286_m1), *CD8* (Rn00580577_m1), *CD3* (Rn00565890_m1), *CD19* (Rn01507619_g1), and *CD68* (Rn01495634_g1), and *18s* (4319413E, ThermoFisher, Waltham, MA, USA) as a housekeeping gene.

RNA Sequencing and Analysis

Sequencing of mRNA was performed by BGI (Hong Kong). Prior to sequencing, RNA quality was assessed by RIN analysis on a 2100 Bioanalyzer (Agilent, Santa Clara, CA, USA). TruSeq transcriptom libraries were prepared for 3 samples per group following established protocols from Illumina and then sequenced with HiSeq2000 using 90bp paired-end reads. The sequencing reads were aligned to the rat genome (Rnor_6.0.96) using STAR (34) and the read counts corresponding to the Ensembl-annotated genes were identified using RSEM (35). Differential gene expression was analyzed using DEseq (36) after within-lane GC normalization by EDAseq (37). The sharing mode parameter was set to "fit-only" for the estimateDispersions method in DEseq. Benjamini-Hochberg false discovery rate (FDR) procedure was applied to correct for multiple testing. Additionally, the gene filtering procedure developed by Bourgon et al. (38) was applied to improve the detection power. mRNAs with FDR-adjusted $P < 0.05$ were considered significantly differentially expressed. Volcano plots were created in R using the ggplot2 and ggrepel packages. Heatmaps were created in Excel. The gene set enrichment analysis was performed using the pre-ranked analysis option in GSEA (39, 40). The ranking was based on the expression score calculated as Log2(fold change)* [-Log10(q-value)] from every gene with a $P < 0.05$. GSEA was run on the complete hallmark gene set collection from the Molecular Signatures Database (MSigDB, h.all.v7.4.symbols.gmt) (41), the hepatic stellate cell signature, quiescent and activated gene sets derived from Zhang et al. (42), and the KEGG pathway gene sets used by the nCounter® Fibrosis Panel (Nanostring Technologies, Seattle, WA, USA), using the Rat_ENSEMBLE_Gene_ID_Human_Orthologs_MSigDB.v 7.4.chip platform to apply the "collapse/remap to gene symbols" option. The RNA sequencing data have been deposited with links to BioProject accession number PRJNA 807371 in the NCBI BioProject database (https://www.ncbi.nlm.nih.gov/bioproject/).

Human Tissue Specimen and nCounter® Fibrosis Panel

We screened patients treated at Hannover Medical School with underlying heart failure and clinical or laboratory suspicion of advanced liver disease who underwent transjugular liver biopsy for further diagnostic. A total of seven patients were identified with the histological diagnosis of hepatic venous congestion and no evidence for viral hepatitis, genetic or metabolic liver disease. As controls, we used five patients with autoimmune hepatitis in clinical remission with absent liver fibrosis. Grading and staging of liver biopsies was performed by Ishak score (43). Liver elastography was determined by acoustic radiation force impulse (ARFI) elastography (44). Detailed patient characteristics are provided in the Supporting Information (**Supplementary Table 1**). RNA extraction from formalin-fixed paraffin-embedded (FFPE) sections was carried out using the Maxwell® RSC RNA FFPE Kit (Promega, Madison, WI, USA). Of the purified RNA, 200 ng were loaded on the nCounter® Digital Analyzer and analyzed by nSolver software v4.0 with the nCounter® Fibrosis Panel (Nanostring

Technologies, Seattle, WA, USA). The study was approved by the Ethics Committees at the Hannover Medical School (No. 3381-2016).

Statistical Analysis

Statistical analysis was done using Prism version 8 (GraphPad, San Diego, CA) and R 4.0.5 (The R Project for Statistical Computing). Shapiro-Wilk test was used to test for normal distribution. Differences between two groups were calculated by Welch's *t*-test and assessment of differences of multiple groups was performed by one-way ANOVA and Bonferroni's multiple comparisons test. For correlation analysis between hemodynamic data and gene expression, data was tested for normality by multivariate Shapiro test followed by two-tailed Pearson or Spearman correlation, depending on normality. All data are expressed as mean ± SEM.

RESULTS

Exposure to SU5416/Hypoxia (SuHx) Leads to Severe, Sustained PAH and RV Failure in Rats

To investigate the effects of severe PAH and RV failure on the development of liver fibrosis, we employed the SU5416/hypoxia rat model (**Figure 1A**). In this well-accepted PAH model, hypoxia alone (ConHx; +DMSO s.c. = vehicle of SU5416) did not induce sustained pulmonary hypertension or even right heart failure 6 weeks after the end of hypoxia. However, rats exposed to a single injection of SU5416, a VEGFR 2 inhibitor, and subsequent chronic hypoxia for 3 weeks, developed a near-systemic increase of right ventricular systolic pressure (RVSP; **Figure 1B**), indicating PAH, elevated right ventricular end-diastolic pressure (RVEDP; **Figure 1C**) as surrogate of RV diastolic dysfunction, and increased RV mass (**Figure 1D**) indicating RV hypertrophy, compared to animals in the ConNx or ConHx control groups. Moreover, pulmonary artery (PA) acceleration time (PAAT) as an inverse echocardiographic indicator of PA pressure was decreased (**Figure 1E**). Consequently, RV ejection fraction (RV EF) by MRI (**Figure 1F**), and tricuspid annular peak systolic excursion by ECHO (TAPSE; **Figure 1G**), both established markers for RV systolic function, were decreased vs. controls. Taken together these results demonstrate, that SuHx-exposed rats developed severe PAH, right ventricular hypertrophy (RVH), and consecutive right ventricular failure.

Rats With Severe PAH and RV Failure Develop Hepatic Congestion and Liver Fibrosis

Next, we explored whether severe PAH and systolic RV dysfunction may lead to hepatic congestion. We therefore analyzed MRI scans and observed a significantly increased mean diameter of hepatic veins in rats with PAH (**Figure 2A**). To evaluate whether congestive vessel dilatation is also observed on the microscopic level, we performed H&E staining and found that rats from the SuHx group with severe PAH also showed a significant increase in sinusoidal dilatation

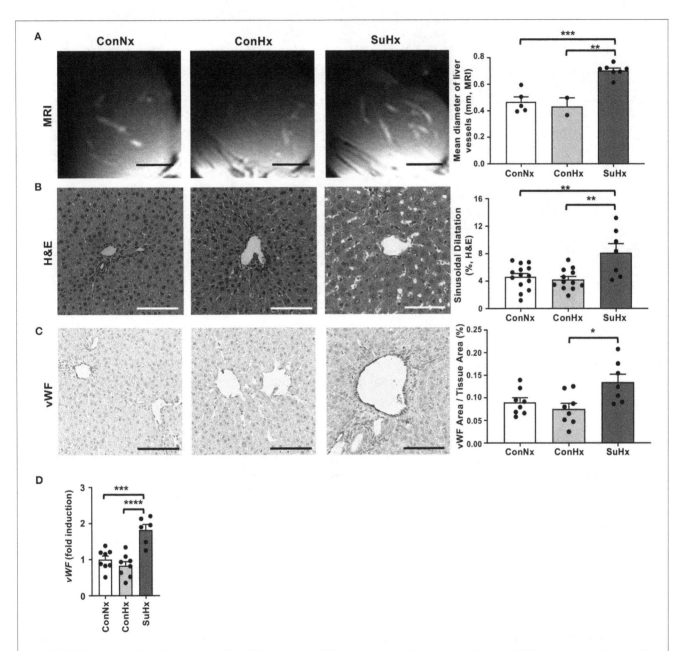

FIGURE 2 | PAH rats show signs of hepatic congestion. **(A)** Representative MRI images and quantification of mean diameter of visible liver vessels in the livers of the different treatment groups. Scale bars 5 mm **(B)** Representative pictures and quantification of vessel area of Hematoxylin and Eosin (H&E) stained livers of analyzed rats. **(C)** Representative pictures and quantification of IHC for vascularization marker von Willebrand factor (vWF). **(D)** Relative expression of von Willebrand factor (vWF) determined by qPCR from whole livers. Means ± SEM, ConNx $n = 8–13$, ConHx $n = 8–12$, SuHx $n = 7$, ANOVA-Bonferroni post-hoc test, $*p < 0.05$, $**p < 0.01$, $***p < 0.001$, $****p < 0.0001$, Scale bars 100 μm.

(**Figure 2B**). In line with these results, immunohistochemical staining (IHC) and qPCR analysis revealed increased expression of von Willebrand Factor (vWF), a glycoprotein secreted by endothelial cells to mediate platelet adhesion, and associated with thrombosis and liver fibrosis, in the SuHx vs. controls (**Figures 2C,D**). To assess whether animals with PAH also develop liver fibrosis under these conditions, we performed picrosirius red and Masson's trichrome staining and observed an increase of fibrotic area by 72 and 142%, respectively,

in SuHx treated rats (**Figures 3A,B**) vs. controls. To confirm these results, we performed quantitative real-time PCR analysis and unraveled an increased expression of profibrotic genes, including collagen 1a1 (Col1a1), alpha smooth muscle actin (Acta2), tissue inhibitor of metalloproteinase metallopeptidase inhibitor 1 (Timp1), and desmin (Des) (**Figures 3C–F**). To rule out that SU5416 alone - without exposure to chronic hypoxia - causes liver fibrosis, we treated six to eight-week old male Sprague Dawley rats with SU5416 or vehicle control (DMSO)

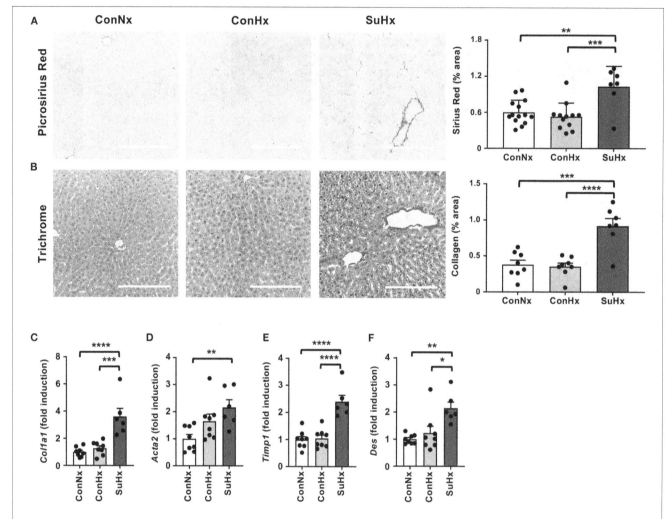

FIGURE 3 | PAH leads to increased liver fibrosis in the SU5416/hypoxia model. **(A)** Representative pictures and quantification of picrosirius red stained livers of the analyzed rats. ConNx $n = 13$, ConHx $n = 12$, SuHx $n = 7$. **(B)** Representative pictures and quantification of Masson's trichrome staining. **(C–F)** Relative expression of fibrogenic markers collagen 1a1 (*Col1a1*), alpha smooth muscle actin (*Acta2*), TIMP metallopeptidase inhibitor 1 (*Timp1*) and desmin (*Des*) determined by qPCR from whole livers. Means ± SEM, ConNx $n = 8$, ConHx $n = 8$, SuHx $n = 7$, ANOVA-Bonferroni *post-hoc* test, *$p < 0.05$, **$p < 0.01$, ***$p < 0.001$, ****$p < 0.0001$, Scale bars: 100 μm.

and kept these animals at normoxia for 9 weeks. There was no significant difference in liver fibrosis and inflammation between both groups (**Supplementary Figures 1, 2**), excluding VEGFR2 inhibition as a possible confounder or cause of liver fibrosis in our model.

Microthrombosis and Inflammation Are Evident in the Congested Livers of PAH Rats

To investigate whether inflammation and intrahepatic thrombosis play a role in the development of liver fibrosis in rats with PAH, we next performed IHC for the coagulatory marker fibrin and the immune cell markers CD3 (T-cells), CD19 (B-cells) and CD68 (macrophages). SuHx rats showed significantly increased fibrin deposition in the liver vessels (**Figure 4A**), as well as increased numbers of CD3 and CD68

positive cells compared to the control groups, while CD19 staining showed no significant difference between the three groups (**Figures 4B–D**). Validation by qPCR revealed a markedly increased expression of CD4 and CD8 T cells as well as macrophage marker CD68 whereas CD19 and TNFα showed a lower yet still significant increase in the SuHx group compared to controls (**Figures 4E–J**).

Severe PAH and RV Dysfunction Are Associated With a Proinflammatory Hepatic Gene Program and a Hepatic Stellate Cell-Specific Gene Signature in the Liver

To confirm the results of IHC and qPCR, we performed whole liver RNA sequencing on animals of each treatment group (ConNx, ConHx, SuHx) (**Supplementary Figure 3**). Gene

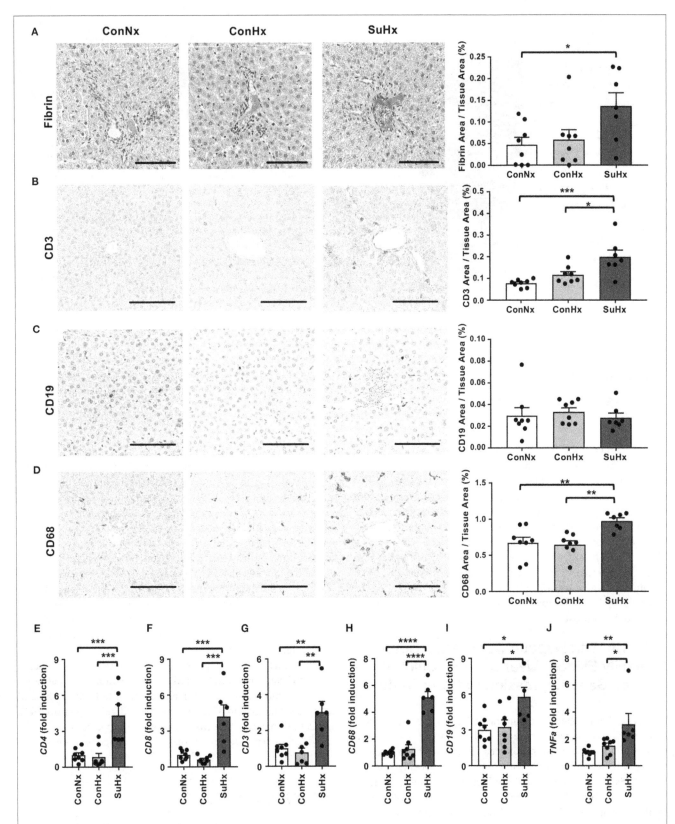

FIGURE 4 | PAH livers show increased coagulation and liver immune cell infiltration is mainly comprised of T-cells and macrophages. **(A–D)** Representative pictures and quantification of IHC for coagulation marker fibrin, as well as immune cell markers of T-cells (CD3), B-cells (CD19) and macrophages (CD68). **(E–J)** Relative expression of immune cell markers CD4, CD8, CD3, CD68, CD19 and TNFa determined by qPCR from whole liver. Means ± SEM, ConNx $n = 8$, ConHx $n = 8$, SuHx $n = 7$, ANOVA-Bonferroni *post-hoc* test, *$p < 0.05$, **$p < 0.01$, ***$p < 0.001$, ****$p < 0.0001$, Scale bars: 100 μm.

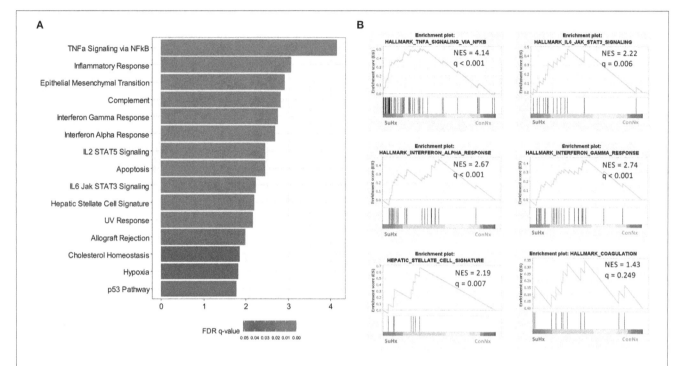

FIGURE 5 | RNA Sequencing reveals inflammatory and fibrotic gene expression in livers of PAH rats. **(A)** GSEA analysis of differentially regulated genes in SuHx treated rats compared with ConNx control group. Shown are all pathways with FDR adjusted q-values < 0.05. **(B)** Enrichment plots of select pathways from the GSEA analysis. ConNx $n = 3$, SuHx $n = 3$.

Set Enrichment Analysis (GSEA) showed an enrichment of pathways associated with inflammation and liver fibrosis in SuHx animals, in particular TNFα signaling, IL6-JAK-STAT3 signaling, Interferon alpha (IFNα) and gamma (IFNγ) response (**Figures 5A,B**). Additionally, in accordance with the results of the fibrin staining, we found the Hallmark Coagulation pathway slightly enriched in SuHx compared to ConNx, although the FDR adjusted p-value in this case was not significant (**Figure 5B**). Lastly, we detected an enrichment of a hepatic stellate cell (HSC) specific gene signature (42), indicating that activation of HSC, the major fibrogenic cell population in the liver, contributes to the observed liver fibrosis.

Patients With Hepatic Congestion but No Clinically Evident Liver Disease Display Fibrotic Gene Expression Patterns in the Liver

To assess whether the findings in the SU5416/hypoxia rat model of PAH/RV failure could have clinical relevance, we analyzed patients with confirmed histological diagnosis of congestive hepatopathy and underlying heart/lung disease. Detailed patient characteristics are shown in **Supplementary Table 1**. Patients with autoimmune hepatitis in biochemical and histological remission without evidence for liver fibrosis (Ishak F0) were used as controls (43). Liver function test showed no significant differences in ALT or AST levels, but a significant elevation of AP and gGT in patients with heart failure and hepatic congestion (**Supplementary Figure 4**). Next, we performed gene

expression analysis of liver biopsies using nCounter® Fibrosis Panel (Nanostring Technologies, Seattle, WA, USA). At first, we performed an analysis using the Nanostring nSolver software and revealed an induction of pathways associated with liver fibrosis (**Figure 6**). When correlating the relative expression of different fibrogenic pathways with mean pulmonary arterial pressure (mPAP) or mean right atrial pressure (mRAP), we observed a significant positive correlation with mRAP while mPAP did not show any association (**Figures 7A,B**). In order to compare the gene expression patterns of patients with both heart failure and hepatic congestion with the SuHx rat model, we performed GSEA and compared the signaling pathways that are activated in both models (**Figure 8**). Importantly, a total of seven out of 12 significantly enriched signaling pathways were evident in both SuHx rats and patients with congestive hepatopathy: The enriched pathways included proinflammatory pathways such as tumor necrosis factor alpha and interferon alpha and gamma signaling and a hepatic stellate cell gene signature (42), indicating that HSC are the fibrogenic cell type responsible for the development of liver fibrosis in hepatic congestion in rats and human.

DISCUSSION

The development of liver fibrosis or cirrhosis in patients with congestive heart disease and heart failure is well-known (10, 19–21, 45–51). However, an adequate *in vivo* model recapitulating both, heart failure and liver fibrosis which would

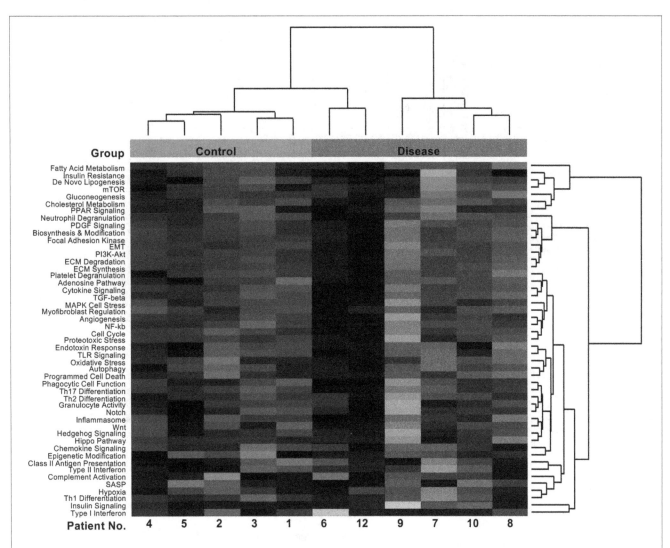

FIGURE 6 | Patients with underlying heart/lung disease display upregulated fibrotic pathways in liver biopsies. Pathway score heatmap of fibrogenic gene sets detected via nCounter® Fibrosis Panel in RNA isolated from FFPE tissues of patients with confirmed histological diagnosis of congestive hepatopathy and underlying heart disease (Disease) and patients with autoimmune hepatitis in remission as control (Control).

allow to study therapeutic interventions in the heart or lung as well as in the liver is lacking. A previous study using a murine model of pulmonary stenosis observed a higher liver to body-weight ratio in animals with severe pulmonary stenosis (28), but liver fibrosis was not evaluated. Another study applied a model of congestive hepatopathy through partial ligation of the inferior vena cava and showed that chronic hepatic congestion leads to sinusoidal thrombosis and mechanical forces resulting in liver fibrosis (29). However, in none of the aforementioned models heart failure was shown to be the cause liver fibrosis.

Here, we studied the development of liver fibrosis in a rat model of PAH-driven right heart failure (33, 52). We also performed gene expression analysis both in the *in vivo* rat model as well as in liver biopsies from patients with histological diagnosis of hepatic congestion secondary to heart failure. Using the rodent model and human samples, we made several important findings and conclude: (1) rats with severe PAH

develop hepatic congestion and liver fibrosis; (2) severe PAH induces hepatic inflammation and microthrombosis; (3) heart failure patients with hepatic congestion but no clinical evidence for underlying liver disease display a fibrotic gene expression pattern in the liver; (4) similar fibrogenic pathways are activated in SuHx-exposed PAH rats on the one hand and patients with hepatic congestion on the other; (5) gene expression data indicates that HSC contribute to the development of liver fibrosis both in PAH rats and in patients with hepatic congestion.

Multiple small animal models of right (27, 53) or left heart failure (26) have been published over the last decades but in none of these models, presence and development of hepatic fibrosis has been systematically studied. Here, we used the SU5416/hypoxia rat model (33, 52) as it features severe PAH and right heart failure (33). In our study, cardiac catheterization, echocardiography and MRI confirmed that animals treated once with the VEGFR2 inhibitor SU5416, followed by subsequent

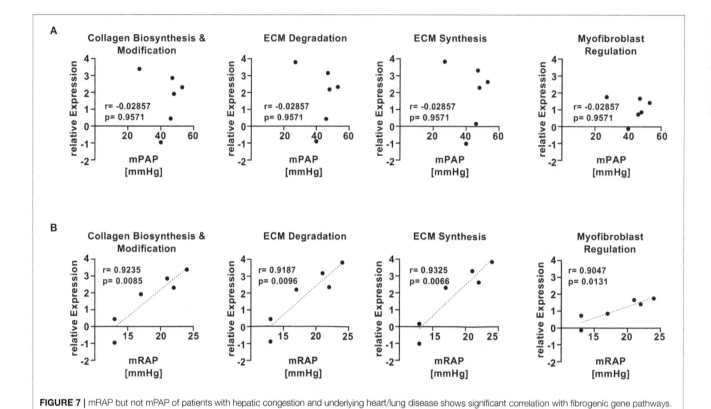

FIGURE 7 | mRAP but not mPAP of patients with hepatic congestion and underlying heart/lung disease shows significant correlation with fibrogenic gene pathways. **(A)** Two-tailed Spearman correlation plots of mean pulmonary arterial pressure (mPAP) vs. relative expression of different fibrogenic pathways from Nanostring analysis. **(B)** Two-tailed Pearson correlation plots of mean right atrial pressure (mRAP) vs. relative expression of different fibrogenic pathways from Nanostring analysis.

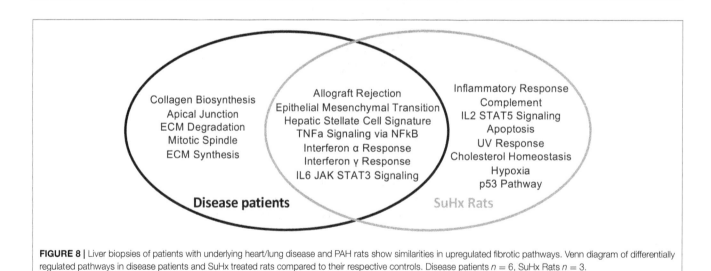

FIGURE 8 | Liver biopsies of patients with underlying heart/lung disease and PAH rats show similarities in upregulated fibrotic pathways. Venn diagram of differentially regulated pathways in disease patients and SuHx treated rats compared to their respective controls. Disease patients $n = 6$, SuHx Rats $n = 3$.

hypoxia for 3 weeks, developed severe PAH and right heart failure. Notably, animals with PAH and RV failure, as judged by greatly increased systolic and end-diastolic RV (filling) pressures, also developed liver fibrosis vs. controls. We propose that the congestion detected in MRI scans and the sinusoidal dilatation observed in liver histology, and the increased fibrin deposits in the liver vessels and immune cell infiltration, likely represent the pathobiological mechanisms of liver fibrosis.

Additional mechanisms have been suggested by another group that studied liver fibrosis development in IVC ligated mice; the authors identified mechanosensitive signals released by liver sinusoidal endothelial cells which promoted portal hypertension by recruiting sinusoidal neutrophils and promoting formation of neutrophil extracellular traps and microthrombi (30).

In our study, liver tissue RNA sequencing revealed an altered cholesterol metabolism compared to controls, in addition with major mechanisms others postulated for development of liver fibrosis in congestive heart failure: hypoxic cell death, caused by insufficient arterial perfusion or the generation of microthrombi, triggering hepatic inflammation resulting in activation of fibroblasts, deposition of extracellular matrix, and finally liver fibrosis (21, 29, 50).

The detection of fibrin deposits and expression of vWF suggested thrombosis as another mechanism of liver fibrosis, which has been described by others (29). Furthermore, GSEA showed enrichment of different immune pathways in SuHx livers: increased IFNγ and TNFα signaling point to NK cell activity (54) and that likely induced the observed IL6 and IL2 signaling by macrophages, T cells and fibroblasts detected in IHC stainings of the SuHx livers (55, 56).

Moreover, we found activation of hepatic stellate cells (HSC), the primary precursors to myofibroblasts in liver fibrosis (57), by detecting a signature gene set derived from the findings of Zhang et al. (42). Although alterations in cholesterol metabolism in the liver has not been commonly described in congestive heart failure, it is a major driving factor of fibrosis in non-alcoholic fatty liver disease (NAFLD) (58, 59).

To validate the clinical relevance of the SU5416/hypoxia model, we performed a fibrosis tissue microarray of liver biopsies from patients with hepatic congestion and underlying heart disease and compared the results with the RNA sequencing data from the rat model. Four of the six patients with heart failure and very high mean right atrial pressure (mRAP) (17–24 mmHg) showed markedly enhanced fibrotic gene expression compared to the control patients, while gene expression of the other two patients (#6 and #12) with the lowest mRAP had a RNA expression profile similar to controls, indicating that mRAP drives hepatic congestion and consecutive liver fibrosis. Laboratory diagnostic revealed significant elevation of alkaline phosphatase (AP) and gamma-glutamyl transferase (gGT) in patients with hepatic congestion, while there was no difference in aminotransferases between patients and controls. The elevation of AP and gGT indicates congestive injury rather than ischemic hepatic injury (4, 60). In line with these results, liver stiffness values of heart failure patients were elevated indicating increased liver stiffness caused by hepatic congestion (61).

Our study has several limitations. The degree of fibrosis in the examined animals was comparatively mild, compared to the IVC ligation model published by Simonetto et al. (29), but it has to be considered that IVC ligation is a non-physiological strong congestion, that rather imitates acute Budd Chiari Syndrome than congestive hepatopathy. Moreover, liver fibrosis in humans develops over years and decades and our rodent model covered only several weeks. It is therefore likely, that a longer duration of the SuHx rat experiment could have led to more severe liver fibrosis.

In future studies, it will be important to explore whether moderate or advanced liver fibrosis is common in PAH patients, patients with HFpEF, and those with heart failure and combined pre- and postcapillary pulmonary hypertension (CpcPH) since in these patients, liver fibrosis possibly represents an unrecognized risk factor relevant for mid to long-term outcome, including non-cardiopulmonary surgical or interventional procedures.

Accordingly, when patients with end stage heart or liver disease are evaluated for heart and/or lung transplantation, evaluation of liver fibrosis is mandatory (5, 62, 63), because liver cirrhosis is associated with increased mortality thereafter (63, 64). Therefore, advanced liver fibrosis is an exclusion criterion for heart transplantation in patients with Ebstein's malformation or those with single ventricles and a Fontan circulation (45, 46). In these patients, the underlying liver disease may require simultaneous heart-liver transplantation in expert centers (65).

In conclusion, our study demonstrates that severe PAH with concomitant right heart failure leads to liver fibrosis in the SU5416/hypoxia PAH rat model. We also identified a HSC specific gene signature in PAH rats that was recapitulated in liver of patients with histological evidence of hepatic congestion and underlying heart disease, indicating HSC being involved in the increase in liver fibrosis. No liver tissue from patients with different severity of PAH or Fontan patients was available, so that the validity of our findings in these patients needs to be recapitulated. However, our results suggest that it could be beneficial to recognize liver fibrosis in patients with PAH.

Therefore, we propose that patients with PAH should be screened for unrecognized liver fibrosis.

AUTHOR CONTRIBUTIONS

FH performed experiments, analyzed data, performed statistical analyses, and drafted the manuscript. EL performed animal experiments, analyzed data, and critically reviewed the manuscript. PC performed the bioinformatics analysis and critically reviewed the manuscript. YSM collected patient data, contributed to data analysis, and critically reviewed the manuscript. RT provided patients samples and critically reviewed the manuscript. MM performed and analyzed MRI imaging. DJ performed experiments, analyzed data, and critically reviewed the manuscript. GH and IM designed and supervised the study, oversaw the statistical analysis, drafted the manuscript, and generated funding. FH, GH, and IM had unrestricted access to all data. All authors contributed to the article and approved the submitted version.

FUNDING

IM was supported by a grant from the German Research Foundation (DFG, ME 3723/2-1) and the Lower Saxony Ministry for Science and Culture (REBIRTH Innovation-/Synergy Grant). GH received research grants from the German Research Foundation (DFG KFO311; HA4348/6-2), the European Pediatric Pulmonary Vascular Disease Network (www.pvdnetwork.org), and the Federal Ministry of Education and Research (BMBF 01KC2001B; ViP+ program 03VP08053). YSM was supported by the Young Faculty program of the Hannover Medical School. RT received funding from the German Research Foundation (KFO250) and the CORE100Pilot–Advanced Clinician Scientist program. DJ received a research grant from the German Research Foundation (DFG KFO311; project Z2 to DJ).

ACKNOWLEDGMENTS

We thank Annette Müller Brechlin, Christina Petzold and Regina Engelhardt (Institute of Pathology, Hannover Medical School, Hannover, Germany) for technical assistance.

REFERENCES

Xanthopoulos A, Starling RC, Kitai T, Triposkiadis F. Heart failure and liver disease: cardiohepatic interactions. *JACC Heart Fail.* (2019) 7:87– 97. doi: 10.1016/j.jchf.2018.10.007

Samsky MD, Patel CB, DeWald TA, Smith AD, Felker GM, Rogers JG, et al. Cardiohepatic interactions in heart failure: an overview and clinical implications. *J Am Coll Cardiol.* (2013) 61:2397–405. doi: 10.1016/j.jacc.2013.03.042

Dai DF, Swanson PE, Krieger EV, Liou IW, Carithers RL, Yeh MM. Congestive hepatic fibrosis score: a novel histologic assessment of clinical severity. *Mod Pathol.* (2014) 27:1552–8. doi: 10.1038/modpathol.2014.79

Nikolaou M, Parissis J, Yilmaz MB, Seronde MF, Kivikko M, Laribi S, et al. Liver function abnormalities, clinical profile, and outcome in acute decompensated heart failure. *Eur Heart J.* (2013) 34:742–9. doi: 10.1093/eurheartj/ehs332

Louie CY, Pham MX, Daugherty TJ, Kambham N, Higgins JP. The liver in heart failure: a biopsy and explant series of the histopathologic and laboratory findings with a particular focus on pre-cardiac transplant evaluation. *Mod Pathol.* (2015) 28:932–43. doi: 10.1038/modpathol.2015.40

Hilscher M, Sanchez W. Congestive hepatopathy. *Clin Liver Dis.* (2016) 8:68–71. doi: 10.1002/cld.573

Lowe MD, Harcombe AA, Grace AA, Petch MC. Lesson of the week: restrictive-constrictive heart failure masquerading as liver disease. *BMJ.* (1999) 318:585–6. doi: 10.1136/bmj.318.7183.585

Sheth AA, Lim JK. Liver disease from asymptomatic constrictive pericarditis. *J Clin Gastroenterol.* (2008) 42:956–8. doi: 10.1097/MCG.0b013e318 031915c

Emamaullee J, Zaidi AN, Schiano T, Kahn J, Valentino PL, Hofer RE, et al. Fontan-associated liver disease: screening, management, and transplant considerations. *Circulation.* (2020) 142:591–604. doi: 10.1161/CIRCULATIONAHA.120. 045597

Hansmann G, Koestenberger M, Alastalo TP, Apitz C, Austin ED, Bonnet D, et al. 2019 Updated consensus statement on the diagnosis and treatment of pediatric pulmonary hypertension: the european pediatric pulmonary vascular disease network (Eppvdn), endorsed by Aepc, Espr and Ishlt. *J Heart Lung Transplant.* (2019) 38:879–901. doi: 10.1016/j.healun.2019. 06.022

Simonneau G, Montani D, Celermajer DS, Denton CP, Gatzoulis MA, Krowka M, et al. Haemodynamic definitions and updated clinical classification of pulmonary hypertension. *Eur Respir J.* (2019) 53:1801913. doi: 10.1183/13993003.01913-2018

Myers RP, Cerini R, Sayegh R, Moreau R, Degott C, Lebrec D, et al. Cardiac hepatopathy: clinical, hemodynamic, and histologic characteristics and correlations. *Hepatology.* (2003) 37:393–400. doi: 10.1053/jhep.2003. 50062

Pandey A, Shah SJ, Butler J, Kellogg DL Jr, Lewis GD, Forman DE, et al. Exercise intolerance in older adults with heart failure with preserved ejection fraction: JACC state-of-the-art review. *J Am Coll Cardiol.* (2021) 78:1166– 87. doi: 10.1016/j.jacc.2021.07.014

Galie N, Humbert M, Vachiery JL, Gibbs S, Lang I, Torbicki A, et al. 2015 Esc/Ers guidelines for the diagnosis and treatment of pulmonary hypertension: the joint task force for the diagnosis and treatment of pulmonary hypertension of the European Society of Cardiology (Esc) and the European Respiratory Society (Ers): endorsed by: Association for European Paediatric and Congenital Cardiology (Aepc), International Society for Heart and Lung Transplantation (Ishlt). *Eur Heart J.* (2016) 37:67– 119. doi: 10.1093/eurheartj/ehv317

Lam CSP, Voors AA, de Boer RA, Solomon SD, van Veldhuisen DJ. Heart failure with preserved ejection fraction: from mechanisms to therapies. *Eur Heart J.* (2018) 39:2780–92. doi: 10.1093/eurheartj/ehy301

Omote K, Verbrugge FH, Borlaug BA. Heart failure with preserved ejection fraction: mechanisms and treatment strategies. *Annu Rev Med.* (2021) 73:321–337. doi: 10.1253/circj.CJ-21-0795

Adir Y, Guazzi M, Offer A, Temporelli PL, Cannito A, Ghio S. Pulmonary hemodynamics in heart failure patients with reduced or preserved ejection fraction and pulmonary hypertension: similarities and disparities. *Am Heart J.* (2017) 192:120–7. doi: 10.1016/j.ahj.2017.06.006

Gerges M, Gerges C, Pistritto AM, Lang MB, Trip P, Jakowitsch J, et al. Pulmonary hypertension in heart failure. epidemiology, right ventricular function, and survival. *Am J Respir Crit Care Med.* (2015) 192:1234– 46. doi: 10.1164/rccm.201503-0529OC

Chen Q, Li Q, Li D, Chen XC, Liu ZM, Hu G, et al. Association between liver fibrosis scores and the risk of mortality among patients with coronary artery disease. *Atherosclerosis.* (2020) 299:45–52. doi: 10.1016/j.atherosclerosis.2020.03.010

Yoshihisa A, Sato Y, Yokokawa T, Sato T, Suzuki S, Oikawa M, et al. Liver fibrosis score predicts mortality in heart failure patients with preserved ejection fraction. *ESC Heart Fail.* (2018) 5:262–70. doi: 10.1002/ehf2.12222

Wanless IR, Liu JJ, Butany J. Role of thrombosis in the pathogenesis of congestive hepatic fibrosis (Cardiac Cirrhosis). *Hepatology.* (1995) 21:1232– 7. doi: 10.1002/hep.1840210504

Anstee QM, Goldin RD, Wright M, Martinelli A, Cox R, Thursz MR. Coagulation status modulates murine hepatic fibrogenesis: implications for the development of novel therapies. *J Thromb Haemost.* (2008) 6:1336– 43. doi: 10.1111/j.1538-7836.2008.03015.x

Anstee QM, Dhar A, Thursz MR. The role of hypercoagulability in liver fibrogenesis. *Clin Res Hepatol Gastroenterol.* (2011) 35:526–33. doi: 10.1016/j.clinre.2011.03.011

Brill A, Fuchs TA, Chauhan AK, Yang JJ, De Meyer SF, Kollnberger M, et al. Von willebrand factor-mediated platelet adhesion is critical for deep vein thrombosis in mouse models. *Blood.* (2011) 117:1400– 7. doi: 10.1182/blood-2010-05-287623

Joshi N, Kopec AK, Ray JL, Cline-Fedewa H, Groeneveld DJ, Lisman T, et al. Von willebrand factor deficiency reduces liver fibrosis in mice. *Toxicol Appl Pharmacol.* (2017) 328:54–9. doi: 10.1016/j.taap.2017.05.018

Riehle C, Bauersachs J. Small animal models of heart failure. *Cardiovasc Res.* (2019) 115:1838–49. doi: 10.1093/cvr/cvz161

Andersen A, van der Feen DE, Andersen S, Schultz JG, Hansmann G, Bogaard HJ. Animal models of right heart failure. *Cardiovasc Diagn Ther.* (2020) 10:1561–79. doi: 10.21037/cdt-20-400

Urashima T, Zhao M, Wagner R, Fajardo G, Farahani S, Quertermous T, et al. Molecular and physiological characterization of Rv remodeling in a murine model of pulmonary stenosis. *Am J Physiol Heart Circ Physiol.* (2008) 295:H1351–68. doi: 10.1152/ajpheart.91526.2007

Simonetto DA, Yang HY, Yin M, de Assuncao TM, Kwon JH, Hilscher M, et al. Chronic passive venous congestion drives hepatic fibrogenesis via sinusoidal thrombosis and mechanical forces. *Hepatology.* (2015) 61:648– 59. doi: 10.1002/hep.27387

Hilscher MB, Sehrawat T, Arab JP, Zeng Z, Gao J, Liu M, et al. Mechanical stretch increases expression of Cxcl1 in liver sinusoidal endothelial cells to recruit neutrophils, generate sinusoidal microthrombi, and promote portal hypertension. *Gastroenterology.* (2019) 157:193–209.e9. doi: 10.1053/j.gastro.2019.03.013

Copple BL, Ganey PE, Roth RA. Liver inflammation during monocrotaline hepatotoxicity. *Toxicology.* (2003) 190:155– 69. doi: 10.1016/S0300-483X(03)00164-1

Bonnet S, Provencher S, Guignabert C, Perros F, Boucherat O, Schermuly RT, et al. Translating research into improved patient care in pulmonary arterial hypertension. *Am J Respir Crit Care Med.* (2017) 195:583– 95. doi: 10.1164/rccm.201607-1515PP

Legchenko E, Chouvarine P, Borchert P, Fernandez-Gonzalez A, Snay E, Meier M, et al. Ppargamma agonist pioglitazone reverses pulmonary hypertension and prevents right heart failure via fatty acid oxidation. *Sci Transl Med.* (2018) 10:eaao0303. doi: 10.1126/scitranslmed.aao0303

Dobin A, Davis CA, Schlesinger F, Drenkow J, Zaleski C, Jha S, et al. Star: ultrafast universal Rna-Seq aligner. *Bioinformatics.* (2013) 29:15– 21. doi: 10.1093/bioinformatics/bts635

Li B, Dewey CN. Rsem: accurate transcript quantification from Rna-Seq data with or without a reference genome. *BMC Bioinformatics.* (2011) 12:323. doi: 10.1186/1471-2105-12-323

Anders S, Huber W. Differential expression analysis for sequence count data. *Genome Biol.* (2010) 11:R106. doi: 10.1186/gb-2010-11-10-r106

Risso D, Schwartz K, Sherlock G, Dudoit S. Gc-content normalization for Rna-Seq data. *BMC Bioinformatics*. (2011) 12:480. doi: 10.1186/1471-2105- 12-480

Bourgon R, Gentleman R, Huber W. Independent filtering increases detection power for high-throughput experiments. *Proc Natl Acad Sci U S A*. (2010) 107:9546–51. doi: 10.1073/pnas.0914 005107

Mootha VK, Lindgren CM, Eriksson KF, Subramanian A, Sihag S, Lehar J, et al. Pgc-1alpha-responsive genes involved in oxidative phosphorylation are coordinately downregulated in human diabetes. *Nat Genet*. (2003) 34:267– 73. doi: 10.1038/ng1180

Subramanian A, Tamayo P, Mootha VK, Mukherjee S, Ebert BL, Gillette MA, et al. Gene set enrichment analysis: a knowledge-based approach for interpreting genome-wide expression profiles. *Proc Natl Acad Sci U S A*. (2005) 102:15545–50. doi: 10.1073/pnas.0506 580102

Liberzon A, Birger C, Thorvaldsdottir H, Ghandi M, Mesirov JP, Tamayo P. The molecular signatures database (Msigdb) hallmark gene set collection. *Cell Syst*. (2015) 1:417–25. doi: 10.1016/j.cels.2015. 12.004

Zhang DY, Goossens N, Guo J, Tsai MC, Chou HI, Altunkaynak C, et al. A hepatic stellate cell gene expression signature associated with outcomes in hepatitis C cirrhosis and hepatocellular carcinoma after curative resection. *Gut*. (2016) 65:1754–64. doi: 10.1136/gutjnl-2015- 309655

Ishak K, Baptista A, Bianchi L, Callea F, De Groote J, Gudat F, et al. Histological grading and staging of chronic hepatitis. *J Hepatol*. (1995) 22:696–9. doi: 10.1016/0168-8278(95)80226-6

Bota S, Herkner H, Sporea I, Salzl P, Sirli R, Neghina AM, et al. Meta-analysis: arfi elastography versus transient elastography for the evaluation of liver fibrosis. *Liver Int*. (2013) 33:1138–47. doi: 10.1111/liv. 12240

Baumgartner H, De Backer J, Babu-Narayan SV, Budts W, Chessa M, Diller GP, et al. 2020 Esc guidelines for the management of adult congenital heart disease. *Eur Heart J*. (2021) 42:563–645. doi: 10.15829/1560-4071- 2021-4702

Rychik J, Atz AM, Celermajer DS, Deal BJ, Gatzoulis MA, Gewillig MH, et al. Evaluation and management of the child and adult with fontan circulation: a scientific statement from the American Heart Association. *Circulation*. (2019) 140:e234–e284. doi: 10.1161/CIR.0000000000000696

McDonagh TA, Metra M, Adamo M, Gardner RS, Baumbach A, Bohm M, et al. 2021 Esc guidelines for the diagnosis and treatment of acute and chronic heart failure. *Eur Heart J*. (2021) 42:3599–726. doi: 10.1093/eurheartj/ehab368

Olsson KM, Delcroix M, Ghofrani HA, Tiede H, Huscher D, Speich R, et al. Anticoagulation and survival in pulmonary arterial hypertension: results from the comparative, prospective registry of newly initiated therapies for pulmonary hypertension (Compera). *Circulation*. (2014) 129:57–65. doi: 10.1161/CIRCULATIONAHA.113. 004526

Dunn GD, Hayes P, Breen KJ, Schenker S. The liver in congestive heart failure: a review. *Am J Med Sci*. (1973) 265:174–89. doi: 10.1097/00000441-197303000-00001

Naschitz JE, Slobodin G, Lewis RJ, Zuckerman E, Yeshurun D. Heart diseases affecting the liver and liver diseases affecting the heart. *Am Heart J*. (2000) 140:111–20. doi: 10.1067/mhj.2000.107177

Sherlock S. The liver in heart failure; relation of anatomical, functional, and circulatory changes. *Br Heart J*. (1951) 13:273–93. doi: 10.1136/hrt. 13.3.273

Nicolls MR, Mizuno S, Taraseviciene-Stewart L, Farkas L, Drake JI, Al Husseini A, et al. New models of pulmonary hypertension based on vegf receptor blockade-induced endothelial cell apoptosis. *Pulm Circ*. (2012) 2:434–42. doi: 10.4103/2045-8932.105031

Stenmark KR, Meyrick B, Galie N, Mooi WJ, McMurtry IF. Animal models of pulmonary arterial hypertension: the hope for etiological discovery and pharmacological cure. *Am J Physiol Lung Cell Mol Physiol*. (2009) 297:L1013– 32. doi: 10.1152/ajplung.00217.2009

Ramadori G, Saile B. Inflammation, damage repair, immune cells, and liver fibrosis: specific or nonspecific, this is the question. *Gastroenterology*. (2004) 127:997–1000. doi: 10.1053/j.gastro.2004.07.041

Schmidt-Arras D, Rose-John S. Il-6 Pathway in the liver: from physiopathology to therapy. *J Hepatol*. (2016) 64:1403– 15. doi: 10.1016/j.jhep.2016.02.004

Wittlich M, Dudek M, Bottcher JP, Schanz O, Hegenbarth S, Bopp T, et al. Liver sinusoidal endothelial cell cross-priming is supported by Cd4 T cell-derived Il-2. *J Hepatol*. (2017) 66:978–86. doi: 10.1016/j.jhep.2016. 12.015

Mederacke I, Hsu CC, Troeger JS, Huebener P, Mu X, Dapito DH, et al. Fate tracing reveals hepatic stellate cells as dominant contributors to liver fibrosis independent of its aetiology. *Nat Commun*. (2013) 4:2823. doi: 10.1038/ncomms3823

Tomita K, Teratani T, Suzuki T, Shimizu M, Sato H, Narimatsu K, et al. Free cholesterol accumulation in hepatic stellate cells: mechanism of liver fibrosis aggravation in nonalcoholic steatohepatitis in mice. *Hepatology*. (2014) 59:154–69. doi: 10.1002/hep.26604

Kohjima M, Enjoji M, Higuchi N, Kato M, Kotoh K, Yoshimoto T, et al. Re-evaluation of fatty acid metabolism-related gene expression in nonalcoholic fatty liver disease. *Int J Mol Med*. (2007) 20:351–8. doi: 10.3892/ijmm. 20.3.351

Auer J. What does the liver tell us about the failing heart? *Eur Heart J*. (2013) 34:711–4. doi: 10.1093/eurheartj/ehs440

Potthoff A, Schettler A, Attia D, Schlue J, Schmitto JD, Fegbeutel C, et al. Liver stiffness measurements and short-term survival after left ventricular assist device implantation: a pilot study. *J Heart Lung Transplant*. (2015) 34:1586–94. doi: 10.1016/j.healun.2015.05.022

Dhall D, Kim SA, Mc Phaul C, Kransdorf EP, Kobashigawa JA, Sundaram V, et al. Heterogeneity of fibrosis in liver biopsies of patients with heart failure undergoing heart transplant evaluation. *Am J Surg Pathol*. (2018) 42:1617–24. doi: 10.1097/PAS.0000000000001163

Weill D. Lung transplantation: indications and contraindications. *J Thorac Dis*. (2018) 10:4574–87. doi: 10.21037/jtd.2018.06.141

Hsu RB, Chang CI, Lin FY, Chou NK, Chi NH, Wang SS, et al. Heart transplantation in patients with liver cirrhosis. *Eur J Cardiothorac Surg*. (2008) 34:307–12. doi: 10.1016/j.ejcts.2008.05.003

6

The Role of NADPH Oxidases (NOXs) in Liver Fibrosis and the Activation of Myofibroblasts

Shuang Liang[1,2]*, Tatiana Kisseleva[1] and David A. Brenner[2]*

[1] Department of Surgery, University of California, San Diego, La Jolla, CA, USA, [2] Department of Medicine, University of California, San Diego, La Jolla, CA, USA

Correspondence:
Shuang Liang
shl067@ucsd.edu;
David A. Brenner
dbrenner@ucsd.edu

Chronic liver injury, resulted from different etiologies (e.g., virus infection, alcohol abuse, nonalcoholic steatohepatitis (NASH) and cholestasis) can lead to liver fibrosis characterized by the excess accumulation of extracellular matrix (ECM) proteins (e.g., type I collagen). Hepatic myofibroblasts that are activated upon liver injury are the key producers of ECM proteins, contributing to both the initiation and progression of liver fibrosis. Hepatic stellate cells (HSCs) and to a lesser extent, portal fibroblast, are believed to be the precursor cells that give rise to hepatic myofibroblasts in response to liver injury. Although, much progress has been made toward dissecting the lineage origin of myofibroblasts, how these cells are activated and become functional producers of ECM proteins remains incompletely understood. Activation of myofibroblasts is a complex process that involves the interactions between parenchymal and non-parenchymal cells, which drives the phenotypic change of HSCs from a quiescent stage to a myofibroblastic and active phenotype. Accumulating evidence has suggested a critical role of NADPH oxidase (NOX), a multi-component complex that catalyzes reactions from molecular oxygen to reactive oxygen species (ROS), in the activation process of hepatic myofibroblasts. NOX isoforms, including NOX1, NOX2 and NOX4, and NOX-derived ROS, have all been implicated to regulate HSC activation and hepatocyte apoptosis, both of which are essential steps for initiating liver fibrosis. This review highlights the importance of NOX isoforms in hepatic myofibroblast activation and the progression of liver fibrosis, and also discusses the therapeutic potential of targeting NOXs for liver fibrosis and associated hepatic diseases.

Keywords: NADPH oxidase (NOX), liver fibrosis, myofibroblasts, reactive oxygen species (ROS), hepatic stellate cells (HSCs), hepatocytes

INTRODUCTION

The main causes of hepatic fibrosis are chronic hepatitis B and C infection, autoimmune and biliary diseases, alcoholic steatohepatitis (ASH) and, increasingly, nonalcoholic steatohepatitis (NASH) (Bataller and Brenner, 2005). Liver fibrosis results from a sustained wound healing process in response to chronic liver injuries, and is characterized by accumulation of excessive extracellular matrix (ECM) proteins. Prolonged and excessive buildup of ECM proteins leads to pronounced distortion of hepatic vascular architecture due to formation of the fibrous scar, which promotes subsequent hepatocyte regeneration and hepatic endothelial dysfunction

(Friedman, 2000). These processes facilitate the transition from liver fibrosis to cirrhosis, which may ultimately progress to more serious complications, such as portal hypertension due to increased resistance to portal blood flow, spontaneous bacterial peritonitis, and hepatic encephalopathy. Liver fibrosis is reversible, whereas cirrhosis, the end-stage consequence of fibrosis, is often irreversible and results in liver failure or the development of hepatocellular carcinoma (HCC) and death unless liver transplantation is done (Tsochatzis et al., 2014). Thus, it is of utmost importance to investigate the molecular and cellular mechanisms involved in the fibrogenic processes in order to design novel therapeutic interventions for liver fibrosis.

The major source of excessive ECM and fibrogenic mediators, such as collagen, is myofibroblasts. Recent studies indicate that the origin of myofibroblasts is liver intrinsic, and activated hepatic stellate cells (HSCs) and portal fibroblasts are believed to be the main precursors that give rise to hepatic myofibroblasts (Brenner et al., 2012). Upon liver injury, HSCs and portal fibroblasts undergo dramatic phonotypical changes by acquiring profibrogenic properties. In the normal liver, quiescent HSCs positive for adipocytes markers (PPARγ, SREBP-1c, and leptin) are the major cell type responsible for vitamin A storage (Bataller and Brenner, 2005). Upon activation by fibrogenic cytokines such as TGF-β1, angiotensin II, and leptin, quiescent HSCs trans-differentiate into myofibroblasts, possessing the properties of contractile, proinflammatory, and profibrogenic (Friedman, 2000). Activated HSCs express myogenic markers, such as α smooth muscle actin, c-myc, and myocyte enhancer factor–2 (Bataller and Brenner, 2005).

Accumulating clinical and pre-clinical data suggest that chronic liver injury results in the generation of oxidative stress, which disrupts lipids, proteins and DNA, induces necrosis/apoptosis of hepatocytes and amplifies the inflammatory response. Moreover, reactive oxygen species (ROS) mediate the progression of hepatic fibrosis by stimulating the production of profibrogenic mediators from Kupffer cells and circulating inflammatory cells and by directly activating HSCs to induce their trans-differentiation into myofibroblasts (Sánchez-Valle et al., 2012). Emerging evidence indicate that the nicotinamide adenine dinucleotide phosphate (NADPH) oxidases (NOXs) are sources of ROS, which play crucial roles in the progression of hepatic fibrosis (Aoyama et al., 2012; Paik et al., 2014). Seven NOXs isoforms have been identified in mammals so far. The major NOX isoforms expressed in the liver are NOX1, NOX2, and NOX4. NOX2 was the first discovered NOX in phagocytes, which plays important role in inflammation and host immune defense. HSCs and hepatocytes express NOX1, NOX2, and NOX4. It becomes increasingly clear that NOX-dependent ROS production is not limited to phagocytes because NOX enzymes are widely expressed and active in many different cell types from varies of tissues and organs. This review will focus on summarizing the roles of NOX isoforms that are distinctly expressed in different cell types in the liver.

NADPH OXIDASES

ROS are defined as oxygen radicals, including reactive molecules, such as peroxide, superoxide, hydroxide, and singlet oxygen. In physiological conditions, ROS are generated during normal oxygen metabolism and play important roles in maintaining cellular homeostasis by orchestrating host defense, cell growth and signaling. However, ROS can also rapidly accumulate in large quantities during oxidative stress when cells encounter either endogenous or exogenous challenges. This, if not properly controlled, might lead to adverse cellular events, including irreversible cellular damage and death which may ultimately results in tissue damage and organ dysfunction (Devasagayam et al., 2004). ROS mediated oxidative stress is strongly associated with varieties of human diseases, including Parkinson's (Smeyne and Smeyne, 2013), Alzheimer (Aliev et al., 2014), cardiovascular (Robert and Robert, 2014), immunological (De Deken et al., 2014), pulmonary (Wong et al., 2013), renal (Ozbek, 2012), as well as liver diseases (Jaeschke, 2011).

In chronic liver diseases, pathological insults, such as ischemia-reperfusion, cholestasis or drug toxicity, induce hepatocyte death, which activates immune cells and promotes HSC transdifferentiation into collagen-producing myofibroblasts, which ultimately drives the development of hepatic fibrosis and cirrhosis. ROS accumulation in hepatocytes can cause cell death, which release damage-associated molecular patterns (DAMPs) that stimulates liver resident Kupffer cells and newly recruited immune cells to produce profibrogenic mediators. ROS is vital for HSC activation, resulting in the initiation of fibrosis. In the liver, several cellular machineries can generate ROS, including the mitochondrial respiratory chain, cytochrome P450 (CYP) family members, peroxisomes, xanthine oxidase, and NADPH oxidases. NADPH oxidase that produces ROS was first discovered in phagocytes, referred as gp91^{phox} (also known as NOX2), and serves as an important inflammatory mediator against invading bacteria. Recently, other NOX2 like molecules have been identified in various tissues. Due to the sequential and functional similarities of these enzymes to NOX2, these enzymes, together with NOX2 are collectively referred to as the NOX family. The NOX family genes encode proteins responsible for a transmembrane electron transport chain containing a flavocytochrome b, which transfers electrons donated by NADPH across biological membranes to form superoxide (O_2^-) and hydrogen peroxide (H_2O_2) from molecular oxygen (Cross and Segal, 2004). Seven NOX family members have been identified so far, including NOX1, NOX2 (formerly known as gp91^{phox}), NOX3, NOX4, NOX5, and dual oxidase Duox proteins (DUOX1 and DUOX2).

The phagocytic NOX (NOX2) core enzyme comprises several different subunits that interact with each other to form an active enzyme complex, including NOX2 (gp91^{phox}), p40^{phox} (PHOX for phagocyte oxidase), p47^{phox}, p67^{phox}, p22^{phox}, Rac2, and Rap1A, which is responsible for superoxide production upon agonist stimulation. In the resting stage, two integral membrane proteins—gp91phox and p22phox, form a large heterodimeric subunit flavocytochrome b$_{558}$ (cyt b$_{558}$). Three of the regulatory proteins, p40^{phox}, p47^{phox}, and p67^{phox} form a complex in the cytosol (Groemping and Rittinger, 2005; Sumimoto et al., 2005). Upon stimulation (e.g., exposure of cells to microorganisms or inflammatory mediators), p40^{phox} is highly phosphorylated, resulting in the entire cytosolic complex translocation to plasma membrane and association with flavocytochrome b$_{558}$. The whole NOX complex activation also requires the association of two low-molecular-weight guanine nucleotide-binding proteins, Rac2 GTPase and Rap1A (Diebold and Bokoch, 2001). Then the activated complex transfers electrons from the cytosolic NADPH to oxygen on the luminal or extracellular region (Koga et al., 1999). The expression of NOX2 is induced by interferon-γ (IFN-γ) through a transcription factor protein complex, called hematopoiesis-associated factor (HAF1), which is comprised of PU.1, interferon regulatory factor 1 (IRF-1), and interferon consensus sequence-binding protein (ICSBP) (Eklund et al., 1998).

NOX1 is identified as the first homolog of NOX2, and shares 60% amino-acid identity with NOX2 (Suh et al., 1999). NOX1 is widely expressed in many cell types, such as vascular smooth muscle cells (VSMCs), endothelial cells, astrocytes, and microglia. In liver, NOX1 is expressed in HSCs, ECs, and hepatocytes. However, the subcellular localization of NOX1 remains nebulous. It was suggested that NOX1 is a plasma membrane protein, and potentially resides in caveolin 1-containing lipid rafts (Hilenski et al., 2004; Zuo et al., 2005). Similar to NOX2, the activation of NOX1 also requires regulatory subunits, known as NOX organizer 1 (NOXO1) and NOX activator 1 (NOXA1), which are homologs of p47^{phox} and p67^{phox}, respectively (Bánfi et al., 2003; Cheng and Lambeth, 2004). In addition, p22^{phox} and Rac GTPase are also required for NOX1 activation. Expression of NOX1 is also highly regulated. Its mRNA is induced by the growth factors including platelet-derived growth factor (PDGF), and angiotensin and phorbol esters (Suh et al., 1999; Lassègue et al., 2001).

NOX4, which is first discovered in kidney, shares 39% sequence homology with NOX2 (Geiszt et al., 2000). Its activity requires direct interaction with p22^{phox}, but independent of the interaction with any cytosolic regulatory subunits (Ambasta et al., 2004). Moreover, Poldip2, a polymerase delta-interacting protein, has been shown to be associated with p22^{phox}, which ultimately increases NOX4 enzymatic activity in VSMCs (Lyle et al., 2009). Similar to NOX1, NOX4 expression can also be regulated by angiotensin II. Moreover, TGFβ is also a potent regulator of NOX4 mRNA (Sturrock et al., 2006; Bondi et al., 2010).

ORIGINS AND ACTIVATION OF HEPATIC MYOFIBROBLASTS

Chronic liver injury of all etiologies can promote liver fibrosis, a wound healing process whose hallmark is the formation of fibrous scar constituted by ECM. The main producer of extracellular matrix proteins in the liver is myofibroblast, a terminally differentiated cell type that plays a critical role in wound healing and connective tissue remodeling. Not only possessing the ECM synthesizing features of fibroblasts,

myofibroblast also has the contractile functions similar to the smooth muscle cells (Hinz et al., 2012). Under the self-limiting and homeostatic tissue repair processes, such as wound healing, myofibroblasts are induced and differentiated from their precursors, migrate to the site of injury, function to produce ECM proteins to contract the wound, and finally undergo apoptosis once injury is resolved. However, these processes can become uncontrolled when the myofibroblasts activities become excessive and persist due to the inability to undergo apoptosis, for example. This will lead to overwhelming ECM deposition, resulting in fibrosis and eventually cirrhosis (Watsky et al., 2010). In addition to the normal tissue repair and wound healing responses, myofibroblasts also contribute to regeneration, inflammation, angiogenesis, and stromal reaction during tumorigenesis. Although, myofibroblasts differ from fibroblasts by their ability of the former to de novo synthesize of α-smooth muscle actin (α-SMA), this is not an absolute requirement to define a cell as myofibroblast. Instead, the most reliable features of myofibroblasts are secretion of extracellular matrix, development of adhesion structures, and formation of contractile bundles (Hinz, 2010). Several novel markers of myofibroblasts, such as endosialin for tumor-associated myofibroblasts (Christian et al., 2008), P311 for hypertrophic scar myofibroblasts (Tan et al., 2010), and integrin α11β1 for human corneal myofibroblasts (Carracedo et al., 2010), have been recently identified. However, none of these markers are specific for myofibroblasts, and they play distinct roles in various types of fibroblasts, therefore affecting myofibroblasts differentiation in a tissue- and context- dependent manner. Nonetheless, reliable and unique markers for myofibroblasts remain to be defined.

Myofibroblasts are absent in healthy liver, but they are induced and activated from their precursor cells in response to hepatic injury. Although, the origin of myofibroblasts is yet unclear, three possible sources of myofibroblasts precursors in the liver have been proposed. The first possible source is the group of resident cells from the mesodermal origin that can potentially become myofibroblasts. This includes HSCs, portal fibroblasts, smooth muscle cells, and fibroblast around the central veins, which are different from hepatocytes, Kupffer cells, and sinusoidal endothelial cells. The second group of possible precursors of myofibroblasts are hepatocytes, cholangiocytes, and endothelial cells that can undergo epithelial or endothelial mesenchymal transition (EMT). However, several fate tracing and genetic labeling studies argued that hepatocytes or cholangiocytes did not undergo EMT in liver fibrosis models (Humphreys et al., 2010; Scholten et al., 2010; Taura et al., 2010). As for renal fibrosis, recent two studies argued that renal epithelial cells can undergo EMT, relaying signals to the interstitium to promote myofibroblast differentiation and fibrogenesis rather than directly giving rise to myofibroblasts population (Grande et al., 2015; Lovisa et al., 2015). Finally, bone marrow (BM)-derived cells consisting of fibrocytes and circulating mesenchymal cells can migrate into fibrotic liver tissue, transform into myofibroblasts and may contribute in the progression of liver fibrosis (Russo et al., 2006). Thus, these cells could also be possible precursors of myofibroblasts. However, a recent study using bone marrow (BM) chimeric mice reconstituted from transgenic collagen reporter mice suggested that BM cells had negligible contribution in collagen production during hepatic fibrosis (Higashiyama et al., 2009).

Among different mesenchymal cell types, the vitamin A-containing lipocytes (HSCs) capable of producing type III collagen was the first identified myofibroblast precursor in the liver (Kent et al., 1976). Since then, much focus has been put on HSCs to identify the origin of myofibroblasts. Upon liver injury, HSCs are activated, and converted from quiescent vitamin-A rich cells to proliferative, fibrogenic, and contractile myofibroblasts (Friedman, 2008). HSCs are regarded as the "warehouse" of retinoid droplets that exhibit blue-green autofluorescence when excited by UV light. However, cells that are absent of retinoid droplets are distinct from HSCs, which undergo a PDGF-mediated conversion into myofibroblasts (Kinnman et al., 2003). These cells are thought to be portal fibroblasts that are accumulated around bile ducts, and might play a critical role in the early stage of bile duct ligation (BDL) induced fibrosis (Tuchweber et al., 1996). Moreover, liver fibrosis seems to develop predominantly from the portal area and progress from there, irrespectively of the underlying etiology. Therefore the role of portal fibroblasts in the development of fibrosis may be more important than generally assumed.

NOXS IN HSC ACTIVATION

Upon liver injury, quiescent HSC become activated. The activation process is characterized by the loss of vitamin-A containing droplets, de novo synthesis of a-SMA, collagen and ECM proteins, and increased contractile and cell survival. The activation of HSC is a complex process, which involves the contribution of extracellular stimuli and different cell types, including parenchymal cells, immune cells. NOX proteins and NOX-derived ROS play a key role during HSC activation (**Figure 1**). ROS are produced in defined cellular compartments, but diffuse throughout the cell (e.g., superoxide) or across the plasma membranes (e.g., H_2O_2). ROS, when present at low levels, could serve as secondary messengers in response to a variety of cellular stimuli. For instance, it has been shown that low amount of hydrogen peroxide (H_2O_2) can act as second messenger that plays a critical role in the initiation and amplification of signaling during lymphocyte activation (Reth, 2002). In contrast, high level of ROS can be toxic and may lead to cell death. Although, low levels of ROS promote HSC to produce collagen and proliferate, while high-level toxic amount of ROS can induce death of HSCs (Novo et al., 2006).

NOXs are highly upregulated in patients with organ fibrosis, such as heart, lung, kidney, and pancreas. In consistence with their role in human fibrosis, NOX-derived ROS is also essential for multiple organ fibrosis in mice (Paik et al., 2006). In addition, during HSC activation, NOX mediates a number of fibrogenic responses induced by different agonists, including Ang II, PDGF, leptin, and TGFβ. Moreover, phagocytosis of apoptotic bodies by HSC leads to NOX activation and procollagen α1 (I) expression (Zhan et al., 2006). The expression of NOX isoforms is different among different types of liver resident cells. Kupffer cells only express phagocytic NOX2, whereas hepatocytes and HSC express

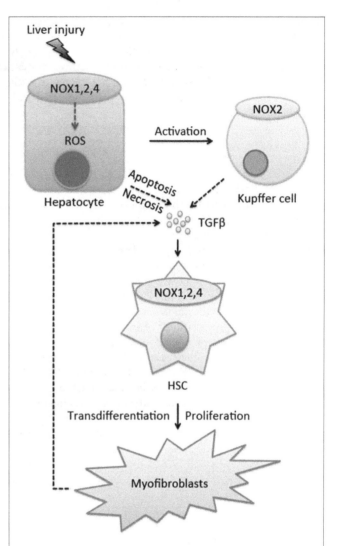

FIGURE 1 | The role of NOXs in myofibroblasts activation. The interactions between hepatocytes, Kupffer cells and HSCs promotes myofibroblast activation. Various NOX isoforms expressed in different cell types in the liver play crucial roles during this process. After exposure to hepatic insults, such as ischaemia/reperfusion (IR) injuries, alcohol abuse, viral infection, hyper-nutrition, and cholestasis, ROS is produced through NOXs in hepatocytes. Increased oxidative stress also induces hepatocyte apoptosis/necrosis, resulting in release of DAMPs that activate Kupffer cells. Injured hepatocytes and activated Kupffer cells secrete proinflammatory and profibrogenic cytokine TGFβ, which promotes the differentiation of HSCs into myofibroblasts (see text for further details).

various NOX isoforms, including phagocytic NOX2 and non-phagocytic NOX1, NOX4, DUOX1, and DUOX2. Endothelial cells mainly express NOX1, NOX2, and NOX4. Upon liver injury, NOX isoforms in HSC are strongly upregulated when quiescent HSC become activated myofibroblasts (Paik et al., 2011; Aoyama et al., 2012). HSCs can also fine-tune ROS production by expressing the regulatory subunits of NOX complexes, including $p22^{phox}$, $p40^{phox}$, $p47^{phox}$, $p67^{phox}$, NOXO1, NOXOA1, and Rac1. It has been shown that the p47phox regulatory subunit is induced in HSCs activated upon BDL-mediated fibrosis (De Minicis et al.,

2010). At resting stage, human HSCs express low levels of both catalytic and regulatory NOX components, including NOX1, NOX2, and p47^{phox}. However, these NOX subunits are highly upregulated in HSCs from patients with fibrotic liver diseases (Bataller et al., 2003). Moreover, NOX1 and NOX4 protein levels were increased in human livers with cirrhosis compared with normal controls (Lan et al., 2015).

NOX4 IN HSCS

A complex network involving paracrine/autocrine signals in parenchymal and nonparenchymal cells is required for HSCs activation and differentiation into myofibroblasts. Accumulating evidence has suggested that NOXs are the key mediators in HSC activation, which promotes hepatic fibrosis. TGFβ is the most potent regulator promoting collagen production and α-SMA expression in myofibroblasts from various organs, including liver (Gressner et al., 2002), kidney (Desmoulière et al., 2003), lung (Hardie et al., 2009), and heart (Kuwahara et al., 2002). During the initiation and progression of liver fibrosis, TGFβ plays a crucial role in regulating HSC activation, as well as inducing hepatocyte apoptosis, which leads to the secretion of cytokines, chemokines and microparticles that are critical for HSC and Kupffer cell activation. A number of studies have shown that NOX4 is essential for TGFβ-induced myofibroblast activation and fibrogenic responses such as collagen production in different organs, including lung (Hecker et al., 2009), kidney (Bondi et al., 2010), heart (Cucoranu et al., 2005; Chan et al., 2013), and prostate (Sampson et al., 2011). Moreover, although NOX4 can be induced by TGFβ in several different organs (Cucoranu et al., 2005; Sturrock et al., 2006; Bondi et al., 2010; Boudreau et al., 2012), the mechanism involved is controversial among different organs. In kidney and lung myofibroblasts, TGFβ induces NOX4 expression and ROS generation through the classical Smad2/3 pathway (Sturrock et al., 2006; Bondi et al., 2010), whereas NOX4 ugregulation is upstream of Smad2/3 activation in cardiac myofibroblasts (Cucoranu et al., 2005). In liver fibrosis, TGFβ induces NOX activity and ROS production during HSC activation, which plays key role in hepatic myofibroblasts activation (Proell et al., 2007). In BDL- or CCl4-mediated liver fibrosis, NOX4 expression and its activity are upregulated via a TGFβ-Smad3 dependent manner in HSCs (Jiang et al., 2012; Sancho et al., 2012). In addition, NOX4 expression correlates with the fibrotic scores in patients with hepatitis C virus infection or NASH (Sancho et al., 2012; Bettaieb et al., 2015). ROS production and the expression of fibrogenic markers are dramatically reduced in HSCs deficient in NOX4 (Jiang et al., 2012). Moreover, experiments using siRNA against NOX4 attenuated HSC activation, and more importantly, knocking down NOX4 in activated myofibroblasts could reverse the fibrotic phenotypes. Knocking down NOX4 in activated HSCs decreased the expression a-SMA and collagen production with no influence on TGFβ1 expression and phosphorylation of Smad2/3. These indicate that NOX4 activation and the following ROS production are downstream of TGFβ-Smad2/3 signaling pathway (Sancho et al., 2012).

Patients with hepatic fibrosis as a result of various chronic liver injuries, including viral infection, toxin, metabolic disorders, alcohol abuse, and cholestasis, have a breach in gut barrier function. This leads to compromised intestinal permeability that allows the entry of bacteria-derived components (e.g., LPS and CpG-containing DNAs through portal circulation and eventually into the liver, where they activates liver immune cells via acting on toll-like receptors (TLRs) (Seki and Brenner, 2008; Yang and Seki, 2012). TLRs are a group of pattern recognition receptors that recognize their cognate ligands with as either pathogen-associated molecular patterns (PAMPs) or DAMPs. Although, both murine and human HSCs express multiple TLRs (Wang et al., 2009), they respond poorly to TLR ligands, such as Gram-positive bacterial products peptidoglycan (PGN) and lipoteichoic acid (LTA) (Paik et al., 2006). Upon ligand engagement, TLRs are activated and transduce signals through downstream adaptor molecules MyD88 and TRIF to induce the expression of proinflammatory cytokines and chemokines. These inflammatory mediators then recruit KCs and circulating monocytes/macrophages, which produce TGFβ1 to drive the differentiation of HSC into myofibroblast (Seki and Brenner, 2008; Aoyama et al., 2010). Although, the LPS-TLR4 axis is crucial for hepatic fibrogenesis and liver fibrosis is dramatically attenuated in germ-free mice (Seki et al., 2007), the roles of NOX and ROS have not been extensively studied in the context of regulating LPS-TLR4 mediated inflammatory or fibrogenic responses in HSCs. In macrophages, NOX inhibitor DPI or siRNA against p22^{phox} significantly decreased LPS-TLR4-mediated activation of endoplasmic reticulum (ER)-stress sensor kinase IRE1α and its downstream target, the transcription factor XBP1 (Martinon et al., 2010). Moreover, it has been shown that the C-terminal domains of NOX4 and TLR4 directly interact with each other in HEK293T cells (Park et al., 2004). Consistently, in human aortic endothelial cell (HAECs), overexpression of the C-terminal region of NOX4 inhibited nuclear factor-kappaB (NF-κB) activation in response to LPS. NOX4 downregulation using siRNA resulted in reduced ROS production and less expression of adhesion molecule (ICAM-1) and chemokines such as CXCL8 and MCP-1 in response to LPS (Park et al., 2006). Therefore, NOX4 and NOX4-mediated ROS generation may regulate LPS induced NF-κB activation and its downstream signaling pathway in HSC activation and profibrogenic effects of myofibroblasts.

NOX1/NOX2 IN HSCS

In addition to the TGFβ-NOX4 axis-mediated activation of HSC and expression of fibrogenic factors, other NOX isoforms, including NOX1, NOX2, and NOX2 regulatory subunit p47^{phox}, are also reported to orchestrate the progression of hepatic fibrosis (Aram et al., 2009; Jiang et al., 2010; Paik et al., 2011). p47$^{phox-/-}$ mouse was the first genetic model of NOX inhibition in the study of HSC function in liver fibrosis. After BDL-induced liver injury, p47$^{phox-/-}$ mice showed attenuated liver injury and fibrosis compared with WT mice. HSCs produce more type I collagen and TGFβ when treated with Angiotensin II (Ang II) (Yoshiji et al., 2001). Ang II also stimulates ROS production, and activates intracellular signaling pathways involving PKC, PI3K-Akt, MAPKs, ERK, and c-Jun, which presumably promotes HSC migration and proliferation. Consistent with this notion, HSC isolated from p47$^{phox-/-}$ mice had reduced cell motility and expansion capacity, and displayed a reduced fibrogenic response to Ang II (Bataller et al., 2003). Although the detailed molecular mechanism underlying Ang II-induced NOX activation and ROS production is still unclear, studies have indicated that Ang II induces ROS production through two consecutive events in vascular smooth muscle cells: the first event, which occurs within 30 s after Ang II stimulation, is dependent on PKC-mediated phosphorylation of p47^{phox}. Phosphorylated p47^{phox} then translocates to the membrane where it binds to and facilitates the activation of NOX1 and/or NOX2. The second event that leads to sustained NOX activation and the following ROS production induced by Ang II (peaked at 30 min) requires the activation of Rac GTPase. Ang II-mediated Rac activation is PI3K, EGFR, and c-Src dependent (Seshiah et al., 2002). In order to keep the prolonged signal induced by Ang II, the expression levels of NADPH catalytic subunits, as well as the regulatory subunits p47phox and p22phox are also upregualted during Ang II stimulation (Fukui et al., 1997; Lassègue et al., 2001; Touyz et al., 2002). Similarly in HSCs, the mRNA levels of both NOX1 and NOX4 are increased upon Ang II treatment (Aoyama et al., 2012).

Proliferation of HSCs is a prerequisite that mediates the proper function of HSC-derived myofibroblasts and fibrogenic response in general. It has been suggested that NOX1 is crucial for promoting HSC proliferation and ROS production in bile duct ligated mouse liver. The underlying molecular mechanism is proposed to involve oxidation and inactivation of phosphatase and tensin homolog (PTEN), leading to the activation of AKT/FOXO4/p27(kip) signaling pathway that promotes HSC proliferation and fibrogenesis following BDL-induced liver injury (Cui et al., 2011). Platelet-derived growth factor (PDGF) is considered the most potent mitogen that promotes HSC proliferation (Pinzani et al., 1989). It has been shown that NOXs play a crucial role in this process (Adachi et al., 2005). PDGF induces HSC proliferation through ROS production, and NOX inhibitor (DPI) or p38 MAPK inhibitor suppressed PDGF-induced ROS production and HSC proliferation (Adachi et al., 2005). Similarly, PDGF stimulates NOX-dependent proliferation of activated pancreatic stellate cells (PaSCs) in chronic alcoholic pancreatitis/fibrosis (Hu et al., 2007). Mechanistically, PDGF stimulation promotes NOX1 expression and ROS production. In line with this, NOX1 is critical in PDGF stimulated vascular hypertrophy through activation of PKCδ (Fan et al., 2005) and inducing transcription factor (ATF)-1 (Katsuyama et al., 2005). Additionally, it has been shown that the transcription factor AP1 binding site is critical for the promoter activity of NOX1 (Cevik et al., 2008). Recently, it has also been shown NOX1/NOX4 inhibitor suppressed PDGF mediated ROS production and proliferative gene expression in primary mouse HSCs (Lan et al., 2015).

NOXS IN HEPATOCYTES

Hepatocytes injury and death are important triggers of myofibroblasts activation. Dying hepatocyte can release DAMPs that induce the secretion of cytokines and chemokines from KCs/macrophage that eventually results in HSC activation and liver fibrosis. TGFβ1, secreted by active KCs/macrophage upon liver injury, can promote hepatocyte apoptosis (Oberhammer et al., 1992). The classical TGFβ mediated signaling pathway requires the binding of TGFβ1 to the TGFβ receptor (TGFβRI and II), leading to the phosphorylation and activation of Smad2/Smad3. Smad2/3 then interact with Smad4 to form an active Smad complex that enters the nucleus and binds to the promoter regions of TGFβ target genes to initiate their transcription. NOX4 is one of the TGFβ target genes. A key finding is that the expression of NOX4 is increased in NASH patients compared with healthy controls (Bettaieb et al., 2015). In hepatocytes, NOX4 expression is induced by TGFβ, and the activity of NOX4 is crucial for TGFβ mediated apoptosis of hepatocytes (Carmona-Cuenca et al., 2008). For instance, knocking down NOX4 in human hepatocytes cell lines (HepG2 and Hep3B) resulted in impaired NOX activity, caspase activation and cell death induced by TGFβ1 (Carmona-Cuenca et al., 2008). In rat fetal hepatocytes, TGFβ1 induces apoptosis through upregulating NOX4-mediated ROS production, followed by down-regulation of pro-survival protein Bcl-x$_L$, which ultimately results in the loss of mitochondrial membrane potential and initiation of cytochrome C release (Herrera et al., 2001). Additionally, TGFβ1-induced NOX4 activity also increases the levels of pro-apoptotic proteins BIM and BMF (Ramjaun et al., 2007; Caja et al., 2009), and thus further amplifies apoptotic signals. NOX4-derived ROS regulates the transcription of Bcl-x$_L$ and Bmf, whereas its regulation of BIM occurs post-transcriptionally (Caja et al., 2009). Moreover, EGF blocks TGFβ-induced NOX4 expression and hepatocytes death in a MEK/ERK and PI3K/Akt dependent manner (Carmona-Cuenca et al., 2006). Interestingly, NOX4 not only contributes to TGFβ-mediated apoptosis, but also to death ligand (such as FasL or TNFα/actinomycin D)-induced hepatocyte apoptosis (Jiang et al., 2012). Hepatocyte-specific deletion of NOX4 reduced oxidative stress, lipid peroxidation and liver fibrosis in mice (Bettaieb et al., 2015). NOX4 was suggested to reduce the activity of the phosphatase PP1C, leading to prolonged activation of key stress signaling PKR/PERK pathway (Bettaieb et al., 2015). Therefore, NOX4 promotes myofibroblasts activation and hepatic fibrosis through at least two distinct mechanisms: (1) directly facilitating TGFβ-induced HSC activation and production of profibrogenic targets, (2) indirectly promoting TGFβ or death ligand-induced hepatocytes apoptosis, which contributes to the production of cytokines, chemokines, and microparticles that leads to HSC activation (Aoyama et al., 2012; Jiang et al., 2012).

Different from other NOX family proteins, the activity of NOX4 mainly depends on its expression levels, and not on agonist-induced assembly of a complex (Serrander et al.,

2007). NOX4 predominantly mediates H_2O_2 production instead of superoxide (Martyn et al., 2006; Serrander et al., 2007). Potentially, H_2O_2 generated by NOX4 may contribute to the activation of certain protein tyrosine kinases that play crucial roles in TGFβ downstream signaling pathways (Bae et al., 2011). Hepatocytes and sinusoidal endothelial cells also express all of the components for NOX1 and NOX2 H (Jiang and Török, 2014). Owever, the mechanisms underlying NOX1/2 enzyme activation in these cells and their roles in regulating fibrosis and myofibroblasts activation remain largely unknown.

TARGETING HEPATIC FIBROSIS BY INHIBITING NOXS

Fibrosis is an intrinsic wound healing response that helps to maintain organ integrity upon severe tissue damage. However, fibrosis may also become problematic when persistent injury and sustained inflammation occurs. Unresolved liver fibrosis leads to accumulation of excessive ECM proteins and scarring, which eventually progresses to cirrhosis and HCC. As the key cells that produce fibrotic ECM and other fibrogenic components, hepatic myofibroblasts, and their products are considered primary targets for antifibrotic therapies (Schuppan and Kim, 2013; Tsochatzis et al., 2014). However, there is still no FDA-approved drug for the treatment of liver fibrosis. Accumulating evidence have suggested the critical pathogenic effects of oxidative stress in the development of liver fibrosis, therapies that target ROS using antioxidants have therefore been applied in pre-clinical models of liver diseases. For example, a natural antioxidant Pyrroloquinoline-quinone (PQQ) found in human foods, suppresses oxidative stress, and liver fibrogenesis in mice with attenuated liver damage, hepatic inflammation and activation of HSCs (Jia et al., 2015). Similarly, Silybin, an extract of silymarin with antioxidant and anti-inflammatory properties, has been shown to be hepatoprotective in rat livers with secondary biliary cirrhosis (Serviddio et al., 2014). Additionally, a recent study suggested that blocking chloride channels prevented the increase of intracellular superoxide anion radicals, leading to attenuated activation of HSCs (den Hartog et al., 2014). However, it should also be noted that several antioxidants have failed in clinical trials to demonstrate their efficacy in antifibrotic response, such as polyenylphosphatidylcholine in alcoholic liver disease (Lieber et al., 2003), and Ursodeoxycholic acid (UDCA) and vitamin E in NASH (Lindor et al., 2004; Sanyal et al., 2010).

Given the vital role of NOX and NOX-derived ROS in hepatic fibrogenesis, the use of novel pharmacological NOX inhibitors to treat patients with chronic liver disease is being considered as the most promising antifibrotic therapeutics. However, historical NOX inhibitors, such as apocynin and

diphenylene iodonium (DPI), do not specifically target NOX-derived ROS and are not isoform specialized. Until recently, GenKyoTex (Geneva, Switzerland) has developed a first-in-class small molecule NOX1/NOX4 dual inhibitor (GKT137831), with little affinity for Nox2 isoform (Laleu et al., 2010). Inhibition of NOX1/NOX4 using GKT137831 attenuated CCl4 or BDL-induced ROS production and hepatic fibrosis in mice (Aoyama et al., 2012; Jiang et al., 2012; Lan et al., 2015). Mechanistically, GKT137831 suppressed profibrotic gene expression and ROS production in HSCs (Aoyama et al., 2012; Lan et al., 2015), and also decreased hepatocyte apoptosis (Jiang et al., 2012). GenKyoTex is finalizing Phase II clinical study, and GKT137831 displayed an excellent safety profile and statistically significant reduction in both liver enzyme and inflammatory marker levels. Together with results from pre-clinical animal models of various fibrotic disorders, NOX inhibition shows strong potential as an effective treatment for hepatic fibrosis. However, chronic liver diseases of different etiologies may require specific and/or combination antifibrotic treatment approaches, based on the fact that the crosstalk between different cell types is critical for myofibroblasts activation. Future, studies on the components and functions of specific NOX isoforms in specific cell types and specific liver diseases will provide deeper insights for designing more specific and potent NOX inhibitors for the treatment of hepatic fibrosis.

CONCLUSIONS

Oxidative stress and inflammation are considered as the main cause of chronic liver diseases. Multiple lines of evidence indicate that NOX-generated ROS plays a pivotal role in the pathogenesis of liver fibrosis. A number of NOX isoforms, including NOX1, NOX2, and NOX4 are involved in the initiation of myofibroblasts activation and progression hepatic fibrosis. However, the intracellular pathways and molecular mechanisms involved in the role of NOX isoforms in specific cell types remain largely unknown. Targeting specific NOX isoforms with specific inhibitors, such as NOX1 and/or NOX4 to prevent HSC activation and protect hepatocyte injury may be promising to treat liver fibrosis, although future work is needed to fully confirm the clinical safety of these compounds. Moreover, the knowledge of molecular pathways involved in NOX-mediated myofibroblasts activation and fibrogenesis can provide new insights for developing novel anti-fibrotic treatments.

AUTHOR CONTRIBUTIONS

SL wrote the manuscript, TK and DB revised the manuscript.

REFERENCES

Adachi, T., Togashi, H., Suzuki, A., Kasai, S., Ito, J., Sugahara, K., et al. (2005). NAD(P)H oxidase plays a crucial role in PDGF-induced proliferation of hepatic stellate cells. *Hepatology* 41, 1272–1281. doi: 10.1002/hep.20719

Aliev, G., Priyadarshini, M., Reddy, V. P., Grieg, N. H., Kaminsky, Y., Cacabelos, R., et al. (2014). Oxidative stress mediated mitochondrial and vascular lesions as markers in the pathogenesis of Alzheimer disease. *Curr. Med. Chem.* 21, 2208–2217. doi: 10.2174/0929867321666131227161303

Ambasta, R. K., Kumar, P., Griendling, K. K., Schmidt, H. H., Busse, R., and Brandes, R. P. (2004). Direct interaction of the novel Nox proteins with p22phox is required for the formation of a functionally active NADPH oxidase. *J. Biol. Chem.* 279, 45935–45941. doi: 10.1074/jbc.M406486200

Aoyama, T., Paik, Y. H., and Seki, E. (2010). Toll-like receptor signaling and liver fibrosis. *Gastroenterol. Res. Pract.* 2010:192543. doi: 10.1155/2010/192543

Aoyama, T., Paik, Y. H., Watanabe, S., Laleu, B., Gaggini, F., Fioraso-Cartier, L., et al. (2012). Nicotinamide adenine dinucleotide phosphate oxidase in experimental liver fibrosis: GKT137831 as a novel potential therapeutic agent. *Hepatology* 56, 2316–2327. doi: 10.1002/hep.25938

Aram, G., Potter, J. J., Liu, X., Wang, L., Torbenson, M. S., and Mezey, E. (2009). Deficiency of nicotinamide adenine dinucleotide phosphate, reduced form oxidase enhances hepatocellular injury but attenuates fibrosis after chronic carbon tetrachloride administration. *Hepatology* 49, 911–919. doi: 10.1002/hep.22708

Bae, Y. S., Oh, H., Rhee, S. G., and Yoo, Y. D. (2011). Regulation of reactive oxygen species generation in cell signaling. *Mol. Cells* 32, 491–509. doi: 10.1007/s10059-011-0276-3

Bánfi, B., Clark, R. A., Steger, K., and Krause, K. H. (2003). Two novel proteins activate superoxide generation by the NADPH oxidase NOX1. *J. Biol. Chem.* 278, 3510–3513. doi: 10.1074/jbc.C200613200

Bataller, R., and Brenner, D. A. (2005). Liver fibrosis. *J. Clin. Invest.* 115, 209–218. doi: 10.1172/JCI24282

Bataller, R., Schwabe, R. F., Choi, Y. H., Yang, L., Paik, Y. H., Lindquist, J., et al. (2003). NADPH oxidase signal transduces angiotensin II in hepatic stellate cells and is critical in hepatic fibrosis. *J. Clin. Invest.* 112, 1383–1394. doi: 10.1172/JCI18212

Bettaieb, A., Jiang, J. X., Sasaki, Y., Chao, T. I., Kiss, Z., Chen, X., et al. (2015). Hepatocyte nicotinamide adenine dinucleotide phosphate reduced oxidase 4 regulates stress signaling, fibrosis, and insulin sensitivity during development of steatohepatitis in mice. *Gastroenterology* 149, 468–480.e410. doi: 10.1053/j.gastro.2015.04.009

Bondi, C. D., Manickam, N., Lee, D. Y., Block, K., Gorin, Y., Abboud, H. E., et al. (2010). NAD(P)H oxidase mediates TGF-beta1-induced activation of kidney myofibroblasts. *J. Am. Soc. Nephrol.* 21, 93–102. doi: 10.1681/ASN.2009020146

Boudreau, H. E., Casterline, B. W., Rada, B., Korzeniowska, A., and Leto, T. L. (2012). Nox4 involvement in TGF-beta and SMAD3-driven induction of the epithelial-to-mesenchymal transition and migration of breast epithelial cells. *Free Radic. Biol. Med.* 53, 1489–1499. doi: 10.1016/j.freeradbiomed.2012.06.016

Brenner, D. A., Kisseleva, T., Scholten, D., Paik, Y. H., Iwaisako, K., Inokuchi, S., et al. (2012). Origin of myofibroblasts in liver fibrosis. *Fibrog. Tiss. Repair* 5:S17. doi: 10.1186/1755-1536-5-S1-S17

Caja, L., Sancho, P., Bertran, E., Iglesias-Serret, D., Gil, J., and Fabregat, I. (2009). Overactivation of the MEK/ERK pathway in liver tumor cells confers resistance to TGF-{beta}-induced cell death through impairing up-regulation of the NADPH oxidase NOX4. *Cancer Res.* 69, 7595–7602. doi: 10.1158/0008-5472.CAN-09-1482

Carmona-Cuenca, I., Herrera, B., Ventura, J. J., Roncero, C., Fernandez, M., and Fabregat, I. (2006). EGF blocks NADPH oxidase activation by TGF-beta in fetal rat hepatocytes, impairing oxidative stress, and cell death. *J. Cell Physiol.* 207, 322–330. doi: 10.1002/jcp.20568

Carmona-Cuenca, I., Roncero, C., Sancho, P., Caja, L., Fausto, N., Fernandez, M., et al. (2008). Upregulation of the NADPH oxidase NOX4 by TGF-beta in hepatocytes is required for its pro-apoptotic activity. *J. Hepatol.* 49, 965–976. doi: 10.1016/j.jhep.2008.07.021

Carracedo, S., Lu, N., Popova, S. N., Jonsson, R., Eckes, B., and Gullberg, D. (2010). The fibroblast integrin alpha11beta1 is induced in a mechanosensitive manner involving activin A and regulates myofibroblast differentiation. *J. Biol. Chem.* 285, 10434–10445. doi: 10.1074/jbc.M109.078766

Cevik, M. O., Katsuyama, M., Kanda, S., Kaneko, T., Iwata, K., Ibi, M., et al. (2008). The AP-1 site is essential for the promoter activity of NOX1/NADPH oxidase, a vascular superoxide-producing enzyme: possible involvement of the ERK1/2-JunB pathway. *Biochem. Biophys. Res. Commun.* 374, 351–355. doi: 10.1016/j.bbrc.2008.07.027

Chan, E. C., Peshavariya, H. M., Liu, G. S., Jiang, F., Lim, S. Y., and Dusting, G. J. (2013). Nox4 modulates collagen production stimulated by transforming growth factor beta1 *in vivo* and *in vitro*. *Biochem. Biophys. Res. Commun.* 430, 918–925. doi: 10.1016/j.bbrc.2012.11.138

Cheng, G., and Lambeth, J. D. (2004). NOXO1, regulation of lipid binding, localization, and activation of Nox1 by the Phox homology (PX) domain. *J. Biol. Chem.* 279, 4737–4742. doi: 10.1074/jbc.M305968200

Christian, S., Winkler, R., Helfrich, I., Boos, A. M., Besemfelder, E., Schadendorf, D., et al. (2008). Endosialin (Tem1) is a marker of tumor-associated myofibroblasts and tumor vessel-associated mural cells. *Am. J. Pathol.* 172, 486–494. doi: 10.2353/ajpath.2008.070623

Cross, A. R., and Segal, A. W. (2004). The NADPH oxidase of professional phagocytes–prototype of the NOX electron transport chain systems. *Biochim. Biophys. Acta* 1657, 1–22. doi: 10.1016/j.bbabio.2004.03.008

Cucoranu, I., Clempus, R., Dikalova, A., Phelan, P. J., Ariyan, S., Dikalov, S., et al. (2005). NAD(P)H oxidase 4 mediates transforming growth factor-beta1-induced differentiation of cardiac fibroblasts into myofibroblasts. *Circ. Res.* 97, 900–907. doi: 10.1161/01.RES.0000187457.24338.3D

Cui, W., Matsuno, K., Iwata, K., Ibi, M., Matsumoto, M., Zhang, J., et al. (2011). NOX1/nicotinamide adenine dinucleotide phosphate, reduced form (NADPH) oxidase promotes proliferation of stellate cells and aggravates liver fibrosis induced by bile duct ligation. *Hepatology* 54, 949–958. doi: 10.1002/hep.24465

De Deken, X., Corvilain, B., Dumont, J. E., and Miot, F. (2014). Roles of DUOX-mediated hydrogen peroxide in metabolism, host defense, and signaling. *Antioxid. Redox Signal.* 20, 2776–2793. doi: 10.1089/ars.2013.5602

De Minicis, S., Seki, E., Paik, Y. H., Osterreicher, C. H., Kodama, Y., Kluwe, J., et al. (2010). Role and cellular source of nicotinamide adenine dinucleotide phosphate oxidase in hepatic fibrosis. *Hepatology* 52, 1420–1430. doi: 10.1002/hep.23804

den Hartog, G. J., Qi, S., Van Tilburg, J. H., Koek, G. H., and Bast, A. (2014). Superoxide anion radicals activate hepatic stellate cells after entry through chloride channels: a new target in liver fibrosis. *Eur. J. Pharmacol.* 724, 140–144. doi: 10.1016/j.ejphar.2013.12.033

Desmoulière, A., Darby, I. A., and Gabbiani, G. (2003). Normal and pathologic soft tissue remodeling: role of the myofibroblast, with special emphasis on liver and kidney fibrosis. *Lab. Invest.* 83, 1689–1707. doi: 10.1097/01.LAB.0000101911.53973.90

Devasagayam, T. P., Tilak, J. C., Boloor, K. K., Sane, K. S., Ghaskadbi, S. S., and Lele, R. D. (2004). Free radicals and antioxidants in human health: current status and future prospects. *J. Assoc. Phys. India* 52, 794–804.

Diebold, B. A., and Bokoch, G. M. (2001). Molecular basis for Rac2 regulation of phagocyte NADPH oxidase. *Nat. Immunol.* 2, 211–215. doi: 10.1038/85259

Eklund, E. A., Jalava, A., and Kakar, R. (1998). PU.1, interferon regulatory factor 1, and interferon consensus sequence-binding protein cooperate to increase gp91(phox) expression. *J. Biol. Chem.* 273, 13957–13965. doi: 10.1074/jbc.273.22.13957

Fan, C. Y., Katsuyama, M., and Yabe-Nishimura, C. (2005). PKCdelta mediates up-regulation of NOX1, a catalytic subunit of NADPH oxidase, via transactivation of the EGF receptor: possible involvement of PKCdelta in vascular hypertrophy. *Biochem. J.* 390, 761–767. doi: 10.1042/BJ20050287

Friedman, S. L. (2000). Molecular regulation of hepatic fibrosis, an integrated cellular response to tissue injury. *J. Biol. Chem.* 275, 2247–2250. doi: 10.1074/jbc.275.4.2247

Friedman, S. L. (2008). Hepatic stellate cells: protean, multifunctional, and enigmatic cells of the liver. *Physiol. Rev.* 88, 125–172. doi: 10.1152/physrev.00013.2007

Fukui, T., Ishizaka, N., Rajagopalan, S., Laursen, J. B., Capers, Q. T., Taylor, W. R., et al. (1997). p22phox mRNA expression and NADPH oxidase activity are increased in aortas from hypertensive rats. *Circ. Res.* 80, 45–51. doi: 10.1161/01.RES.80.1.45

Geiszt, M., Kopp, J. B., Várnai, P., and Leto, T. L. (2000). Identification of renox, an NAD(P)H oxidase in kidney. *Proc. Natl. Acad. Sci. U.S.A.* 97, 8010–8014. doi: 10.1073/pnas.130135897

Grande, M. T., Sánchez-Laorden, B., López-Blau, C., De Frutos, C. A., Boutet, A., Arévalo, M., et al. (2015). Snail1-induced partial epithelial-to-mesenchymal transition drives renal fibrosis in mice and can be targeted to reverse established disease. *Nat. Med.* 21, 989–997. doi: 10.1038/nm.3901

Gressner, A. M., Weiskirchen, R., Breitkopf, K., and Dooley, S. (2002). Roles of TGF-beta in hepatic fibrosis. *Front. Biosci.* 7, d793–d807. doi: 10.2741/gressner

Groemping, Y., and Rittinger, K. (2005). Activation and assembly of the NADPH oxidase: a structural perspective. *Biochem. J.* 386, 401–416. doi: 10.1042/BJ20041835

Hardie, W. D., Glasser, S. W., and Hagood, J. S. (2009). Emerging concepts in the pathogenesis of lung fibrosis. *Am. J. Pathol.* 175, 3–16. doi: 10.2353/ajpath.2009.081170

Hecker, L., Vittal, R., Jones, T., Jagirdar, R., Luckhardt, T. R., Horowitz, J. C., et al. (2009). NADPH oxidase-4 mediates myofibroblast activation and fibrogenic responses to lung injury. *Nat. Med.* 15, 1077–1081. doi: 10.1038/nm.2005

Herrera, B., Fernández, M., Alvarez, A. M., Roncero, C., Benito, M., Gil, J., et al. (2001). Activation of caspases occurs downstream from radical oxygen species production, Bcl-xL down-regulation, and early cytochrome C release in apoptosis induced by transforming growth factor beta in rat fetal hepatocytes. *Hepatology* 34, 548–556. doi: 10.1053/jhep.2001.27447

Higashiyama, R., Moro, T., Nakao, S., Mikami, K., Fukumitsu, H., Ueda, Y., et al. (2009). Negligible contribution of bone marrow-derived cells to collagen production during hepatic fibrogenesis in mice. *Gastroenterology* 137, 1459–1466.e1451. doi: 10.1053/j.gastro.2009.07.006

Hilenski, L. L., Clempus, R. E., Quinn, M. T., Lambeth, J. D., and Griendling, K. K. (2004). Distinct subcellular localizations of Nox1 and Nox4 in vascular smooth muscle cells. *Arterioscler. Thromb. Vasc. Biol.* 24, 677–683. doi: 10.1161/01.ATV.0000112024.13727.2c

Hinz, B. (2010). The myofibroblast: paradigm for a mechanically active cell. *J. Biomech.* 43, 146–155. doi: 10.1016/j.jbiomech.2009.09.020

Hinz, B., Phan, S. H., Thannickal, V. J., Prunotto, M., Desmoulière, A., Varga, J., et al. (2012). Recent developments in myofibroblast biology: paradigms for connective tissue remodeling. *Am. J. Pathol.* 180, 1340–1355. doi: 10.1016/j.ajpath.2012.02.004

Hu, R., Wang, Y. L., Edderkaoui, M., Lugea, A., Apte, M. V., and Pandol, S. J. (2007). Ethanol augments PDGF-induced NADPH oxidase activity and proliferation in rat pancreatic stellate cells. *Pancreatology* 7, 332–340. doi: 10.1159/000105499

Humphreys, B. D., Lin, S. L., Kobayashi, A., Hudson, T. E., Nowlin, B. T., Bonventre, J. V., et al. (2010). Fate tracing reveals the pericyte and not epithelial origin of myofibroblasts in kidney fibrosis. *Am. J. Pathol.* 176, 85–97. doi: 10.2353/ajpath.2010.090517

Jaeschke, H. (2011). Reactive oxygen and mechanisms of inflammatory liver injury: present concepts. *J. Gastroenterol. Hepatol.* 26 (Suppl. 1), 173–179. doi: 10.1111/j.1440-1746.2010.06592.x

Jia, D., Duan, F., Peng, P., Sun, L., Ruan, Y., and Gu, J. (2015). Pyrroloquinoline-quinone suppresses liver fibrogenesis in mice. *PLoS ONE* 10:e0121939. doi: 10.1371/journal.pone.0121939

Jiang, J. X., Chen, X., Serizawa, N., Szyndralewiez, C., Page, P., Schröder, K., et al. (2012). Liver fibrosis and hepatocyte apoptosis are attenuated by GKT137831, a novel NOX4/NOX1 inhibitor *in vivo*. *Free Radic. Biol. Med.* 53, 289–296. doi: 10.1016/j.freeradbiomed.2012.05.007

Jiang, J. X., and Török, N. J. (2014). NADPH oxidases in chronic liver Diseases. *Adv. Hepatol.* 2014:742931. doi: 10.1155/2014/742931

Jiang, J. X., Venugopal, S., Serizawa, N., Chen, X., Scott, F., Li, Y., et al. (2010). Reduced nicotinamide adenine dinucleotide phosphate oxidase 2 plays a key role in stellate cell activation and liver fibrogenesis *in vivo*. *Gastroenterology* 139, 1375–1384. doi: 10.1053/j.gastro.2010.05.074

Katsuyama, M., Fan, C., Arakawa, N., Nishinaka, T., Miyagishi, M., Taira, K., et al. (2005). Essential role of ATF-1 in induction of NOX1, a catalytic subunit of NADPH oxidase: involvement of mitochondrial respiratory chain. *Biochem. J.* 386, 255–261. doi: 10.1042/BJ20041180

Kent, G., Gay, S., Inouye, T., Bahu, R., Minick, O. T., and Popper, H. (1976). Vitamin A-containing lipocytes and formation of type III collagen in liver injury. *Proc. Natl. Acad. Sci. U.S.A.* 73, 3719–3722. doi: 10.1073/pnas.73.10.3719

Kinnman, N., Francoz, C., Barbu, V., Wendum, D., Rey, C., Hultcrantz, R., et al. (2003). The myofibroblastic conversion of peribiliary fibrogenic cells distinct from hepatic stellate cells is stimulated by platelet-derived growth factor during liver fibrogenesis. *Lab. Invest.* 83, 163–173. doi: 10.1097/01.LAB.0000054178.01162.E4

Koga, H., Terasawa, H., Nunoi, H., Takeshige, K., Inagaki, F., and Sumimoto, H. (1999). Tetratricopeptide repeat (TPR) motifs of p67(phox) participate in interaction with the small GTPase Rac and activation of the phagocyte NADPH oxidase. *J. Biol. Chem.* 274, 25051–25060. doi: 10.1074/jbc.274.35.25051

Kuwahara, F., Kai, H., Tokuda, K., Kai, M., Takeshita, A., Egashira, K., et al. (2002). Transforming growth factor-beta function blocking prevents myocardial

fibrosis and diastolic dysfunction in pressure-overloaded rats. *Circulation* 106, 130–135. doi: 10.1161/01.CIR.0000020689.12472.E0

Laleu, B., Gaggini, F., Orchard, M., Fioraso-Cartier, L., Cagnon, L., Houngninou-Molango, S., et al. (2010). First in class, potent, and orally bioavailable NADPH oxidase isoform 4 (Nox4) inhibitors for the treatment of idiopathic pulmonary fibrosis. *J. Med. Chem.* 53, 7715–7730. doi: 10.1021/jm100773e

Lan, T., Kisseleva, T., and Brenner, D. A. (2015). Deficiency of NOX1 or NOX4 prevents liver inflammation and fibrosis in mice through inhibition of hepatic stellate cell activation. *PLoS ONE* 10:e0129743. doi: 10.1371/journal.pone.0129743

Lassègue, B., Sorescu, D., Szöcs, K., Yin, Q., Akers, M., Zhang, Y., et al. (2001). Novel gp91(phox) homologues in vascular smooth muscle cells: nox1 mediates angiotensin II-induced superoxide formation and redox-sensitive signaling pathways. *Circ. Res.* 88, 888–894. doi: 10.1161/hh0901.090299

Lieber, C. S., Weiss, D. G., Groszmann, R., Paronetto, F., Schenker, S., and Veterans Affairs Cooperative Study 391 Group (2003). II. Veterans Affairs Cooperative Study of polyenylphosphatidylcholine in alcoholic liver disease. *Alcohol Clin. Exp. Res.* 27, 1765–1772. doi: 10.1097/01.ALC.0000093743.03049.80

Lindor, K. D., Kowdley, K. V., Heathcote, E. J., Harrison, M. E., Jorgensen, R., Angulo, P., et al. (2004). Ursodeoxycholic acid for treatment of nonalcoholic steatohepatitis: results of a randomized trial. *Hepatology* 39, 770–778. doi: 10.1002/hep.20092

Lovisa, S., Lebleu, V. S., Tampe, B., Sugimoto, H., Vadnagara, K., Carstens, J. L., et al. (2015). Epithelial-to-mesenchymal transition induces cell cycle arrest and parenchymal damage in renal fibrosis. *Nat. Med.* 21, 998–1009. doi: 10.1038/nm.3902

Lyle, A. N., Deshpande, N. N., Taniyama, Y., Seidel-Rogol, B., Pounkova, L., Du, P., et al. (2009). Poldip2, a novel regulator of Nox4 and cytoskeletal integrity in vascular smooth muscle cells. *Circ. Res.* 105, 249–259. doi: 10.1161/CIRCRESAHA.109.193722

Martinon, F., Chen, X., Lee, A. H., and Glimcher, L. H. (2010). TLR activation of the transcription factor XBP1 regulates innate immune responses in macrophages. *Nat. Immunol.* 11, 411–418. doi: 10.1038/ni.1857

Martyn, K. D., Frederick, L. M., von Loehneysen, K., Dinauer, M. C., and Knaus, U. G. (2006). Functional analysis of Nox4 reveals unique characteristics compared to other NADPH oxidases. *Cell Signal.* 18, 69–82. doi: 10.1016/j.cellsig.2005.03.023

Novo, E., Marra, F., Zamara, E., Valfrè di Bonzo, L., Caligiuri, A., Cannito, S., et al. (2006). Dose dependent and divergent effects of superoxide anion on cell death, proliferation, and migration of activated human hepatic stellate cells. *Gut* 55, 90–97. doi: 10.1136/gut.2005.069633

Oberhammer, F. A., Pavelka, M., Sharma, S., Tiefenbacher, R., Purchio, A. F., Bursch, W., et al. (1992). Induction of apoptosis in cultured hepatocytes and in regressing liver by transforming growth factor beta 1. *Proc. Natl. Acad. Sci. U.S.A.* 89, 5408–5412. doi: 10.1073/pnas.89.12.5408

Ozbek, E. (2012). Induction of oxidative stress in kidney. *Int. J. Nephrol.* 2012:465897. doi: 10.1155/2012/465897

Paik, Y. H., Iwaisako, K., Seki, E., Inokuchi, S., Schnabl, B., Osterreicher, C. H., et al. (2011). The nicotinamide adenine dinucleotide phosphate oxidase (NOX) homologues NOX1 and NOX2/gp91(phox) mediate hepatic fibrosis in mice. *Hepatology* 53, 1730–1741. doi: 10.1002/hep.24281

Paik, Y. H., Kim, J., Aoyama, T., De Minicis, S., Bataller, R., and Brenner, D. A. (2014). Role of NADPH oxidases in liver fibrosis. *Antioxid. Redox Signal.* 20, 2854–2872. doi: 10.1089/ars.2013.5619

Paik, Y. H., Lee, K. S., Lee, H. J., Yang, K. M., Lee, S. J., Lee, D. K., et al. (2006). Hepatic stellate cells primed with cytokines upregulate inflammation in response to peptidoglycan or lipoteichoic acid. *Lab. Invest.* 86, 676–686. doi: 10.1038/labinvest.3700422

Park, H. S., Chun, J. N., Jung, H. Y., Choi, C., and Bae, Y. S. (2006). Role of NADPH oxidase 4 in lipopolysaccharide-induced proinflammatory responses by human aortic endothelial cells. *Cardiovasc. Res.* 72, 447–455. doi: 10.1016/j.cardiores.2006.09.012

Park, H. S., Jung, H. Y., Park, E. Y., Kim, J., Lee, W. J., and Bae, Y. S. (2004). Cutting edge: direct interaction of TLR4 with NAD(P)H oxidase 4 isozyme is essential for lipopolysaccharide-induced production of reactive oxygen species and activation of NF-kappa B. *J. Immunol.* 173, 3589–3593. doi: 10.4049/jimmunol.173.6.3589

Pinzani, M., Gesualdo, L., Sabbah, G. M., and Abboud, H. E. (1989). Effects of platelet-derived growth factor and other polypeptide mitogens on DNA synthesis and growth of cultured rat liver fat-storing cells. *J. Clin. Invest.* 84, 1786–1793. doi: 10.1172/JCI114363

Proell, V., Carmona-Cuenca, I., Murillo, M. M., Huber, H., Fabregat, I., and Mikulits, W. (2007). TGF-beta dependent regulation of oxygen radicals during transdifferentiation of activated hepatic stellate cells to myofibroblastoid cells. *Comp. Hepatol.* 6:1. doi: 10.1186/1476-5926-6-1

Ramjaun, A. R., Tomlinson, S., Eddaoudi, A., and Downward, J. (2007). Upregulation of two BH3-only proteins, Bmf and Bim, during TGF beta-induced apoptosis. *Oncogene* 26, 970–981. doi: 10.1038/sj.onc.1209852

Reth, M. (2002). Hydrogen peroxide as second messenger in lymphocyte activation. *Nat. Immunol.* 3, 1129–1134. doi: 10.1038/ni1202-1129

Robert, A. M., and Robert, L. (2014). Xanthine oxido-reductase, free radicals and cardiovascular disease. A critical review. *Pathol. Oncol. Res.* 20, 1–10. doi: 10.1007/s12253-013-9698-x

Russo, F. P., Alison, M. R., Bigger, B. W., Amofah, E., Florou, A., Amin, F., et al. (2006). The bone marrow functionally contributes to liver fibrosis. *Gastroenterology* 130, 1807–1821. doi: 10.1053/j.gastro.2006.01.036

Sampson, N., Koziel, R., Zenzmaier, C., Bubendorf, L., Plas, E., Jansen-Durr, P., et al. (2011). ROS signaling by NOX4 drives fibroblast-to-myofibroblast differentiation in the diseased prostatic stroma. *Mol. Endocrinol.* 25, 503–515. doi: 10.1210/me.2010-0340

Sánchez-Valle, V., Chávez-Tapia, N. C., Uribe, M., and Méndez-Sánchez, N. (2012). Role of oxidative stress and molecular changes in liver fibrosis: a review. *Curr. Med. Chem.* 19, 4850–4860. doi: 10.2174/092986712803341520

Sancho, P., Mainez, J., Crosas-Molist, E., Roncero, C., Fernández-Rodriguez, C. M., Pinedo, F., et al. (2012). NADPH oxidase NOX4 mediates stellate cell activation and hepatocyte cell death during liver fibrosis development. *PLoS ONE* 7:e45285. doi: 10.1371/journal.pone.0045285

Sanyal, A. J., Chalasani, N., Kowdley, K. V., Mccullough, A., Diehl, A. M., Bass, N. M., et al. (2010). Pioglitazone, vitamin E, or placebo for nonalcoholic steatohepatitis. *N. Engl. J. Med.* 362, 1675–1685. doi: 10.1056/NEJMoa0907929

Scholten, D., Osterreicher, C. H., Scholten, A., Iwaisako, K., Gu, G., Brenner, D. A., et al. (2010). Genetic labeling does not detect epithelial-to-mesenchymal transition of cholangiocytes in liver fibrosis in mice. *Gastroenterology* 139, 987–998. doi: 10.1053/j.gastro.2010.05.005

Schuppan, D., and Kim, Y. O. (2013). Evolving therapies for liver fibrosis. *J. Clin. Invest.* 123, 1887–1901. doi: 10.1172/JCI66028

Seki, E., and Brenner, D. A. (2008). Toll-like receptors and adaptor molecules in liver disease: update. *Hepatology* 48, 322–335. doi: 10.1002/hep.22306

Seki, E., De Minicis, S., Osterreicher, C. H., Kluwe, J., Osawa, Y., Brenner, D. A., et al. (2007). TLR4 enhances TGF-beta signaling and hepatic fibrosis. *Nat. Med.* 13, 1324–1332. doi: 10.1038/nm1663

Serrander, L., Cartier, L., Bedard, K., Banfi, B., Lardy, B., Plastre, O., et al. (2007). NOX4 activity is determined by mRNA levels and reveals a unique pattern of ROS generation. *Biochem. J.* 406, 105–114. doi: 10.1042/BJ20061903

Serviddio, G., Bellanti, F., Stanca, E., Lunetti, P., Blonda, M., Tamborra, R., et al. (2014). Silybin exerts antioxidant effects and induces mitochondrial biogenesis in liver of rat with secondary biliary cirrhosis. *Free Radic. Biol. Med.* 73, 117–126. doi: 10.1016/j.freeradbiomed.2014.05.002

Seshiah, P. N., Weber, D. S., Rocic, P., Valppu, L., Taniyama, Y., and Griendling, K. K. (2002). Angiotensin II stimulation of NAD(P)H oxidase activity: upstream mediators. *Circ. Res.* 91, 406–413. doi: 10.1161/01.RES.0000033523.08033.16

Smeyne, M., and Smeyne, R. J. (2013). Glutathione metabolism and Parkinson's disease. *Free Radic. Biol. Med.* 62, 13–25. doi: 10.1016/j.freeradbiomed.2013.05.001

Sturrock, A., Cahill, B., Norman, K., Huecksteadt, T. P., Hill, K., Sanders, K., et al. (2006). Transforming growth factor-beta1 induces Nox4 NAD(P)H oxidase and reactive oxygen species-dependent proliferation in human pulmonary artery smooth muscle cells. *Am. J. Physiol. Lung. Cell. Mol. Physiol.* 290, L661–L673. doi: 10.1152/ajplung.00269.2005

Suh, Y. A., Arnold, R. S., Lassegue, B., Shi, J., Xu, X., Sorescu, D., et al. (1999). Cell transformation by the superoxide-generating oxidase Mox1. *Nature* 401, 79–82. doi: 10.1038/43459

Sumimoto, H., Miyano, K., and Takeya, R. (2005). Molecular composition and regulation of the Nox family NAD(P)H oxidases. *Biochem. Biophys. Res. Commun.* 338, 677–686. doi: 10.1016/j.bbrc.2005.08.210

Tan, J., Peng, X., Luo, G., Ma, B., Cao, C., He, W., et al. (2010). Investigating the role of P311 in the hypertrophic scar. *PLoS ONE* 5:e9995. doi: 10.1371/journal.pone.0009995

Taura, K., Miura, K., Iwaisako, K., Osterreicher, C. H., Kodama, Y., Penz-Osterreicher, M., et al. (2010). Hepatocytes do not undergo epithelial-mesenchymal transition in liver fibrosis in mice. *Hepatology* 51, 1027–1036. doi: 10.1002/hep.23368

Touyz, R. M., Chen, X., Tabet, F., Yao, G., He, G., Quinn, M. T., et al. (2002). Expression of a functionally active gp91phox-containing neutrophil-type NAD(P)H oxidase in smooth muscle cells from human resistance arteries: regulation by angiotensin II. *Circ. Res.* 90, 1205–1213. doi: 10.1161/01.RES.0000020404.01971.2F

Tsochatzis, E. A., Bosch, J., and Burroughs, A. K. (2014). Liver cirrhosis. *Lancet* 383, 1749–1761. doi: 10.1016/S0140-6736(14)60121-5

Tuchweber, B., Desmouliere, A., Bochaton-Piallat, M. L., Rubbia-Brandt, L., and Gabbiani, G. (1996). Proliferation and phenotypic modulation of portal fibroblasts in the early stages of cholestatic fibrosis in the rat. *Lab. Invest.* 74, 265–278.

Wang, B., Trippler, M., Pei, R., Lu, M., Broering, R., Gerken, G., et al. (2009). Toll-like receptor activated human and murine hepatic stellate cells are potent regulators of hepatitis C virus replication. *J. Hepatol.* 51, 1037–1045. doi: 10.1016/j.jhep.2009.06.020

Watsky, M. A., Weber, K. T., Sun, Y., and Postlethwaite, A. (2010). New insights into the mechanism of fibroblast to myofibroblast transformation and associated pathologies. *Int. Rev. Cell. Mol. Biol.* 282, 165–192. doi: 10.1016/S1937-6448(10)82004-0

Wong, C. M., Bansal, G., Pavlickova, L., Marcocci, L., and Suzuki, Y. J. (2013). Reactive oxygen species and antioxidants in pulmonary hypertension. *Antioxid. Redox Signal.* 18, 1789–1796. doi: 10.1089/ars.2012.4568

Yang, L., and Seki, E. (2012). Toll-like receptors in liver fibrosis: cellular crosstalk and mechanisms. *Front. Physiol.* 3:138. doi: 10.3389/fphys.2012.00138

Yoshiji, H., Kuriyama, S., Yoshii, J., Ikenaka, Y., Noguchi, R., Nakatani, T., et al. (2001). Angiotensin-II type 1 receptor interaction is a major regulator for liver fibrosis development in rats. *Hepatology* 34, 745–750. doi: 10.1053/jhep.2001.28231

Zhan, S. S., Jiang, J. X., Wu, J., Halsted, C., Friedman, S. L., Zern, M. A., et al. (2006). Phagocytosis of apoptotic bodies by hepatic stellate cells induces NADPH oxidase and is associated with liver fibrosis *in vivo*. *Hepatology* 43, 435–443. doi: 10.1002/hep.21093

Zuo, L., Ushio-Fukai, M., Ikeda, S., Hilenski, L., Patrushev, N., and Alexander, R. W. (2005). Caveolin-1 is essential for activation of Rac1 and NAD(P)H oxidase after angiotensin II type 1 receptor stimulation in vascular smooth muscle cells: role in redox signaling and vascular hypertrophy. *Arterioscler. Thromb. Vasc. Biol.* 25, 1824–1830. doi: 10.1161/01.ATV.0000175295.09607.18

7

The Role of miRNAs in Stress-Responsive Hepatic Stellate Cells during Liver Fibrosis

Joeri Lambrecht, Inge Mannaerts and Leo A. van Grunsven *

Liver Cell Biology Lab, Department of Biomedical Sciences, Vrije Universiteit Brussel, Brussels, Belgium

*Correspondence:
Leo A. van Grunsven,
Liver Cell Biology Lab, Department of
Biomedical Sciences, Vrije Universiteit
Brussel, Laarbeeklaan 103, Fac. G&F,
Brussel B-1090, Belgium
leo.van.grunsven@vub.ac.be

The progression of liver fibrosis and cirrhosis is associated with the persistence of an injury causing agent, leading to changes in the extracellular environment and a disruption of the cellular homeostasis of liver resident cells. Recruitment of inflammatory cells, apoptosis of hepatocytes, and changes in liver microvasculature are some examples of changing cellular environment that lead to the induction of stress responses in nearby cells. During liver fibrosis, the major stresses include hypoxia, oxidative stress, and endoplasmic reticulum stress. When hepatic stellate cells (HSCs) are subjected to such stress, they modulate fibrosis progression by induction of their activation toward a myofibroblastic phenotype, or by undergoing apoptosis, and thus helping fibrosis resolution. It is widely accepted that microRNAs are import regulators of gene expression, both during normal cellular homeostasis, as well as in pathologic conditions. MicroRNAs are short RNA sequences that regulate the gene expression by mRNA destabilization and inhibition of mRNA translation. Specific microRNAs have been identified to play a role in the activation process of HSCs on the one hand and in stress-responsive pathways on the other hand in other cell types (**Table 2**). However, so far there are no reports for the involvement of miRNAs in the different stress responses linked to HSC activation. Here, we review briefly the major stress response pathways and propose several miRNAs to be regulated by these stress responsive pathways in activating HSCs, and discuss their potential specific pro-or anti-fibrotic characteristics.

Keywords: miRNAs, hepatic stellate cells, fibrosis, ER stress, hypoxia, oxidative stress

Introduction

Liver fibrosis is the pathological condition of the liver resulting from sustained wound healing in response to chronic liver injury. Multiple factors can lead to such injury, including genetic (the accumulation of misfolded alpha1-antitrypsin), cholestatic (sclerosing cholangitis), metabolic (non-alcoholic fatty liver disease and non-alcoholic steatohepatitis), drug induced (paracetamol-intoxication and alcohol) and viral diseases (hepatitis B and C) (Friedman, 2003; Wallace et al., 2008). Liver fibrosis can eventually progress toward cirrhosis, which is characterized by the loss of endothelial fenestrations, excessive scar formation in the space of Disse, and the presence of vascularized fibrotic septa. These distortions of liver architecture and subsequent cellular homeostasis lead to impaired organ function, ascites, encephalopathy, variceal hemorrhage, portal hypertension and the development of hepatocellular carcinoma (Schuppan and Afdhal, 2008).

Role of miRNAs during Hepatic Stellate Cell Activation

One of the key features in the development of liver fibrosis is the augmenting presence of myofibroblasts in the liver. Myofibroblasts are characterized by their stellate shape, the expression of some specific proteins, such as alpha-smooth muscle actin (α-SMA), and the excessive production of extracellular matrix proteins, including fibronectin and collagen type I, III, and IV. Hepatic stellate cells (HSCs) transdifferentiate upon injury into myofibroblasts, and can be considered as the major origin of myofibroblasts (Mederacke et al., 2013). During initiation and progression of the liver fibrosis process, the liver is subjected to various kinds of stress including hypoxia (Nath and Szabo, 2012), oxidative stress (Parola and Robino, 2001), and endoplasmic reticulum (ER) stress (Li et al., 2015). HSCs will respond by activating into myofibroblasts, which is characterized by a change in gene (Jiang et al., 2006; De Minicis et al., 2007) and microRNA expression (Guo et al., 2009a), as reviewed in He et al. (2012a); Huang et al. (2014a) and Coll et al. (2015). Numerous detailed reports on gene expression changes during HSC activation are available, but information regarding their regulation by specific miRNAs remains rather vague.

MiRNAs are short non-protein coding RNA sequences of 20–23 nucleotides that are evolutionary conserved and are encoded in the genome. The human genome is supposed to encode for approximately 1000 miRNAs, which can be expressed in an ubiquitous or a tissue/cell-type specific way (Lee, 2013), and each of these miRNAs is thought to have a great range of potential targets, thus indicating its importance in gene regulation (Bartel and Chen, 2004). MiRNA-encoding genes are transcribed by RNA polymerase II, with the generation of primary miRNA, which will then be processed in the nucleus by activity of a microprocessor complex, named Drosha. The activity of this Drosha containing complex leads to the production of a hairpin-shaped premature miRNA defined by a length of approximately 70 nucleotides and the presence of a stem-loop structure (Lee et al., 2003; Gregory et al., 2004). Correctly processed premature miRNAs are then bound by Exportin-5 in a Ran guanosine triphosphate (RanGTP)-dependent manner, leading to the transport of these pre-miRNAs toward the cytoplasm (Lund et al., 2004). In the cytoplasm, the pre-miRNAs undergo processing by Dicer, another ribonuclease III enzyme, resulting in the production of double stranded RNA (dsRNA) of 20–23 nucleotides (Bernstein et al., 2001). In this double stranded nucleotide-complex, a mature miRNA strand, known as the guide strand, and a miRNA* strand, known as the passenger strand can be identified. The mature miRNA strand will be loaded into the Argonaute 2 (Ago2)-containing RNA-induced silencing complex (RISC), which is the effector of miRNA-mediated activities (Gregory et al., 2005). It is believed that the RISC complex can cause down-regulation of gene expression through 2 mechanisms; by an inhibition of mRNA translation or by reducing the mRNA stability and thus facilitating the degradation (**Figure 1**) (Bagga et al., 2005; Orban and Izaurralde, 2005; Pillai et al., 2005).

Since the discovery of miRNAs in 1993 (Wightman et al., 1993), researchers continuously tried to evoke the role of miRNAs in cellular homeostasis and in development of pathological conditions, including liver fibrosis. There are many miRNAs expressed during, and described to be involved in, HSC activation (**Table 1**), making them the topic of concise reviews (He et al., 2012a; Huang et al., 2014a). Here, we only briefly highlight some key miRNAs to illustrate the possible roles a miRNA could have in quiescent or activated HSCs. When evaluating these miRNA-studies it is important to keep in mind that although many miRNAs are conserved among eukaryotic organisms, it is possible that they do not display the same expression patterns in specific (pathological) processes, and thus can display interspecies differences in expression (Ha et al., 2008).

miR-29

miR-29 is the first and most thoroughly investigated miRNA-family in HSCs. miR-29a, miR-29b, and miR-29c are all down-regulated during the *in vitro* activation of isolated rat and mouse HSCs, and in liver biopsies from patients with advanced liver fibrosis. This down-regulation is promoted by transforming growth factor-β (TGF-β) and factors like inflammatory signals including lipopolysaccharide (LPS) and nuclear factor kappa B (NF-κB) (Roderburg et al., 2011). The miR-29 family is of importance for HSC activation, as they can bind to 3′-UTR collagen types I and IV (Kwiecinski et al., 2011). Consequently, miR-29 overexpression in HSCs reduces Collagen I and IV synthesis (Roderburg et al., 2011) and maintenance of the quiescent morphology (Sekiya et al., 2011). In addition to collagen targeting, PDGF-C and IGF-I are identified as targets of miR-29, with PDGF-C having pro-mitogenic and migratory capacities, and IGF-I being an important mitogenic factor when present in an autocrine manner in combination with PDGF-BB (Kwiecinski et al., 2012). In support with these findings, miR-29a/b levels were found to decrease in CCl4-treated male mice. Interestingly, female mice do not show this decrease, most likely due to differences in E2, which can induce miR-29a/b levels (Zhang et al., 2012). Not only collagen production, but also other aspects of HSC activation such as inflammatory response and cell proliferation can be regulated by miRNAs such as is the case for miR-146a and miR-16, respectively.

miR-146

miR-146 is also down-regulated during TGF-β-induced HSC activation (He et al., 2012b), while overexpression of miR-146a in HSCs leads to up-regulation of tissue inhibitor of metalloproteinase 3 (TIMP-3) and down-regulation of IL-6 mRNA (Maubach et al., 2011). In another study, overexpression of miR-146a lead to inhibition of proliferation of activated HSCs. This would be the result of direct binding to the promoter region of the SMAD4 mRNA, which regulates TGF-β1-mediated gene expression, thus leaving the cell insensitive to TGF-β1 stimulation (He et al., 2012b), demonstrating its importance in the inflammatory response, and its link with liver fibrosis. In addition, miR-146a is known to have a role in the inflammatory response during liver reperfusion injury, as it negatively regulates IL-1 receptor-associated kinase 1 (IRAK1)

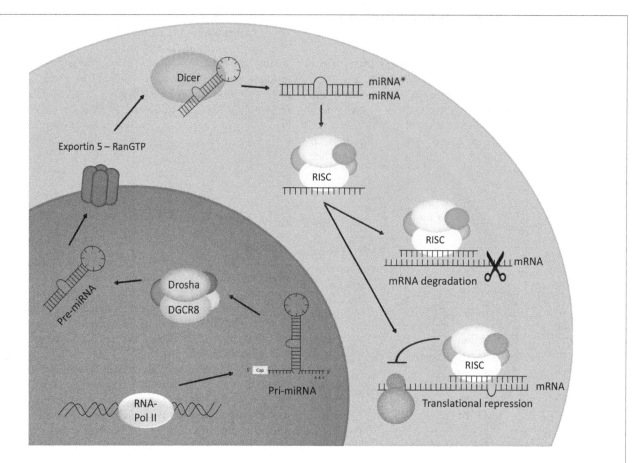

FIGURE 1 | MiRNA biogenesis. Transcription of the genes coding for miRNAs leads to the generation of primary miRNAs, which will be cleaved in the nucleus by Drosha, a ribonuclease III complex. The produced ribonucleic structure is called premature miRNA, and will be transported to the cytoplasm by Exportin 5, where it will undergo cleaving by Dicer, another ribonuclease III enzyme. One strain of the double-stranded obtained structure will integrate in the RISC-complex, leading to translational repression, or degradation of the target mRNA.

and Toll-like receptor-associated factor 6 (TRAF6), leading to a decrease in pro-inflammatory cytokine production, and by inhibiting the pro-inflammatory NF-κB pathway (Jiang et al., 2014). MiR-126 represents another miRNA that can regulate the NF-κB pathway by suppressing the expression of NF-κB inhibitor alpha (IκBα), thus leading to NF-κB activation (Feng et al., 2015).

MiR-16

miR-16 is another down-regulated miRNA during HSC activation. This miRNA has been shown to inhibit the expression of Cyclin D1, an important regulator of the cell cycle pathway. Expression levels of miR-16 and Cyclin D1 are inversely correlated in activating HSCs. Overexpression of this miRNA in activated HSCs leads to accumulation of the cells in the G0/G1-phase or G0/G1 to S-phase of cell cycle progression (Guo et al., 2009c). In HSCs, miR-16 also acts as an anti-apoptotic regulator in HSCs, by inhibition of B-cell lymphoma 2 (Bcl-2) translation, a known anti-apoptotic gene, leading to the enhanced expression levels of the underlying caspase-pathway consisting of caspases 3, 8, and 9, and thus induction of apoptosis (Guo et al., 2009b).

Function of Stress-Responsive Pathways and Possible Contribution of miRNAs during HSC Activation

As mentioned before, HSCs will undergo an activation process in the presence of different (fibrogenic) stimuli like liver injury, paracrine stimulation and autocrine regulation. This activation changes the quiescent fat storing cells into fibrogenic, proliferative and contractile myofibroblasts characterized by their expression of abundant intracellular filaments like α-SMA and vimentin, secretion of ECM including collagen type I and III and fibronectin and their high contractility (Kisseleva and Brenner, 2013). The contribution of stress response pathways in liver fibrosis, cirrhosis and to the HSC activation is generally accepted (Parola and Robino, 2001; Nath and Szabo, 2012; Li et al., 2015), but cannot be interpreted as a simple cause and consequence reaction. As literature mainly describes the contribution of hypoxia (Nath and Szabo, 2012), oxidative stress (Parola and Robino, 2001), and ER stress (Li et al., 2015) pathways during liver fibrosis and cirrhosis progression (**Figure 2**), we will focus on these three pathways.

TABLE 1 | Significantly regulated miRNAs during HSC-activation.

References	Up-regulated	Down-regulated
MiRNAs REGULATED DURING HSC ACTIVATION		
Guo et al., 2009b	miR−29c*, −138, −140, **−143**, **−193**, −207, −325 − 5p, −328, −349, −501, −872, −874	miR−15, **−16**, −20b − 3p, −92b, −122, **−126**, **−146a**, −341, −375
Ji et al., 2009	miR-27a, −27b, −30a, −30c, −30d, −130a, −130b, −450, −455	miR-9, **−19b**, −301, −520b, −520c, −721
Maubach et al., 2011	Let-7b, −7c, −7e, miR-**125b**, −21, −22, −31, −132, **−143**, **−145**, **−152**, **−199a**, −210, **−214**, **−221**, **−222**	Let-7f, miR-**10a**, **−16**, −26b, **−29a**, −30a − 5p, −30b, −30c, −30d, −99a, −122a, −125a, **−126**, **−146a**, **−150**, −151*, −181a, **−192**, **−194**, **−195**, −207, −296, **−335**, −422b, −483
Chen et al., 2011	miR-31, −34b, **−34c**, **−125b−5p**, **−143**, **−145**, **−152**, **−193**, **−199a** **−5p**, −199a−3p, **−214**, −218, **−221**, **−222**, −301a,−345−5p, −425	miR-**10a−5p**, −101a, **−126**, −126*, −139−5p, **−150**, **−192**, **−195**, **−335**, −338, −378*, −450a, −497, −877
Lakner et al., 2012	miR-**34c**, −184, **−221**	miR−**16**, −19a, **−19b**, **−29a**, −29c, −92a, **−150**, **−194**

*Summary of published data regarding microRNA microarray profiling of activating primary rat HSCs. MiRNAs which display an overlap in different published data sets are displayed in bold. *Mature miRNA derived from the 5' arm of the precursor RNA also known as passenger strand.*

Specific stress-related genes can be quickly switched on and off in presence or absence of environmental stress-inducing factors and this can be mediated by miRNAs (Babar et al., 2008; Leung and Sharp, 2010) (**Table 2**, right panel). So far there are no reports describing the functionality of specific miRNAs in these stress response pathways of activating HSCs during liver fibrosis. However, assumptions about miRNAs forming the link in stress-responsive HSCs (**Table 2**) and their potential functions in these conditions can be made based on the available data and will be discussed here. We should keep in mind that the presence or lack of overlap in miRNA expression pattern can be due to cell-type and species-specificity and is no proof for actual involvement of the miRNA in stress responsive HSCs, and should be elucidated in future research.

Hypoxia Regulated miRNAs

In the process of liver fibrosis and cirrhosis, hypoxia in the liver cells can be due to disruption of the normal hepatic blood flow, damage of the microvasculature, and excessive deposition of extracellular matrix in the sinusoidal space (Copple et al., 2006). Cellular hypoxia leads to the activation of several Hypoxia Inducible Factors (HIFs), a family of transcriptional factors that work as key regulators for the maintenance of cellular homeostasis when confronted with low oxygen levels (Paternostro et al., 2010). At normal cellular oxygen levels, the oxygen-dependent hypoxia inducible factor HIF-1α (HIF-1α) is hydroxylated by members of the prolyl hydroxylase family (PHD), leading to the rapid degradation of this protein. Decrease of the cellular oxygen levels leads to loss of function of PHD, and subsequent accumulation and translocation of HIF-1α/HIF-2α to the nucleus. In the nucleus, the functional HIF transcription factor complex is formed consisting of HIF-α, HIF-1β and some hypoxic responsive elements (Semenza, 2007). HIF regulates certain processes such as angiogenesis, iron metabolism, glycolysis, and pH control (Jiang et al., 1996; Rosmorduc et al., 1999; Moon et al., 2009). Hypoxic conditions lead to activation of the HSC cell line LX-2 as illustrated by an

up-regulation of α-SMA and collagen I protein levels, possibly through activation of the Smad/TGF-β pathway (Shi et al., 2007). HIF is proposed as a main regulator of hypoxia-mediated HSC activation, since it can act as a regulator and stimulator of profibrogenic mediators such as platelet-derived growth factor (PDGF) A and B, plasminogen activator inhibitor-1, and vascular epithelial growth factor (VEGF) (Forsythe et al., 1996; Moon et al., 2009; Wang et al., 2013). The essential role of HIF-1α during hypoxia-induced HSC activation was confirmed *in vitro* by inhibition of HSC-activation due to silencing of HIF-1α (Wang et al., 2013), and the reduced expression of activation genes in HIF-1α-deficient HSCs undergoing hypoxia (Copple et al., 2011). *In vivo* experiments using bile duct ligated (BDL) Hif-1α-deficient and control mice, showed less fibrosis in Hif-1α-deficient mice, as observed by lower levels of α-SMA and type I collagen, thus further indicating its importance during liver fibrosis (Moon et al., 2009).

MiRNAs can act down-stream and up-stream of the HIF pathway. For example, miR-210 expression is directly regulated by HIF-1α as it can bind to the hypoxia responsive element (HRE) located up-stream of the transcription start site of miR-210, leading to its enhanced transcription (Huang et al., 2009). It is suggested, that HIF-2α would mediate miR-210 expression in the absence of HIF-1α, also by interaction with consensus HREs in the miR-210 promoter region (Zhang et al., 2009). MiR-210 effects a broad variety of cellular processes such as fine-tuning cell proliferation by targeting e2f transcription factor 3 (E2f3) (Giannakakis et al., 2008) and MNT, a known MYC antagonist, and a member of the Myc/Max/Mad network (Zhang et al., 2009) while regulating apoptosis by controlling expression of the pro-apoptotic FLICE-associated huge protein (FLASH)/caspase-8-associated protein 2 (Casp8ap2) (Kim et al., 2009). Genes such as Nptx1, Rad52, Acvr1b, Fgrl, Hoxa1, and Hoxa9 associated with pathways like angiogenesis, tumor invasion, regulation of the mitochondrial metabolism, and DNA damage repair were also found to be miR-210 targets (Fasanaro et al., 2009; Huang et al., 2009). The hypoxia-induced up-regulation of miR-210 in various cancer cell lines (Huang et al., 2009) displays an overlap with its

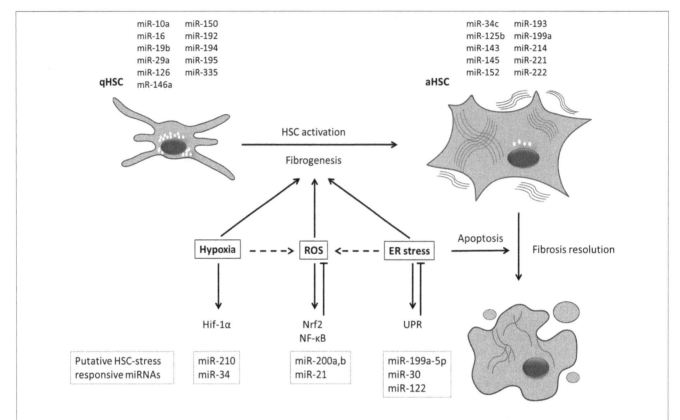

FIGURE 2 | Dynamic contribution of stress stimuli and miRNAs to liver fibrosis progression and resolution. HSCs are major contributors to the myofibroblastic cell pool in the fibrotic liver. In the presence of various activation stimuli, HSCs will undergo a myofibroblastic transdifferentiation process toward an activated state, which is characterized by a change in miRNA and mRNA expression pattern. It is widely accepted that the presence of hypoxia, oxidative stress (ROS), and endoplasmic reticulum (ER) stress most likely supports this activation process. However, ER stress could have a potential dual role in the process, as it can also lead to induction of apoptosis in activated HSCs, and thus could contribute to resolution of fibrosis. Simplified representation of some of the signaling cascades and potential miRNAs involved in these stress responses are given. MiRNAs depicted above the HSCs have been reported to be enriched in either qHSC or aHSCs. Putative HSC-stress responsive miRNAs that are discussed in the text are depicted below the signaling cascades.

enhanced expression during the activation process of HSCs, thus suggesting a potential role of this miRNA in hypoxia-mediated HSC activation.

Another potential link in hypoxia-mediated regulation of HSC activation is presented by miR-31. MiR-31 is up-regulated in both *in vivo* and *in vitro* activated rat HSCs (Maubach et al., 2011). This was confirmed in humans, where miR-31 was not changed in whole liver samples of fibrotic livers, but an increased expression of miR-31 was detected in HSCs during fibrogenesis. Functional studies showed repression of HSC activation by miR-31 inhibition, while miR-31 overexpression revealed its promoting role in cell migration (Hu et al., 2015). Interestingly it has been suggested that the biological function of miR-31 in activating HSCs would be obtained through its effect on Factor-inhibiting HIF-1(FIH) (Mahon et al., 2001; Hu et al., 2015). In head and neck carcinoma, miR-31 negatively regulates the expression of FIH and can thus regulate the expression of FIH in a hypoxia-independent manner (Liu et al., 2010). In cancer models this miRNA is up-regulated under hypoxic conditions (Hebert et al., 2007), suggesting a very complicated and diverse functionality of miR-31 during the reach for cellular homeostasis.

Previous research identified a direct link between the increased nuclear levels of HIF-1α protein and an increased activated status of HSCs in a hypoxic environment. HIF-1α has an indirect activating effect on the expression of pro-fibrogenic genes such as TGF-β, IL-6 and CTGF (Copple et al., 2011; Wang et al., 2013). The exact role of miR-31 in this hypoxia-induced HSC activation remains to be elucidated. We speculate on two possible scenarios that are perhaps not exclusive. Due to pro-activating signals from surrounding liver cells, HSCs will up-regulate miR-31 expression, leading to inhibition of FIH function, and thus enhanced HIF-1α expression, thereby favoring HSC activation in normoxic conditions. Hypoxic regions appear in the liver due to injury, what could favor the (further) induction of miR-31 expression, boosting the already enhanced HIF-1α expression, further leading to progression or maintenance of HSC activation.

Oxidative Stress Regulated miRNAs

Cells in aerobic organisms have a continuous balance between the production of pro-oxidants, such as reactive oxygen species (ROS), and anti-oxidants. When a cell is subjected to oxidative

TABLE 2 | Potential miRNAs involved in stress responsive HSC activation.

	miRNAs INVOLVED IN HSC ACTIVATION			STRESS RESPONSIVE miRNAs IN OTHER CELL TYPES				
miRNA	Expression during in vitro HSC activation	Species	References	Stress	Expression during stress	Cell type	Challenge or treatment	References
miR-214	Up-regulated	Rat, mouse	Maubach et al., 2011; Iizuka et al., 2012	Hypoxia	Up-regulated	Squamous cell carcinoma-cell line	1% oxygen for 1 h or 5% oxygen for 8 h	Hebert et al., 2007
miR-15b	Down-regulated	Rat	Guo et al., 2009b	Hypoxia	Down-regulated	CNE cells: a human naso-pharyngeal carcinoma cell line	Deferoxamine Mesylate	Hua et al., 2006
miR-422b	Down-regulated	Rat	Maubach et al., 2011	Hypoxia	Down-regulated	Squamous cell carcinoma-cell line	1% O_2 for 1 h or 5% O_2 for 8 h	Hebert et al., 2007
miR-125b	Up-regulated	Rat	Maubach et al., 2011; Chen et al., 2011	Hypoxia	Up-regulated	Colon and breast cancer cell lines	Culture in 0.2% O_2	Kulshreshtha et al., 2007
miR-101a	Down-regulated	Rat, mouse	Chen et al., 2011; Tu et al., 2014a	Hypoxia	Down-regulated	Neonatal rat cardiofibroblasts	Culture in 2% O_2	Zhao et al., 2015
miR-27a	Up-regulated	Rat	Ji et al., 2009	Hypoxia	Up-regulated	Colon-, breast-, human bladder-, and human colon-cancer cell lines	Culture in 3% O_2, $CoCl_2$	Kulshreshtha et al., 2007; Xu et al., 2014
miR-195	Down-regulated	Rat	Maubach et al., 2011	Hypoxia	Down-regulated	Chondrocytes	Culture in 5% O_2	Bai et al., 2015
miR-210	Up-regulated	Rat	Maubach et al., 2011	Hypoxia	Up-regulated	Pancreatic, breast, head and neck, lung, colon, renal cell lines	2% O_2 for 24 h	Huang et al., 2009
miR-31	Up-regulated	Rat	Maubach et al., 2011	Hypoxia	Up-regulated	Squamous cell carcinoma-cell line	1% O_2 for 1 h or 5% O_2 for 8 h	Hebert et al., 2007
miR-9	Down-regulated	Rat	Ji et al., 2009	Oxidative stress	Down-regulated	ARPE-19: human retinal pigment cells	4-hydroxynonenal and tert-butyl hydroperoxide	Yoon et al., 2014
miR-92a	Down-regulated	Rat	Lakner et al., 2012	Oxidative stress	Down-regulated	TK6: human lymphoblast cell line, endothelial cells (HUVEC)	Irradiation, H_2O_2	Chaudhry et al., 2013; Zhang et al., 2014
miR-21	Up-regulated	Rat	Maubach et al., 2011	Oxidative stress	Up-regulated	Neonatal cardiomyocytes	H_2O_2	Wei et al., 2014
miR-200a	Up-regulated	HSC-T6 cell line	Sun et al., 2014	Oxidative stress	Up-regulated	Mouse fibroblasts	H_2O_2	Mateescu et al., 2011
miR-199a-5p	Up-regulated	Rat	Maubach et al., 2011	ER stress	Up-regulated	Human hepatocyte line	Thapsigargin and deoxycholic acid	Dai et al., 2013
miR-30a	Up-regulated	Rat	Ji et al., 2009	ER stress	Down-regulated	Neonatal rat ventricular cells and rat aorta vascular smooth muscle cells	H_2O_2	Chen et al., 2014
miR-122	Down-regulated	Rat	Guo et al., 2009b	ER stress	Down-regulated	Huh7, HepG2 cell lines	Thapsigargin	Yang et al., 2011
miR-30c-2*	Down-regulated	Rat	Ji et al., 2009	ER stress	Up-regulated	NIH-3T3 fibroblasts	Tunicamycin and thapsigargin	Byrd et al., 2012
miR-34a	Up-regulated	Rat	Chen et al., 2011	ER stress	Down-regulated	Mouse embryonic fibroblasts	Brefeldin A	Upton et al., 2012
miR-455	Up-regulated	Rat	Ji et al., 2009	ER stress	Down-regulated	Neonatal rat ventricular myocytes	Tunicamycin	Belmont et al., 2012
miR-181a	Up-regulated	Human HSC cell line	Zheng et al., 2015	ER stress	Down-regulated	Various cell lines	Thapsigargin treatment	Su et al., 2013

*MiRNAs which display an overlap in expression profile between activating HSCs and in specific stress responses are displayed in green, those with a contradictory expression profile are displayed in red. *Mature miRNA derived from the 5′ arm of the precursor RNA also known as passenger strand.*

stress, this normal balance fades by excessive production of pro-oxidants. Various types of ROS are known, such as the singlet molecular oxygen, hydrogen peroxide and the hydrogen radical, which all have a specific half-life and mechanism of action (Sies, 1991).

There are several possible sources of ROS in the cell. Mitochondria, the main site of oxygen consumption in aerobic cells, are the main producers of ROS derived mainly through the leakage of electrons and formation of superoxide (Guarente, 2008). Cytochrome P450 (CYP) acts in the detoxification of metabolic as well as xenobiotic compounds by means of oxidation (Aubert et al., 2011) making it also an important source of ROS. Specifically the form CYP2E1, which is highly expressed in hepatocytes, has been demonstrated to be a key source of ROS in the liver (Poli, 2000). Another major source of ROS in several cell types and HSCs is nicotinamide adenine dinucleotide phosphate-oxidase (NADPH oxidase) (De Minicis and Brenner, 2007; Sergey, 2011).

Oxidative stress and the subsequent decreased levels of anti-oxidants during liver fibrosis has been shown for a broad variety of etiologies (Poli, 2000). ROS are produced by various cell types, but it is thought that the major contributors of ROS production in this pathology are apoptotic hepatocytes. HSCs express a non-phagocytic form of NADPH oxidase, which presents a basal level of activity, producing constitutively low levels of ROS and increasing production upon different stimuli (Bataller et al., 2003). NADPH oxidase of HSCs is activated upon phagocytosis of these apoptotic bodies of hepatocytes (Shan-Shan et al., 2006). Furthermore, NADPH oxidase-generated ROS in HSCs is also induced by advanced glycation end-products (AGEs) which are products of a non-enzymatic reaction of sugars with molecules such as proteins, lipids and nucleic acids that accumulate in diseases related to the metabolic syndrome (Yan et al., 2010). Liver fibrosis is correlated with accumulation of systemic AGEs and ROS in HSCs has been show to participate during the development of liver diseases (Šebeková et al., 2002; Hyogo et al., 2007; Guimarães et al., 2010).

Activated Kupffer cells and neutrophils are also described as important producers of ROS during early stages of liver fibrosis (Kisseleva and Brenner, 2007). The most important result of oxidative stress is lipid peroxidation. As example, liver fibrosis caused by excessive alcohol intake leads to injury of the different liver cell types and consecutive excessive oxidation of polyunsaturated membrane lipids due to enhanced generation of ROS due to the elevated levels of cytochrome CYP2E1 (Nieto et al., 1999). The products of such lipid peroxidation could further catalyze the progression of fibrosis by activation of the production of collagen α2 (I) in HSCs in a paracrine manner (Bedossa et al., 1994). Furthermore, exposure of HSCs to ROS can promote their proliferation and invasiveness. It is thought that it would obtain these effects by an induction of MMP-2 expression, and the enhancement of MT1-MMP and TIMP-2 protein levels, in an ERK1/2 and PI3K dependent manner (Galli et al., 2005).

Several miRNAs have already been linked to the regulation of the oxidative stress pathway, including members of the miR-200 family. From this miRNA-family, especially miR-200c has been shown to display an increased expression after cellular exposure to H_2O_2. This miRNA would lead to down-regulation of zinc finger E-box binding homeobox 1 (Zfhx1a, aka Zeb1, or TCF8), a transcriptional repressor, both on mRNA and protein level, leading to cellular senescence and inhibition of cell proliferation. Interestingly, an inhibitory loop was found between miR-200c and Zeb1, as the promoter region of miR-200c contains two conserved Zeb1 binding sites (Magenta et al., 2011). MiR-200c can also regulate apoptosis, as it inhibits the translation of FAS associated phosphatase (FAP-1) mRNA. Decreased expression of FAP-1 leads to a greater sensitivity to CD95-mediated apoptosis (Schickel et al., 2010). Some of the other identified targets of miR-200c include Moesin (MSN), Fibronectin 1 (FN1), and Rho GTPase activating protein 19 (ARHGAP19), important regulators of the migratory and invasive capacity of cancer cells (Howe et al., 2011). Another miRNA associated with oxidative stress is miR-21. Cells exposed to ROS would up-regulate miR-21, which can directly interact with the 3'UTR of the programmed cell death 4 (PDCD4) gene, a known tumor suppressor and apoptosis-regulator, thereby preventing cell death. Oxidative stress mediated up-regulation of miR-21 can be induced by NF-κB activation through five NF-κB binding sites in the 5' miR-21 promoter region (Tu et al., 2014b; Wei et al., 2014). Up-regulation of miR-21 would be a down-stream effect of NADPH oxidase activity (Dattaroy et al., 2015), as this induces NF-κB translocation to the nucleus (Yao et al., 2007) and its subsequent binding to the miR-21 promotor (Sheedy et al., 2010). This enhanced expression of miR-21 also leads to a suppression of SMAD7 expression and therefore favors assembly of SMAD2/3-SMAD4 heterodimers, a crucial event in the pro-fibrogenic TGF-β signaling pathway (Dattaroy et al., 2015).

A potential link in oxidative stress-induced HSC activation could be represented by miR-200a, which is down-regulated during the process of liver fibrosis in rat, and in TGF-β1-mediated activation of a rat HSC cell line (Sun et al., 2014). MiR-200a also regulates proliferation of these activating HSCs, shown by an accumulation of cells in the G0/G1 phase upon miR-200a overexpression. Targets of miR-200a include pro-fibrogenic factors TGF-β2 and β-catenin (Sun et al., 2014). Another important miRNA-200a target gene is Kelch-like ECH-associated protein 1 (Keap1), which negatively regulates the stability of nuclear factor-erythroid-2-related factor 2 (Nrf2), a known regulator of the expression of antioxidants involved in the protection against oxidative damage (Yang et al., 2014). While no information is available for miR-200c, in rat, miR-200a seems to be down-regulated upon HSC activation while during liver fibrosis progression in human and mouse, miR-200a and miR-200b undergo a significant up-regulation (Murakami et al., 2011). This is in line with the up-regulation in expression of the miR-200 family after induction of oxidative stress in mouse fibroblasts where miR-200a can target p38α mitogen-activated protein kinase (MAPK) (Mateescu et al., 2011), which is downstream of the oxidative stress stimulus, and leads to an inhibition of cell division (Kurata, 2000). Despite opposing expression patterns observed in different species, the involvement of miR-200a in both HSC activation and oxidative stress response is clear. It is therefore tempting to speculate that miR-200a could participate in the anti-oxidant response of HSCs during liver injury.

Endoplasmic Reticulum Stress Regulated miRNAs

The generation of mediators that lead to a perturbation of the ER homeostasis can be evoked by various stimuli associated with the initiation or progression of the liver fibrosis process, such as repeated cycles of ischemia and reperfusion due to distorted hepatic flow, genetic mutations of proteins involved in ER constitution and function, excessive exposure to certain drugs (paracetamol, ethanol), obesity-linked enhanced presence of lipids, and viral infections (HCV, HBV). These stimuli can lead to oxidative stress, formation of protein aggregates, altered membrane lipid-composition, and hyperhomocysteinemia with resulting N-homocysteinylation, all leading to the dysfunction of the ER, and accumulation of unfolded and misfolded proteins (Malhi and Kaufman, 2011). Cells will try to counteract this accumulation of misfolded proteins by diverse mechanisms such as the unfolded protein response (UPR). The activation of the UPR pathway, due to ER-resident stress sensors such as ATF-6, IRE1, and PERK (Asselah et al., 2010), will lead to an enhanced and more stringent folding and degradation of proteins in the ER, and an overall diminishment of protein synthesis. When the UPR fails to diminish the ER stress, the cells go into apoptosis. Persistent ER stress has several consequences including the excessive energy depletion due to the enhanced utilization of energy for translocation of misfolded proteins; ASK1/JNK mediated signaling leading to activation of caspases, and the activation of the pro-apoptotic pathway of CHOP/GADD153 transcription factor, which all direct the cell toward apoptosis (Xu et al., 2005). It will also lead to the release of the stored calcium in the ER, which affects mitochondria; moreover it will lead to the induction of oxidative stress, activation of the pro-inflammatory NF-κB pathway and apoptosis of the cell. ER stress will also lead to translocation and activation of SREBP, causing an enhanced synthesis of lipids such as fatty acids and cholesterol, and an enhanced cellular uptake of lipoproteins (Ji and Kaplowitz, 2006; Ji, 2008).

Cultured HSCs, which are known to be relatively apoptosis-insensitive, have been shown to undergo apoptosis in response to persistent ER stress due to an increase of the amount of intracellular calcium, and activation of JNK/p38 MAPK and Calpain/Caspase pathways (Huang et al., 2014b). Activation of the latter pathway can be explained by the decrease of Calpastatin expression, which works as an inhibitor of the pro-apoptotic Calpain. During the activation of HSCs, Calpastatin levels become elevated, leading to the desensitization of the HSCs toward apoptotic stimuli. ER-stress mediated decrease of Calpastatin expression can thus lead to higher Calpain levels, and consequent sensitization toward apoptotic stimuli (De Minicis et al., 2012). The fibrosis counteracting effect of ER stress was further supported by the decrease in α-SMA and Col1a1-expression in ER-stress responsive activating HSCs (Huang et al., 2014b). However, it is found that when HSCs are exposed to oxidative stress-induced ER stress, the UPR will lead to the up-regulation of different pathways leading to enhanced autophagy and consequent HSC activation in vitro (Hernandez-Gea et al., 2013). All described ER stress could thus be considered as a complex mechanism of fibrosis regulation, with a possible stimulatory role in HSC activation and a possible role in fibrosis resolution due to its pro-apoptotic effects in activated HSCs.

The role of miRNAs during ER-stress remains largely unknown. One of the miRNAs that has been studied in this process is miR-199a-5p, which displays an up-regulation in hepatocytes undergoing ER stress. This miRNA would have several ER-stress related targets including the chaperone protein GRP78 (which is also known as Bip and HSPA5), activating transcription factor 6 (ATF6), and inositol-requiring enzyme 1α (IRE1α), with the latter two being UPR transducers. As IRE1α activated ER stress can induce cell death, activation of miR-199a-5p, and thus subsequent down-regulation of IRE1α, would work as a rescue mechanism to prevent the induction of apoptosis. In silico target prediction identified DNA-damage regulated autophagy modulator 1 (DRAM1) and cyclin-dependent kinase inhibitor 1B (p27), both pro-apoptotic genes, as additional potential targets of miR-199a-5p, thus further underlining its pro-survival role (Dai et al., 2013). miR-199a-5p could also have some effect on cell proliferation, as it has been shown to target frizzles type 7 receptor (FZD7), and thus regulates the expression of its downstream genes including β-catenin, Jun, Cyclin D1, and Myc (Song et al., 2014). A second class of miRNAs linked with ER stress includes members of the miR-30 family, which are being down-regulated due to this specific stress responsive pathway. This miRNA family contains six members (from a to e), which contain all an identical seed sequence motif, but are located at different sites of the genome. GRP78 is targeted by miR-30a, which further underlines the importance of this miRNA in this stress response. Knockdown of miR-30 in cardiac cells identified ATF6, CHOP, and caspase-12 as indirect targets of this miRNA, thus revealing its role in regulation of cell death (Chen et al., 2014).

MiR-122 could perhaps represent a regulator of ER-stress-modulated HSC activation. MiR-122 is described as liver-specific and the most abundant miRNA in the liver (Lagos-Quintana et al., 2002). It has been shown that miR-122 is down-regulated in total liver samples during the progression of liver disease in mouse, rat (Li et al., 2013) and human (Padgett et al., 2009), and this down-regulation was furthermore observed in activating HSCs (Li et al., 2013). Overexpression of this miRNA in LX-2 cells leads to a decrease in cell proliferation and maturation of Col1a1, most likely through regulation of P4HA1 by miR-122. The expression of P4HA1 is up-regulated during fibrosis progression, and encodes a component of prolyl 4-hydroxylase, which is necessary for collagen maturation (Li et al., 2013). Overexpression of miR-122 in LX2 further identified FN1, which is involved in the assembly of collagen fibrils, and serum response factor (SRF) as direct targets, and confirmed its inhibitory effect on TGF-β-induced HSC activation (Zeng et al., 2015). Further target identification studies in hepatocytes identified mitogen-activated protein kinase kinase kinase 3 (MAP3K3), which plays a role in cell survival and proliferation, the intermediate filament vimentin, and HIF-1α (Csak et al., 2015). MiR-122 inhibition in hepatoma cells suggests a role in the UPR. Moreover its inhibition leads to an up-regulation of the 26S proteasome non-ATPase regulatory subunit 10 (PMSD10), which can enhance the protein folding-capacity and thus promoting recovery, by up-regulation of GRP78. MiR-122 would have this effect on PMSD10 in an indirect manner through targeting of cyclin dependent kinase 4 (CDk4) which interacts with PMSD10. Other miR-122 targets include the ER stress chaperones calreticulin (CALR), ER protein 29 (ERP29) and SET nuclear oncogene (SET), which help in the correct folding of malfunctional proteins (Yang et al., 2011). Taken together, even though miR-122 is not abundantly expressed in HSCs, it is tempting to speculate that down-regulation of miR-122 is involved in the UPR in HSCs.

Discussion

MiRNAs have been proposed as key regulators of gene expression and dysregulated patterns of miRNA expression were observed in various diseases (Tufekci et al., 2014), including the progression of liver fibrosis and cirrhosis (Wang et al., 2012; Xin et al., 2014). Studying miRNAs is very popular and raised a lot of expectations in their use as biomarkers for diseases and therapeutic interventions using miRNA mimics and antagomirs. Unfortunately, so far this has not turned out to be easy, partly because of their cell type-specific and species-specific activity and wide range of targets.

Diagnosis of liver fibrosis could be facilitated by identification of blood-circulating biomarkers representative for HSC activation, as the current golden standard for diagnosis remains the invasive and harmful liver biopsy (Piccinino et al., 1986; Friedman, 2003). Circulating miRNAs, both protein-bound and packaged into extracellular vesicles (Turchinovich et al., 2011), have been proposed as such a potential biomarker, and various research groups already tried to identify circulating miRNAs that could be linked with progression and regression of liver disease (Roderburg and Luedde, 2014). To date, this has not yet led to a diagnostic protocol that is used in clinic.

It is tempting to speculate that perhaps stress-responsive miRNAs of activating HSCs secreted in the blood could also be used as a liquid biopsy to document the stress present in the liver.

We discussed several miRNAs with a potential role in stress-mediated regulation of HSC activation. Experimental validation of these suggested links between stress-related miRNAs and HSCs should address a number of issues. First, are specific miRNAs dysregulated in HSCs in response to specific stress signals and does this lead to an imbalance of the cellular homeostasis and consequent HSC apoptosis or activation? *In vivo*, paracrine stimulation of quiescent HSCs by stress-undergoing surrounding cells is likely to create a warning for the quiescent cell, leading to its activation and reducing its responsiveness to more stress-signals. Secondly, responding to stress is necessary to counteract short term challenges to restore cell homeostasis. Thus the question is, whether there are miRNAs that specifically respond to prolonged stresses present in the fibrotic liver, and if so, could a targeted mimic/antagomir approach inhibit HSC activation or promote HSC apoptosis or inactivation?

In conclusion, HSC activation *in vivo* can be seen as a very complicated and multifactorial process in which hypoxia (Cannito et al., 2014), oxidative stress (Poli, 2000), and ER stress (Malhi and Kaufman, 2011) are surely involved. This suggests a potential role for stress-related miRNAs during HSC activation and disease development and opens perspectives for new therapeutic approaches.

Acknowledgments

IM is supported by a Fund of Scientific Research Flanders FWO-V post-doctoral fellowships (12N5415N LV) and JL and LV are supported by the Vrije Universiteit Brussel (GOA78, OZR1930).

References

Asselah, T., Bieche, I., Mansouri, A., Laurendeau, I., Cazals-Hatem, D., Feldmann, G., et al. (2010). *In vivo* hepatic endoplasmic reticulum stress in patients with chronic hepatitis C. *J. Pathol.* 221, 264–274. doi: 10.1002/path.2703

Aubert, J., Begriche, K., Knockaert, L., Robin, M. A., and Fromenty, B. (2011). Increased expression of cytochrome P450 2E1 in nonalcoholic fatty liver disease: mechanisms and pathophysiological role. *Clin. Res. Hepatol. Gastroenterol.* 35, 630–637. doi: 10.1016/j.clinre.2011.04.015

Babar, I. A., Slack, F. J., and Weidhaas, J. B. (2008). miRNA modulation of the cellular stress response. *Future Oncol.* 4, 289–298. doi: 10.2217/14796694.4.2.289

Bagga, S., Bracht, J., Hunter, S., Massirer, K., Holtz, J., Eachus, R., et al. (2005). Regulation by let-7 and lin-4 miRNAs results in target mRNA degradation. *Cell* 122, 553–563. doi: 10.1016/j.cell.2005.07.031

Bai, R., Zhao, A. Q., Zhao, Z. Q., Liu, W. L., and Jian, D. M. (2015). MicroRNA-195 induced apoptosis in hypoxic chondrocytes by targeting hypoxia-inducible factor 1 alpha. *Eur. Rev. Med. Pharmacol. Sci.* 19, 545–551.

Bartel, D. P., and Chen, C. Z. (2004). Micromanagers of gene expression: the potentially widespread influence of metazoan microRNAs. *Nat. Rev. Genet.* 5, 396–400. doi: 10.1038/nrg1328

Bataller, R., Schwabe, R. F., Choi, Y. H., Yang, L., Paik, Y. H., Lindquist, J., et al. (2003). NADPH oxidase signal transduces angiotensin II in hepatic stellate cells and is critical in hepatic fibrosis. *J. Clin. Invest.* 112, 1383–1394. doi: 10.1172/JCI18212

Bedossa, P., Houglum, K., Trautwein, C., Holstege, A., and Chojkier, M. (1994). Stimulation of collagen alpha 1(I) gene expression is associated with lipid peroxidation in hepatocellular injury: a link to tissue fibrosis? *Hepatology* 19, 1262–1271. doi: 10.1002/hep.1840190527

Belmont, P. J., Chen, W. J., Thuerauf, D. J., and Glembotski, C. C. (2012). Regulation of microRNA expression in the heart by the ATF6 branch of the ER stress response. *J. Mol. Cell. Cardiol.* 52, 1176–1182. doi: 10.1016/j.yjmcc.2012.01.017

Bernstein, E., Caudy, A. A., Hammond, S. M., and Hannon, G. J. (2001). Role for a bidentate ribonuclease in the initiation step of RNA interference. *Nature* 409, 363–366. doi: 10.1038/35053110

Byrd, A. E., Aragon, I. V., and Brewer, J. W. (2012). MicroRNA-30c-2* limits expression of proadaptive factor XBP1 in the unfolded protein response. *J. Cell Biol.* 196, 689–698. doi: 10.1083/jcb.201201077

Cannito, S., Paternostro, C., Busletta, C., Bocca, C., Colombatto, S., Miglietta, A., et al. (2014). Hypoxia, hypoxia-inducible factors and fibrogenesis in chronic liver diseases. *Histol. Histopathol.* 29, 33–44.

Chaudhry, M. A., Omaruddin, R. A., Brumbaugh, C. D., Tariq, M. A., and Pourmand, N. (2013). Identification of radiation-induced microRNA transcriptome by next-generation massively parallel sequencing. *J. Radiat. Res.* 54, 808–822. doi: 10.1093/jrr/rrt014

Chen, C., Wu, C. Q., Zhang, Z. Q., Yao, D. K., and Zhu, L. (2011). Loss of expression of miR-335 is implicated in hepatic stellate cell migration and activation. *Exp. Cell Res.* 317, 1714–1725. doi: 10.1016/j.yexcr.2011.05.001

Chen, M., Ma, G., Yue, Y., Wei, Y., Li, Q., Tong, Z., et al. (2014). Downregulation of the miR-30 family microRNAs contributes to endoplasmic reticulum stress in cardiac muscle and vascular smooth muscle cells. *Int. J. Cardiol.* 173, 65–73. doi: 10.1016/j.ijcard.2014.02.007

Coll, M., Taghdouini, A. E., Perea, L., Mannaerts, I., Vila-Casadesús, M., Blaya, D., et al. (2015). Integrative miRNA and gene expression profiling analysis of human quiescent hepatic stellate cells. *Sci. Rep.* 5:11549. doi: 10.1038/srep11549

Copple, B. L., Bai, S., Burgoon, L. D., and Moon, J. O. (2011). Hypoxia-inducible factor-1alpha regulates the expression of genes in hypoxic hepatic stellate cells important for collagen deposition and angiogenesis. *Liver Int.* 31, 230–244. doi: 10.1111/j.1478-3231.2010.02347.x

Copple, B. L., Roth, R. A., and Ganey, P. E. (2006). Anticoagulation and inhibition of nitric oxide synthase influence hepatic hypoxia after monocrotaline exposure. *Toxicology* 225, 128–137. doi: 10.1016/j.tox.2006.05.016

Csak, T., Bala, S., Lippai, D., Satishchandran, A., Catalano, D., Kodys, K., et al. (2015). microRNA-122 regulates hypoxia-inducible factor-1 and vimentin in hepatocytes and correlates with fibrosis in diet-induced steatohepatitis. *Liver Int.* 35, 532–541. doi: 10.1111/liv.12633

Dai, B. H., Geng, L., Wang, Y., Sui, C. J., Xie, F., Shen, R. X., et al. (2013). microRNA-199a-5p protects hepatocytes from bile acid-induced sustained endoplasmic reticulum stress. *Cell Death Dis.* 4, e604. doi: 10.1038/cddis.2013.134

Dattaroy, D., Pourhoseini, S., Das, S., Alhasson, F., Seth, R. K., Nagarkatti, M., et al. (2015). Micro-RNA 21 inhibition of SMAD7 enhances fibrogenesis via leptin-mediated NADPH oxidase in experimental and human nonalcoholic steatohepatitis. *Am. J. Physiol. Gastrointest. Liver Physiol.* 308, G298–G312. doi: 10.1152/ajpgi.00346.2014

De Minicis, S., and Brenner, D. A. (2007). NOX in liver fibrosis. *Arch. Biochem. Biophys.* 462, 266–272. doi: 10.1016/j.abb.2007.04.016

De Minicis, S., Candelaresi, C., Agostinelli, L., Taffetani, S., Saccomanno, S., Rychlicki, C., et al. (2012). Endoplasmic Reticulum stress induces hepatic stellate cell apoptosis and contributes to fibrosis resolution. *Liver Int.* 32, 1574–1584. doi: 10.1111/j.1478-3231.2012.02860.x

De Minicis, S., Seki, E., Uchinami, H., Kluwe, J., Zhang, Y., Brenner, D. A., et al. (2007). Gene expression profiles during hepatic stellate cell activation in culture and *in vivo. Gastroenterology* 132, 1937–1946. doi: 10.1053/j.gastro.2007.02.033

Fasanaro, P., Greco, S., Lorenzi, M., Pescatori, M., Brioschi, M., Kulshreshtha, R., et al. (2009). An integrated approach for experimental target identification of hypoxia-induced miR-210. *J. Biol. Chem.* 284, 35134–35143. doi: 10.1074/jbc.M109.052779

Feng, X., Tan, W., Cheng, S., Wang, H., Ye, S., Yu, C., et al. (2015). Upregulation of microRNA-126 in hepatic stellate cells may affect pathogenesis of liver fibrosis through the NF-kappaB pathway. *DNA Cell Biol.* 34, 470–480. doi: 10.1089/dna.2014.2760

Forsythe, J. A., Jiang, B. H., Iyer, N. V., Agani, F., Leung, S. W., Koos, R. D., et al. (1996). Activation of vascular endothelial growth factor gene transcription by hypoxia-inducible factor 1. *Mol. Cell. Biol.* 16, 4604–4613.

Friedman, S. L. (2003). Liver fibrosis – from bench to bedside. *J. Hepatol.* 38, 38–53. doi: 10.1016/S0168-8278(02)00429-4

Galli, A., Svegliati-Baroni, G., Ceni, E., Milani, S., Ridolfi, F., Salzano, R., et al. (2005). Oxidative stress stimulates proliferation and invasiveness of hepatic stellate cells via a MMP2-mediated mechanism. *Hepatology* 41, 1074–1084. doi: 10.1002/hep.20683

Giannakakis, A., Sandaltzopoulos, R., Greshock, J., Liang, S., Huang, J., Hasegawa, K., et al. (2008). miR-210 links hypoxia with cell cycle regulation and is deleted in human epithelial ovarian cancer. *Cancer Biol. Ther.* 7, 255–264. doi: 10.4161/cbt.7.2.5297

Gregory, R. I., Chendrimada, T. P., Cooch, N., and Shiekhattar, R. (2005). Human RISC couples microRNA biogenesis and posttranscriptional gene silencing. *Cell* 123, 631–640. doi: 10.1016/j.cell.2005.10.022

Gregory, R. I., Yan, K. P., Amuthan, G., Chendrimada, T., Doratotaj, B., Cooch, N., et al. (2004). The microprocessor complex mediates the genesis of microRNAs. *Nature* 432, 235–240. doi: 10.1038/nature03120

Guarente, L. (2008). Mitochondria–a nexus for aging, calorie restriction, and sirtuins? *Cell* 132, 171–176. doi: 10.1016/j.cell.2008.01.007

Guimarães, E. L. M., Empsen, C., Geerts, A., and van Grunsven, L. A. (2010). Advanced glycation end products induce production of reactive oxygen species via the activation of NADPH oxidase in murine hepatic stellate cells. *J. Hepatol.* 52, 389–397. doi: 10.1016/j.jhep.2009.12.007

Guo, C. J., Pan, Q., Cheng, T., Jiang, B., Chen, G. Y., and Li, D. G. (2009a). Changes in microRNAs associated with hepatic stellate cell activation status identify signaling pathways. *FEBS J.* 276, 5163–5176. doi: 10.1111/j.1742-4658.2009.07213.x

Guo, C. J., Pan, Q., Jiang, B., Chen, G. Y., and Li, D. G. (2009c). Effects of upregulated expression of microRNA-16 on biological properties of culture-activated hepatic stellate cells. *Apoptosis* 14, 1331–1340. doi: 10.1007/s10495-009-0401-3

Guo, C. J., Pan, Q., Li, D. G., Sun, H., and Liu, B. W. (2009b). miR-15b and miR-16 are implicated in activation of the rat hepatic stellate cell: an essential role for apoptosis. *J. Hepatol.* 50, 766–778. doi: 10.1016/j.jhep.2008.11.025

Ha, M., Pang, M., Agarwal, V., and Chen, Z. J. (2008). Interspecies regulation of microRNAs and their targets. *Biochim. Biophys. Acta* 1779, 735–742. doi: 10.1016/j.bbagrm.2008.03.004

He, Y., Huang, C., Sun, X., Long, X. R., Lv, X. W., and Li, J. (2012b). MicroRNA-146a modulates TGF-beta1-induced hepatic stellate cell proliferation by targeting SMAD4. *Cell. Signal.* 24, 1923–1930. doi: 10.1016/j.cellsig.2012.06.003

He, Y., Huang, C., Zhang, S.-P., Sun, X., Long, X.-R., and Li, J. (2012a). The potential of microRNAs in liver fibrosis. *Cell. Signal.* 24, 2268–2272. doi: 10.1016/j.cellsig.2012.07.023

Hebert, C., Norris, K., Scheper, M. A., Nikitakis, N., and Sauk, J. J. (2007). High mobility group A2 is a target for miRNA-98 in head and neck squamous cell carcinoma. *Mol. Cancer* 6, 5. doi: 10.1186/1476-4598-6-5

Hernandez-Gea, V., Hilscher, M., Rozenfeld, R., Lim, M. P., Nieto, N., Werner, S., et al. (2013). Endoplasmic reticulum stress induces fibrogenic activity in hepatic stellate cells through autophagy. *J. Hepatol.* 59, 98–104. doi: 10.1016/j.jhep.2013.02.016

Howe, E. N., Cochrane, D. R., and Richer, J. K. (2011). Targets of miR-200c mediate suppression of cell motility and anoikis resistance. *Breast Cancer Res.* 13, R45. doi: 10.1186/bcr2867

Hu, J., Chen, C., Liu, Q., Liu, B., Song, C., Zhu, S., et al. (2015). The role of miR-31/FIH1 pathway in TGFbeta-induced liver fibrosis. *Clin. Sci.* 129, 305–317. doi: 10.1042/CS20140012

Hua, Z., Lv, Q., Ye, W., Wong, C. K., Cai, G., Gu, D., et al. (2006). MiRNA-directed regulation of VEGF and other angiogenic factors under hypoxia. *PLoS ONE* 1:e116. doi: 10.1371/journal.pone.0000116

Huang, J., Yu, X., Fries, J. W., Zhang, L., and Odenthal, M. (2014a). MicroRNA function in the profibrogenic interplay upon chronic liver disease. *Int. J. Mol. Sci.* 15, 9360–9371. doi: 10.3390/ijms15069360

Huang, X., Ding, L., Bennewith, K. L., Tong, R. T., Welford, S. M., Ang, K. K., et al. (2009). Hypoxia-inducible mir-210 regulates normoxic gene expression involved in tumor initiation. *Mol. Cell* 35, 856–867. doi: 10.1016/j.molcel.2009.09.006

Huang, Y., Li, X., Wang, Y., Wang, H., Huang, C., and Li, J. (2014b). Endoplasmic reticulum stress-induced hepatic stellate cell apoptosis through calcium-mediated JNK/P38 MAPK and Calpain/Caspase-12 pathways. *Mol. Cell. Biochem.* 394, 1–12. doi: 10.1007/s11010-014-2073-8

Hyogo, H., Yamagishi, S.-i., Iwamoto, K., Arihiro, K., Takeuchi, M., Sato, T., et al. and Tazuma, S. (2007). Elevated levels of serum advanced glycation end products in patients with non-alcoholic steatohepatitis. *J. Gastroenterol. Hepatol.* 22, 1112–1119. doi: 10.1111/j.1440-1746.2007.04943.x

Iizuka, M., Ogawa, T., Enomoto, M., Motoyama, H., Yoshizato, K., Ikeda, K., et al. (2012). Induction of microRNA-214-5p in human and rodent liver fibrosis. *Fibrogenesis Tissue Repair* 5, 12. doi: 10.1186/1755-1536-5-12

Ji, C. (2008). Dissection of endoplasmic reticulum stress signaling in alcoholic and non-alcoholic liver injury. *J. Gastroenterol. Hepatol.* 23(Suppl. 1), S16–S24. doi: 10.1111/j.1440-1746.2007.05276.x

Ji, C., and Kaplowitz, N. (2006). ER stress: can the liver cope? *J. Hepatol.* 45, 321–333. doi: 10.1016/j.jhep.2006.06.004

Ji, J., Zhang, J., Huang, G., Qian, J., Wang, X., and Mei, S. (2009). Over-expressed microRNA-27a and 27b influence fat accumulation and cell proliferation during rat hepatic stellate cell activation. *FEBS Lett.* 583, 759–766. doi: 10.1016/j.febslet.2009.01.034

Jiang, B. H., Semenza, G. L., Bauer, C., and Marti, H. H. (1996). Hypoxia-inducible factor 1 levels vary exponentially over a physiologically relevant range of O2 tension. *Am. J. Physiol.* 271, C1172–C1180.

Jiang, F., Parsons, C. J., and Stefanovic, B. (2006). Gene expression profile of quiescent and activated rat hepatic stellate cells implicates Wnt signaling pathway in activation. *J. Hepatol.* 45, 401–409. doi: 10.1016/j.jhep.2006.03.016

Jiang, W., Kong, L., Ni, Q., Lu, Y., Ding, W., Liu, G., et al. (2014). miR-146a ameliorates liver ischemia/reperfusion injury by suppressing IRAK1 and TRAF6. *PLoS ONE* 9:e101530. doi: 10.1371/journal.pone.0101530

Kim, H. W., Haider, H. K., Jiang, S., and Ashraf, M. (2009). Ischemic preconditioning augments survival of stem cells via miR-210 expression by targeting caspase-8-associated protein 2. *J. Biol. Chem.* 284, 33161–33168. doi: 10.1074/jbc.M109.020925

Kisseleva, T., and Brenner, D. A. (2007). Role of hepatic stellate cells in fibrogenesis and the reversal of fibrosis. *J. Gastroenterol. Hepatol.* 22(Suppl. 1), S73–S78. doi: 10.1111/j.1440-1746.2006.04658.x

Kisseleva, T., and Brenner, D. A. (2013). Inactivation of myofibroblasts during regression of liver fibrosis. *Cell Cycle* 12, 381–382. doi: 10.4161/cc.23549

Kulshreshtha, R., Ferracin, M., Wojcik, S. E., Garzon, R., Alder, H., Agosto-Perez, F. J., et al. (2007). A microRNA signature of hypoxia. *Mol. Cell. Biol.* 27, 1859–1867. doi: 10.1128/MCB.01395-06

Šebeková, K. N., Kupèová, V., Schinzel, R., and Heidland, A. (2002). Markedly elevated levels of plasma advanced glycation end products in patients with liver cirrhosis – amelioration by liver transplantation. *J. Hepatol.* 36, 66–71. doi: 10.1016/S0168-8278(01)00232-X

Kurata, S. (2000). Selective activation of p38 MAPK cascade and mitotic arrest caused by low level oxidative stress. *J. Biol. Chem.* 275, 23413–23416. doi: 10.1074/jbc.C000308200

Kwiecinski, M., Elfimova, N., Noetel, A., Tox, U., Steffen, H. M., Hacker, U., et al. (2012). Expression of platelet-derived growth factor-C and insulin-like growth factor I in hepatic stellate cells is inhibited by miR-29. *Lab. Invest.* 92, 978–987. doi: 10.1038/labinvest.2012.70

Kwiecinski, M., Noetel, A., Elfimova, N., Trebicka, J., Schievenbusch, S., Strack, I., et al. (2011). Hepatocyte growth factor (HGF) inhibits collagen I and IV synthesis in hepatic stellate cells by miRNA-29 induction. *PLoS ONE* 6:e24568. doi: 10.1371/journal.pone.0024568

Lagos-Quintana, M., Rauhut, R., Yalcin, A., Meyer, J., Lendeckel, W., and Tuschl, T. (2002). Identification of tissue-specific microRNAs from mouse. *Curr. Biol.* 12, 735–739. doi: 10.1016/S0960-9822(02)00809-6

Lakner, A. M., Steuerwald, N. M., Walling, T. L., Ghosh, S., Li, T., McKillop, I. H., et al. (2012). Inhibitory effects of microRNA 19b in hepatic stellate cell-mediated fibrogenesis. *Hepatology* 56, 300–310. doi: 10.1002/hep.25613

Lee, H. J. (2013). Exceptional stories of microRNAs. *Exp. Biol. Med.* 238, 339–343. doi: 10.1258/ebm.2012.012251

Lee, Y., Ahn, C., Han, J., Choi, H., Kim, J., Yim, J., et al. (2003). The nuclear RNase III Drosha initiates microRNA processing. *Nature* 425, 415–419. doi: 10.1038/nature01957

Leung, A. K., and Sharp, P. A. (2010). MicroRNA functions in stress responses. *Mol. Cell* 40, 205–215. doi: 10.1016/j.molcel.2010.09.027

Li, J., Ghazwani, M., Zhang, Y., Lu, J., Li, J., Fan, J., et al. (2013). miR-122 regulates collagen production via targeting hepatic stellate cells and suppressing P4HA1 expression. *J. Hepatol.* 58, 522–528. doi: 10.1016/j.jhep.2012.11.011

Li, X., Wang, Y., Wang, H., Huang, C., Huang, Y., and Li, J. (2015). Endoplasmic reticulum stress is the crossroads of autophagy, inflammation, and apoptosis signaling pathways and participates in liver fibrosis. *Inflamm. Res.* 64, 1–7. doi: 10.1007/s00011-014-0772-y

Liu, C. J., Tsai, M. M., Hung, P. S., Kao, S. Y., Liu, T. Y., Wu, K. J., et al. (2010). miR-31 ablates expression of the HIF regulatory factor FIH to activate the HIF pathway in head and neck carcinoma. *Cancer Res.* 70, 1635–1644. doi: 10.1158/0008-5472.CAN-09-2291

Lund, E., Guttinger, S., Calado, A., Dahlberg, J. E., and Kutay, U. (2004). Nuclear export of microRNA precursors. *Science* 303, 95–98. doi: 10.1126/science.1090599

Magenta, A., Cencioni, C., Fasanaro, P., Zaccagnini, G., Greco, S., Sarra-Ferraris, G., et al. (2011). miR-200c is upregulated by oxidative stress and induces

endothelial cell apoptosis and senescence via ZEB1 inhibition. *Cell Death Differ.* 18, 1628–1639. doi: 10.1038/cdd.2011.42

Mahon, P. C., Hirota, K., and Semenza, G. L. (2001). FIH-1: a novel protein that interacts with HIF-1alpha and VHL to mediate repression of HIF-1 transcriptional activity. *Genes Dev.* 15, 2675–2686. doi: 10.1101/gad.924501

Malhi, H., and Kaufman, R. J. (2011). Endoplasmic reticulum stress in liver disease. *J. Hepatol.* 54, 795–809. doi: 10.1016/j.jhep.2010.11.005

Mateescu, B., Batista, L., Cardon, M., Gruosso, T., de Feraudy, Y., Mariani, O., et al. (2011). miR-141 and miR-200a act on ovarian tumorigenesis by controlling oxidative stress response. *Nat. Med.* 17, 1627–1635. doi: 10.1038/nm.2512

Maubach, G., Lim, M. C., Chen, J., Yang, H., and Zhuo, L. (2011). miRNA studies in *in vitro* and *in vivo* activated hepatic stellate cells. *World J. Gastroenterol.* 17, 2748–2773. doi: 10.3748/wjg.v17.i22

Mederacke, I., Hsu, C. C., Troeger, J. S., Huebener, P., Mu, X., Dapito, D. H., et al. (2013). Fate tracing reveals hepatic stellate cells as dominant contributors to liver fibrosis independent of its aetiology. *Nat. Commun.* 4, 2823. doi: 10.1038/ncomms3823

Moon, J. O., Welch, T. P., Gonzalez, F. J., and Copple, B. L. (2009). Reduced liver fibrosis in hypoxia-inducible factor-1alpha-deficient mice. *Am. J. Physiol. Gastrointest. Liver Physiol.* 296, G582–G592. doi: 10.1152/ajpgi.90368.2008

Murakami, Y., Toyoda, H., Tanaka, M., Kuroda, M., Harada, Y., Matsuda, F., et al. (2011). The progression of liver fibrosis is related with overexpression of the miR-199 and 200 families. *PLoS ONE* 6:e16081. doi: 10.1371/journal.pone.0016081

Nath, B., and Szabo, G. (2012). Hypoxia and hypoxia inducible factors: diverse roles in liver diseases. *Hepatology* 55, 622–633. doi: 10.1002/hep.25497

Nieto, N., Friedman, S. L., Greenwel, P., and Cederbaum, A. I. (1999). CYP2E1-mediated oxidative stress induces collagen type, I., expression in rat hepatic stellate cells. *Hepatology* 30, 987–996. doi: 10.1002/hep.510300433

Orban, T. I., and Izaurralde, E. (2005). Decay of mRNAs targeted by RISC requires XRN1, the Ski complex, and the exosome. *RNA* 11, 459–469. doi: 10.1261/rna.7231505

Padgett, K. A., Lan, R. Y., Leung, P. C., Lleo, A., Dawson, K., Pfeiff, J., et al. (2009). Primary biliary cirrhosis is associated with altered hepatic microRNA expression. *J. Autoimmun.* 32, 246–253. doi: 10.1016/j.jaut.2009.02.022

Parola, M., and Robino, G. (2001). Oxidative stress-related molecules and liver fibrosis. *J. Hepatol.* 35, 297–306. doi: 10.1016/S0168-8278(01)00142-8

Paternostro, C., David, E., Novo, E., and Parola, M. (2010). Hypoxia, angiogenesis and liver fibrogenesis in the progression of chronic liver diseases. *World J. Gastroenterol.* 16, 281–288. doi: 10.3748/wjg.v16.i3.281

Piccinino, F., Sagnelli, E., Pasquale, G., and Giusti, G. (1986). Complications following percutaneous liver biopsy. A multicentre retrospective study on 68,276 biopsies. *J. Hepatol.* 2, 165–173. doi: 10.1016/S0168-8278(86)80075-7

Pillai, R. S., Bhattacharyya, S. N., Artus, C. G., Zoller, T., Cougot, N., Basyuk, E., et al. (2005). Inhibition of translational initiation by Let-7 MicroRNA in human cells. *Science* 309, 1573–1576. doi: 10.1126/science.1115079

Poli, G. (2000). Pathogenesis of liver fibrosis: role of oxidative stress. *Mol. Aspects Med.* 21, 49–98. doi: 10.1016/S0098-2997(00)00004-2

Roderburg, C., and Luedde, T. (2014). Circulating microRNAs as markers of liver inflammation, fibrosis and cancer. *J. Hepatol.* 61, 1434–1437. doi: 10.1016/j.jhep.2014.07.017

Roderburg, C., Urban, G. W., Bettermann, K., Vucur, M., Zimmermann, H., Schmidt, S., et al. (2011). Micro-RNA profiling reveals a role for miR-29 in human and murine liver fibrosis. *Hepatology* 53, 209–218. doi: 10.1002/hep.23922

Rosmorduc, O., Wendum, D., Corpechot, C., Galy, B., Sebbagh, N., Raleigh, J., et al. (1999). Hepatocellular hypoxia-induced vascular endothelial growth factor expression and angiogenesis in experimental biliary cirrhosis. *Am. J. Pathol.* 155, 1065–1073. doi: 10.1016/S0002-9440(10)65209-1

Schickel, R., Park, S. M., Murmann, A. E., and Peter, M. E. (2010). miR-200c regulates induction of apoptosis through CD95 by targeting FAP-1. *Mol. Cell* 38, 908–915. doi: 10.1016/j.molcel.2010.05.018

Schuppan, D., and Afdhal, N. H. (2008). Liver cirrhosis. *Lancet* 371, 838–851. doi: 10.1016/S0140-6736(08)60383-9

Sekiya, Y., Ogawa, T., Yoshizato, K., Ikeda, K., and Kawada, N. (2011). Suppression of hepatic stellate cell activation by microRNA-29b. *Biochem. Biophys. Res. Commun.* 412, 74–79. doi: 10.1016/j.bbrc.2011.07.041

Semenza, G. L. (2007). Hypoxia-inducible factor 1 (HIF-1) pathway. *Sci. STKE* 2007:cm8. doi: 10.1126/stke.4072007cm8

Sergey, D. (2011). Cross talk between mitochondria and NADPH oxidases. *Free Radic. Biol. Med.* 51, 1289–1301. doi: 10.1016/j.freeradbiomed.2011.06.033

Shan-Shan, Z., Joy, X. J., Jian, W., Charles, H., Scott, L. F., Mark, A. Z., et al. (2006). Phagocytosis of apoptotic bodies by hepatic stellate cells induces NADPH oxidase and is associated with liver fibrosis *in vivo*. *Hepatology* 43, 435–443. doi: 10.1002/hep.21093

Sheedy, F. J., E., Palsson-McDermott, Hennessy, E. J., Martin, C., O'Leary, J. J., Ruan, Q., et al. (2010). Negative regulation of TLR4 via targeting of the proinflammatory tumor suppressor PDCD4 by the microRNA miR-21. *Nat. Immunol.* 11, 141–147. doi: 10.1038/ni.1828

Shi, Y. F., Fong, C. C., Zhang, Q., Cheung, P. Y., Tzang, C. H., Wu, R. S., et al. (2007). Hypoxia induces the activation of human hepatic stellate cells LX-2 through TGF-beta signaling pathway. *FEBS Lett.* 581, 203–210. doi: 10.1016/j.febslet.2006.12.010

Sies, H. (1991). Oxidative stress: from basic research to clinical application. *Am. J. Med.* 91, 31S–38S. doi: 10.1016/0002-9343(91)90281-2

Song, J., Gao, L., Yang, G., Tang, S., Xie, H., Wang, Y., et al. (2014). MiR-199a regulates cell proliferation and survival by targeting FZD7. *PLoS ONE* 9:e110074. doi: 10.1371/journal.pone.0110074

Su, S. F., Chang, Y. W., Andreu-Vieyra, C., Fang, J. Y., Yang, Z., Han, B., et al. (2013). miR-30d, miR-181a and miR-199a-5p cooperatively suppress the endoplasmic reticulum chaperone and signaling regulator GRP78 in cancer. *Oncogene* 32, 4694–4701. doi: 10.1038/onc.2012.483

Sun, X., He, Y., Ma, T. T., Huang, C., Zhang, L., and Li, J. (2014). Participation of miR-200a in TGF-beta1-mediated hepatic stellate cell activation. *Mol. Cell. Biochem.* 388, 11–23. doi: 10.1007/s11010-013-1895-0

Tu, H., Sun, H., Lin, Y., Ding, J., Nan, K., Li, Z., et al. (2014b). Oxidative stress upregulates PDCD4 expression in patients with gastric cancer via miR-21. *Curr. Pharm. Des.* 20, 1917–1923. doi: 10.2174/13816128113199990547

Tu, X., Zhang, H., Zhang, J., Zhao, S., Zheng, X., Zhang, Z., et al. (2014a). MicroRNA-101 suppresses liver fibrosis by targeting the TGFbeta signalling pathway. *J. Pathol.* 234, 46–59. doi: 10.1002/path.4373

Tufekci, K. U., Oner, M. G., Meuwissen, R. L., and Genc, S. (2014). The role of microRNAs in human diseases. *Methods Mol. Biol.* 1107, 33–50. doi: 10.1007/978-1-62703-748-8_3

Turchinovich, A., Weiz, L., Langheinz, A., and Burwinkel, B. (2011). Characterization of extracellular circulating microRNA. *Nucleic Acids Res.* 39, 7223–7233. doi: 10.1093/nar/gkr254

Upton, J. P., Wang, L., Han, D., Wang, E. S., Huskey, N. E., Lim, L., et al. (2012). IRE1alpha cleaves select microRNAs during ER stress to derepress translation of proapoptotic Caspase-2. *Science* 338, 818–822. doi: 10.1126/science.1226191

Wallace, K., Burt, A. D., and Wright, M. C. (2008). Liver fibrosis. *Biochem. J.* 411, 1–18. doi: 10.1042/BJ20071570

Wang, X. W., Heegaard, N. H., and Orum, H. (2012). MicroRNAs in liver disease. *Gastroenterology* 142, 1431–1443. doi: 10.1053/j.gastro.2012.04.007

Wang, Y., Huang, Y., Guan, F., Xiao, Y., Deng, J., Chen, H., et al. (2013). Hypoxia-inducible factor-1alpha and MAPK co-regulate activation of hepatic stellate cells upon hypoxia stimulation. *PLoS ONE* 8:e74051. doi: 10.1371/journal.pone.0074051

Wei, C., Li, L., Kim, I. K., Sun, P., and Gupta, S. (2014). NF-kappaB mediated miR-21 regulation in cardiomyocytes apoptosis under oxidative stress. *Free Radic. Res.* 48, 282–291. doi: 10.3109/10715762.2013.865839

Wightman, B., Ha, I., and Ruvkun, G. (1993). Posttranscriptional regulation of the heterochronic gene lin-14 by lin-4 mediates temporal pattern formation in *C. elegans*. *Cell* 75, 855–862. doi: 10.1016/0092-8674(93)90530-4

Xin, X., Zhang, Y., Liu, X., Xin, H., Cao, Y., and Geng, M. (2014). MicroRNA in hepatic fibrosis and cirrhosis. *Front. Biosci.* 19, 1418–1424. doi: 10.2741/4292

Xu, C., Bailly-Maitre, B., and Reed, J. C. (2005). Endoplasmic reticulum stress: cell life and death decisions. *J. Clin. Invest.* 115, 2656–2664. doi: 10.1172/JCI26373

Xu, Y., Zhou, M., Wang, J., Zhao, Y., Li, S., Zhou, B., et al. (2014). Role of microRNA-27a in down-regulation of angiogenic factor AGGF1 under hypoxia associated with high-grade bladder urothelial carcinoma. *Biochim. Biophys. Acta* 1842, 712–725. doi: 10.1016/j.bbadis.2014.01.007

Yan, S. F., Ramasamy, R., and Schmidt, A. M. (2010). The RAGE axis: a fundamental mechanism signaling danger to the vulnerable vasculature. *Circ. Res.* 106, 842–853. doi: 10.1161/CIRCRESAHA.109.212217

Yang, F., Zhang, L., Wang, F., Wang, Y., Huo, X. S., Yin, Y. X., et al. (2011). Modulation of the unfolded protein response is the core of microRNA-122-involved sensitivity to chemotherapy in hepatocellular carcinoma. *Neoplasia* 13, 590–600. doi: 10.1593/neo.11422

Yang, J. J., Tao, H., Hu, W., Liu, L. P., Shi, K. H., Deng, Z. Y., et al. (2014). MicroRNA-200a controls Nrf2 activation by target Keap1 in hepatic stellate cell proliferation and fibrosis. *Cell. Signal.* 26, 2381–2389. doi: 10.1016/j.cellsig.2014.07.016

Yao, H., Yang, S. R., Kode, A., Rajendrasozhan, S., Caito, S., Adenuga, D., et al. (2007). Redox regulation of lung inflammation: role of NADPH oxidase and NF-kappaB signalling. *Biochem. Soc. Trans.* 35, 1151–1155. doi: 10.1042/BST0351151

Yoon, C., Kim, D., Kim, S., Park, G. B., Hur, D. Y., Yang, J. W., et al. (2014). MiR-9 regulates the post-transcriptional level of VEGF165a by targeting SRPK-1 in ARPE-19 cells. *Graefes Arch. Clin. Exp. Ophthalmol.* 252, 1369–1376. doi: 10.1007/s00417-014-2698-z

Zeng, C., Wang, Y. L., Xie, C., Sang, Y., Li, T. J., Zhang, M., et al. (2015). Identification of a novel TGF-beta-miR-122-fibronectin 1/serum response factor signaling cascade and its implication in hepatic fibrogenesis. *Oncotarget* 6, 12224–12233. doi: 10.1074/jbc.M111.314922

Zhang, L., Zhou, M., Qin, G., Weintraub, N. L., and Tang, Y. (2014). MiR-92a regulates viability and angiogenesis of endothelial cells under oxidative stress. *Biochem. Biophys. Res. Commun.* 446, 952–958. doi: 10.1016/j.bbrc.2014.03.035

Zhang, Y., Wu, L., Wang, Y., Zhang, M., Li, L., Zhu, D., et al. (2012). Protective role of estrogen-induced miRNA-29 expression in carbon tetrachloride-induced mouse liver injury. *J. Biol. Chem.* 287, 14851–14862. doi: 10.1074/jbc.M111.314922

Zhang, Z., Sun, H., Dai, H., Walsh, R. M., Imakura, M., Schelter, J., et al. (2009). MicroRNA miR-210 modulates cellular response to hypoxia through the MYC antagonist MNT. *Cell Cycle* 8, 2756–2768. doi: 10.4161/cc.8.17.9387

Zhao, X., Wang, K., Liao, Y., Zeng, Q., Li, Y., Hu, F., et al. (2015). MicroRNA-101a inhibits cardiac fibrosis induced by hypoxia via targeting TGFbetaRI on cardiac fibroblasts. *Cell. Physiol. Biochem.* 35, 213–226. doi: 10.1159/000369689

Zheng, J., Wu, C., Xu, Z., Xia, P., Dong, P., Chen, B., et al. (2015). Hepatic stellate cell is activated by microRNA-181b via PTEN/Akt pathway. *Mol. Cell. Biochem.* 398, 1–9. doi: 10.1007/s11010-014-2199-8

8

Circular RNA CREBBP Suppresses Hepatic Fibrosis *Via* Targeting the hsa-miR-1291/ LEFTY2 Axis

Ya-Ru Yang[1†], Shuang Hu[2,3†], Fang-Tian Bu[2,3], Hao Li[2,3], Cheng Huang[2,3], Xiao-Ming Meng[2,3], Lei Zhang[2,3], Xiong-Wen Lv[2,3] and Jun Li[2,3]*

[1]Department of Clinical Pharmacology, Second Hospital of Anhui Medical University, Hefei, China, [2]Inflammation and Immune Mediated Diseases Laboratory of Anhui Province, School of Pharmacy, Anhui Institute of Innovative Drugs, Anhui Medical University, Hefei, China, [3]Institute for Liver Diseases of Anhui Medical University, Anhui Medical University, Hefei, China

*Correspondence:
Jun Li
ayefyyy@126.com

[†]These authors have contributed equally to this work

CircRNAs (circRNAs) are commonly dysregulated in a variety of human diseases and are involved in the development and progression of cancer. However, the role of circRNAs in hepatic fibrosis (HF) is still unclear. Our previous high throughput screen revealed changes in many circRNAs in mice with carbon tetrachloride (CCl4)-induced HF. For example, circCREBBP was significantly down-regulated in primary hepatic stellate cells (HSCs) and liver tissue of HF mice induced by CCl4 compared to those in the vehicle group. Overexpression of circCREBBP with AAV8-circCREBBP *in vivo* prevented CCl4-induced HF worsening by reducing serum alanine aminotransferase (ALT) and aspartate aminotransferase (AST) contents, liver hydroxyproline levels, collagen deposition, and levels of pro-fibrosis genes and pro-inflammatory cytokines. Furthermore, *in vitro* function loss and function gain analysis showed that circCREBBP inhibited HSCs activation and proliferation. Mechanically, circCREBBP acts as a sponge for hsa-miR-1291 and subsequently promotes LEFTY2 expression. In conclusion, our current results reveal a novel mechanism by which circCREBBP alleviates liver fibrosis by targeting the hsa-miR-1291/LEFTY2 axis, and also suggest that circCREBBP may be a potential biomarker for heart failure.

Keywords: biomarker, HF, circCREBBP, miR-17-5p, hsa-miR-1291, LEFTY2

INTRODUCTION

Chronic liver disease is a global health problem due to its high incidence and limited treatment options worldwide. They can be caused by a variety of causes, including communicable and non-communicable diseases (Poilil Surendran et al., 2017). Fibrosis is the final common pathway of chronic liver disease of various etiologies, including toxic damage, viral infections, autoimmune conditions, and metabolic and genetic diseases (Campana and Iredale, 2017). Hepatic stellate cells (HSCs) receive the signals secreted by the damaged liver cells and immune cells to transdifferentiate into activated myofibroblast-like cells characterized by the expression of α-smooth muscle actin (α-SMA) and the production of extracellular matrix (ECM) (He et al., 2015). Excessive accumulation of ECM distorts the liver architecture by forming fibrous scars, and hepatocytes are replaced by abundant ECM (Chen et al., 2020). Although hepatic fibrosis (HF) is reversible, if left untreated, it will develop into cirrhosis, which is an important cause of death and disease (Zhao et al., 2019). Thus, understanding the mechanisms of HF regression will lead to the identification of new therapeutic targets for HF.

Noncoding RNAs, represented by circRNAs, microRNAs and lncRNAs, lack the ability to transform into proteins and account for nearly 98% of the transcriptome (Zhang et al., 2017). As important

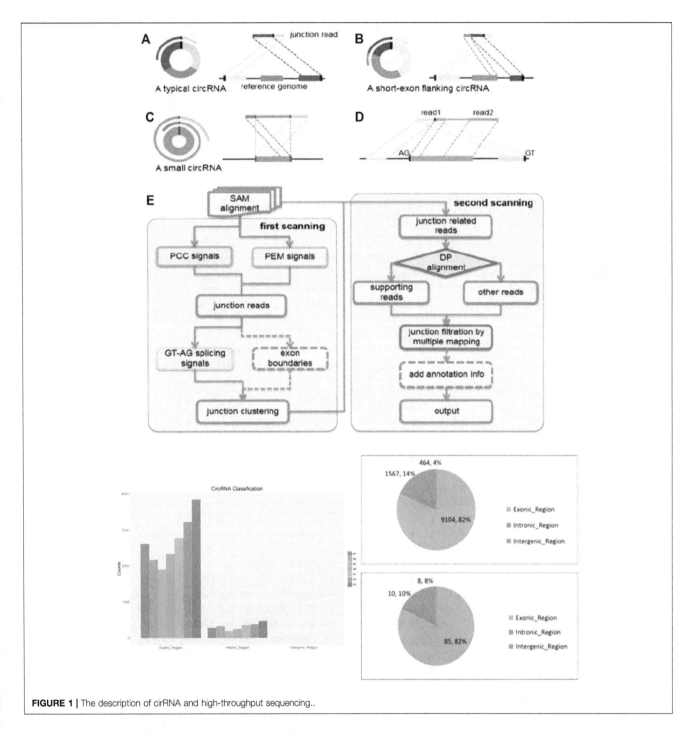

FIGURE 1 | The description of cirRNA and high-throughput sequencing..

members of ncRNAs, circRNAs have attracted extensive attention in recent decades. Different from linear RNA, circRNA is a covalently linked single stranded RNA without 5 'and 3′ ends (**Figure 1**) (Xia et al., 2019). In recent years, next-generation sequencing and bioinformatics technologies have revealed the vital role of circRNAs in the diagnosis and prognosis of various diseases (Pamudurti et al., 2017). Therefore, circRNAs may play a key role in gene regulation, including acting as microRNA "sponges" to isolate and inhibit miRNA targeting messenger RNAs, regulating RNA polymerase II (Pol-II) transcription and splicing of parent genes (Wang et al., 2019). Of note, various circRNAs are dysregulated in pathophysiological processes and regulate gene expression through miRNA sponges, known as the competitive endogenous RNA (ceRNA) mechanism (Zheng et al., 2016). In recent years, our research group has devoted itself to the effects of ncRNAs in liver diseases. Although there are reports that several circRNAs are dysregulated in HF (Zhou et al., 2018; Zhu et al., 2018), the expression profile, biological functions and molecular mechanisms of circRNAs in HF, especially HSC, are still unclear and require further research.

In this study, we analyzed the expression profile of circRNAs, miRNAs and mRNAs in HF patients in order to identify biomarkers associated with the course of HF and regression to pathological stage. We found a novel dysregulated circRNAs circCREBBP (hsa_circ_0007673, mmu_circ_0006288) which derived from CREB-binding protein n (CREBBP, hereafter CBP) gene locus. Interestingly, circCREBBP significantly downregulated in the HF compared with healthy controls. Functionally, the overexpression of circCREBBP inhibits the activation of HSCs, reduces the transdifferentiation of myofibroblasts, alleviates liver fibrosis injury in mice, and reduces collagen deposition, suggesting that circCREBBP has an anti-fibrosis effect in HF. In terms of mechanism, we confirmed that circCREBBP, as a miRNA sponge, binds to hsa-miR-1291 and regulates the expression of left-right determinant cluster 2 (LEFTY2), revealing that circCREBBP/ha-miR-1291/LEFTY2 axis plays a key role in HSCs activation and HF. Therefore, our study suggests that circCREBBP may be a promising biomarker for the treatment of HF. To our knowledge, this is the first report to investigate the expression profile, regulatory function and mechanism of circCREBBP in HF.

METHODS

Animal Experiments

C57BL/6 male mice (6–8 weeks old) were purchased from Anhui Medical University, and all animal experiments were approved by the Animal Care and Use Committee of Anhui Medical University (Hefei, China). HF was induced using intraperitoneal injection of 10% CCl4 (CCl4:olive oil = 1:4; dose, 0.001 ml/g/mouse biweekly for 4 weeks). Mice in the vehicle group were injected with the same volume of olive oil for the same time. All animal procedures were approved by the Animal Experiment Ethics Committee of Anhui Medical University.

CircRNA Expression Profile Analysis

RNA Extraction and Quality Control Total RNA was prepared from HSCs using the Mirneasy microkit (QIAGEN, Germany). The RNA was then purified using the RNA Clean XP kit (Beckman Coulter, United States) and the RNA-enzyme free DNA asome (Qiagen, Germany). Next, RNA count and integrity were measured using Nanodrop 2000 (Thermo Fisher Scientific, MA) and Agilent BioAnalyzer 2100 (Agilent Technologies, United States), respectively. Library Preparation and High-throughput Sequencing ® The RNA-Seq library was constructed using the Stranged Total RNA Sample Preparation Kit (Illumina, United States) as per the manufacturer's instructions. The RNA-Seq library was then quantified with a ® 2.0 fluorimeter using Qubit (Life Technologies, United States). In addition, the RNA-Seq library was validated by the Agilent 2100 BioAnalyzer (Agilent Technologies, Inc., United States). Insertion size and molar concentration were measured, and clusters were generated using CBOT. The libraries were diluted to 10 μm and sequenced in the Illumina HiSeq 2500 system (Illumina, United States). The library was constructed,

Antibodies	Dilution ratio	Species
α-SMA	1:2000	Rabbit
COL1A1	1:1000	Rabbit
Cyclin D1	1:500	Rabbit
c-Myc	1:1000	Rabbit
CDK4	1:500	Mouse
LEFTY2	1:1000	Rabbit

validated and sequenced by OriginBiotech (Shanghai, China) (**Table 1**).

Data Analysis

FASTQC1 software (v. 0.11.3) Test the quality control of RNA sequence readings. In addition to the known Illumina TruSeq adapter sequences, error reads, and ribosomal RNA reads, the RNA sequences were first pruned using SEQTK2 software. The deleted fragment was then mapped to the mouse reference genome using BWA-Mem software (v.2.0.4). Furthermore, circRNA was predicted with circI software, matched with circBase and known circRNAs, and the count was normalized with SRPBM. The deleted gene fragment is also passed by Hisat2 (v. 2.0.4). Pull rod. 1.3.0) Perform pruning to read each gene count. In the Perl script, the gene count is standardized by the pruning mean (TMM) of the M value and the number of fragments per kilobase transcript (FPKM). The differentially expressed circRNAs (DECs) among the three groups were analyzed by EDGER software. The main inclusion criteria for Decs were FC≥2. CircRNAs were predicted by analyzing significantly disregulated circRNAs-miRNAs interactions according to Origin Biotech's custom software based on miRanda software.

Microarray Analysis

Affymetrix ® miRNA 4.0 Array (Affymetrix, United States) is used under the manufacturer's agreement. The FlashtagTM Biotin HSR Labeling Kit (Affymetrix) is used for poly (A) biotin labeling and hybridization. Next, the array and images were stained using a gene-chip hybridization cleaning and staining kit (Thermo Fisher, Inc., United States) and scanned to obtain the raw data. The miRNAs (DEMs) differentially expressed between HREE groups were identified by volcano map filtering and folding change filtering (Log2FCL >1). Two databases, TargetScan and IRANDA, were used to predict miRNAs targets, and common targets were obtained. Next, he used Venny to screen for intersections between the target gene and DEM. Pathway analysis was performed, followed by enrichment analysis based on genetic information from GO and KEGG pathways.

Analysis of the ceRNA Network

CircRNAs-miRNAs-mRNAs-cernet is constructed based on the negative regulatory relationship between differentially expressed miRNAs and their differentially expressed target genes mRNAs and circRNAs. Interactive CERNET is built using Cytoscape.

Human Liver Samples

All liver specimens were obtained from the First An Affiliated Hospital of Anhui Province (China City) from March 2016 to

TABLE 1 | Sequences of PCR primers.

circRNA ID	Product length	Forward	Reverse
hsa_circ_0072309	115	5′-GGAACGACAGGGGTTCAGTT-3′	5′-TCATCTGTGCAATGCAGTCAG-3′
hsa_circ_0023919	110	5′-CAGGTAGCAAGTACATGGGGA-3′	5′-ACCTGCTTGCAGCTGTAGAAT-3′
hsa_circ_0008267	89	5′-GTCAGTGGTGGAAGTGAGAC-3′	5′-TGTGTGTGATGTGTTGTCCT-3′
hsa_circ_0007637	100	5′-GGACTGAACACCGCACAGG-3′	5′-TCTCCTCCATTGGGTATCAGC-3′
hsa_circ_0006117	120	5′-CACTCCAGAAACTTTCCCTCCT-3′	5′-CAAATGACAATTTACCTGTGGTAGC-3′
hsa_circ_0003502	78	5′-TAGTGGGCATCTGTCTCATCTTG-3′	5′-GAGCATCCCTATGGAGAGCAG-3′
hsa_circ_0003441	105	5′-CAGTTCTTGGTGGTGAAGTGG-3′	5′-GACTTTGTCTGGAGAGCTTGT-3′

June 2019. The study was approved by the Biomedical Ethics Committee of Anhui Medical University. All patients and volunteers in this study were given written informed consent. Liver tissues were collected from 14 patients with liver fibrosis caused by hepatitis B virus (HBV) and hepatitis C virus (HCV) infection. Ten normal liver tissue samples were obtained from transplant donors. The samples were immediately frozen in liquid nitrogen, then stored at −80°C, and part of the tissue samples were fixed and embedded for pathological staining. Patient characteristics.

AAV2/8-Mediated Overexpression of circCREBBP in Mice

Luciferase-labelled specific liver tissue location of AAV2/8-mmu_circ_0006288 and vector were designed and synthesized by Hanbio Biotechnology (Shanghai, China). AAV2/8-mmu_circ_0006288 and vector (1 × 10 12 vg/ml), diluted in saline, were injected into the tail vein of mice, respectively. One week later, mouse HF model was established for 4 weeks after AAV2/8-mmu_circ_0006288 administration. Mice exposed to AAV2/8-mmu_circ_0006288 delivery were anaesthetized, effect of AAV2/8-mmu_circ_0006288 on liver tissue location was confirmed using an IVIS Lumina III Imaging System (Caliper Life Sciences, United States). For miR-Up-agomir treated mice, 1 week after HF modeling, mice received tail vein injection of miR-1291 agomir or NC agomir (10 mmol/kg, 4 times injections) synthesized by Genepharma (Shanghai, China). After administration, mice were sacrificed and liver tissue was fixed and paraffin-embedded or primary hepatocytes were isolated.

Histology and Immunohistochemistry

Paraffin-embedded liver tissue sections (4 μm) were immobilized with paraformaldehyde for H&E fixation, Sirius red staining and Masson staining have been described previously (Huang et al., 2019). The slides were scanned by an automated digital slide scanner (Pannoramic MIDI, 3DHISTECH, Hungary) and analyzed by CaseViewer software. The positive staining area was measured with IPWIN32 software.

DNA Sequencing

RNA was reverse-transcribed into cDNA using PrimeScript RT Master Mix (Takara, Japan). Polymerase chain reaction (PCR) was performed using a 2×Taq master mixture (Takara, Japan) in accordance with the manufacturer's protocol. PCR products were identified by DNA sequencer (ABI3730XL, United States).

TABLE 2 | Clinical characteristics of patients.

Parameters	Patients	Healthy donor
Case, n	4	3
Sex, n (%)		
Male	1(25.0%)	1(33.3%)
Female	3(75.0%)	2(66.7%)
Age, n (±SD)	62.7(±10.0)	65.0(±10.0)
Aetiology, n (%)		
Hepatocellular carcinoma		
	4	–
Hepatic cirrhosis		
Hepatic hemangioma	–	3
Others	0	–
HCC, n(%)		
With	4(100.0%)	–
Without	0(0.0%)	–
Serum ALT, U/L	39.5(±15.97)	16.5(±15.3)
Serum AST, U/L	42.0(±27.04)	21.5(±15.8)

Fluorescence *in situ* Hybridization

CircCREBBP and miR-1291 were hybridized *in situ* with a specific probe. A 5 'CY3 labeled miR-1291 probe and a 5′ FAM labeled probe were designed and synthesized, and the probe was linked to circCREBBP through the splicing junction. Hybridization analysis was performed using a fluorescence *in situ* hybridization kit (GenePharma, China) according to the manufacturer's protocol. Liver sections were processed and incubated with a probe at 37°C for 16 h. The nuclei were stained with DAPI. The signal was detected with an inverted fluorescence microscope (Olympus Japan IX83).

Cell Culture

LX-2 cells are a human immortalized HSC cell line that was cultured at 37°C in a humidified atmosphere of 5% CO_2 in Dulbecco modified Eagle medium (Gibco, United States) supplemented with 10% fetal bovine serum (Gibco, United States) and 1% penicillin/streptomycin.

Construction of Stable circCREBBP

The lentivirus circCREBBP and its vector were designed and constructed by Hanson Biotech (Shanghai) Co., Ltd. LX-2 cells were transfected with lentivirus circCREBBP or vector (multiple infection, MOI = 10).

circCREBBP Knockdown

Small interfering RNAs (siRNAs) of circCREBBP were synthesized to target the junction site of circCREBBP. Si-circCREBBP was

TABLE 3 | Comparison of hepatic fibrosis(HF) versus the control for the top 5 up-regulated and 5 down-regulated expression of circRNAs(FC ≥ 2.0, p < 0.05) sorted by their FC.

circRNA	Symbol	Log2FC	p-value	MRE1	MRE2	MRE3	MRE4	MRE5
Up regulation								
hsa_circ_0072437	ENSG00000151883(PARP8: poly(ADP-ribose) Polymerase family member 8 [Source:HGNC Symbol;Acc:HGNC:26124]),	3.194124543	0.039305686	hsa-mi R-638	hsa-mi R-6798 -5p	hsa-mi R-6791 -5p	hsa-mi R-596	hsa-mi R-671- 5p
hsa_circ_0001147	ENSG00000131051(RBM39 :RNA binding motif protein 39 [Source:HGNC Symbol;Acc:HGNC:15923]),	3.191561937	0.00442684	hsa-mi R-7109 -3p	hsa-mi R-6841 -3p	hsa-mi R-5196 -3p	hsa-mi R-4660	hsa-mi R-369- 5p
hsa_circ_0047086	ENSG00000158201(ABHD3: Abhydrolase domain Containing 3 [Source:HGNC Symbol;Acc:HGNC:18718]),	2.882623733	0.043746065	hsa-mi R-1301 -3p	hsa-mi R-5047	hsa-mi R-6736 -5p	hsa-mi R-3917	hsa-mi R-140- 5p
hsa_circ_0010117	ENSG00000065526(SPEN:s Pen family transcriptional repressor [Source:HGNC Symbol;Acc:HGNC:17575]),	2.619363616	0.022660121	hsa-mi R-6721 -5p	hsa-mi R-4763 -3p	hsa-mi R-4640 -5p	hsa-mi R-1207 -5p	hsa-mi R-6779 -5p
hsa_circ_0005325	ENSG00000126261(UBA2:u biquitin-like modifier [Source:HGNC Symbol;Acc:HGNC:30661]),	2.546078796	0.033936649	hsa-mi R-6859 -5p	hsa-mi R-509- 3-5p	hsa-mi R-302c -5p	hsa-mi R-6823 -5p	hsa-mi R-548a v-3p
Down regulation								
hsa_circ_0066631	ENSG00000057019(DCBLD 2:discoidin, CUB and LCCL domain containing 2 [Source:HGNC Symbol;Acc:HGNC:24627]),	−3.91682969	0.007456996	hsa-mi R-664b -3p	hsa-mi R-6874 -3p	hsa-mi R-6777 -3p	hsa-mi R-1266 -5p	hsa-mi R-7110 -3p
hsa_circ_0000647	ENSG00000140612(SEC11A :SEC11 homolog A, signal peptidase complex subunit [Source:HGNC	−3.094896056	0.045355691	hsa-mi R-3663 -3p	hsa-mi R-145-5p	hsa-mi R-4252	hsa-mi R-29a-3p	hsa-mi R-29c-3p
hsa_circ_0072547	ENSG00000062194(GPBP1: GC-rich promoter binding Protein 1 [Source:HGNC Symbol;Acc:HGNC:29520]),	−2.873901282	0.033122459	hsa-mi R-4646 -5p	hsa-mi R-5196 -5p	hsa-mi R-362- 5p	hsa-mi R-4686	hsa-mi R-4653 -5p
hsa_circ_0002663	ENSG00000189376(C8orf7 6:chromosome 8 open reading frame 76 [Source:HGNC Symbol;Acc:HGNC:25924]), ENSG00000259305(ZHX1-C 8orf76:ZHX1-C8orf76 Readthrough [Source:HGNC Symbol;Acc:HGNC:42975]),	−2.710010664	0.042511698	hsa-mi R-3135 b	hsa-mi R-6877 -3p	hsa-mi R-7109 -3p	hsa-mi R-615- 3p	hsa-mi R-6511 b-5p
hsa_circ_0074362	ENSG00000145819(ARHGA P26:Rho GTPase activating Protein 26 [Source:HGNC Symbol;Acc:HGNC:17073]),	−2.714094405	0.041240882	hsa-mi R-4436 b-5p	hsa-mi R-378a -5p	hsa-mi R-3614 -5p	hsa-mi R-2467 -3p	hsa-mi R-632

transfected into LX-2 cells using Lipofectamine rNAIMAX (Life Technologies, Inc.) according to the manufacturer's protocol. After transfection for 6 h, fresh medium was substituted for transfection for another 48 h. The silencing efficiency of circCREBBP was confirmed by qRT-PCR after transfection.

RNA Extraction and qRT-PCR

Total RNA was isolated using TRIzol reagent (Invitrogen, CA) according to the manufacturer's protocol (Yang et al., 2020). Concentration and quality of RNA were measured by NanoDrop 2000 (Thermo Fisher Scientific, MA), paired samples were adjusted to the similar concentration for used. Divergent primers were designed for circRNAs. qRT-PCR assay was performed using CFX96 RT-PCR system (Bio-Rad, CA) with SYBR Premix Ex Taq™ II (Takara, Japan).

Western Blotting

As mentioned earlier, Western blotting was performed using RIPA lysis buffer [39]. The same amount of protein was separated by SDS-PAGE electrophoresis, then transferred to

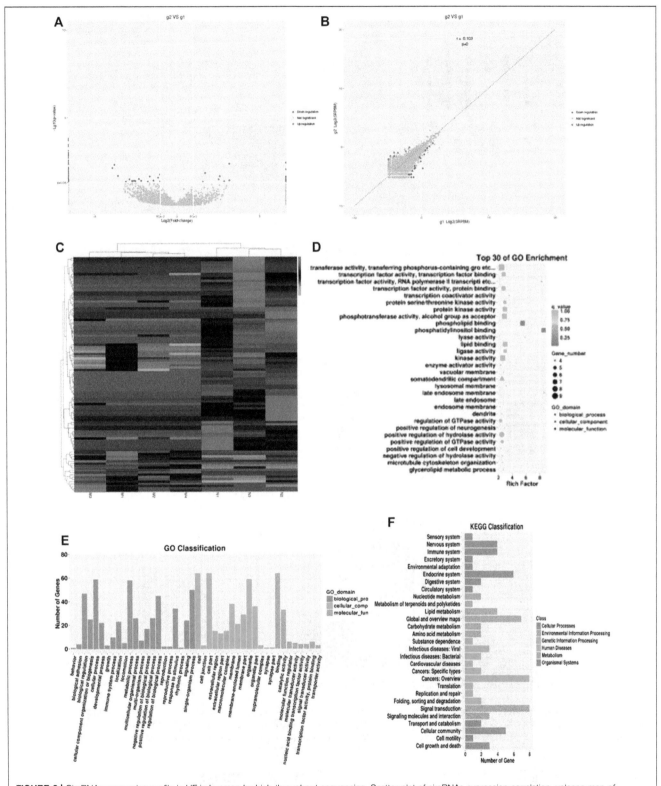

FIGURE 2 | CircRNAs expression profile in HF in huaman by high-throughput sequencing. Scatter plot of circRNAs expression correlation, volcano map of differentially expressed circRNAs and Heatmap among samples **(A–C)**. the scatter plot of GO enrichment of differentially expressed circRNAs parental gene **(D and E)**. the analysis results of KEGG pathway in differentially expressed circRNAs parental gene **(F)**.

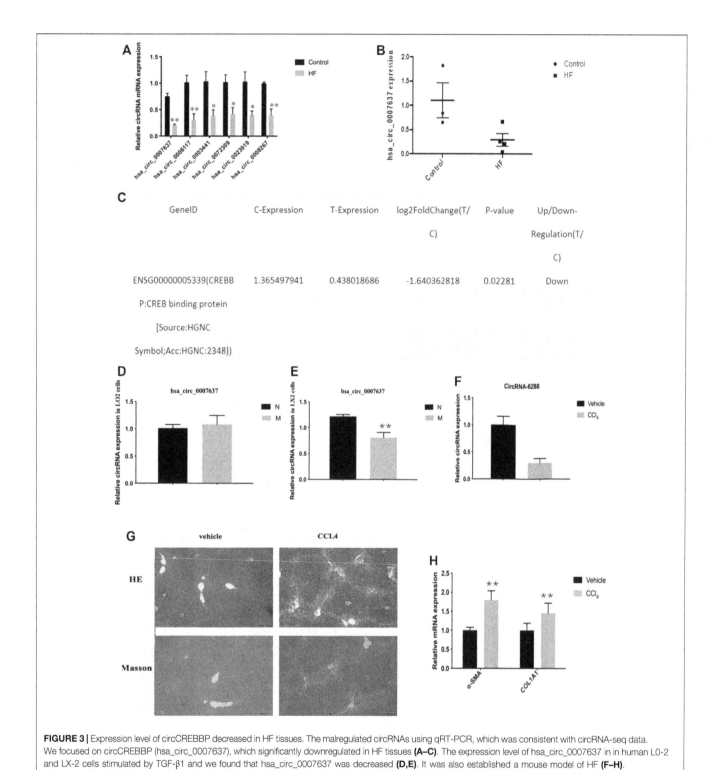

FIGURE 3 | Expression level of circCREBBP decreased in HF tissues. The malregulated circRNAs using qRT-PCR, which was consistent with circRNA-seq data. We focused on circCREBBP (hsa_circ_0007637), which significantly downregulated in HF tissues **(A–C)**. The expression level of hsa_circ_0007637 in in human L0-2 and LX-2 cells stimulated by TGF-β1 and we found that hsa_circ_0007637 was decreased **(D,E)**. It was also established a mouse model of HF **(F–H)**.

PVDF membrane in Malipoli, United States, and sealed. The bands were visualized using the Enhanced Chemiluminescence Detection System (Bio-Rad, CA), and then quantified using ImageJ software (NIH, Bethesda, United States) and standardized β-actin for internal control. The related antibodies information is following:

Statistical Analysis

Data collected in this study were presented as mean ± analyzed using one-way analysis of variance (ANOVA), followed by Newman-Keuls post facto test (Prism 5.0 GraphPad Software, Inc., San Diego, CA, United States).

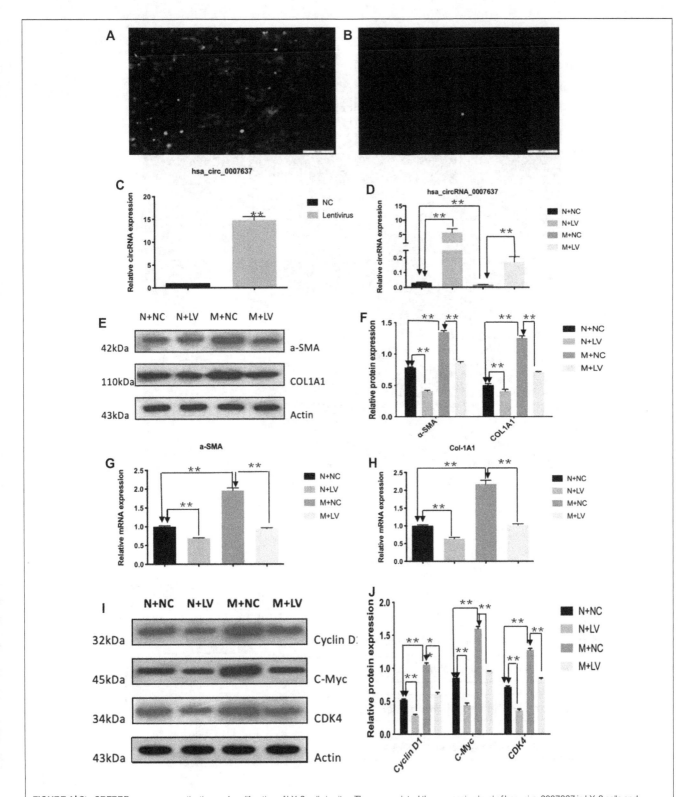

FIGURE 4 | CircCREBBP suppresses activation and proliferation of LX-2 cells in vitro. The up-regulated the expression level of hsa_circ_0007637 in LX-2 cells and the efficiency of overexpression hsa_circ_0007637 **(A–C)**. The up-regulated expression of circCREBBP subsequently decreased the mRNA and protein levels of α-SMA and Col1A1 **(D–H)**. CircCREBBP could arrest cycle and inhibit cell proliferation **(I,J)**.

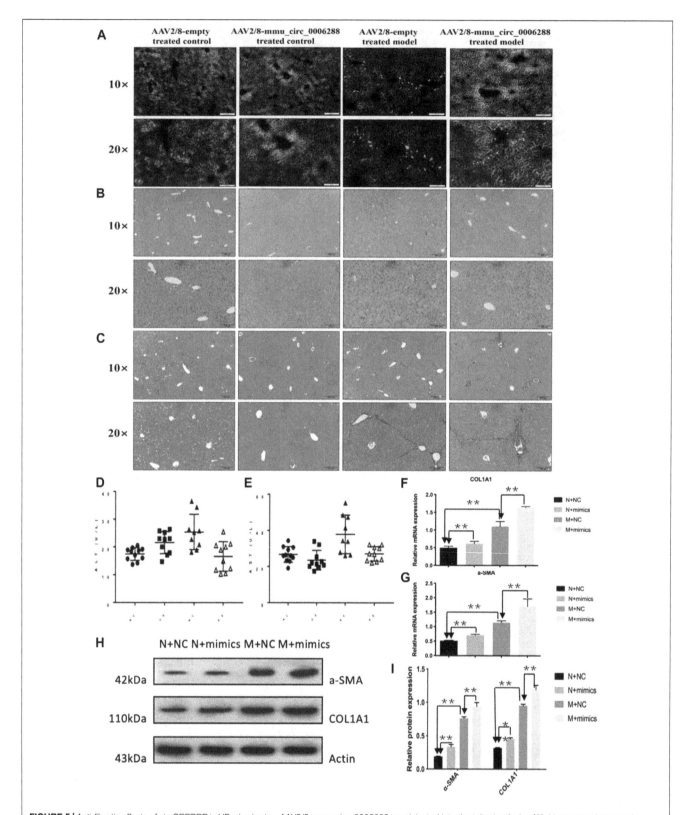

FIGURE 5 | Anti-fibrotic effects of circCREBBP in HF mice in vivo. AAV2/8-mmu_circ_0006288 was injected into the tail vein of mice **(A)**. Liver parenchyma and vascular architecture distortion, collagen deposition were consistently reduced in HF mice following AAV2/8-mmu-circ-0006288 administration **(B,C)**. The expression levels of ALT and AST in serum were reduced in AAV2/8-mmu-circ-0006288-treated HF mice **(D,E)**. The fibrosis factor (α-SMA and COL1A1) were down-regulated after circCREBBP was overexpressed **(F–I)**.

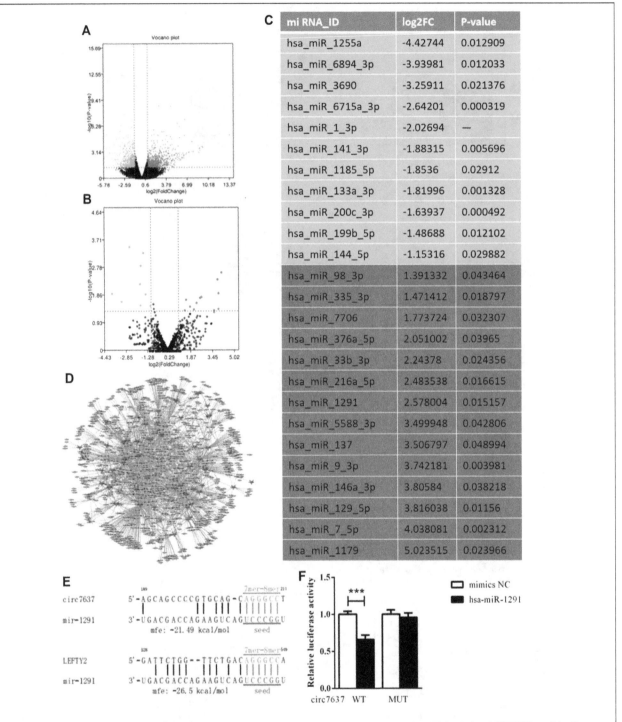

FIGURE 6 | Microarray analysis and identification of circCREBBP-hsa-miR-1291 connectivity. To assess the potential miRNAs bind to circCREBBP, and identify promising novel miRNAs relate to HF, miRNA expression profile in HF tissues was analyzed by microarray. Importantly, we found 14 miRNAs downregulated in HF mice, along with 11 miRNAs upregulated in HF mice **(A–C)**. Network based on the correlations between differentially expressed miRNAs and their differentially expressed circRNA targets was showed in a diagram **(D)**. Based on sequence pairing, binding sites of hsa-miR-1291 were identified within the circCREBBP sequences **(E,F)**.

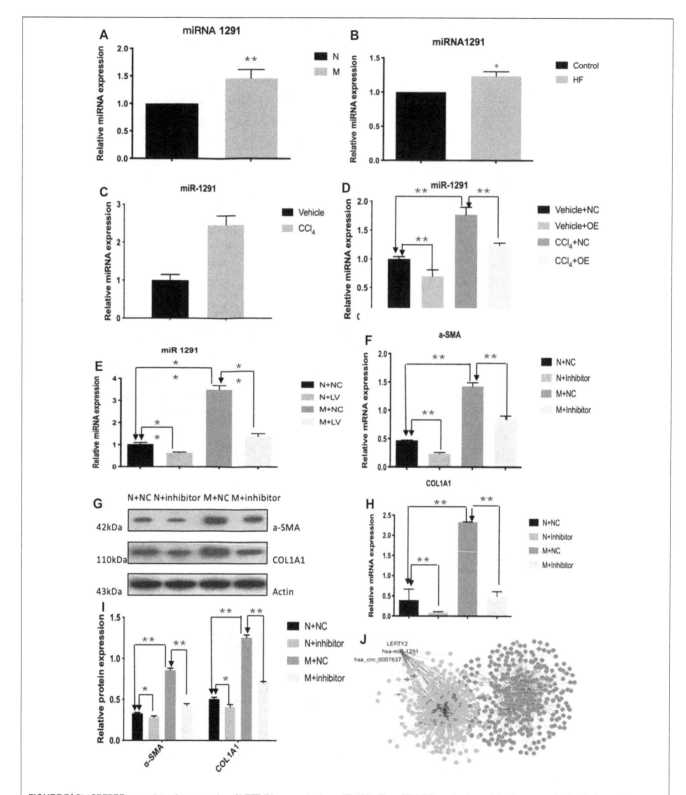

FIGURE 7 | CircCREBBP upregulates the expression of LEFTY2 by sponging hsa-miR-1291. The qRT-PCR results showed that the expression level of hsa-miR-1291 were up-regulated in TGF-β1-indcued LX-2 cells, HF patients and mouse tissues **(A–C)**. When circCREBBP expression was increased, hsa-miR-1291 expression level was down-regulated **(D,E)**. α-SMA and Col1A1 protein and mRNA expression levels in LX-2 cells transfected with over-expressed hsa-miRNA-1291 were decreased **(F–I)**. An interaction network of circRNAs-miRNAs-mRNAs was established based on the negative regulatory relationship between differentially expressed miRNAs and their differentially expressed target circRNAs and mRNAs **(J)**.

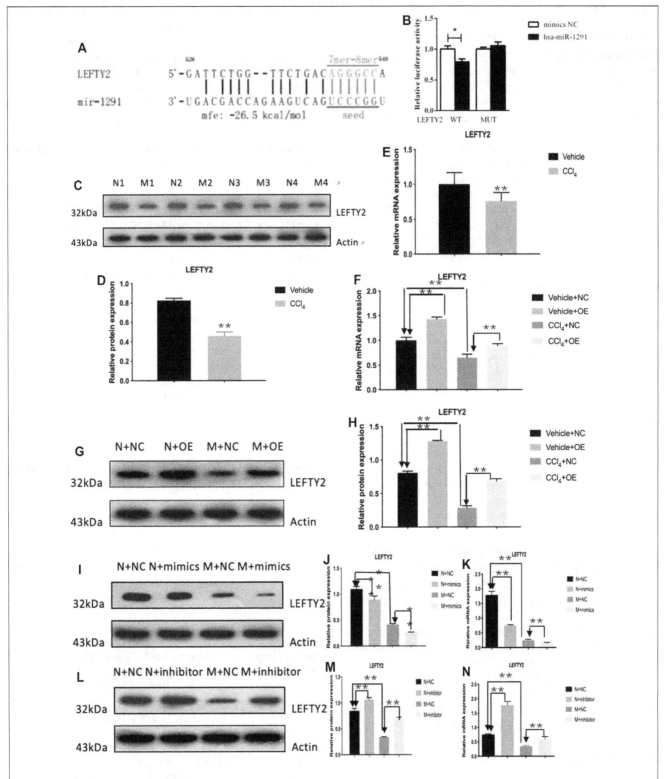

FIGURE 8 | LEFTY2 is one of the target genes of hsa-miR-1291 **(A,B)**. The expression level of LEFTY2 was down-regulated in HF mouse tissues **(C–E)**. The expression level of LEFTY2 was increased in AAV2/8-mmu_circ_0006288-treated HF mice **(F–H)**. When hsa-miRNA-1291 expression was increased or decreased, LEFTY2 expression level was down-regulated or up-regulated **(I–N)**.

RESULTS

CircRNAs Expression Profile in HF in Huaman by High-Throughput Sequencing

To investigate the expression profile of circRNAs involved in HF, HF tissues were analyzed by circular RNA high-throughput sequencing (Seq) (the clinical characteristics of patients were shown in **Table 2**). Results showed that 103 circRNAs were differentially expressed in HF tissues compared with non-HF tissues, and the expression levels of 18 circRNAs were up-regulated, 85 circRNAs expression levels were down-regulated in HF tissues (**Table 3**). Moreover, Scatter plot of circRNAs expression correlation, volcano map of differentially expressed circRNAs and Heatmap among samples were showed in **Figures 2A–C**. Meanwhile, the scatter plot of GO enrichment of differentially expressed circRNAs parental gene was showed in **Figures 2D,E** the analysis results of KEGG pathway in differentially expressed circRNAs parental gene were presented in **Figure 2F**.

Expression of circCREBBP Decreased in HF Tissues

Most circRNAs are obtained from exon regions of known protein-coding genes by unsplicing 28. By classifying circRNAs based on their expression intensity and screening for exon types, we identified malregulated circRNAs using qRT-PCR, which was consistent with circRNA-seq data. We focused on circCREBBP (hsa_circ_0007637), which significantly downregulated in HF tissues (**Figures 3A–C**). Additionally, we also detected the expression level of hsa_circ_0007637 in human L0-2 and LX-2 cells stimulated by TGF-β1 and we found that hsa_circ_0007637 was decrease (**Figures 3D,E**). Next, we also established a mouse model of HF (**Figures 3G,H**), suggested that the expression of circCREBBP is related to the pathology of HF, and its potential value as a diagnostic and prognostic indicator of HF.

circCREBBP Suppresses Activation and Proliferation of LX-2 Cells *in vitro*

To assess the functional roles of circCREBBP (hsa_circ_0007637) in LX-2 cells (a human HSC line with the key features of activated HSCs), loss-of-function and gain-of-function assays were performed, respectively. First, we up-regulated the expression level of hsa_circ_0007637 in LX-2 cells and the efficiency of overexpression hsa_circ_0007637 were shown in **Figures 4A–C**. Functionally, up-regulated expression of circCREBBP (**Figure 4D**) subsequently decreased the mRNA and protein levels of α-SMA and Col1A1 (**Figures 4E–H**). Moreover, up-regulated expression of circCREBBP could arrest cycle and inhibit cell proliferation (**Figures 4I,J**).

Anti-Fibrotic Effects of circCREBBP in HF Mice *in vivo*

Next, we further investigated the effects of circCREBBP (mmu_circ_0006288) on HF mice. We injected rAAV2/8-mmu_circ_0006288-eGFP into the tail vein of mice (**Figure 5A**). Functionally, liver parenchyma and vascular architecture distortion, collagen deposition were consistently reduced in HF mice following rAAV2/8-mmu_circ_0006288-eGFP administration (**Figures 5B,C**). Both expression levels of ALT and AST in serum were reduced in rAAV2/8-mmu_circ_0006288-eGFP-treated HF mice (**Figures 5D,E**). In addition, fibrosis factor (α-) was down-regulated in SMA and type I collagen after CIRCREBBP overexpression (**Figures 5F–I**). Taken together, these results suggest that liver specific raAV2/8-mmu \u circ\u 0006288-EGFP can significantly inhibit liver fibrosis injury and fibrosis marker expression in HF mice overexpressed with circCREBBP.

Microarray Analysis and Identification of circCREBBP-Hsa-miR-1291 Connectivity

A feature of circRNAs is acts as miRNAs sponges. To assess the potential miRNAs bind to circCREBBP, and identify promising novel miRNAs relate to HF, miRNA expression profile in HF tissues was analyzed by microarray. Importantly, we found 14 miRNAs downregulated in HF mice, along with 11 miRNAs upregulated in HF mice (**Figures 6A–C**). Network based on the correlations between differentially expressed miRNAs and their differentially expressed circRNA targets was showed in a diagram (**Figure 6D**). Based on sequence pairing, binding sites of hsa-miR-1291 were identified within the circCREBBP sequences (**Figures 6E,F**). Therefore, a focus was placed on the interaction between circCREBP and hsa-miR-1291 for further investigation.

circCREBBP Upregulates the Expression of LEFTY2 by Sponging Hsa-miR-1291

The qRT-PCR results showed that the expression level of hsa-miR-1291 were up-regulated in TGF-β1-indcued LX-2 cells, HF patients and mouse tissues (**Figures 7A–C**). When circCREBBP expression was increased, hsa-miR-1291 expression level was down-regulated (**Figures 7D,E**). Meanwhile, α-SMA and Col1A1 protein and mRNA expression levels in LX-2 cells transfected with over-expressed hsa-miRNA-1291 were decreased (**Figures 7F–I**). Next, an interaction network of circRNAs-miRNAs-mRNAs was established based on the negative regulatory relationship between differentially expressed miRNAs and their differentially expressed target circRNAs and mRNAs (**Figure 7J**). We found that LEFTY2 is one of the target genes of hsa-miR-1291. Binding sites of LEFTY2 were identified within the hsa-miRNA-1291 sequences (**Figures 8A,B**). Importantly, expression level of LEFTY2 was down-regulated in HF mouse tissues (**Figures 8C–E**). At the same time, expression level of LEFTY2 was increased in rAAV2/8-mmu_circ_0006288-eGFP-treated HF mice (**Figures 8F–H**). What's more, when hsa-miRNA-1291 expression was increased or decreased, LEFTY2 expression level was down-regulated or up-regulated (**Figures 8I–N**). These results demonstrated that circCREBBP acted as a sponge of hsa-miR-1291 to eliminate the effects of LEFTY2 on HF through circCREBBP/hsa-miR-1291/LEFTY2 axis.

DISCUSSION

CircRNA-seq showed that circCREBBP was significantly down-regulated in HF mice compared with the vector. CIRCREBBP continued to decline in patients with heart failure compared to healthy controls. Dysregulation of circCREBBP in patients with heart failure prompted us to investigate the functional role of circCREBBP (Jimenez-Castro et al., 2015). First, we identified the characteristics and stability of circCREBBP, which is derived from the CREBBP gene and is involved in the development of target protein 41 through specific ubiquitination and subsequent proteolysis. CREBBP is mutated and lost in human cancers and plays a tumor suppressor role in pathophysiological processes (Jia et al., 2018; Menke et al., 2018). In this study, the overexpression of circCREBBP significantly inhibited HSCs activation, reduced the transdifferentiation of myofibroblasts, alleviated hepatic fibrosis injury, reduced collagen deposition, and inhibited the expression of fibrosis factors. Taken together, these findings suggest that circCREBBP has an anti-fibrosis effect in HF, and that circCREBBP could be a potential biomarker for the treatment of HF.

CircRNAs containing multiple miRNA binding sites or miRNA response elements 15 act as miRNA sponges (Liu et al., 2019; Wang et al., 2020). Based on miRNA-mediated mRNA cleavage, circRNAs essentially regulate the expression of target genes. To evaluate miRNA candidate genes that may be associated with circCREBBP and associated with HF, we selected miRNAs targeted by circCREBBP that are malregulated in the development of liver fibrosis. Mechanically, circCREBBP plays a regulatory role by secreting miRNAs. Increased expression of hsa-miRNA-1291 has been reported to be associated with liver cancer and chronic hepatitis 42. In particular, we confirmed that hsa-miRNA-1291 expression is increased during liver fibrosis and that the expression pattern of hsa-miRNA-1291 is contrary to circCREBBP. In addition, the overexpression of circCREBBP directly reduced the level of hsa-miRNA-1291 in HSC. In addition, we confirmed that hSA-miRNA-1291 was bound to the 3'UTR of LEFTY2, and the expression of LEFTY2 was decreased and increased in liver fibrosis after the overexpression of circCREBBP. However, after increasing the level of hsa-miRNA-1291, the effect of circCREBBP on LEFTY2 was partially eliminated.

In conclusion, this study reveals a novel regulatory axis of circCREBBP/hsa-miRNA-1291/LEFTY2 in HF. We investigated the expression pattern, function and mechanism of circCREBBP in heart failure. We further confirmed the expression of circCREBBP in the fading stage of HF, but its mechanism remains unclear and needs further verification. In addition, circCREBBP provides a platform for candidate miRNA genes associated with liver or fibrosis, and the role of circCREBBP in the ceRNA mechanism remains to be studied.

AUTHOR CONTRIBUTIONS

All authors listed have made a substantial, direct, and intellectual contribution to the work and approved it for publication.

REFERENCES

Campana, L., and Iredale, J. P. (2017). Regression of Liver Fibrosis. *Semin. Liver Dis.* 37, 1–10. doi:10.1055/s-0036-1597816

Chen, X., Li, H. D., Bu, F. T., Li, X. F., Chen, Y., Zhu, S., et al. (2020). Circular RNA circFBXW4 Suppresses Hepatic Fibrosis via Targeting the miR-18b-3p/FBXW7 axis. *Theranostics* 10, 4851–4870. doi:10.7150/thno.42423

He, Y., Jin, L., Wang, J., Yan, Z., Chen, T., and Zhao, Y. (2015). Mechanisms of Fibrosis in Acute Liver Failure. *Liver Int.* 35, 1877–1885. doi:10.1111/liv.12731

Huang, X. Y., Huang, Z. L., Zhang, P. B., Huang, X. Y., Huang, J., Wang, H. C., et al. (2019). CircRNA-100338 Is Associated with mTOR Signaling Pathway and Poor Prognosis in Hepatocellular Carcinoma. *Front. Oncol.* 9, 392. doi:10.3389/fonc.2019.00392

Jia, D., Augert, A., Kim, D. W., Eastwood, E., Wu, N., Ibrahim, A. H., et al. (2018). Crebbp Loss Drives Small Cell Lung Cancer and Increases Sensitivity to HDAC Inhibition. *Cancer Discov.* 8, 1422–1437. doi:10.1158/2159-8290.CD-18-0385

Jiménez-Castro, M. B., Gracia-Sancho, J., and Peralta, C. (2015). Brain Death and Marginal Grafts in Liver Transplantation. *Cell Death Dis.* 6, e1777. doi:10.1038/cddis.2015.147

Liu, J., Song, S., Lin, S., Zhang, M., Du, Y., Zhang, D., et al. (2019). Circ-SERPINE2 Promotes the Development of Gastric Carcinoma by Sponging miR-375 and Modulating YWHAZ. *Cell Prolif.* 52, e12648. doi:10.1111/cpr.12648

Menke, L. A., study, D. D. D., Gardeitchik, T., Hammond, P., Heimdal, K. R., Houge, G., et al. (2018). Further Delineation of an Entity Caused by CREBBP and EP300 Mutations but Not Resembling Rubinstein-Taybi Syndrome. *Am. J. Med. Genet. A.* 176, 862–876. doi:10.1002/ajmg.a.38626

Pamudurti, N. R., Bartok, O., Jens, M., Ashwal-Fluss, R., Stottmeister, C., Ruhe, L., et al. (2017). Translation of CircRNAs. *Mol. Cel.* 66, 9–e7. doi:10.1016/j.molcel.2017.02.021

Poilil Surendran, S., George Thomas, R., Moon, M. J., and Jeong, Y. Y. (2017). Nanoparticles for the Treatment of Liver Fibrosis. *Int. J. Nanomedicine* 12, 6997–7006. doi:10.2147/IJN.S145951

Wang, J., Zhao, X., Wang, Y., Ren, F., Sun, D., Yan, Y., et al. (2020). circRNA-002178 Act as a ceRNA to Promote PDL1/PD1 Expression in Lung Adenocarcinoma. *Cel Death Dis.* 11, 32. doi:10.1038/s41419-020-2230-9

Wang, T., Chen, N., Ren, W., Liu, F., Gao, F., Ye, L., et al. (2019). Integrated Analysis of circRNAs and mRNAs Expression Profile Revealed the Involvement of Hsa_circ_0007919 in the Pathogenesis of Ulcerative Colitis. *J. Gastroenterol.* 54, 804–818. doi:10.1007/s00535-019-01585-7

Xia, X., Tang, X., and Wang, S. (2019). Roles of CircRNAs in Autoimmune Diseases. *Front. Immunol.* 10, 639. doi:10.3389/fimmu.2019.00639

Yang, Y. R., Bu, F. T., Yang, Y., Li, H., Huang, C., Meng, X. M., et al. (2020). LEFTY2 Alleviates Hepatic Stellate Cell Activation and Liver Fibrosis by Regulating the TGF-β1/Smad3 Pathway. *Mol. Immunol.* 126, 31–39. doi:10.1016/j.molimm.2020.07.012

Zhang, J., Wang, P., Wan, L., Xu, S., and Pang, D. (2017). The Emergence of Noncoding RNAs as Heracles in Autophagy. *Autophagy* 13, 1004–1024. doi:10.1080/15548627.2017.1312041

Zhao, Z., Lin, C. Y., and Cheng, K. (2019). siRNA- and miRNA-Based Therapeutics for Liver Fibrosis. *Transl Res.* 214, 17–29. doi:10.1016/j.trsl.2019.07.007

Zheng, Q., Bao, C., Guo, W., Li, S., Chen, J., Chen, B., et al. (2016). Circular RNA Profiling Reveals an Abundant circHIPK3 that Regulates Cell Growth by Sponging Multiple miRNAs. *Nat. Commun.* 7, 11215. doi:10.1038/ncomms11215

Zhou, Y., Lv, X., Qu, H., Zhao, K., Fu, L., Zhu, L., et al. (2018). Preliminary Screening and Functional Analysis of Circular RNAs Associated with Hepatic Stellate Cell Activation. *Gene* 677, 317–323. doi:10.1016/j.gene.2018.08.052

Zhu, L., Ren, T., Zhu, Z., Cheng, M., Mou, Q., Mu, M., et al. (2018). Thymosin-β4 Mediates Hepatic Stellate Cell Activation by Interfering with CircRNA-0067835/miR-155/FoxO3 Signaling Pathway. *Cell Physiol. Biochem.* 51, 1389–1398. doi:10.1159/000495556

9

Molecular Mechanisms and Potential New Therapeutic Drugs for Liver Fibrosis

*Fa-Da Wang, Jing Zhou and En-Qiang Chen **

Center of Infectious Diseases, West China Hospital, Sichuan University, Chengdu, China

Correspondence:
En-Qiang Chen
chenenqiang1983@hotmail.com

Liver fibrosis is the pathological process of excessive extracellular matrix deposition after liver injury and is a precursor to cirrhosis, hepatocellular carcinoma (HCC). It is essentially a wound healing response to liver tissue damage. Numerous studies have shown that hepatic stellate cells play a critical role in this process, with various cells, cytokines, and signaling pathways engaged. Currently, the treatment targeting etiology is considered the most effective measure to prevent and treat liver fibrosis, but reversal fibrosis by elimination of the causative agent often occurs too slowly or too rarely to avoid life-threatening complications, especially in advanced fibrosis. Liver transplantation is the only treatment option in the end-stage, leaving us with an urgent need for new therapies. An in-depth understanding of the mechanisms of liver fibrosis could identify new targets for the treatment. Most of the drugs targeting critical cells and cytokines in the pathogenesis of liver fibrosis are still in pre-clinical trials and there are hardly any definitive anti-fibrotic chemical or biological drugs available for clinical use. In this review, we will summarize the pathogenesis of liver fibrosis, focusing on the role of key cells, associated mechanisms, and signaling pathways, and summarize various therapeutic measures or drugs that have been trialed in clinical practice or are in the research stage.

Keywords: liver fibrosis, hepatic stellate cells, cytokines, extracellular matrix, traditional Chinese medicine

INTRODUCTION

Hepatic fibrosis is a universal pathological process that occurs in various types of chronic liver disease, including viral hepatitis, alcoholic hepatitis, fatty liver disease, nonalcoholic fatty liver disease (NAFLD), wilson's disease, and cholangitis. When hepatocytes are damaged, the release of signals such as reactive oxygen species (ROS) and intercellular interactions lead to the differentiation of HSCs towards myofibroblasts, and the latter is the primary source of the extracellular matrix (ECM) (Casini et al., 1997; Novo et al., 2009; Ghatak et al., 2011; Mederacke et al., 2013). Damaged hepatocytes also activate inflammatory cells such as macrophages and lymphocytes to generate multiple types of cytokines, including transforming growth factor-β (TGF-β) and platelet-derived growth factor (PDGF). These cytokines would result in dysregulation of ECM degradation and synthesis, leading to the development of liver fibrosis (Luedde et al., 2014; Seki and Schwabe, 2015). Suppose the injury persists and therapeutic interventions are not taken in time, the liver parenchyma will gradually be replaced by scar tissue formed by excessive ECM, leading to the loss of standard structure and the formation of cirrhosis. Additionally, the risk of hepatocellular carcinoma (HCC) and serious complications such as gastrointestinal bleeding increased.

Over the past decades, we have made some important progress in the mechanism study of liver fibrosis, but the complex pathogenesis of liver fibrosis poses certain difficulties for the development of anti-hepatic fibrosis drugs. Many therapeutic interventions are effective in

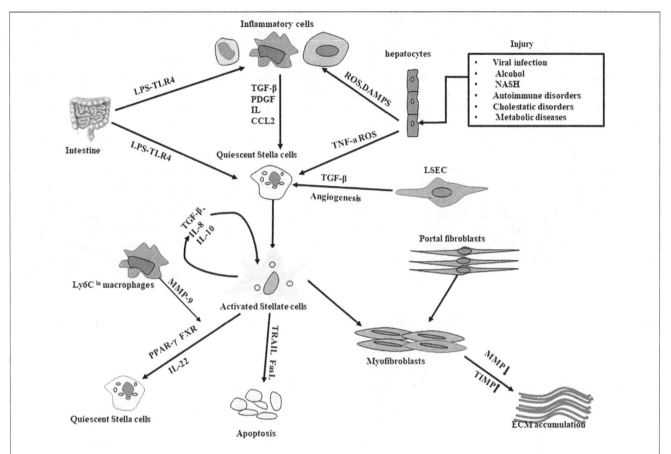

FIGURE 1 | Mechanisms of liver fibrosis. Liver injury is caused by a variety of stimuli that result in hepatocyte damage and the release of substances such as ROS; in response to persistent hepatocyte injury, HSCs and macrophages (including Kupffer cells) are activated, activated myofibroblasts increase and excessive ECM is produced, leading to the progression of liver fibrosis. The activation of hepatic stellate cells is a key step in the process of liver fibrosis. Many influential factors regulating HSC activation, proliferation, function, and survival have emerged as important therapeutic targets; likewise, protection of hepatocytes from damage and degradation of excessive ECM deposition provide therapeutic options. HSCs: Hepatic stellate cells CCL2:C-C chemokine ligands types 2; LPS: Lipopolysaccharide LSEC : Liver sinusoidal endothelial cells TIMP: inhibitors of matrix metalloproteinase; MMP: matrix metalloproteinase; DAMPS:damage-associated molecular patterns; ECM: extracellular matrix; ROS: reactive oxygen species.

experimental models, but their efficacy and safety in humans are unknown and cannot be applied in the clinic for the time being. Though still lack of specific anti-fibrosis agents in clinical, numerous studies have shown that the etiological treatment of primary liver disease is effective and even partially reversible for liver fibrosis (Dienstag et al., 2003; Czaja and Carpenter, 2004; Schiff et al., 2008; Chang et al., 2010). In addition, it is worth mentioning that traditional Chinese medicine (TCM) has a beneficial effect on anti-fibrosis (Chen et al., 2015). In this review, we will summarize the various therapeutic measures or drugs that have been trialed in clinical practice or are in the research stage.

OVERVIEW OF THE MECHANISMS OF LIVER FIBROSIS

Liver fibrosis is caused by an excessive accumulation of scar tissue, accompanied by angiogenesis (Lin et al., 2021), which ultimately leads to changes in the architecture of the liver. The mechanisms of liver fibrosis can be generalized as follows, multiple stimuli (such as toxins, viruses, cholestasis, hypoxia, and insulin resistance, etc.) attack the liver cells and induce the formation of reactive oxygen species (such as hydrogen peroxide, hydroxyl radicals, and aldehyde end products, etc.), which in turn cause hepatocyte damage, apoptosis, steatosis, and immune cell infiltration, especially kupffer cells (KCs) (Wehr et al., 2013; Pradere et al., 2013). At the same time, sinusoidal endothelial cells experience the loss of fenestrae, known as capillarization of the sinusoids (Marrone et al., 2016). Chronic damage to hepatocytes is the initiator of the fibrotic cascade, it induces the production of pro-fibrotic cytokines/growth factors (e.g., TNF-a, IL-6, TGF-β, and PDGF) indirectly through interactions with hepatic macrophages and natural killer (NK) cells. Meanwhile, it directly activates primary response cells (e.g., hepatic stellate cells) through the release of cellular contents, ultimately leading to the activation of HSCs and the fibrotic network and excessive deposition of ECM (**Figure 1**) (Canbay et al., 2002; Elpek, 2014). Based on the pathogenesis, we can regress liver fibrosis by protecting hepatocytes, inhibiting the activation of hepatic stellate cells, and fibrotic scar evolution.

The ECM is a complex network of macromolecular substances that can regulate various physiological functions such as cell growth, proliferation, migration, differentiation, adhesion, metabolism, damage repair, and tissue remodeling through various signaling systems. In the normal liver, it is a highly dynamic substrate that maintains an exact balance between synthesis and degradation (Theocharis et al., 2016; Villesen et al., 2020). However, in chronic liver disease, the balance is disturbed due to the involvement of multiple cells and cytokines, leading to a greater synthesis than degradation. But most of these changes can be reversed if the liver injury is transient (Hernandez-Gea and Friedman, 2011). The process of liver fibrosis is complicated, involving both hepatic parenchymal and non-parenchymal cells as well as immune cells, and the main functions of different cells and cytokines in liver fibrosis are described in detail below.

KEY CELL TYPES IN LIVER FIBROSIS

Hepatic Stellate Cells and Myofibroblasts

In normal liver, HSCs exhibit a quiescent state, whose physiological functions are related to fat storage and the metabolism of vitamin A. Another function of the quiescent HSC is to secrete adequate amounts of ECM proteins such as type III collagen, type IV collagen, and laminin. Besides, HSC secretes a variety of degradative enzymes called matrix metalloproteinases (MMPs), such as MMP-1, which promote the degradation of ECM. HSC also produces tissue inhibitors of matrix metalloproteinases (TIMPs), such as the TIMP-1 and TIMP-2. The TIMP1 can prevent ECM degradation by blocking MMPs and can inhibit HSC apoptosis (Carloni et al., 1996; Roeb et al., 1997; Benyon and Arthur, 2001; Geerts, 2001; Yoneda et al., 2016). The highly regulated interaction between MMPs and TIMPs is responsible for the renewal of the liver matrix and the maintenance of homeostasis and healthy liver architectures *in vivo* (Murphy et al., 2002). When the liver injury occurs, numerous key cells and inflammatory mediators are involved, including inflammatory stimuli, fibrogenic cytokines TGF-β, ROS, produced by activating macrophages, platelets, and products of damaged hepatocytes drive HSC activation. Quiescent HSCs become activated and TIMP-1 expression is upregulated, which is an essential and central step of liver fibrogenesis. The activated HSCs can not only transform into myofibroblasts and secrete enough ECM, but also secret cytokines such as TGF-β to maintain a constant state of activation, ultimately resulting in the deposition of mature collagen fibers in the space of the Disse and leading to the formation of scars (Tsuchida and Friedman, 2017).

In past, our understanding of HSCs has been dominated by their crucial role in liver fibrosis, thus generating anti-fibrotic strategies that target this cell. As research has progressed and understanding of the role of HSCs in disease has increased, we have found that HSCs have a role in promoting liver cell regeneration (Yang et al., 2008), which may be achieved mainly through the following mechanisms, secretion of cytokines that promote liver cell proliferation, promote the migration of stem cells to the liver, and promote the epithelial transformation of mesenchymal cells into hepatocytes. Therefore, we need to consider their role in liver regeneration when targeting HSCs in liver fibrosis (Ge et al., 2020).

Myofibroblasts (MFs) are key cells in fibrotic diseases, including lung, kidney, and liver disease (Friedman et al., 2013). It is the major cell that produces ECM in the process of liver fibrosis, such as collagen I and III. The origin of myofibroblasts has been controversial, but experiments and data now demonstrate that the main sources are HSCs and portal myofibroblasts. Following an injury to liver tissue, myofibroblasts are transformed from activated HSCs in response to a large number of cytokines and inflammatory cells. The overproduced cytokines can continue to act on myofibroblasts to keep them activated, which in turn produces large aggregates of ECM. In biliary disease, the main source of myofibroblasts is portal myofibroblasts (Iwaisako et al., 2014; Wells et al., 2015). Besides, animal experiments have shown that HSCs and myofibroblasts can be converted from mesothelial cells via mesothelial-mesenchymal transition after liver injury (Li et al., 2013).

Hepatocytes

Hepatocytes make up 80% of the total cell population and volume of the human liver, and under physiological conditions perform a variety of functions such as detoxification, secretion of bile, proteins, and lipids (Schulze et al., 2019). It is also a primary target for toxic substances that attack the liver. Hepatocyte death is an important initial event in all liver diseases. Dead hepatocytes release intracellular compounds called damage-associated molecular patterns (DAMPs) that signal to surround hepatic stellate cells and Kuffer's cells and therefore play an important role in the development of fibrosis and inflammation (An et al., 2020; Gaul et al., 2021). Therefore, protecting hepatocytes from damage is an important therapeutic intervention.

Inflammatory Cells

Inflammation is a fundamental characteristic of chronic liver disease, cell death is typically the precipitating event. The release of signals such as reactive oxygen species (ROS) from the damaged cells can activate the inflammatory cells, including macrophages, lymphocytes, and NK cells etc (Jaeschke, 2011). Among them, hepatic macrophages (Kupffer cells) play major roles and are known as regulators in the process of liver fibrosis (Wynn and Barron, 2010). KCs are an essential component of the innate immune mononuclear phagocytic system and play critical functions in homeostasis, and act as first responders following liver injury. In response to tissue damage, numerous Ly-6Chi macrophages are recruited to the liver, releasing cytokines and attracting NK cells and other immune cells (Karlmark et al., 2009; Reid et al., 2016). These macrophages could induce the transdifferentiation of HSCs into collagen-producing myofibroblasts by secreting TGF-β1 and PDGF. Dendritic cells (DCs) increase fibrosis regression, mainly through the production of MMP-9 (Jiao et al., 2012). NK cells directly kill target cells and are capable of producing a variety of cytokines that play various roles in liver injury, fibrosis, and hepatocarcinogenesis, activated NKT cells have a role in killing activated HSCs (Radaeva et al., 2006). However, in chronic liver disease, NKT cells have a pro-inflammatory function, recruit neutrophils and myeloid cells, and promote the activation of hepatic stellate, leading to hepatocyte necrosis, fibrosis, and even HCC (Jin et al., 2011; Wolf et al., 2014).

Activated inflammatory cells are the primary source of cytokines, such as C-C chemokine ligands types 2 and 5 (CCL2 and CCL5), IL, TGF-β1, PDGF, etc. The role of inflammatory cells is double-sided, which could promote the regression of liver fibrosis and accelerate the deterioration of fibrosis. For example, hepatic macrophages can not only relieve inflammation and fibrosis by degrading the ECM and releasing anti-inflammatory cytokines but also promote liver fibrosis by activating HSCs (Duffield et al., 2005; Tacke and Zimmermann, 2014). The Ly6Chi macrophages can differentiate into restorative Ly6Clo macrophages to engulf cell debris and secrete MMP-9 and MMP-1/MMP-2 to promote scar regression (Ramachandran et al., 2012).

Liver Sinusoidal Endothelial Cells

In normal liver tissue, liver sinusoidal endothelial cells (LSECs) have characteristics of vasodilatory, anti-inflammatory, anti-thrombotic, anti-angiogenic, anti-fibrotic, and regeneration-promoting effects (Ding et al., 2010), so LSECs are considered to be the gatekeepers of hepatic homeostasis. At the same time, LSECs are the main source of endothelium-derived nitric oxide (NO), which keeps HSCs in a resting state. In the presence of liver injury, LSECs become capillarized, which can not only reduce the production of vasodilators (such as NO, cyclooxygenase, and prostaglandin I2 [PGI2]) but also increase the production of vasoconstrictors (endothelin 1, thromboxane A2, angiotensin II). This imbalance not only alters the phenotype of LSECs but also contributes to the activation of HSCs and promotes inflammation and liver fibrosis (Deleve et al., 2008; Xie et al., 2012; Poisson et al., 2017). It also secretes TGF-β, PDGF or activates signaling pathways such as Wntβcatenin, which can activate HSCs in a paracrine and autocrine manner. Due to the unique properties of LSECs, selective LSEC-targeted therapy appears to be an attractive strategy for the treatment of liver fibrosis (Gracia-Sancho et al., 2021).

MOLECULAR SIGNALING PATHWAYS INVOLVED IN LIVER FIBROGENESIS

TGF-β Signaling and Platelet-Derived Growth Factor Signaling

Transforming growth factors (TGF) have the function of regulating the growth and development of various cells, which are essential for the homeostasis of tissues and organs. In the liver, they are mainly produced by HSCs, LSECs, KCs, and DCs as well as NKT cells, and can act on themselves or other cells through autocrine or paracrine secretion (Schon and Weiskirchen, 2014). The functions of TGF-β vary between different types and stages of

liver disease. During liver fibrosis, TGF-β is up-regulated, the main function of TGF-β is to activate HSCs, which are considered to be the main pro-fibrotic factor in the process of liver fibrosis. It also enhances the expression of TIMPs and directly promotes the synthesis of interstitial fibrillar collagens (García-Trevijano et al., 1999; Hellerbrand et al., 1999; Dewidar et al., 2019). Due to its important function in liver fibrosis, blocking the signaling pathway of TGF-β is now a potential target for the treatment of liver fibrosis (Guo et al., 2012).

The platelet-derived growth factor (PDGF) is a member of the family of growth factors whose biological functions include angiogenesis, regulation of cell proliferation and survival, cell migration, and stimulation of the synthesis of major components of the connective tissue matrix (Heldin and Westermark, 1999). In the context of liver disease, the expression of PDGF and its receptors have now been shown to be significantly upregulated (Pinzani et al., 1996). It has been regarded as the most effective growth factor for HSC proliferation in hepatic fibrosis, and the receptors of PDGF have become a new promising direction in the treatment of liver fibrosis (Pinzani et al., 1989; Borkham-Kamphorst et al., 2007).

Inflammatory Cytokines Pathways

The progression and regression of liver fibrosis are regulated by a complex signaling pathway consisting of cytokines, growth factors, and chemokines. IL-6, TNF-a, Interleukins, PDGF, and TGF-β are the key pro-inflammatory and profibrogenic cytokines that drive liver fibrosis. Interleukins (ILs) are important immunomodulatory cytokines. During liver injury, it is produced by various cell types and exerts pro-inflammatory (such as IL-13, IL-17, and IL-33) as well as anti-inflammatory effects (such as IL-22 and IL-10) in hepatic cells (Hu et al., 2016; Xu et al., 2016; Liu et al., 2019). For instance, An animal study has shown that the IL-6/gp130 pathway plays a protective role for non-parenchymal hepatocytes in the progression of fibrosis (Streetz et al., 2003). But a recent study has demonstrated that IL-6 can induce differentiation of HSCs towards myofibroblast via MAPK and JAK/STAT signaling pathways (Kagan et al., 2017). In addition, IL-22 has been shown to attenuate liver fibrosis by binding to cell receptors, attenuating the activation of HSCs and down-regulating levels of inflammatory cytokines (Lu et al., 2015). This suggests that a strategy using blocking pro-inflammatory interleukins or inducing anti-inflammatory interleukin production to treat liver fibrosis can be effective.

Tumour necrosis factor (TNF) and related receptor pathways can activate apoptosis in hepatocytes via the caspases pathway and exert anti-apoptotic effects via the NF-κB pathway (Osawa et al., 2018). TNF also plays a vital role in the activation of HSCs and the synthesis of ECM (Osawa et al., 2013). TNF reduces apoptosis of activated rat HSCs through upregulation of the anti-apoptotic factor NF-κB. However, the effects of TNF-a on HSCs and fibrosis are multiple. In animal experiments, it has shown an anti-fibrotic effect by reducing glutathione and inhibiting the secretion of pro-collagen a1 (Hernandez-Munoz et al., 1997; Varela-Rey et al., 2007).

TABLE 1 | Targets and main mechanisms of some of existing anti-fibrotic drugs and novel therapeutic approaches.

Agent	Anti-fibrotic target	Mechanism	Refs
Etiological treatment	Etiology	Removal of causative factors	(Powell and Klatskin, 1968; Marcellini et al., 2005; Takahashi et al., 2014; Rockey, 2016; Lens et al., 2017; Tada et al., 2018; Bardou-Jacquet et al., 2020; Ye et al., 2020)
Glucocorticoids	HSC lymphocytes	Reducing the transmission of transforming growth factors Weakening the activity of hepatic stellate cells Inhibiting the proliferation of lymphocytes	(Bolkenius et al., 2004; Czaja, 2014)
Curcumin	Inflammation cell and inflammation response	Anti-inflammatory and antioxidant effects Blocking the epithelial-mesenchymal transition of hepatocytes Inhibiting the activation of Kuffer cells Inhibiting NF-κB upregulation and reducing sinusoidal angiogenesis	(Zhang et al., 2014; Zhao et al., 2018; Kong et al., 2020)
YCHD	TGF-β and RAS system	Reduction of RAS pathway components and down-regulation of TGF expression	Wu et al. (2015)
XCHT	Nrf2	Inhibition of hepatic stellate cell activation	Li et al. (2017)
Baicalein	PDGF receptors	Inhibit the activation and value-added of hepatic stellate cells by down-regulating PDGF receptors	Sun et al. (2010)
FFBJ	HSC	Inhibition of hepatic stellate cell proliferation and activation, as well as limiting the expression of TGF-β1 and PDGF	Yang et al. (2016)
GW570	HSC	A PPARγ receptor agonism, simulating PPARγ mediated gene transcription	Yang et al. (2010)
Obeticholic acid		An FXR agonist, FXR expressed in hepatic stellate cells has an anti-fibrotic effect	Mudaliar et al. (2013)
Pioglitazone		A PPARγ receptor agonism	Musso et al. (2017)
Nilotinib		Inhibition of TK, TK activation transforms HSC into an activated state	(Ma et al., 2017) (Shaker et al., 2013)
Sorafenib			
β-aminopropionitrile	ECM	Inhibits LOX, LOX-mediated cross-linking of collagen limits MMP degradation of ECM	Georges et al. (2007)
CVC	Cytokines	Dual antagonist of the CCR type 2 and 5	Friedman et al. (2018)
TG101348		JAK2 receptor antagonist	Akcora et al. (2019)
E5564	TLR4	Inhibitors of TLR4	(Fort et al., 2005; Kitazawa et al., 2009; Takashima et al., 2009)
P13			
CRX526			
vitamin E	ROS	Antioxidant effects	(Sanyal et al., 2010; Bril et al., 2019; Miyazawa et al., 2019)
losartan/candesartan	AT1 receptor	Angiotensin II may exert its pro-fibrotic effects, Blocking or attenuating the role of Angiotensin II.	(Colmenero et al., 2009; Kim et al., 2012)
RNA interference	target genes	Downregulation of genes of critical cytokines in activated HSCs	(Chen et al., 2008; Cong et al., 2013; Zhou and Yang, 2014; Jiménez Calvente et al., 2015)
MiRNAs	mRNAs	Trigger the degradation of target mRNAs about liver fibrosis	(Chen et al., 2018; Wang et al., 2019)
MSC	Inflammation	Modulation of the hepatic immune response	
	HSC	Secretion of trophic cytokines to reduce hepatocyte apoptosis	(Eom et al., 2015)
	MMPs/TIMP-1	Antioxidant effects Inhibition of HSC appreciation Increased expression of MMPs Reduced expression of TIMP-1	

Abbreviations: PPAR, proliferator-activated receptor; HSCs, Hepatic stellate cells; FXR, farnesoid X receptor; ECM, extracellular matrix; ROS, reactive oxygen species; TK, Tyrosine kinase; JAK, Janus kinase; TLR, Toll-like receptor; P13, a peptide called P13; YCHD, Yinchenhao Decoction; XCHT, Xiaochaihutang; FFBJ, Fufang Biejia Ruangan Tablets; MSC, Mesenchymal stem cell; PDGF, platelet growth factor RAS, renin-angiotensin system.

Toll-Like Receptors in Liver Fibrosis

The liver is exposed to venous blood from the small and large intestines through the portal vein. Due to this unique blood supply system, the liver is easily exposed to bacterial products that are transferred from the lumen of the intestine *via* the portal vein. The small and large intestines are rich in flora. In healthy organisms, due to the barrier effect of the intestinal mucosa, only a small amount of translocated bacterial products reach the liver, and the liver immune system tolerates these bacterial products to avoid harmful reactions. After the injury to the liver or the intestinal mucosa, the flora becomes disturbed, and intestinal bacteria can translocate to the liver. Its metabolites such as lipopolysaccharide (LPS) can conjugate with functional toll-like receptor 4 (TLR4) to activate reactive cells such as HSCs and Kupffer cells, and also enhance the activity of transforming growth factors thus leading to the development of liver fibrosis (Seki et al., 2007; Schnabl and Brenner, 2014). In the liver, both hepatocytes and non-parenchymal cells (NPCs) have expressed TLR4. Compared to other organs, healthy livers have a low level of TLR4. However, damaged livers increase the expression of TLR4 and its co-receptors, thus making TLR4 signaling-mediated inflammatory responses more sensitive (Kitazawa et al., 2008; Guo and Friedman, 2010).

POTENTIALLY EFFECTIVE TREATMENTS FOR LIVER FIBROSIS

Recently, it has been shown that fibrosis can reverse after the removal of pathogenic conditions. Although no drugs are currently approved for the treatment of liver fibrosis, some treatment modalities have shown effectiveness in patients, such as antiviral therapy for patients with viral hepatitis, zinc for wilson's disease, phlebotomy for hemochromatosis, alcohol withdrawal for alcoholic liver disease and ursodeoxycholic acid (UDCA) in the treatment of primary biliary cholangitis (Powell and Klatskin, 1968; Marcellini et al., 2005; Takahashi et al., 2014; Bardou-Jacquet et al., 2020; Ye et al., 2020). glucocorticoids, vitamin E, and angiotensin receptor antagonists have gradually been shown to have antifibrotic effects as well. In addition, TCM appears to have an increasingly prominent role in the treatment of liver fibrosis and its efficacy is promising (Fujiwara et al., 2010; He et al., 2013), but more clinical trials are needed to confirm its effectiveness. In the following, we will describe these potential treatments in detail below (**Table 1**).

Antiviral Therapy

Among all the factors that contribute to chronic liver disease, hepatitis virus infection is the most common, primarily hepatitis B and C. Chronic hepatitis B virus infection is a worldwide public health problem, with approximately 250 million people chronically infected and at high risk of developing cirrhosis and liver cancer. When liver cells are infected with the virus, cellular damage induces an inflammatory response, at the same time the virus itself can directly induce activation of the immune system, leading to activation of HSCs and progress to liver fibrosis. Clearing hepatitis viruses or inhibiting hepatitis virus replication is the most effective way to reduce liver cell damage. With the advent of antiviral drugs, we have now made considerable progress in the fight against the hepatitis B and C virus. Through effective antiviral therapy, most liver fibrosis can be reversed, and liver cirrhosis and its related complications can be reduced (Rockey, 2016; Lens et al., 2017; Tada et al., 2018).

Drugs Targeting Inflammation

Glucocorticoids have immunomodulatory and anti-inflammatory effects. As we mentioned earlier, the inflammatory response and immune cells play critical roles in the process of liver fibrosis. Thus glucocorticoids may have some therapeutic effects in liver fibrosis. It has been shown that glucocorticoids can reduce liver fibrosis by reducing the transmission of transforming growth factors, weakening the activity of HSCs, and inhibiting the proliferate of lymphocytes,

but the efficacy of glucocorticoids differently in different diseases (Bolkenius et al., 2004; Czaja, 2014). Glucocorticoids or immunosuppressive agents are the most significant treatment options for chronic autoimmune liver disease, and liver fibrosis can be reversed with adequate management (Valera et al., 2011). Early glucocorticoid treatment is effective for prognosis in hepatitis and liver failure due to viral hepatitis B (Fujiwara et al., 2010; He et al., 2013). Nevertheless, the use of corticosteroids for alcohol-related acute liver failure or slow-onset acute liver failure is still controversial in clinical practice, although the AASLD and EASL guidelines recommend treatment with corticosteroids. Studies have shown that the use of glucocorticoids improves short-term survival but does not significantly improve long-term prognosis and carries risks such as infection (Thursz et al., 2015; Sersté et al., 2018; Gustot and Jalan, 2019). Similarly, the use of glucocorticoids to treat a drug-induced liver injury is also in dispute (Andrade et al., 2019). Consequently, there is still a need for extensive trials and data to evaluate the safety and efficacy of glucocorticoids in liver disease.

Traditional Chinese Medicine With Multiple Effects on Liver Fibrosis

Notably, there is growing evidence that TCM is effective in the prevention and treatment of liver fibrosis (Pan et al., 2020). TCM can suppress liver fibrosis activity through different mechanisms, including inhibition of cytokine production and suppression of HSCs activation, as well as regulating the progression of liver fibrosis through other molecular mechanisms (Shan et al., 2019). Turmeric is an herb that grows in Asia and has been widely used as a spice in food and for therapeutic applications. In China, it is also an ingredient in TCM and recently its extract curcumin has received much attention. Curcumin has been widely used in anti-fibrotic models due to its anti-inflammatory and antioxidant effects. It has been shown to alleviate liver fibrosis by blocking the epithelial-mesenchymal transition of hepatocytes through the regulation of oxidative stress and autophagy (Cai et al., 2018; Cai et al., 2019), and to weaken the role of Ly6C^{hi} cells in liver fibrosis by inhibiting the activation of Kuffer cells, thereby reducing the secretion of chemokines (Cai et al., 2018; Cai et al., 2019). In addition, it also has the effect of inhibiting NF-κB upregulation and reducing sinusoidal angiogenesis (Cai et al., 2018; Cai et al., 2019). More research is underway on the mechanism of curcumin against liver fibrosis.

YCHD (Yinchenhao Decoction) is a traditional Chinese herbal formulation used to treat liver fibrosis and has been experimentally shown to have multiple active ingredients targeting various targets of liver fibrosis (Cai et al., 2018; Cai et al., 2019). Recent studies have indicated RAS system in liver fibrosis/cirrhosis may exert pro-fibrotic effects, and the antifibrotic effects of the YCHD fibrosis effect may be related to the reduction of RAS pathway components and down-regulation of TGF expression (Bataller et al., 2000; Yoshiji et al., 2007). XCHT (Xiaochaihutang) is a water decoction traditionally used in china for the treatment of liver diseases, and the mechanism for its anti-fibrosis is not completely clear.

Nrf2 is an important redox-sensitive transcription factor *in vivo*, which can promote cell survival, as well as maintain the redox state of cells. Animal experiments have shown that XCHT is an effective drug for the treatment of liver fibrosis, and its therapeutic effect is mainly through upregulation of the Nrf2 pathway thus resulting in the inhibition of HSCs activation (Bataller et al., 2000; Yoshiji et al., 2007). In addition, baicalein, the main component of XCHT, can inhibit the activation and proliferation of HSCs by down-regulating PDGF receptors, thus exerting an anti-fibrotic effect (Bataller et al., 2000; Yoshiji et al., 2007). It has been reported that ETV combined with FFBJ (Fufang Biejia Ruangan Tablets) showed significant anti-fibrotic effects in CHB patients. The mechanism of action may be related to the inhibition of HSCs proliferation and activation, as well as limiting the expression of TGF-β1 and PDGF (Bataller et al., 2000; Yoshiji et al., 2007).

Similar TCMs also include Huangqi Decoction Dahuang Zhechong Pills, Fuzheng Huayu Formula, Anluo Huaxian Pills (Li, 2020), etc. Although TCM has been used for thousands of years, its clinical effectiveness in liver fibrosis needs further evaluation due to the lack of rigorous randomized controlled trials.

Vitamin E and Renin-Angiotensin System Inhibitor

Vitamin E, angiotensin-converting enzyme inhibitors (ACE-I), and angiotensin II type 1 (AT1) receptor blockers have recently drawn attention to the treatment of liver fibrosis. Vitamin E is an important nutrient with antioxidant effects, it can inhibit the production of singlet free radicals, oxygen, lipid hydroperoxides, and lipid radicals. Since products such as free radicals play an important role in the development of liver fibrosis, it may be a potential option for the treatment of liver fibrosis. However, in patients with non-alcoholic liver disease, vitamin E could not significantly reduce the severity of fibrosis (Sanyal et al., 2010; Bril et al., 2019; Miyazawa et al., 2019).

Recent studies have also shown that the production of angiotensin II type 1 receptor is increased in activated HSCs and enhanced the activity of the renin-angiotensin system (RAS) in liver fibrosis/cirrhosis. Angiotensin II may exert its pro-fibrotic effects through increased oxidative stress, activation and proliferation of HSCs, upregulation of TGF-β and TIMP1, and accelerated deposition of collagen (Bataller et al., 2000; Yoshiji et al., 2007). Based on these mechanisms, ACE-I and AT1 receptor blockers are potential treatment options for liver fibrosis. A clinical study evaluating the efficacy of angiotensin II receptor blocker (ARB) losartan in patients with HCV showed that it can reduce inflammation and decrease fibrosis gene expression (Colmenero et al., 2009).In patients with chronic alcoholic liver diseases, the combination of UDCA and ARB candesartan improved patients' fibrosis scores compared to UDCA treatment alone (Kim et al., 2012). However, as no clear effects have been shown in other clinical trials, further studies are needed to demonstrate the benefit of RAS antagonists in liver fibrosis.

CANDIDATE THERAPEUTIC TARGETS IN CLINICAL TRIALS

There are no directly effective anti-fibrotic drugs in clinical practice and most of them are still in clinical trials and in the research stage. Although etiological treatment has proven to be effective, some etiologies cannot be eliminated. In addition, even with effective etiological treatment, reversal of advanced liver fibrosis cannot completely avoid complications such as gastrointestinal bleeding and HCC, so we urgently need direct anti-fibrotic drugs.

The main pathogenesis of liver fibrosis can be summarized as follows: Following the chronic injury to hepatocytes, the multitude of cellular and cytokine interactions lead to the activation of key cells such as HSCs and MFs, which in turn leads to the overproduction of ECM and the development of liver fibrosis (Parola and Pinzani, 2019; Kisseleva and Brenner, 2021). Based on the pathogenesis of liver fibrosis, the drugs we are exploring focus on the following aspects: protecting hepatocytes from damage, inhibiting cytokine activity and cell proliferation, promoting apoptosis of key cells, reducing ECM synthesis, and promoting its degradation. Many relevant drugs are already in clinical trials, including FXR agonists, PPAR agonists, and TAK agonists, which inhibit hepatic stellate cell activation and promote ECM degradation, TLR4 receptor antagonists, and novel therapeutic approaches such as miRNA and mesenchymal stem cell therapy. Below we describe in detail the novel treatments and drugs according to the different targets (**Table 1**).

Inhibition and Reversal of the Activation of Hepatic Stellate Cells

Because of its important role in liver fibrosis, HSCs become a major target for anti-fibrotic drugs (Elpek, 2014). Reversing liver fibrosis by converting activated HSCs to a quiescent state or promoting their apoptosis is our main goal. Experimental models of fibrosis consistently demonstrate that elimination of activated HSCs by apoptosis or other pathways can lead to regression of fibrosis (Iredale et al., 1998; Troeger et al., 2012). Recent studies have shown that activated HSCs can be transformed into non-fibrotic cells by transcriptional reprogramming, such as ectopic expression of GATA4, FOXA3, HNF1a, and HNF4a *in vivo* (Song et al., 2016). Besides, cellular senescence may be an anti-fibrotic strategy. Expression of nuclear receptors PPAR and FXR in HSCs suppress HSCs activation, as studies have shown that HSC senescence can be invoked by PPARγ, FXR agonist, such as GW570 (Krützfeldt et al., 2005; Janssen et al., 2013; Thakral and Ghoshal, 2015), pioglitazone (Krützfeldt et al., 2005; Janssen et al., 2013; Thakral and Ghoshal, 2015), obeticholic acid (Krützfeldt et al., 2005; Janssen et al., 2013; Thakral and Ghoshal, 2015), thereby alleviating liver fibrosis degree. TK (Tyrosine kinase) is expressed in HSCs and its activation transforms them into an activated state, thus inhibition of TK may be a potential target for the treatment of liver fibrosis. Sorafenib has been used as a treatment for patients with HCC, where complications of cirrhosis (such as portal hypertension) have been reduced, and its anti-fibrotic activity has been confirmed in numerous trials (Ma et al., 2017). Nilotinib triggers apoptosis and autophagic cell death via inhibition of histone deacetylase in activated HSC cells (Krützfeldt et al., 2005; Janssen et al., 2013; Thakral and Ghoshal, 2015). Unfortunately, most of these drugs are in animal studies and are not yet available for clinical use, their safety and efficacy deserve to be evaluated.

Reduction of Fibrotic Scar Evolution

The removal of the excess ECM is one of our goals for treating liver fibrosis. Collagen is the most abundant ECM protein in liver fibrosis. Specific inhibition of type 1 collagen fibrils synthesis has now been achieved in animals by miRNA, and this miRNA leads to a significant reduction in collagen 1 synthesis in fibrosis models (Jiménez Calvente et al., 2015). Besides, LOX is a copper-dependent amine oxidase (Perepelyuk et al., 2013), and LOX-mediated cross-linking of collagen limits MMP degradation of ECM. The β-aminopropionitrile inhibits LOX, reduces liver stiffness, decreases the number of fibroblasts, and attenuates cell injury-induced liver fibrosis (Georges et al., 2007). However, the clinical trial did not demonstrate significant efficacy (Loomba et al., 2018). Similar to LOX, transglutaminase (TGs) forms a covalent isopeptide bond by covalently linking a glutamine residue of one protein chain to a lysine residue of another protein chain. Intercross-linking of TGs can promote liver fibrosis, and therefore invoking specific inhibitors of TGs could be a potential target for the treatment of liver fibrosis (Van Herck et al., 2010).

Drugs Targeting Cytokines and Signaling Pathways

Cytokines are involved in the entire process of liver fibrosis, blocking their signaling pathways, and receptors may inhibit the production of the ECM and accelerate its degradation. Cenicriviroc (CVC), an oral dual antagonist of the CCR type 2 and 5, has been shown to have antifibrotic effects in animal studies. A clinical trial has shown amelioration of liver fibrosis in patients with nonalcoholic steatohepatitis (NASH) after 1 year of treatment with CVC (Krützfeldt et al., 2005; Janssen et al., 2013; Thakral and Ghoshal, 2015), and further clinical trials on CVC are currently underway, and we hope that it will become an anti-fibrotic option in the future. The Janus kinases (JAK) signaling pathway plays an important role in the pathogenesis of hepatic fibrosis and can be activated by a variety of cytokines such as IL. Studies have shown that the use of the JAK2 receptor antagonist TG101348 can reduce hepatic fibrosis in animal models (Krützfeldt et al., 2005; Janssen et al., 2013; Thakral and Ghoshal, 2015). However, cytokine function is also important for maintaining the immune response, tissue repair, etc. Long-term targeting of these cytokines is challenging due to the severe adverse effects. A great deal of research has been done on cytokine antagonism (Gressner and Weiskirchen, 2006).

Drugs Targeting TLR4

As we mentioned earlier that intestinal microbiota is closely associated with the development of liver fibrosis. the main mechanism by which liver fibrosis occurs, in this case, is the combination of the bacterial metabolites LPS and TLR4, further activating key cells in the liver fibrosis process. Therefore, inhibition of TLR4-related intracellular signaling may be effective in reducing TLR4-mediated inflammation and inhibiting liver fibrosis (Beutler, 2004). It was shown that a peptide called P13, which was previously shown to be a potent inhibitor of TLR signaling in vitro. Using this peptide to treat mice effectively inhibited LPS-induced inflammatory mediator production and significantly limited liver damage, enhancing survival in a mouse model of inflammation (Tsung et al., 2007). Several small-molecule inhibitors of TLR4 are currently being tested, including lipid A mimetics, e.g., E5564 and CRX526 (Fort et al., 2005; Kitazawa et al., 2009; Takashima et al., 2009), soluble fusion proteins with extracellular structural domains. However, these are still in animal studies and may become targets for anti-fibrotic drugs in the future.

siRNA and miRNA in Liver Fibrosis

Liver fibrosis is highly related to activated HSCs, and the activation of HSCs is regulated by a variety of cytokines. Downregulation of these cytokines in activated HSCs using RNA interference (RNAi) is a promising strategy for reversing liver fibrosis. RNA interference is a new technique that uses small interfering RNAs (siRNAs) of 21–23 nucleotides to specifically knock out target genes, and this new technique is based on the high specificity of siRNAs and their ability to downregulate genes associated with liver fibrosis (Kim and Rossi, 2007). Many therapies for siRNA are currently in clinical trials to translocate siRNA into HSC or other hepatic parenchymal cells, for example, lipid nanoparticles containing HSP47 siRNA for the treatment of liver fibrosis (Kulkarni et al., 2018). The main mechanism of siRNA action is to cause homologous degradation of the targeted mRNA (Aagaard and Rossi, 2007). It has been shown that siRNA can address liver fibrosis by regulating collagen expression in HSC (Krützfeldt et al., 2005; Janssen et al., 2013; Thakral and Ghoshal, 2015). Meanwhile, it has been reported that direct knockdown of TGF-β expression using siRNA can exert antifibrotic effects in a rat model (Krützfeldt et al., 2005; Janssen et al., 2013; Thakral and Ghoshal, 2015). Similarly, the use of PDGF siRNA suppressed the advancement of liver fibrosis in mice (Krützfeldt et al., 2005; Janssen et al., 2013; Thakral and Ghoshal, 2015). Besides, MMP2-specific siRNA and TIMP-specific siRNAs also exert an anti-fibrotic effect on the liver (Krützfeldt et al., 2005; Janssen et al., 2013; Thakral and Ghoshal, 2015).

MiRNAs are endogenous small non-coding RNAs that can post-transcriptionally regulate the expression of mRNAs and ultimately trigger the degradation of target mRNAs. miRNAs are associated with a variety of liver diseases, including liver fibrosis, and therefore miRNAs are an alternative treatment for liver fibrosis. It has been found that miRNAs can be both up and down-regulated during liver fibrosis. Up-regulated miRNA can be reverted by anti-miRNA oligonucleotides, and miRNA masking (Krützfeldt et al., 2005; Janssen et al., 2013; Thakral and Ghoshal, 2015), unlike the upregulated miRNA, some downregulation of miRNA inhibiting liver fibrosis has been found (Chen et al., 2018; Wang et al., 2019), down-regulated MiRNA can be restored by MiRNA mimics or plasmids expressing miRNA (Cheng and Mahato, 2011). Similar to siRNAs, the biggest challenge for miRNAs is to overcome degradation and targeted transport in the blood. To date, there are no clinical trials on MiRNA about the treatment of liver fibrosis. A lot of effort has been spent on siRNA with MiRNA and viral and non-viral transport systems have been developed, which also still face significant challenges. There are already anti-fibrotic siRNAs in clinical trials, and in the future siRNA with miRNA may become a novel treatment for liver disease.

Mesenchymal Stem Cell Therapy for Liver Fibrosis

Recently, MSC therapy has been regarded as an effective alternative for the treatment of liver disease. MSCs possess the ability to self-renew and differentiate into many types of cells, and differentiation of MSCs into hepatocytes is the prospect of liver regeneration (Hu et al., 2020). The main mechanisms of the anti-fibrotic effects of MSCs can be generalized as follows, modulation of the hepatic immune response, secretion of trophic cytokines to reduce hepatocyte apoptosis, antioxidant effects, inhibition of HSC proliferation, and increased expression of MMPs or reduced expression of TIMP-1 (Hernandez-Munoz et al., 1997; Varela-Rey et al., 2007). Mesenchymal stem cells are now widely used in clinical and preclinical studies of liver fibrosis, Jang and others showed the beneficial effects of autologous bone marrow MSC transplantation for the treatment of alcoholic cirrhosis (Jang et al., 2014), Kharaziha et al. (2009) showed that liver function improved in patients with cirrhosis after injected autologous mesenchymal stem cells. However, due to their multi-differentiation potential, MSCs can differentiate into myofibroblasts rather than hepatocytes (Baertschiger et al., 2009; di Bonzo et al., 2008). Besides, another risk of MSC transplantation is that they are susceptible to malignant transformation and promote the growth of existing tumors (Zhu et al., 2006). MSCs have the potential to differentiate into hepatocytes, immunomodulatory properties, and the ability to secrete trophic cytokines, making them a potential treatment for liver disease. however, with both their fibrotic potential and their ability to promote the growth of pre-existing tumor cells, MSC therapy needs to be evaluated further.

CONCLUSION

Recently, with our greater understanding of the mechanisms of liver fibrosis, a plethora of therapeutic strategies have been generated. but the treatment of liver fibrosis remains a difficult clinical problem that we face today and etiological treatment is currently recognized as the most effective anti-fibrotic approach. Multiple interactions between ECM, hepatic stellate, endothelial cells, and immune cells have been demonstrated during liver fibrosis, but the central event in fibrosis is the activation of HSCs. Due to multiple cells and cytokines being involved in the progression of liver fibrosis, it is crucial for us to fully understand the biology of critical cells such as HSCs, myofibroblasts, and macrophages, including their activation and inactivation, to facilitate the development of specific targeted drugs. In addition, the inflammatory response is one of the fundamental features of liver fibrosis, so controlling liver inflammation and inflammatory cells is also a viable strategy for treating liver fibrosis. Besides, novel therapies targeting intestinal microecology, mRNA, and mesenchymal stem cells are also becoming available for clinical trials, and several drugs have been successful in regressing liver fibrosis in experimental models.

A growing number of potential drugs are in phase II and III trials, and we expect that some of these drugs may soon be approved for use in patients. These new drugs target multiple pathways in the pathogenesis of chronic liver disease, but the mechanisms of liver fibrosis are complex. With certain cells having a dual role in the development and regression of liver fibrosis, and targeted therapies may have some side effects. Therefore we must understand the mechanisms more clearly so that we can establish scientific treatments that are safe and effective in achieving long-term results. In the future, a better understanding of the molecular mechanisms involved in the regression of liver fibrosis may provide new preventive and therapeutic strategies for patients with fibrosis and even cirrhosis.

AUTHOR CONTRIBUTIONS

F-DW, JZ conceived this review and collected the literature, E-QC conducted the study supervision and revised the manuscript. All authors contributed to the article and approved the submitted version.

REFERENCES

Aagaard, L., and Rossi, J. J. (2007). RNAi Therapeutics: Principles, Prospects and Challenges. *Adv. Drug Deliv. Rev.* 59 (2-3), 75–86. doi:10.1016/j.addr.2007.03.005

Akcora, B. Ö., Dathathri, E., Ortiz-Perez, A., Gabriël, A. V., Storm, G., Prakash, J., et al. (2019). TG101348, a Selective JAK2 Antagonist, Ameliorates Hepatic Fibrogenesis *In Vivo. Faseb j* 33 (8), 9466–9475. doi:10.1096/fj.201900215RR

An, P., Wei, L. L., Zhao, S., Sverdlov, D. Y., Vaid, K. A., Miyamoto, M., et al. (2020). Hepatocyte Mitochondria-Derived Danger Signals Directly Activate Hepatic Stellate Cells and Drive Progression of Liver Fibrosis. *Nat. Commun.* 11 (1), 2362. doi:10.1038/s41467-020-16092-0

Andrade, R. J., Chalasani, N., Björnsson, E. S., Suzuki, A., Kullak-Ublick, G. A., Watkins, P. B., et al. (2019). Drug-induced Liver Injury. *Nat. Rev. Dis. Primers* 5 (1), 58. doi:10.1038/s41572-019-0105-0

Baertschiger, R. M., Serre-Beinier, V., Morel, P., Bosco, D., Peyrou, M., Clément, S., et al. (2009). Fibrogenic Potential of Human Multipotent Mesenchymal Stromal Cells in Injured Liver. *PLoS One* 4 (8), e6657. doi:10.1371/journal.pone.0006657

Bardou-Jacquet, E., Morandeau, E., Anderson, G. J., Ramm, G. A., Ramm, L. E., Morcet, J., et al. (2020). Regression of Fibrosis Stage with Treatment Reduces Long-Term Risk of Liver Cancer in Patients with Hemochromatosis Caused by Mutation in HFE. *Clin. Gastroenterol. Hepatol.* 18 (8), 1851–1857. doi:10.1016/

j.cgh.2019.10.010

Bataller, R., Ginès, P., Nicolás, J. M., Görbig, M. N., Garcia-Ramallo, E., Gasull, X., et al. (2000). Angiotensin II Induces Contraction and Proliferation of Human Hepatic Stellate Cells. *Gastroenterology* 118 (6), 1149–1156. doi:10.1016/s0016-5085(00)70368-4

Benyon, R. C., and Arthur, M. J. (2001). Extracellular Matrix Degradation and the Role of Hepatic Stellate Cells. *Semin. Liver Dis.* 21 (3), 373–384. doi:10.1055/s-2001-17552

Beutler, B. (2004). Inferences, Questions and Possibilities in Toll-like Receptor Signalling. *Nature* 430 (6996), 257–263. doi:10.1038/nature02761

Bolkenius, U., Hahn, D., Gressner, A. M., Breitkopf, K., Dooley, S., and Wickert, L. (2004). Glucocorticoids Decrease the Bioavailability of TGF-Beta Which Leads to a Reduced TGF-Beta Signaling in Hepatic Stellate Cells. *Biochem. Biophys. Res. Commun.* 325 (4), 1264–1270. doi:10.1016/j.bbrc.2004.10.164

Borkham-Kamphorst, E., van Roeyen, C. R., Ostendorf, T., Floege, J., Gressner, A. M., and Weiskirchen, R. (2007). Pro-fibrogenic Potential of PDGF-D in Liver Fibrosis. *J. Hepatol.* 46 (6), 1064–1074. doi:10.1016/j.jhep.2007.01.029

Bril, F., Biernacki, D. M., Kalavalapalli, S., Lomonaco, R., Subbarayan, S. K., Lai, J., et al. (2019). Role of Vitamin E for Nonalcoholic Steatohepatitis in Patients with Type 2 Diabetes: A Randomized Controlled Trial. *Diabetes Care* 42 (8), 1481–1488. doi:10.2337/dc19-0167

Cai, F. F., Bian, Y. Q., Wu, R., Sun, Y., Chen, X. L., Yang, M. D., et al. (2019). Yinchenhao Decoction Suppresses Rat Liver Fibrosis Involved in an Apoptosis Regulation Mechanism Based on Network Pharmacology and Transcriptomic Analysis. *Biomed. Pharmacother.* 114, 108863. doi:10.1016/j.biopha.2019.108863

Cai, F. F., Wu, R., Song, Y. N., Xiong, A. Z., Chen, X. L., Yang, M. D., et al. (2018). Yinchenhao Decoction Alleviates Liver Fibrosis by Regulating Bile Acid Metabolism and TGF-β/Smad/ERK Signalling Pathway. *Sci. Rep.* 8 (1), 15367. doi:10.1038/s41598-018-33669-4

Canbay, A., Higuchi, H., Bronk, S. F., Taniai, M., Sebo, T. J., and Gores, G. J. (2002). Fas Enhances Fibrogenesis in the Bile Duct Ligated Mouse: a Link between Apoptosis and Fibrosis. *Gastroenterology* 123 (4), 1323–1330. doi:10.1053/gast.2002.35953

Carloni, V., Romanelli, R. G., Pinzani, M., Laffi, G., and Gentilini, P. (1996). Expression and Function of Integrin Receptors for Collagen and Laminin in Cultured Human Hepatic Stellate Cells. *Gastroenterology* 110 (4), 1127–1136. doi:10.1053/gast.1996.v110.pm8613002

Casini, A., Ceni, E., Salzano, R., Biondi, P., Parola, M., Galli, A., et al. (1997). Neutrophil-derived Superoxide Anion Induces Lipid Peroxidation and Stimulates Collagen Synthesis in Human Hepatic Stellate Cells: Role of Nitric Oxide. *Hepatology* 25 (2), 361–367. doi:10.1053/jhep.1997.v25.pm0009021948

Chang, T. T., Liaw, Y. F., Wu, S. S., Schiff, E., Han, K. H., Lai, C. L., et al. (2010). Long-term Entecavir Therapy Results in the Reversal of Fibrosis/cirrhosis and Continued Histological Improvement in Patients with Chronic Hepatitis B. *Hepatology* 52 (3), 886–893. doi:10.1002/hep.23785

Chen, S. R., Chen, X. P., Lu, J. J., Wang, Y., and Wang, Y. T. (2015). Potent Natural Products and Herbal Medicines for Treating Liver Fibrosis. *Chin. Med.* 10, 7. doi:10.1186/s13020-015-0036-y

Chen, S. W., Zhang, X. R., Wang, C. Z., Chen, W. Z., Xie, W. F., and Chen, Y. X. (2008). RNA Interference Targeting the Platelet-Derived Growth Factor Receptor Beta Subunit Ameliorates Experimental Hepatic Fibrosis in Rats. *Liver Int.* 28 (10), 1446–1457. doi:10.1111/j.1478-3231.2008.01759.x

Chen, Y., Ou, Y., Dong, J., Yang, G., Zeng, Z., Liu, Y., et al. (2018). Osteopontin Promotes Collagen I Synthesis in Hepatic Stellate Cells by miRNA-129-5p Inhibition. *Exp. Cel Res* 362 (2), 343–348. doi:10.1016/j.yexcr.2017.11.035

Cheng, K., and Mahato, R. I. (2011). Biological and Therapeutic Applications of Small RNAs. *Pharm. Res.* 28 (12), 2961–2965. doi:10.1007/s11095-011-0609-0

Colmenero, J., Bataller, R., Sancho-Bru, P., Domínguez, M., Moreno, M., Forns, X., et al. (2009). Effects of Losartan on Hepatic Expression of Nonphagocytic NADPH Oxidase and Fibrogenic Genes in Patients with Chronic Hepatitis C. *Am. J. Physiol. Gastrointest. Liver Physiol.* 297 (4), G726–G734. doi:10.1152/ajpgi.00162.2009

Cong, M., Liu, T., Wang, P., Fan, X., Yang, A., Bai, Y., et al. (2013). Antifibrotic Effects of a Recombinant Adeno-Associated Virus Carrying Small Interfering RNA Targeting TIMP-1 in Rat Liver Fibrosis. *Am. J. Pathol.* 182 (5), 1607–1616. doi:10.1016/j.ajpath.2013.01.036

Czaja, A. J., and Carpenter, H. A. (2004). Decreased Fibrosis during Corticosteroid Therapy of Autoimmune Hepatitis. *J. Hepatol.* 40 (4), 646–652. doi:10.1016/j.jhep.2004.01.009

Czaja, A. J. (2014). Hepatic Inflammation and Progressive Liver Fibrosis in Chronic Liver Disease. *World J. Gastroenterol.* 20 (10), 2515–2532. doi:10.3748/wjg.v20.i10.2515

Deleve, L. D., Wang, X., and Guo, Y. (2008). Sinusoidal Endothelial Cells Prevent Rat Stellate Cell Activation and Promote Reversion to Quiescence. *Hepatology* 48 (3), 920–930. doi:10.1002/hep.22351

Dewidar, B., Meyer, C., Dooley, S., and Meindl-Beinker, A. N. (2019). TGF-β in Hepatic Stellate Cell Activation and Liver Fibrogenesis-Updated 2019. *Cells* 8 (11). doi:10.3390/cells8111419

di Bonzo, L. V., Ferrero, I., Cravanzola, C., Mareschi, K., Rustichell, D., Novo, E., et al. (2008). Human Mesenchymal Stem Cells as a Two-Edged Sword in Hepatic Regenerative Medicine: Engraftment and Hepatocyte Differentiation versus Profibrogenic Potential. *Gut* 57 (2), 223–231. doi:10.1136/gut.2006.111617

Dienstag, J. L., Goldin, R. D., Heathcote, E. J., Hann, H. W., Woessner, M., Stephenson, S. L., et al. (2003). Histological Outcome during Long-Term Lamivudine Therapy. *Gastroenterology* 124 (1), 105–117. doi:10.1053/gast.2003.50013

Ding, B. S., Nolan, D. J., Butler, J. M., James, D., Babazadeh, A. O., Rosenwaks, Z., et al. (2010). Inductive Angiocrine Signals from Sinusoidal Endothelium Are Required for Liver Regeneration. *Nature* 468 (7321), 310–315. doi:10.1038/nature09493

Duffield, J. S., Forbes, S. J., Constandinou, C. M., Clay, S., Partolina, M., Vuthoori, S., et al. (2005). Selective Depletion of Macrophages Reveals Distinct, Opposing Roles during Liver Injury and Repair. *J. Clin. Invest.* 115 (1), 56–65. doi:10.1172/jci22675

Elpek, G. Ö. (2014). Cellular and Molecular Mechanisms in the Pathogenesis of Liver Fibrosis: An Update. *World J. Gastroenterol.* 20 (23), 7260–7276. doi:10.3748/wjg.v20.i23.7260

Eom, Y. W., Shim, K. Y., and Baik, S. K. (2015). Mesenchymal Stem Cell Therapy for Liver Fibrosis. *Korean J. Intern. Med.* 30 (5), 580–589. doi:10.3904/kjim.2015.30.5.580

Fort, M. M., Mozaffarian, A., Stöver, A. G., Correia, Jda. S., Johnson, D. A., Crane, R. T., et al. (2005). A Synthetic TLR4 Antagonist Has Anti-inflammatory Effects in Two Murine Models of Inflammatory Bowel Disease. *J. Immunol.* 174 (10), 6416–6423. doi:10.4049/jimmunol.174.10.6416

Friedman, S. L., Ratziu, V., Harrison, S. A., Abdelmalek, M. F., Aithal, G. P., Caballeria, J., et al. (2018). A Randomized, Placebo-Controlled Trial of Cenicriviroc for Treatment of Nonalcoholic Steatohepatitis with Fibrosis. *Hepatology* 67 (5), 1754–1767. doi:10.1002/hep.29477

Friedman, S. L., Sheppard, D., Duffield, J. S., and Violette, S. (2013). Therapy for Fibrotic Diseases: Nearing the Starting Line. *Sci. Transl Med.* 5 (167), 167sr1. doi:10.1126/scitranslmed.3004700

Fujiwara, K., Yasui, S., Okitsu, K., Yonemitsu, Y., Oda, S., and Yokosuka, O. (2010). The Requirement for a Sufficient Period of Corticosteroid Treatment in Combination with Nucleoside Analogue for Severe Acute Exacerbation of Chronic Hepatitis B. *J. Gastroenterol.* 45 (12), 1255–1262. doi:10.1007/s00535-010-0280-y

García-Trevijano, E. R., Iraburu, M. J., Fontana, L., Domínguez-Rosales, J. A., Auster, A., Covarrubias-Pinedo, A., et al. (1999). Transforming Growth Factor β1induces the Expression of α1(i) Procollagen mRNA by a Hydrogen Peroxide-c/ebpβ-dependent Mechanism in Rat Hepatic Stellate Cells. *Hepatology* 29 (3), 960–970. doi:10.1002/hep.510290346

Gaul, S., Leszczynska, A., Alegre, F., Kaufmann, B., Johnson, C. D., Adams, L. A., et al. (2021). Hepatocyte Pyroptosis and Release of Inflammasome Particles Induce Stellate Cell Activation and Liver Fibrosis. *J. Hepatol.* 74 (1), 156–167. doi:10.1016/j.jhep.2020.07.041

Ge, J. Y., Zheng, Y. W., Tsuchida, T., Furuya, K., Isoda, H., Taniguchi, H., et al. (2020). Hepatic Stellate Cells Contribute to Liver Regeneration through Galectins in Hepatic Stem Cell Niche. *Stem Cel Res Ther* 11 (1), 425. doi:10.1186/s13287-020-01942-x

Geerts, A. (2001). History, Heterogeneity, Developmental Biology, and Functions of Quiescent Hepatic Stellate Cells. *Semin. Liver Dis.* 21 (3), 311–335. doi:10.1055/s-2001-17550

Georges, P. C., Hui, J. J., Gombos, Z., McCormick, M. E., Wang, A. Y., Uemura, M., et al. (2007). Increased Stiffness of the Rat Liver Precedes Matrix Deposition: Implications for Fibrosis. *Am. J. Physiol. Gastrointest. Liver Physiol.* 293 (6), G1147 G1154. doi:10.1152/ajpgi.00032.2007

Ghatak, S., Biswas, A., Dhali, G. K., Chowdhury, A., Boyer, J. L., and Santra, A. (2011). Oxidative Stress and Hepatic Stellate Cell Activation Are Key Events in Arsenic Induced Liver Fibrosis in Mice. *Toxicol. Appl. Pharmacol.* 251 (1), 59–69. doi:10.1016/j.taap.2010.11.016

Gracia-Sancho, J., Caparrós, E., Fernández-Iglesias, A., and Francés, R. (2021). Role of Liver Sinusoidal Endothelial Cells in Liver Diseases. *Nat. Rev. Gastroenterol. Hepatol.* 18 (6), 411–431. doi:10.1038/s41575-020-00411-3

Gressner, A. M., and Weiskirchen, R. (2006). Modern Pathogenetic Concepts of Liver Fibrosis Suggest Stellate Cells and TGF-Beta as Major Players and Therapeutic Targets. *J. Cel Mol Med* 10 (1), 76–99. doi:10.1111/j.1582-4934.2006.tb00292.x

Guo, J., and Friedman, S. L. (2010). Toll-like Receptor 4 Signaling in Liver Injury and Hepatic Fibrogenesis. *Fibrogenesis Tissue Repair* 3, 21. doi:10.1186/1755-1536-3-21

Guo, Y., Xiao, L., Sun, L., and Liu, F. (2012). Wnt/beta-catenin Signaling: a Promising New Target for Fibrosis Diseases. *Physiol. Res.* 61 (4), 337–346. doi:10.33549/physiolres.932289

Gustot, T., and Jalan, R. (2019). Acute-on-chronic Liver Failure in Patients with Alcohol-Related Liver Disease. *J. Hepatol.* 70 (2), 319–327. doi:10.1016/j.jhep.2018.12.008

He, B., Zhang, Y., Lü, M. H., Cao, Y. L., Fan, Y. H., Deng, J. Q., et al. (2013). Glucocorticoids Can Increase the Survival Rate of Patients with Severe Viral Hepatitis B: a Meta-Analysis. *Eur. J. Gastroenterol. Hepatol.* 25 (8), 926–934. doi:10.1097/MEG.0b013e32835f4cbd

Heldin, C. H., and Westermark, B. (1999). Mechanism of Action and *In Vivo* Role of Platelet-Derived Growth Factor. *Physiol. Rev.* 79 (4), 1283–1316. doi:10.1152/physrev.1999.79.4.1283

Hellerbrand, C., Stefanovic, B., Giordano, F., Burchardt, E. R., and Brenner, D. A. (1999). The Role of TGFbeta1 in Initiating Hepatic Stellate Cell Activation *In Vivo*. *J. Hepatol.* 30 (1), 77–87. doi:10.1016/s0168-8278(99)80010-5

Hernandez-Gea, V., and Friedman, S. L. (2011). Pathogenesis of Liver Fibrosis. *Annu. Rev. Pathol.* 6, 425–456. doi:10.1146/annurev-pathol-011110-130246

Hernandez-Munoz, I., de la Torre, P., Sanchez-Alcazar, J., Garcia, I., Santiago, E., Munoz-Yague, M., et al. (1997). Tumor Necrosis Factor Alpha Inhibits Collagen Alpha 1(I) Gene Expression in Rat Hepatic Stellate Cells through a G Protein. *Gastroenterology* 113 (2), 625–640. doi:10.1053/gast.1997.v113.pm9247485

Hu, B. L., Shi, C., Lei, R. E., Lu, D. H., Luo, W., Qin, S. Y., et al. (2016). Interleukin-22 Ameliorates Liver Fibrosis through miR-200a/beta-Catenin. *Sci. Rep.* 6, 36436. doi:10.1038/srep36436

Hu, C., Zhao, L., Zhang, L., Bao, Q., and Li, L. (2020). Mesenchymal Stem Cell-Based Cell-free Strategies: Safe and Effective Treatments for Liver Injury. *Stem Cel Res Ther* 11 (1), 377. doi:10.1186/s13287-020-01895-1

Iredale, J. P., Benyon, R. C., Pickering, J., McCullen, M., Northrop, M., Pawley, S., et al. (1998). Mechanisms of Spontaneous Resolution of Rat Liver Fibrosis. Hepatic Stellate Cell Apoptosis and Reduced Hepatic Expression of Metalloproteinase Inhibitors. *J. Clin. Invest.* 102 (3), 538–549. doi:10.1172/jci1018

Iwaisako, K., Jiang, C., Zhang, M., Cong, M., Moore-Morris, T. J., Park, T. J., et al. (2014). Origin of Myofibroblasts in the Fibrotic Liver in Mice. *Proc. Natl. Acad. Sci. U S A.* 111 (32), E3297–E3305. doi:10.1073/pnas.1400062111

Jaeschke, H. (2011). Reactive Oxygen and Mechanisms of Inflammatory Liver Injury: Present Concepts. *J. Gastroenterol. Hepatol.* 26(Suppl. 1), 173–179. doi:10.1111/j.1440-1746.2010.06592.x

Jang, Y. O., Kim, Y. J., Baik, S. K., Kim, M. Y., Eom, Y. W., Cho, M. Y., et al. (2014). Histological Improvement Following Administration of Autologous Bone Marrow-Derived Mesenchymal Stem Cells for Alcoholic Cirrhosis: a Pilot Study. *Liver Int.* 34 (1), 33–41. doi:10.1111/liv.12218

Janssen, H. L., Reesink, H. W., Lawitz, E. J., Zeuzem, S., Rodriguez-Torres, M., Patel, K., et al. (2013). Treatment of HCV Infection by Targeting microRNA. *N. Engl. J. Med.* 368 (18), 1685–1694. doi:10.1056/NEJMoa1209026

Jiao, J., Sastre, D., Fiel, M. I., Lee, U. E., Ghiassi-Nejad, Z., Ginhoux, F., et al. (2012). Dendritic Cell Regulation of Carbon Tetrachloride-Induced Murine Liver Fibrosis Regression. *Hepatology* 55 (1), 244–255. doi:10.1002/hep.24621

Jiménez Calvente, C., Sehgal, A., Popov, Y., Kim, Y. O., Zevallos, V., Sahin, U., et al. (2015). Specific Hepatic Delivery of Procollagen α1(I) Small Interfering RNA in Lipid-like Nanoparticles Resolves Liver Fibrosis. *Hepatology* 62 (4), 1285–1297. doi:10.1002/hep.27936

Jin, Z., Sun, R., Wei, H., Gao, X., Chen, Y., and Tian, Z. (2011). Accelerated Liver

Fibrosis in Hepatitis B Virus Transgenic Mice: Involvement of Natural Killer T Cells. *Hepatology* 53 (1), 219–229. doi:10.1002/hep.23983

Kagan, P., Sultan, M., Tachlytski, I., Safran, M., and Ben-Ari, Z. (2017). Both MAPK and STAT3 Signal Transduction Pathways Are Necessary for IL-6-dependent Hepatic Stellate Cells Activation. *PLoS One* 12 (5), e0176173. doi:10.1371/journal.pone.0176173

Karlmark, K. R., Weiskirchen, R., Zimmermann, H. W., Gassler, N., Ginhoux, F., Weber, C., et al. (2009). Hepatic Recruitment of the Inflammatory Gr1+ Monocyte Subset upon Liver Injury Promotes Hepatic Fibrosis. *Hepatology* 50 (1), 261–274. doi:10.1002/hep.22950

Kharaziha, P., Hellström, P. M., Noorinayer, B., Farzaneh, F., Aghajani, K., Jafari, F., et al. (2009). Improvement of Liver Function in Liver Cirrhosis Patients after Autologous Mesenchymal Stem Cell Injection: a Phase I-II Clinical Trial. *Eur. J. Gastroenterol. Hepatol.* 21 (10), 1199–1205. doi:10.1097/MEG.0b013e32832a1f6c

Kim, D. H., and Rossi, J. J. (2007). Strategies for Silencing Human Disease Using RNA Interference. *Nat. Rev. Genet.* 8 (3), 173–184. doi:10.1038/nrg2006

Kim, M. Y., Cho, M. Y., Baik, S. K., Jeong, P. H., Suk, K. T., Jang, Y. O., et al. (2012). Beneficial Effects of Candesartan, an Angiotensin-Blocking Agent, on Compensated Alcoholic Liver Fibrosis - a Randomized Open-Label Controlled Study. *Liver Int.* 32 (6), 977–987. doi:10.1111/j.1478-3231.2012.02774.x

Kisseleva, T., and Brenner, D. (2021). Molecular and Cellular Mechanisms of Liver Fibrosis and its Regression. *Nat. Rev. Gastroenterol. Hepatol.* 18 (3), 151–166. doi:10.1038/s41575-020-00372-7

Kitazawa, T., Tsujimoto, T., Kawaratani, H., Fujimoto, M., and Fukui, H. (2008). Expression of Toll-like Receptor 4 in Various Organs in Rats with D-Galactosamine-Induced Acute Hepatic Failure. *J. Gastroenterol. Hepatol.* 23 (8 Pt 2), e494–8. doi:10.1111/j.1440-1746.2007.05246.x

Kitazawa, T., Tsujimoto, T., Kawaratani, H., and Fukui, H. (2009). Therapeutic Approach to Regulate Innate Immune Response by Toll-like Receptor 4 Antagonist E5564 in Rats with D-Galactosamine-Induced Acute Severe Liver Injury. *J. Gastroenterol. Hepatol.* 24 (6), 1089–1094. doi:10.1111/j.1440-1746.2008.05770.x

Kong, D., Zhang, Z., Chen, L., Huang, W., Zhang, F., Wang, L., et al. (2020). Curcumin Blunts Epithelial-Mesenchymal Transition of Hepatocytes to Alleviate Hepatic Fibrosis through Regulating Oxidative Stress and Autophagy. *Redox Biol.* 36, 101600. doi:10.1016/j.redox.2020.101600

Krützfeldt, J., Rajewsky, N., Braich, R., Rajeev, K. G., Tuschl, T., Manoharan, M., et al. (2005). Silencing of microRNAs *In Vivo* with 'antagomirs'. *Nature* 438 (7068), 685–689. doi:10.1038/nature04303

Kulkarni, J. A., Cullis, P. R., and van der Meel, R. (2018). Lipid Nanoparticles Enabling Gene Therapies: From Concepts to Clinical Utility. *Nucleic Acid Ther.* 28 (3), 146–157. doi:10.1089/nat.2018.0721

Lens, S., Alvarado-Tapias, E., Mariño, Z., Londoño, M. C., Martinez, J., LLop, E., et al. (2017). Effects of All-Oral Anti-viral Therapy on HVPG and Systemic Hemodynamics in Patients with Hepatitis C Virus-Associated Cirrhosis. *Gastroenterology* 153 (5), 1273–e1. doi:10.1053/j.gastro.2017.07.016

Li, H. (2020). Advances in Anti Hepatic Fibrotic Therapy with Traditional Chinese Medicine Herbal Formula. *J. Ethnopharmacol* 251, 112442. doi:10.1016/j.jep.2019.112442

Li, J., Hu, R., Xu, S., Li, Y., Qin, Y., Wu, Q., et al. (2017). Xiaochaihutang Attenuates Liver Fibrosis by Activation of Nrf2 Pathway in Rats. *Biomed. Pharmacother.* 96, 847–853. doi:10.1016/j.biopha.2017.10.065

Li, Y., Wang, J., and Asahina, K. (2013). Mesothelial Cells Give Rise to Hepatic Stellate Cells and Myofibroblasts via Mesothelial-Mesenchymal Transition in Liver Injury. *Proc. Natl. Acad. Sci. U S A.* 110 (6), 2324–2329. doi:10.1073/pnas.1214136110

Lin, Y., Dong, M. Q., Liu, Z. M., Xu, M., Huang, Z. H., Liu, H. J., et al. (2021). A Strategy of Vascular-targeted Therapy for Liver Fibrosis. *Hepatology*. doi:10.1002/hep.32299

Liu, J., Yang, Y., Zheng, C., Chen, G., Shen, Z., Zheng, S., et al. (2019). Correlation of Interleukin-33/ST2 Receptor and Liver Fibrosis Progression in Biliary Atresia Patients. *Front. Pediatr.* 7, 403. doi:10.3389/fped.2019.00403

Loomba, R., Lawitz, E., Mantry, P. S., Jayakumar, S., Caldwell, S. H., Arnold, H., et al. (2018). The ASK1 Inhibitor Selonsertib in Patients with Nonalcoholic Steatohepatitis: A Randomized, Phase 2 Trial. *Hepatology* 67 (2), 549–559. doi:10.1002/hep.29514

Lu, D. H., Guo, X. Y., Qin, S. Y., Luo, W., Huang, X. L., Chen, M., et al. (2015).

Interleukin-22 Ameliorates Liver Fibrogenesis by Attenuating Hepatic Stellate Cell Activation and Downregulating the Levels of Inflammatory Cytokines. *World J. Gastroenterol.* 21 (5), 1531–1545. doi:10.3748/wjg.v21.i5.1531

Luedde, T., Kaplowitz, N., and Schwabe, R. F. (2014). Cell Death and Cell Death Responses in Liver Disease: Mechanisms and Clinical Relevance. *Gastroenterology* 147 (4), 765–e4. doi:10.1053/j.gastro.2014.07.018

Ma, R., Chen, J., Liang, Y., Lin, S., Zhu, L., Liang, X., et al. (2017). Sorafenib: A Potential Therapeutic Drug for Hepatic Fibrosis and its Outcomes. *Biomed. Pharmacother.* 88, 459–468. doi:10.1016/j.biopha.2017.01.107

Marcellini, M., Di Ciommo, V., Callea, F., Devito, R., Comparcola, D., Sartorelli, M. R., et al. (2005). Treatment of Wilson's Disease with Zinc from the Time of Diagnosis in Pediatric Patients: a Single-Hospital, 10-year Follow-Up Study. *J. Lab. Clin. Med.* 145 (3), 139–143. doi:10.1016/j.lab.2005.01.007

Marrone, G., Shah, V. H., and Gracia-Sancho, J. (2016). Sinusoidal Communication in Liver Fibrosis and Regeneration. *J. Hepatol.* 65 (3), 608–617. doi:10.1016/j.jhep.2016.04.018

Mederacke, I., Hsu, C. C., Troeger, J. S., Huebener, P., Mu, X., Dapito, D. H., et al. (2013). Fate Tracing Reveals Hepatic Stellate Cells as Dominant Contributors to Liver Fibrosis Independent of its Aetiology. *Nat. Commun.* 4, 2823. doi:10.1038/ncomms3823

Miyazawa, T., Burdeos, G. C., Itaya, M., Nakagawa, K., and Miyazawa, T. (2019). Vitamin E: Regulatory Redox Interactions. *IUBMB Life* 71 (4), 430–441. doi:10.1002/iub.2008

Mudaliar, S., Henry, R. R., Sanyal, A. J., Morrow, L., Marschall, H. U., Kipnes, M., et al. (2013). Efficacy and Safety of the Farnesoid X Receptor Agonist Obeticholic Acid in Patients with Type 2 Diabetes and Nonalcoholic Fatty Liver Disease. *Gastroenterology* 145 (3), 574–e1. doi:10.1053/j.gastro.2013.05.042

Murphy, F. R., Issa, R., Zhou, X., Ratnarajah, S., Nagase, H., Arthur, M. J., et al. (2002). Inhibition of Apoptosis of Activated Hepatic Stellate Cells by Tissue Inhibitor of Metalloproteinase-1 Is Mediated via Effects on Matrix Metalloproteinase Inhibition: Implications for Reversibility of Liver Fibrosis. *J. Biol. Chem.* 277 (13), 11069–11076. doi:10.1074/jbc.M111490200

Musso, G., Cassader, M., Paschetta, E., and Gambino, R. (2017). Thiazolidinediones and Advanced Liver Fibrosis in Nonalcoholic Steatohepatitis: A Meta-Analysis. *JAMA Intern. Med.* 177 (5), 633–640. doi:10.1001/jamainternmed.2016.9607

Novo, E., di Bonzo, L. V., Cannito, S., Colombatto, S., and Parola, M. (2009). Hepatic Myofibroblasts: a Heterogeneous Population of Multifunctional Cells in Liver Fibrogenesis. *Int. J. Biochem. Cel Biol* 41 (11), 2089–2093. doi:10.1016/j.biocel.2009.03.010

Osawa, Y., Hoshi, M., Yasuda, I., Saibara, T., Moriwaki, H., and Kozawa, O. (2013). Tumor Necrosis Factor-α Promotes Cholestasis-Induced Liver Fibrosis in the Mouse through Tissue Inhibitor of Metalloproteinase-1 Production in Hepatic Stellate Cells. *PLoS One* 8 (6), e65251. doi:10.1371/journal.pone.0065251

Osawa, Y., Kojika, E., Hayashi, Y., Kimura, M., Nishikawa, K., Yoshio, S., et al. (2018). Tumor Necrosis Factor-α-Mediated Hepatocyte Apoptosis Stimulates Fibrosis in the Steatotic Liver in Mice. *Hepatol. Commun.* 2 (4), 407–420. doi:10.1002/hep4.1158

Pan, X., Ma, X., Jiang, Y., Wen, J., Yang, L., Chen, D., et al. (2020). A Comprehensive Review of Natural Products against Liver Fibrosis: Flavonoids, Quinones, Lignans, Phenols, and Acids. *Evid. Based Complement. Alternat Med.* 2020, 7171498. doi:10.1155/2020/7171498

Parola, M., and Pinzani, M. (2019). Liver Fibrosis: Pathophysiology, Pathogenetic Targets and Clinical Issues. *Mol. Aspects Med.* 65, 37–55. doi:10.1016/j.mam.2018.09.002

Perepelyuk, M., Terajima, M., Wang, A. Y., Georges, P. C., Janmey, P. A., Yamauchi, M., et al. (2013). Hepatic Stellate Cells and portal Fibroblasts Are the Major Cellular Sources of Collagens and Lysyl Oxidases in normal Liver and Early after Injury. *Am. J. Physiol. Gastrointest. Liver Physiol.* 304 (6), G605–G614. doi:10.1152/ajpgi.00222.2012

Pinzani, M., Gesualdo, L., Sabbah, G. M., and Abboud, H. E. (1989). Effects of Platelet-Derived Growth Factor and Other Polypeptide Mitogens on DNA Synthesis and Growth of Cultured Rat Liver Fat-Storing Cells. *J. Clin. Invest.* 84 (6), 1786–1793. doi:10.1172/jci114363

Pinzani, M., Milani, S., Herbst, H., DeFranco, R., Grappone, C., Gentilini, A., et al. (1996). Expression of Platelet-Derived Growth Factor and its Receptors in normal Human Liver and during Active Hepatic Fibrogenesis. *Am. J. Pathol.* 148 (3), 785–800.

Poisson, J., Lemoinne, S., Boulanger, C., Durand, F., Moreau, R., Valla, D., et al.

(2017). Liver Sinusoidal Endothelial Cells: Physiology and Role in Liver Diseases. *J. Hepatol.* 66 (1), 212–227. doi:10.1016/j.jhep.2016.07.009

Powell, W. J., Jr., and Klatskin, G. (1968). Duration of Survival in Patients with Laennec's Cirrhosis. Influence of Alcohol Withdrawal, and Possible Effects of Recent Changes in General Management of the Disease. *Am. J. Med.* 44 (3), 406–420. doi:10.1016/0002-9343(68)90111-3

Pradere, J. P., Kluwe, J., De Minicis, S., Jiao, J. J., Gwak, G. Y., Dapito, D. H., et al. (2013). Hepatic Macrophages but Not Dendritic Cells Contribute to Liver Fibrosis by Promoting the Survival of Activated Hepatic Stellate Cells in Mice. *Hepatology* 58 (4), 1461–1473. doi:10.1002/hep.26429

Radaeva, S., Sun, R., Jaruga, B., Nguyen, V. T., Tian, Z., and Gao, B. (2006). Natural Killer Cells Ameliorate Liver Fibrosis by Killing Activated Stellate Cells in NKG2D-dependent and Tumor Necrosis Factor-Related Apoptosis-Inducing Ligand-dependent Manners. *Gastroenterology* 130 (2), 435–452. doi:10.1053/j.gastro.2005.10.055

Ramachandran, P., Pellicoro, A., Vernon, M. A., Boulter, L., Aucott, R. L., Ali, A., et al. (2012). Differential Ly-6C Expression Identifies the Recruited Macrophage Phenotype, Which Orchestrates the Regression of Murine Liver Fibrosis. *Proc. Natl. Acad. Sci. U S A.* 109 (46), E3186–E3195. doi:10.1073/pnas.1119964109

Reid, D. T., Reyes, J. L., McDonald, B. A., Vo, T., Reimer, R. A., and Eksteen, B. (2016). Kupffer Cells Undergo Fundamental Changes during the Development of Experimental NASH and Are Critical in Initiating Liver Damage and Inflammation. *PLoS One* 11 (7), e0159524. doi:10.1371/journal.pone.0159524

Rockey, D. C. (2016). Liver Fibrosis Reversion after Suppression of Hepatitis B Virus. *Clin. Liver Dis.* 20 (4), 667–679. doi:10.1016/j.cld.2016.06.003

Roeb, E., Purucker, E., Breuer, B., Nguyen, H., Heinrich, P. C., Rose-John, S., et al. (1997). TIMP Expression in Toxic and Cholestatic Liver Injury in Rat. *J. Hepatol.* 27 (3), 535–544. doi:10.1016/s0168-8278(97)80359-5

Sanyal, A. J., Chalasani, N., Kowdley, K. V., McCullough, A., Diehl, A. M., Bass, N. M., et al. (2010). Pioglitazone, Vitamin E, or Placebo for Nonalcoholic Steatohepatitis. *N. Engl. J. Med.* 362 (18), 1675–1685. doi:10.1056/NEJMoa0907929

Schiff, E., Simsek, H., Lee, W. M., Chao, Y. C., Sette, H., Jr., Janssen, H. L., et al. (2008). Efficacy and Safety of Entecavir in Patients with Chronic Hepatitis B and Advanced Hepatic Fibrosis or Cirrhosis. *Am. J. Gastroenterol.* 103 (11), 2776–2783. doi:10.1111/j.1572-0241.2008.02086.x

Schnabl, B., and Brenner, D. A. (2014). Interactions between the Intestinal Microbiome and Liver Diseases. *Gastroenterology* 146 (6), 1513–1524. doi:10.1053/j.gastro.2014.01.020

Schon, H. T., and Weiskirchen, R. (2014). Immunomodulatory Effects of Transforming Growth Factor-β in the Liver. *Hepatobiliary Surg. Nutr.* 3 (6), 386–406. doi:10.3978/j.issn.2304-3881.2014.11.06

Schulze, R. J., Schott, M. B., Casey, C. A., Tuma, P. L., and McNiven, M. A. (2019). The Cell Biology of the Hepatocyte: A Membrane Trafficking Machine. *J. Cel Biol* 218 (7), 2096–2112. doi:10.1083/jcb.201903090

Seki, E., De Minicis, S., Osterreicher, C. H., Kluwe, J., Osawa, Y., Brenner, D. A., et al. (2007). TLR4 Enhances TGF-Beta Signaling and Hepatic Fibrosis. *Nat. Med.* 13 (11), 1324–1332. doi:10.1038/nm1663

Seki, E., and Schwabe, R. F. (2015). Hepatic Inflammation and Fibrosis: Functional Links and Key Pathways. *Hepatology* 61 (3), 1066–1079. doi:10.1002/hep.27332

Sersté, T., Cornillie, A., Njimi, H., Pavesi, M., Arroyo, V., Putignano, A., et al. (2018). The Prognostic Value of Acute-On-Chronic Liver Failure during the Course of Severe Alcoholic Hepatitis. *J. Hepatol.* 69 (2), 318–324. doi:10.1016/j.jhep.2018.02.022

Shaker, M. E., Ghani, A., Shiha, G. E., Ibrahim, T. M., and Mehal, W. Z. (2013). Nilotinib Induces Apoptosis and Autophagic Cell Death of Activated Hepatic Stellate Cells via Inhibition of Histone Deacetylases. *Biochim. Biophys. Acta* 1833 (8), 1992–2003. doi:10.1016/j.bbamcr.2013.02.033

Shan, L., Liu, Z., Ci, L., Shuai, C., Lv, X., and Li, J. (2019). Research Progress on the Anti-hepatic Fibrosis Action and Mechanism of Natural Products. *Int. Immunopharmacol* 75, 105765. doi:10.1016/j.intimp.2019.105765

Song, G., Pacher, M., Balakrishnan, A., Yuan, Q., Tsay, H. C., Yang, D., et al. (2016). Direct Reprogramming of Hepatic Myofibroblasts into Hepatocytes *In Vivo* Attenuates Liver Fibrosis. *Cell Stem Cell* 18 (6), 797–808. doi:10.1016/j.stem.2016.01.010

Streetz, K. L., Tacke, F., Leifeld, L., Wüstefeld, T., Graw, A., Klein, C., et al. (2003). Interleukin 6/gp130-dependent Pathways Are Protective during Chronic Liver Diseases. *Hepatology* 38 (1), 218–229. doi:10.1053/jhep.2003.50268

Sun, H., Che, Q. M., Zhao, X., and Pu, X. P. (2010). Antifibrotic Effects of Chronic

Baicalein Administration in a CCl4 Liver Fibrosis Model in Rats. *Eur. J. Pharmacol.* 631 (1-3), 53–60. doi:10.1016/j.ejphar.2010.01.002

Tacke, F., and Zimmermann, H. W. (2014). Macrophage Heterogeneity in Liver Injury and Fibrosis. *J. Hepatol.* 60 (5), 1090–1096. doi:10.1016/j.jhep.2013.12.025

Tada, T., Kumada, T., Toyoda, H., Sone, Y., Takeshima, K., Ogawa, S., et al. (2018). Viral Eradication Reduces Both Liver Stiffness and Steatosis in Patients with Chronic Hepatitis C Virus Infection Who Received Direct-Acting Anti-viral Therapy. *Aliment. Pharmacol. Ther.* 47 (7), 1012–1022. doi:10.1111/apt.14554

Takahashi, H., Shigefuku, R., Maeyama, S., and Suzuki, M. (2014). Cirrhosis Improvement to Alcoholic Liver Fibrosis after Passive Abstinence. *BMJ Case Rep.* 2014. doi:10.1136/bcr-2013-201618

Takashima, K., Matsunaga, N., Yoshimatsu, M., Hazeki, K., Kaisho, T., Uekata, M., et al. (2009). Analysis of Binding Site for the Novel Small-Molecule TLR4 Signal Transduction Inhibitor TAK-242 and its Therapeutic Effect on Mouse Sepsis Model. *Br. J. Pharmacol.* 157 (7), 1250–1262. doi:10.1111/j.1476-5381.2009.00297.x

Thakral, S., and Ghoshal, K. (2015). miR-122 Is a Unique Molecule with Great Potential in Diagnosis, Prognosis of Liver Disease, and Therapy Both as miRNA Mimic and Antimir. *Curr. Gene Ther.* 15 (2), 142–150. doi:10.2174/1566523214666141224095610

Theocharis, A. D., Skandalis, S. S., Gialeli, C., and Karamanos, N. K. (2016). Extracellular Matrix Structure. *Adv. Drug Deliv. Rev.* 97, 4–27. doi:10.1016/j.addr.2015.11.001

Thursz, M. R., Richardson, P., Allison, M., Austin, A., Bowers, M., Day, C. P., et al. (2015). Prednisolone or Pentoxifylline for Alcoholic Hepatitis. *N. Engl. J. Med.* 372 (17), 1619–1628. doi:10.1056/NEJMoa1412278

Troeger, J. S., Mederacke, I., Gwak, G. Y., Dapito, D. H., Mu, X., Hsu, C. C., et al. (2012). Deactivation of Hepatic Stellate Cells during Liver Fibrosis Resolution in Mice. *Gastroenterology* 143 (4), 1073–e22. doi:10.1053/j.gastro.2012.06.036

Tsuchida, T., and Friedman, S. L. (2017). Mechanisms of Hepatic Stellate Cell Activation. *Nat. Rev. Gastroenterol. Hepatol.* 14 (7), 397–411. doi:10.1038/nrgastro.2017.38

Tsung, A., McCoy, S. L., Klune, J. R., Geller, D. A., Billiar, T. R., and Hefeneider, S. H. (2007). A Novel Inhibitory Peptide of Toll-like Receptor Signaling Limits Lipopolysaccharide-Induced Production of Inflammatory Mediators and Enhances Survival in Mice. *Shock* 27 (4), 364–369. doi:10.1097/01.shk.0000239773.95280.2c

Valera, J. M., Smok, G., Márquez, S., Poniachik, J., and Brahm, J. (2011). Histological Regression of Liver Fibrosis with Immunosuppressive Therapy in Autoimmune Hepatitis. *Gastroenterol. Hepatol.* 34 (1), 10–15. doi:10.1016/j.gastrohep.2010.10.003

Van Herck, J. L., Schrijvers, D. M., De Meyer, G. R., Martinet, W., Van Hove, C. E., Bult, H., et al. (2010). Transglutaminase 2 Deficiency Decreases Plaque Fibrosis and Increases Plaque Inflammation in Apolipoprotein-E-Deficient Mice. *J. Vasc. Res.* 47 (3), 231–240. doi:10.1159/000255966

Varela-Rey, M., Fontán-Gabás, L., Blanco, P., López-Zabalza, M. J., and Iraburu, M. J. (2007). Glutathione Depletion Is Involved in the Inhibition of Procollagen alpha1(I) mRNA Levels Caused by TNF-Alpha on Hepatic Stellate Cells. *Cytokine* 37 (3), 212–217. doi:10.1016/j.cyto.2007.03.013

Villesen, I. F., Daniels, S. J., Leeming, D. J., Karsdal, M. A., and Nielsen, M. J. (2020). Review Article: the Signalling and Functional Role of the Extracellular Matrix in the Development of Liver Fibrosis. *Aliment. Pharmacol. Ther.* 52 (1), 85–97. doi:10.1111/apt.15773

Wang, Y. Z., Zhang, W., Wang, Y. H., Fu, X. L., and Xue, C. Q. (2019). Repression of Liver Cirrhosis Achieved by Inhibitory Effect of miR-454 on Hepatic Stellate Cells Activation and Proliferation via Wnt10a. *J. Biochem.* 165 (4), 361–367. doi:10.1093/jb/mvy111

Wehr, A., Baeck, C., Heymann, F., Niemietz, P. M., Hammerich, L., Martin, C., et al. (2013). Chemokine Receptor CXCR6-dependent Hepatic NK T Cell Accumulation Promotes Inflammation and Liver Fibrosis. *J. Immunol.* 190 (10), 5226–5236. doi:10.4049/jimmunol.1202909

Wells, R. G., Schwabe, R. F., and Schwabe, R. (2015). Origin and Function of Myofibroblasts in the Liver. *Semin. Liver Dis.* 35 (2), 97–106. doi:10.1055/s-0035-1550061

Wolf, M. J., Adili, A., Piotrowitz, K., Abdullah, Z., Boege, Y., Stemmer, K., et al. (2014). Metabolic Activation of Intrahepatic CD8+ T Cells and NKT Cells Causes Nonalcoholic Steatohepatitis and Liver Cancer via Cross-Talk with Hepatocytes. *Cancer Cell* 26 (4), 549_564. doi:10.1016/j.ccell.2014.09.003

Wu, L., Zhou, P. Q., Xie, J. W., Zhu, R., Zhou, S. C., Wang, G., et al. (2015). Effects of Yinchenhao Decoction on Self-Regulation of Renin-Angiotensin System by Targeting Angiotensin Converting Enzyme 2 in Bile Duct-Ligated Rat Liver. *J. Huazhong Univ. Sci. Technolog Med. Sci.* 35 (4), 519–524. doi:10.1007/s11596-015-1463-9

Wynn, T. A., and Barron, L. (2010). Macrophages: Master Regulators of Inflammation and Fibrosis. *Semin. Liver Dis.* 30 (3), 245–257. doi:10.1055/s-0030-1255354

Xie, G., Wang, X., Wang, L., Wang, L., Atkinson, R. D., Kanel, G. C., et al. (2012). Role of Differentiation of Liver Sinusoidal Endothelial Cells in Progression and Regression of Hepatic Fibrosis in Rats. *Gastroenterology* 142 (4), 918–e6. doi:10.1053/j.gastro.2011.12.017

Xu, Y., Liang, P., Bian, M., Chen, W., Wang, X., Lin, J., et al. (2016). Interleukin-13 Is Involved in the Formation of Liver Fibrosis in Clonorchis Sinensis-Infected Mice. *Parasitol. Res.* 115 (7), 2653–2660. doi:10.1007/s00436-016-5012-7

Yang, L., Jung, Y., Omenetti, A., Witek, R. P., Choi, S., Vandongen, H. M., et al. (2008). Fate-mapping Evidence that Hepatic Stellate Cells Are Epithelial Progenitors in Adult Mouse Livers. *Stem Cells* 26 (8), 2104–2113. doi:10.1634/stemcells.2008-0115

Yang, L., Stimpson, S. A., Chen, L., Wallace Harrington, W., and Rockey, D. C. (2010). Effectiveness of the PPARγ Agonist, GW570, in Liver Fibrosis. *Inflamm. Res.* 59 (12), 1061–1071. doi:10.1007/s00011-010-0226-0

Yang, N. H., Yuan, G. S., Zhou, Y. C., Liu, J. W., Huang, H. P., Hu, C. G., et al. (2016). Entecavir Combined with Fufang Biejia Ruangan Tablet in Treatment of Chronic Hepatitis B Patients with Liver Fibrosis: 96-week Efficacy Analyses. *Nan Fang Yi Ke Da Xue Xue Bao* 36 (6), 775–779.

Ye, H. L., Zhang, J. W., Chen, X. Z., Wu, P. B., Chen, L., and Zhang, G. (2020). Ursodeoxycholic Acid Alleviates Experimental Liver Fibrosis Involving Inhibition of Autophagy. *Life Sci.* 242, 117175. doi:10.1016/j.lfs.2019.117175

Yoneda, A., Sakai-Sawada, K., Niitsu, Y., and Tamura, Y. (2016). Vitamin A and Insulin Are Required for the Maintenance of Hepatic Stellate Cell Quiescence. *Exp. Cel Res* 341 (1), 8–17. doi:10.1016/j.yexcr.2016.01.012

Yoshiji, H., Kuriyama, S., and Fukui, H. (2007). Blockade of Renin-Angiotensin System in Antifibrotic Therapy. *J. Gastroenterol. Hepatol.* 22 (Suppl. 1), S93–S95. doi:10.1111/j.1440-1746.2006.04663.x

Zhang, F., Zhang, Z., Chen, L., Kong, D., Zhang, X., Lu, C., et al. (2014). Curcumin Attenuates Angiogenesis in Liver Fibrosis and Inhibits Angiogenic Properties of Hepatic Stellate Cells. *J. Cel Mol Med* 18 (7), 1392–1406. doi:10.1111/jcmm.12286

Zhao, X. A., Chen, G., Liu, Y., Chen, Y., Wu, H., Xiong, Y., et al. (2018). Curcumin Reduces Ly6Chi Monocyte Infiltration to Protect against Liver Fibrosis by Inhibiting Kupffer Cells Activation to Reduce Chemokines Secretion. *Biomed. Pharmacother.* 106, 868–878. doi:10.1016/j.biopha.2018.07.028

Zhou, X., and Yang, X. F. (2014). Progress of Targeting Transforming Growth Factor-B1 Small Interfering RNA in Liver Fibrosis. *Chin. Med. Sci. J.* 29 (4), 231–235. doi:10.1016/s1001-9294(14)60076-6

Zhu, W., Xu, W., Jiang, R., Qian, H., Chen, M., Hu, J., et al. (2006). Mesenchymal Stem Cells Derived from Bone Marrow Favor Tumor Cell Growth *In Vivo*. *Exp. Mol. Pathol.* 80 (3), 267–274. doi:10.1016/j.yexmp.2005.07.004

10

Kinsenoside Protects against Radiation-Induced Liver Fibrosis *via* Downregulating Connective Tissue Growth Factor through TGF-β1 Signaling

Xiaoqi Nie[1,2], Qianqian Yu[1], Long Li[1], Minxiao Yi[1], Bili Wu[1], Yongbiao Huang[1], Yonghui Zhang[3], Hu Han[1]* and Xianglin Yuan[1]*

[1]Department of Oncology, Tongji Hospital, Huazhong University of Science and Technology, Wuhan, China, [2]Department of Dermatology, Tongji Hospital, Huazhong University of Science and Technology, Wuhan, China, [3]School of Pharmacy, Tongji Medical College, Huazhong University of Science and Technology, Wuhan, China

*Correspondence:
Hu Han
hanhu2007@163.com
Xianglin Yuan
yuanxianglin@hust.edu.cn

Radiation-induced liver fibrosis (RILF) is a serious complication of the radiotherapy of liver cancer, which lacks effective prevention and treatment measures. Kinsenoside (KD) is a monomeric glycoside isolated from *Anoectochilus roxburghii*, which has been reported to show protective effect on the early progression of liver fibrosis. However, the role of KD in affecting RILF remains unknown. Here, we found that KD alleviated RILF via downregulating connective tissue growth factor (CTGF) through TGF-β1 signaling. Sprague-Dawley rats were administered with 20 mg/kg KD per day for 8 weeks after a single 30Gy irradiation on the right part of liver, and tumor-bearing nude mice were administered with 30 mg/kg KD per day after a single fraction of 10Gy on the tumor inoculation site. Twenty-four weeks postirradiation, we found that the administration of KD after irradiation resulted in decreased expression of α-SMA and fibronectin in the liver tissue while had no adverse effect on the tumor radiotherapy. Besides, KD inhibited the activation of hepatic stellate cells (HSCs) postirradiation via targeting CTGF as indicated by the transcriptome sequencing. Results of the pathway enrichment and immunohistochemistry suggested that KD reduced the expression of TGF-β1 protein after radiotherapy, and exogenous TGF-β1 induced HSCs to produce α-SMA and other fibrosis-related proteins. The content of activated TGF-β1 in the supernatant decreased after treatment with KD. In addition, KD inhibited the expression of the fibrosis-related proteins by regulating the TGF-β1/Smad/CTGF pathway, resulting in the intervention of liver fibrosis. In conclusion, this study revealed that KD alleviated RILF through the regulation of TGFβ1/Smad/CTGF pathway with no side effects on the tumor therapy. KD, in combination with blocking the TGF-β1 pathway and CTGF molecule or not, may become the innovative and effective treatment for RILF.

Keywords: radiation-induced liver fibrosis, kinsenoside, hepatic stellate cells, transforming growth factor-β1, connective tissue growth factor

INTRODUCTION

Radiotherapy is an important treatment method for liver cancer. However, the damage to normal tissues caused by radiotherapy often restricts the efficacy of radiotherapy, and the delayed organ damage such as the radiation-induced liver fibrosis (RILF) is inevitable and even lethal in some cases (Du et al., 2010; Han et al., 2019). Radiation-induced liver injury is generally divided into the subacute radiation-induced liver disease stage and the advanced RILF stage (Liang et al., 2018). The loss of liver parenchymal cells, the destruction of liver lobule structure and the hyperplasia of fibrous connective tissue are the main histological characteristics of the RILF (Lee and Friedman 2011; Kim and Jung 2017). The radiation-induced tissue fibrosis was formerly considered to be inevitable and irreversible, while it is currently believed that the radiation-induced fibrosis is caused by the dynamic interaction between multiple cell types in specific organs, suggesting that the RILF may be regulable (Du et al., 2010; Hu et al., 2018). However, the potential regulatory mechanism needs to be further explored. As the number of long-term surviving patients largely increased with the improvement of the therapeutic effect for liver cancer, one of the main directions of the radiobiological research is to reduce and treat the late liver fibrosis caused by the radiotherapy (Jung et al., 2013; Atta 2015; Cheng et al., 2015).

Anoectochilus roxburghii (*A. roxburghii*), a traditional Chinese herbal plant, has a variety of pharmacological effects, including anti-obesity, anti-hyperglycemia, anti-osteoporosis, and so on, among which the liver-protecting effect shows significant effect in clinical use (Ye et al., 2017). Kinsenoside (3-(R)-3-β-D-Glucopyranosyloxybutanolide, KD) is a biologically active compound isolated and extracted from *A. roxburghii* which has been reported to have the anti-hyperglycemic and anti-hyperlipidemic effects, and to alleviate the acute inflammation. In addition, KD has shown a protective effect on the liver in the mice and the patients with liver disease, but the mechanism is not yet clearly understood (Tullius et al., 2014; Zarzycka et al., 2014; Zhang et al., 2014; Qi et al., 2018; Ming et al., 2021). Up to now, there is no research focusing on the roles of KD playing in the RILF.

When activated, myofibroblasts are the most important collagen-producing cells in the fibrosis process, and it is generally believed that hepatic stellate cells (HSCs) are the main source of collagen-producing fibroblasts in the cirrhotic liver (Wei et al., 2013). Studies have shown that HSCs are the critical effector cells in the process of the RILF (Oakley et al., 2005; Hasan et al., 2017; Dewidar et al., 2019b). In the development of the RILF, HSCs are activated and continue to proliferate, which leads to the imbalance and interaction of various fibrosis-related cytokines, ultimately resulting in the accumulation of the extracellular matrix (ECM) (Wang et al., 2013; Chen et al., 2017; Yuan et al., 2019a).

The transforming growth factor-β (TGF-β) signaling pathway family is the core member that maintains the dynamic balance of tissues and organs, and plays a vital role in regulating cell proliferation, differentiation, migration or death (Derynck and Budi 2019; Dituri et al., 2019; Katsuno et al., 2019). As reported, TGF-β is not only a key regulator of liver pathophysiology, but also one of the most important pro-fibrotic cytokines in the process of liver fibrosis (Xu et al., 2016; Wu et al., 2018b; Mu et al., 2018; Dewidar et al., 2019a; Dewidar et al., 2019b).

Based on these existing research results, we studied whether KD could protect the liver after radiation and interfere with the RILF. In addition, to further clarify the mechanism through which KD affected the RILF, we tested the effect of KD on the HSCs and screened the key target molecules and signaling pathways affected by KD.

MATERIALS AND METHODS

Ethics Statement

Male Sprague-Dawley (SD, Experimental Animal Center of Hubei Province, China) rats aged 7–8 weeks and Balb/c nude mice (Hunan SJA Laboratory Animal Co., Ltd., Hunan, China) aged 4 weeks were housed in the specific pathogen-free breeding system. All rats and mice were randomly grouped and adaptively fed for a week. All the experimental designs and procedures were conducted in accordance with the ARRIVE guidelines and the National Institutes of Health guide for the care and use of Laboratory animals (NIH Publications No. 8023, revised 1978).

Irradiation and Kinsenoside Treatment of SD Rats

The SD rats were divided into four groups by randomization (n = 5 per group): Control group (Con), only KD group (KD), irradiation group (IR) and irradiation treated with KD group (IR + KD). The radiation dose was a single 30Gy for the irradiation groups, and the irradiation field was 2.5 × 2.5 cm in the right part of the liver (RS2000 X-ray Biological Research Irradiator, 25 mA, 160 kV; Rad Source Technologies Inc., Suwanee, GA). The KD powder was obtained from the School of Pharmacy, Tongji Medical College, Huazhong University of Science and Technology, and the KD solution was made by dissolving the powder in the pure water. The KD solution was given 20 mg/kg per day by oral gavage, while the Con group and IR group were fed with pure water at the same time. The gavage feeding time for the irradiation groups was 8 weeks postirradiation. The animals used to observe the pathological results were euthanized at the 24th week after irradiation.

Irradiation and Transplantation Tumor Experiment of Nude Mice

The hepatocellular carcinoma cells (HepG2) were injected into the subcutaneous tissue under the left upper limb of nude mice. The diameters of the xenograft tumors were measured and the mice weighed every 3 days. When the mean size of the xenograft tumors reached 85–120 mm³, the tumor-bearing nude mice were divided into four groups by randomization (n = 7 per group): Con group, KD group, IR group and IR + KD group. The radiation dose was a single 10Gy for the irradiation groups, and the irradiation fields were the tumor inoculation sites. The KD solution was given 30 mg/kg per day by oral gavage immediately postirradiation. The gavage feeding time was 12 days until the nude mice were euthanized.

Liver Histology

At the 24th week postirradiation, the rats were euthanized and the liver tissues were cut into pieces. Part of the liver tissues were immersed in 4% paraformaldehyde for paraffin embedding. The liver sections were stained with Masson's trichrome and HE staining (Aspen Biological, Wuhan, China). The Masson's-stained sections were used to assess the degree of liver fibrosis using the METAVIR scoring method. All the scoring work was carried out by two independent senior pathologists that were blinded to the experiment.

Immunohistochemistry and Immunofluorescence

For the immunohistochemistry (IHC) of the liver tissues, the primary antibodies were TGF-β1 (1:200; Cell Signaling Technology Inc., Danvers, MA) and α-smooth muscle actin (α-SMA) (1:200; Servicebio Technology, Wuhan, China). For the immunofluorescence of the liver tissues and HSCs, the primary antibodies were collagen (1:200; BOSTER Biological Technology, Wuhan, China) and α-SMA (1:200; Servicebio Technology, Wuhan, China).

The IHC scores were based on the staining intensity and positive-stained cells. Five fields of each slice were randomly selected and the average value was the final IHC score. All the scoring work was carried out by two independent senior pathologists that were blinded to the experiment.

Western Blot Analysis

Liver tissues (30–100 mg) were homogenized and the protein liquid was extracted. The proteins were separated and transferred to the polyvinylidene difluoride (PVDF) membranes (Millipore, Billerica, MA). The PVDF membranes were incubated with primary antibody overnight at 4°C. The antibodies included: α-SMA (1:1,000; Servicebio Technology, Wuhan, China), fibronectin (FN), collagen I and connective tissue growth factor (CTGF) (1:1,000; BOSTER Biological Technology, Wuhan, China), TGF-β1 and Smad2/3 and P-Smad2/3 (1:1,000; Cell Signaling Technology Inc., Danvers, MA), GAPDH and β-actin (1:1,000; Aspen Biological, Wuhan, China). Then, the PVDF membranes were incubated with the anti-rabbit IgG secondary antibody (1:6,000; Aspen Biological, Wuhan, China) at room temperature for 1 hour. Finally, the proteins were detected with the Super Signal West Pico plus Chemiluminescent Substrate (Thermo Fisher Scientific, Waltham, MA).

Hydroxyproline Content Assay

The content of hydroxyproline in the liver tissues was detected by the hydroxyproline assay kit (Nanjing Jiancheng Bioengineering Institute, Nanjing, China). All the steps were implemented strictly following the instructions.

Cell Culture and Treatment

The immortalized hepatic rat stellate cell line (HSC-T6) was kindly provided by Procell Life Science Technology Co., Ltd.

(Wuhan, China). The HSCs were cultured in Dulbecco's Modified Eagle's Medium (DMEM) supplemented with 10% fetal bovine serum (FBS, Gibco). The culture incubator for the cells was 37°C with constant temperature, constant humidity, and 5% CO_2. The HSCs were seeded in the 6-well plates and cultured for about 24 h before treated with different concentrations of KD and TGF-β1, respectively. After that, cells were cultured for 24 h until further detection.

Real-Time Fluorescence Quantitative PCR

The RNA of the cells was extracted with TRIzol solution, then the concentration of RNA in each group was determined. The cDNA was obtained according to the reverse transcription cDNA synthesis kit (Thermo, United States). The relative expression of genes was finally calculated according to the SYBR Green PCR kit (Thermo, United States) and the $2^{-\Delta\Delta Ct}$ method.

High Throughput mRNA Sequencing

Total RNA was extracted with the TRIzol Reagent kit (Invitrogen), quantified and qualified with NanoDrop (Thermo Fisher Scientific Inc.) and Agilent 2,100 Bioanalyzer (Agilent Technologies). Next generation sequencing library preparation was constructed using 1 µg total RNA with RIN value above 6.5 in accordance with the manufacturer's instructions. The Poly(A) mRNA Magnetic Isolation Module or rRNA Removal Kit was used to isolate the poly(A) mRNA.The mRNA fragmentation and priming was performed using First Strand Synthesis Reaction Buffer and Random Primers. cDNA was synthesized using the ProtoScript II Reverse Transcriptase and the Second Strand Synthesis Enzyme Mix, followed by purification by beads. The End Prep Enzyme Mix and the T-A ligation was used to repair cDNA ends, add a dA-tailing, and add adaptors to both ends. DNA fragments around 420 bp were then recovered in the size selection. The P5 and P7 primers were used for sample amplification by PCR for 13 cycles. The PCR products were then cleaned up, validated and quantified.

The Illumina HiSeq instrument (Illumina, San Diego, CA, United States) was then used in accordance with the manufacturer's instructions. The libraries were multiplexed and loaded. The 2 × 150 bp paired-end (PE) configuration was used for sequencing. The HiSeq Control Software (HCS) + OLB + GAPipeline-1.6 (Illumina) was used for image analysis and base calling. GENEWIZ was used to process and analyze the sequences.

Cell Cycle Detection

The cells were digested and the cell suspension was centrifuged. The cells were resuspended in 1ml of pre-cooled 70% ethanol solution and placed in the −20°C refrigerator for more than 12 h. After the fixation, the cells were washed twice and treated in accordance with the requirements of the cell cycle detection kit (Servicebio Technology, Wuhan, China).

Enzyme Linked Immunosorbent Assay

The cell culture supernatant was separated for testing, and the TGF-β1 content in the supernatant was detected according to the enzyme linked immunosorbent assay (ELISA) kit (ELK Biotechnology, Wuhan, China) instructions.

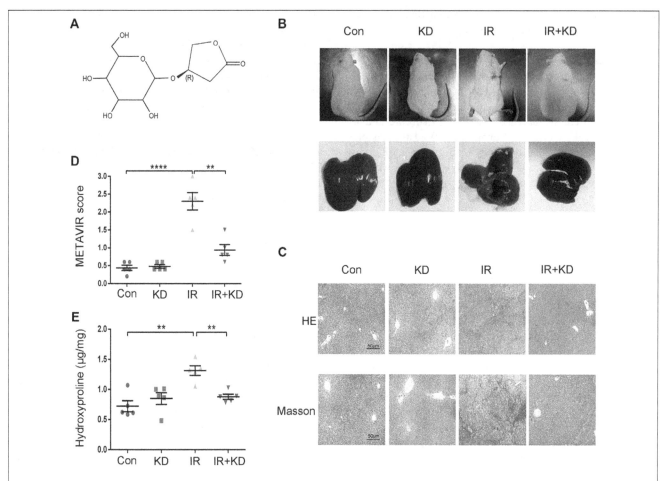

FIGURE 1 | KD alleviates the RILF in the rat model **(A)** Chemical structure of KD **(B)** Photograph of irradiated areas and part of the livers of the rats. The liver was yellowish and rough in the IR group, while in the other groups the livers were ruddy and smooth **(C)** RILF was assessed through the H&E and Masson's trichrome staining of representative liver slices. In the IR group, blue stained collagen deposited in liver tissues, while KD treatment significantly attenuated the radiation induced injury **(D)** METAVIR scores for grading the liver fibrosis. KD treatment attenuated the degree of fibrosis **(E)** The content of hydroxyproline in the liver tissues. Hydroxyproline content increased after irradiation and decreased significantly in the IR + KD group. For all results in this figure, original magnification, ×100. Mean ± SEM. n. s. denotes not significant; **$p < 0.01$, ***$p < 0.001$, ****$p < 0.0001$.

Statistical Analysis

In this study, GraphPad Prism software was used to perform statistical data analysis. The results were expressed as mean ± standard error of mean (SEM). Student's t test was used to analyze continuous variable data. *$p < 0.05$, **$p < 0.01$, ***$p < 0.001$, ****$p < 0.0001$. $p < 0.05$ was statistically significant.

RESULTS

Kinsenoside Attenuates Radiation-Induced Liver Fibrosis in the Rat Model

In order to investigate the effect of KD on the RILF, we established the animal model of the RILF. 24 weeks after irradiation, the partial hair loss and ulceration appeared in the irradiated area. Besides, the liver was yellowish and the surface of the liver was rough and grainy in the IR group, while in the IR + KD group the liver was ruddy and smooth (**Figure 1B**). Next, the pathological analysis results of the HE and Masson staining showed that the rats suffered RILF from irradiation,

and the normal liver lobule structure of the rat liver was destroyed, with the central vein even collapsed. There was obvious fibrous connective tissue deposition in the liver, and the portal area was often more obvious, while KD could attenuate RILF. KD administration significantly reduced the deposition of collagen fibers, and the damage to the liver structure and central veins was also reduced (**Figure 1C**). METAVIR fibrosis score and hydroxyproline content were important indicators for judging the degree of liver fibrosis (Bedossa and Poynard 1996). The liver fibrosis score of the IR group was significantly higher than that of the Con group, while the IR + KD group score decreased (**Figures 1D,E**), indicating that KD administration after irradiation attenuated liver tissue fibrosis caused by radiation.

Kinsenoside Inhibits Expression of the Fibrosis-Related Proteins in the Rat Model

The expression level of α-SMA is an important sign of HSC activation, and it is also one of the important indicators to judge

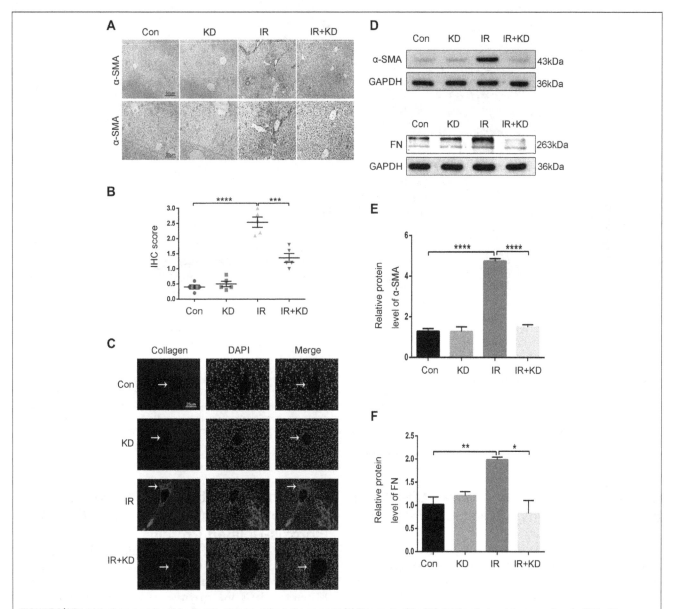

FIGURE 2 | KD inhibits the expression of the fibrosis-related proteins in the rat model **(A)** The results of the IHC staining displayed the expression of α-SMA of the liver histology slices. KD significantly reduced the expression of brown stained α-SMA after irradiation **(B)** The IHC scores for grading the expression of α-SMA **(C)** Expression and localization of collagen in the liver tissue. The red stain represented collagen, which indicated that collagen expression in the IR + KD group was significantly lower than that in the IR group **(D-F)** The results of the western blots showed the expression of α-SMA and FN proteins in the liver tissue. The administration of KD after irradiation resulted in decreased expression of a-SMA and FN. For all results in this figure, original magnification, ×100 and ×200. Mean ± SEM. n. s. denotes not significant; *$p < 0.05$, **$p < 0.01$, ***$p < 0.001$, ****$p < 0.0001$.

the degree of liver fibrosis (Liu et al., 2015). Besides, FN was an important ECM regulatory component in the fibrosis process related to HSCs activation (Zollinger and Smith 2017; Klingberg et al., 2018). At the 24th week postirradiation, the liver tissues of the rats in each group were subjected to α-SMA immunohistochemistry. The expression of α-SMA increased in the liver portal area of the rats in the IR group, and the expression level of a-SMA in the IR + KD group was significantly lower than that of the IR group (**Figures 2A,B**). We performed immunofluorescence staining of liver tissue collagen. The results showed that the expression of collagen in the liver portal area increased in the IR group, and was significantly reduced in the IR + KD group (**Figure 2C**), indicating that the degree of fibrosis was significantly reduced after the administration of KD. Furthermore, the results of Western Blot analysis showed that administration of KD after irradiation resulted in decreased expression of α-SMA (**Figures 2D,E**) and FN (**Figures 2D,F**) in liver tissue. Based on these results, KD inhibited the expression of the fibrosis-related proteins, and alleviated RILF in the rat model.

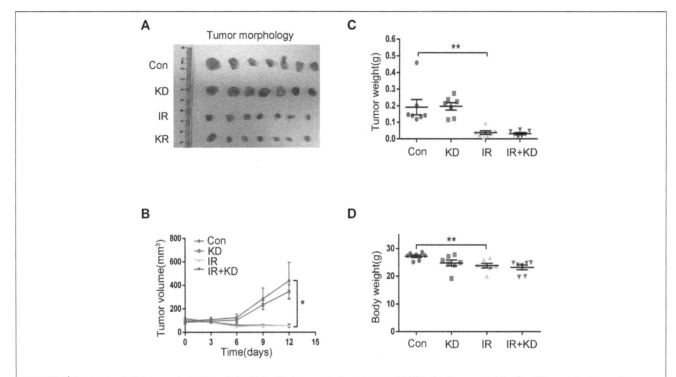

FIGURE 3 | Treatment with KD does not alter the radiosensitivity of liver cancer in the mouse model **(A)** In the IR group and the IR + KD group, the tumor size significantly reduced compared with the Con group and the KD group **(B)** The tumor volume-time curve showed that the tumor volume of the irradiated groups increased slower than the control groups, and there was no statistical difference in the tumor volume between the IR group and the IR + KD group **(C)** Compared with the control group, the tumor weight was significantly reduced after irradiation, but there was no statistical difference in tumor weights between the IR group and the IR + KD group **(D)** There was no statistical difference in the body weights of nude mice between the IR group and the IR + KD group. For all results in this figure, mean ± SEM. n. s. denotes not significant; *$p < 0.05$, **$p < 0.01$.

Kinsenoside Exerts No Adverse Effects on the Radiosensitivity of Liver Cancer in the Mouse Model

In order to test whether KD reduced the efficacy of radiotherapy for liver cancer, we tested the effects of KD after the inoculation of liver cancer cells (HepG2) in the nude mice. The tumor size in the IR and IR + KD groups decreased significantly after irradiation, and the tumor volume-time curve showed that the tumor volume in the irradiated groups increased slowly compared to the control groups, while there was no statistical difference in the tumor volume between the IR group and IR + KD group (**Figures 3A,B**).

In addition, the tumor weight of the IR group and IR + KD group was significantly lower than those of the control groups, but there was no statistical difference in the tumor weight between IR group and IR + KD group (**Figure 3C**). Furthermore, the body weight of nude mice in each group was determined. The body weight after irradiation was reduced compared with the control groups, but there was no difference between the two irradiation groups (**Figure 3D**). Overall, these above results comprehensively showed that the administration of KD after irradiation did not affect the efficacy of tumor radiotherapy, suggesting that KD did not affect the curative effect of radiotherapy on tumors while inhibiting RILF.

Kinsenoside Inhibits Cell Proliferation of Hepatic Stellate Cells and Activation of Fibrosis-Related Proteins

Studies have shown that HSCs are the critical effector cells in the process of liver fibrosis (Wan et al., 2017; Wu et al., 2018a; Dewidar et al., 2019b). In order to study the regulatory effect of KD on the HSCs, we separately detected the cell cycle of each group and found that compared with the IR group, the HSC-T6 cells in the IR + KD group were blocked in the G0/G1 phase (**Figure 4A**), indicating that KD played a role in inhibiting the proliferation of HSCs. We detected the expression of α-SMA gene in each group, and the results showed that radiation exposure caused the activation of HSC-T6 cells at the transcription level, while the administration of KD inhibited this activation (**Figure 4B**). Furthermore, the expression of α-SMA protein in each group was detected by immunofluorescence. The results showed that the fluorescence intensity of α-SMA protein in the IR group was significantly higher than that in the control groups. While the fluorescence intensity of the protein in the IR + KD group decreased significantly, compared with the IR group (**Figure 4C**), indicating that the radiation exposure activated the HSC-T6 cells, while KD administration after irradiation reduced this activation. Subsequently, we tested the marker proteins of RILF. As shown in the Figures, the expression of the marker proteins decreased in the IR + KD group, compared

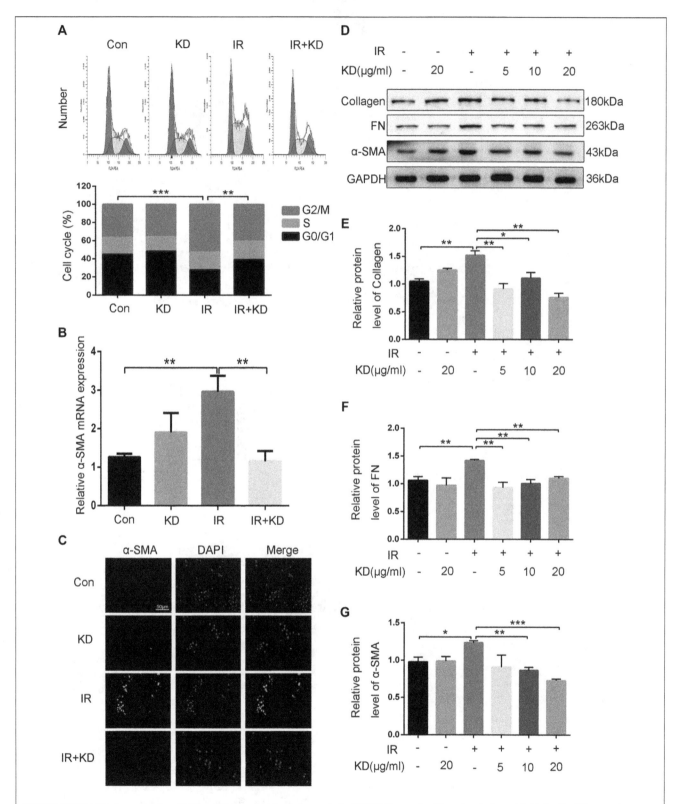

FIGURE 4 | KD inhibits the proliferation of HSCs and the key proteins that promote the RILF **(A)** The results of the cell cycle showed that in the IR + KD group, the cell cycle arrested in the G0/G1 phase compared with the IR group, which indicated the inhibition of the cell proliferation **(B)** The expression of a-SMA mRNA in HSC-T6 cells increased after 6Gy irradiation, while the administration of KD after irradiation inhibited this expression **(C)** The protein fluorescence intensity of α-SMA increased in the IR group compared with the control groups, and the fluorescence intensity decreased in the IR + KD group compared with the IR group **(D-G)** Unirradiated HSC-T6 cells expressed little or did not express fibrosis-related proteins such as collagen, FN and a-SMA protein. The expression of these fibrosis-related proteins increased after 6Gy irradiation, and the administration of KD after irradiation inhibited the expression of these proteins. For all results in this figure, mean ± SEM. n. s. denotes not significant; $^*p < 0.05$, $^{**}p < 0.01$, $^{***}p < 0.001$.

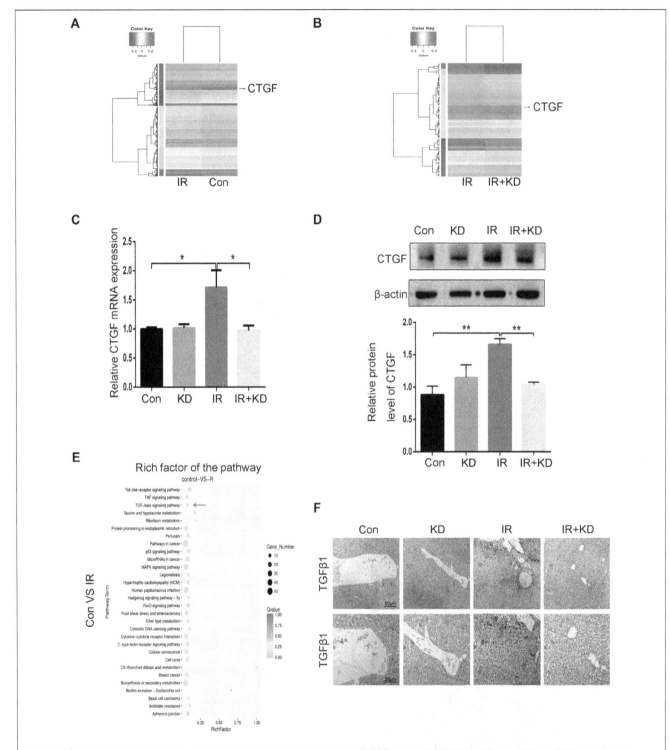

FIGURE 5 | The key fibrosis-related gene and signaling pathway that are inhibited by KD **(A)** The results of high-throughput sequencing of the transcriptome showed that the expression of CTGF gene increased after irradiation **(B)** The results of high-throughput sequencing of the transcriptome showed that the expression of CTGF gene decreased after the administration of KD **(C)** The results of Real-Time PCR were consistent with the results of the sequencing. The expression of CTGF mRNA increased in the IR group, but decreased in the IR + KD group **(D)** The results of western blotting were consistent with the results of sequencing. The expression of CTGF protein increased in the IR group, but decreased in the IR + KD group **(E)** In the transcriptome KEGG gene pathway enrichment map, the TGF-β pathway was closely related to CTGF and RILF **(F)** The results of tissue TGF-β1 immunohistochemistry indicated that in the IR + KD group the expression of TGF-β1 in the liver tissue decreased compared with the IR group. For all results in this figure, original magnification, ×40 and ×100. Mean ± SEM. *$p < 0.05$, **$p < 0.01$.

with the IR group (**Figures 4D–G**). These results indicated that HSCs were activated after irradiation and produced proteins to promote fibrosis, while KD could inhibit the activation of HSCs and inhibit the production of these key fibrosis proteins.

Screening of the Target Gene Connective Tissue Growth Factor and TGF-β1 Signaling Pathway

To find the differential genes that KD targeted in the process of alleviating RILF, we performed transcriptome high-throughput sequencing. Through the differential gene screening and the cluster map analysis, we found that in the IR group, CTGF was a high-expressed gene compared to the control group, while in the IR + KD group, CTGF was low-expressed compared to the IR group (**Figures 5A,B**), indicating that CTGF might be an important target gene for KD to attenuate RILF. CTGF is an important fibrosis-promoting mediator downstream target of TGF-β that plays a key role in the liver fibrosis (Weiskirchen, 2016; Wu et al., 2018b; Alatas et al., 2020). Next, we verified the transcriptome sequencing results by Real-Time PCR and western blot analyses. It was found that CTGF was significantly upregulated both in the mRNA and protein levels after HSC-T6 cells irradiated with 6Gy rays, while the expression of CTGF decreased in the IR + KD group, compared with that in the IR group (**Figures 5C,D**). These results suggested that KD could inhibit the expression of CTGF in HSCs after irradiation.

The signaling pathway enrichment was conducted to screen the pathways upstream of CTGF that played a key role in the process of RILF. The bubble chart of the transcriptome showed a series of enriched signal pathways, among which the TGF-β pathway was closely related to CTGF and the extracellular environment (**Figure 5E**). Based on the results, we speculated that TGF-β pathway was involved in the process that KD alleviated RILF. In order to further verify this, we performed TGF-β immunohistochemical staining on the rat liver tissue. As shown in **Figure 5F**, expression of TGF-β1 increased in the IR group, while there was almost no expression of TGF-β1 in the IR + KD group. These results indicated that the TGF-β1 pathway played a key role in promoting liver fibrosis caused by radiation, and KD administration after irradiation could reduce the expression of TGF-β1.

Kinsenoside Reduces Radiation-Induced Liver Fibrosis by Blocking TGF-β1/Smad/ Connective Tissue Growth Factor Pathway

To further clarify whether TGF-β1 promoted the activation of HSCs and the expression of fibrosis-related proteins, we detected the expression of fibrosis-related proteins after exogenous TGF-β1 acted on the HSC-T6 cells. As the concentration of exogenous TGF-β1 increased, the expression of CTGF protein increased, and the expression of collagen and α-SMA protein both showed a gradient

increase (**Figures 6A,B**). Results showed that the increase in the concentration of TGF-β1 led to the activation of HSCs, which in turn increased the expression of CTGF protein and collagen, thereby producing the effect of promoting fibrosis. In addition, we collected cell supernatants from each group to test the content of activated TGF-β1 by the ELISA. The results showed that the secreted activated TGF-β1 was significantly higher in HSC-T6 cells after 6Gy irradiation than the control groups, while the secreted activated TGF-β1 decreased in the IR + KD group, compared with the IR group (**Figure 6C**). Next, we further analyzed the expression of TGF-β1 and its downstream pathway proteins. The expressions of TGF-β1 and its downstream proteins, total Smad2/3 and phosphorylated Smad2/3, were all increased after irradiation and decreased in the IR + KD group (**Figures 6D–G**). In addition, CTGF is the pro-fibrotic mediator downstream of the TGF-β1 pathway, and we have found that KD could inhibit the expression of CTGF. Based on these results, KD could inhibit the activated TGF-β1/Smad/CTGF pathway postirradiation, thereby inhibiting RILF (**Figure 7**).

DISCUSSION

The RILF is a kind of normal liver tissue damage induced by radiation, lacking effective prevention and treatment methods currently. As reported, the mortality rate of the radiation-induced liver injury in severe cases reaches 75%, and most of these patients eventually suffer from liver failure (Guha and Kavanagh 2011; Chen et al., 2015; Munoz-Schuffenegger et al., 2017). At present, the liver fibrosis is considered to be a healing response to the chronic liver injury. However, if the inducing factors of liver damage are not properly removed, the liver fibrosis will continue and cause serious distortion of the liver tissue structure, which may eventually lead to the liver failure and death (Aydın and Akçalı 2018; Roehlen et al., 2020; Kisseleva and Brenner 2021). In this study, we successfully established the rat model of the RILF, and the results of the HE and Masson staining indicated that KD significantly improved the RILF. In addition, we measured the fibrosis score and the content of hydroxyproline in the liver tissues of each group to further verify the effect of KD on alleviating the RILF. Our research showed that KD reduced the liver fibrosis in rats after radiotherapy, and provided a new method for the prevention and treatment of the RILF.

It's well accepted that the RILF closely related to the continuous overexpression of a variety of inflammatory and fibrotic cytokines, but the underlying specific mechanisms remain to be undiscovered (Chen et al., 2017; Rosenbloom et al., 2017; Yuan et al., 2019b). The main cause of the liver fibrosis is the excessive accumulation of the fibrosis-related proteins such as collagen in the perisinusoidal space, and changes in these ECM components induce the hepatic sinusoidal endothelial cells (LSEC) to form the basement membranes, which interferes with the normal nutrient transport between blood and the surrounding cells, especially the liver cells, and ultimately leads to dysfunction

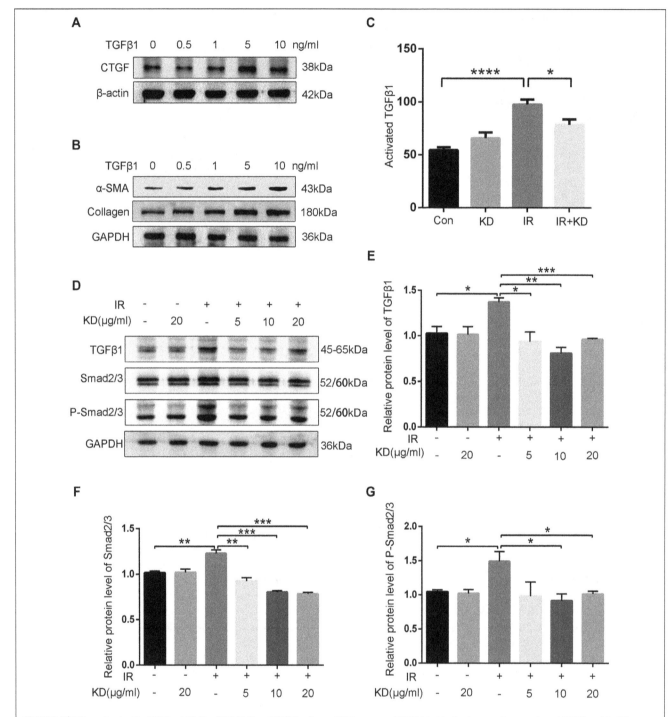

FIGURE 6 | KD ameliorates the RILF by inhibiting TGF-β1/Smad/CTGF pathway **(A)** Exogenous TGF-β1 led to the increased expression of CTGF protein **(B)** Exogenous TGF-β1 induced an increase in the expression of collagen and α-SMA proteins **(C)** The TGF-β1 activity in the conditioned media significantly increased after 6Gy irradiation compared with the control group, while the TGF-β1 activity in the conditioned media in the IR + KD group decreased compared with the IR group **(D-G)** The expressions of TGF-β1 and downstream Smad2/3 as well as phosphorylated Smad2/3 reduced in the IR + KD group compared with the IR group. Mean ± SEM. *$p < 0.05$, **$p < 0.01$, ***$p < 0.001$, ****$p < 0.0001$.

(Natarajan et al., 2017; Ni et al., 2017). Based on the reported studies, we performed the immunohistochemical (IHC) staining of the livers and scored IHC scoring of the α-SMA protein, which was the marker of the liver fibrosis and the

HSCs activation. The results showed that the α-SMA protein in the post-irradiated liver was downregulated when treated with KD. The results of the collagen immunofluorescence showed that the collagen expression in the IR + KD group was

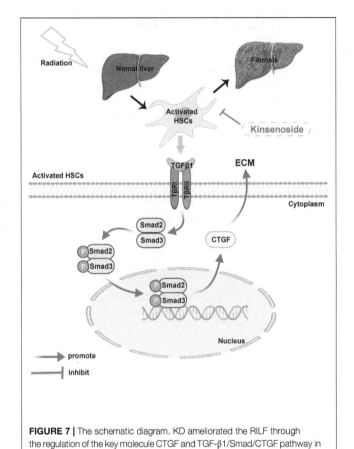

FIGURE 7 | The schematic diagram. KD ameliorated the RILF through the regulation of the key molecule CTGF and TGF-β1/Smad/CTGF pathway in the HSCs.

significantly lower than that in the IR group, which indicated the inhibitory effect of KD on the activation of the HSCs and the subsequent induction of the liver fibrosis. Additionally, we extracted the total protein of the liver tissue and detected the expression of the key proteins involved in the liver fibrosis. The results suggested that KD significantly reduced the expression of α-SMA and FN after radiotherapy.

KD, an extract of the traditional Chinese herbal plant *A. roxburghii*, has a variety of pharmacological effects, among which the liver-protecting effect shows significant importance (Xiang et al., 2016a; Xiang et al., 2016b). Studies have shown that KD can ameliorate the autoimmune hepatitis and protect against the CCl_4-induced liver damage in mice, while the mechanism remains unknown (Xiang et al., 2016b). The results of our studies on the animal model shown that KD had protective effects on the RILF, which provided a theoretical basis for solving the urgent clinical problems on prevention and treatment of the RILF. Importantly, the drugs used to prevent the RILF are supposed not to affect the efficacy of radiotherapy on the malignant liver tumors. In this study, the xenograft tumors were inoculated and irradiated with a single 10Gy radiation after reaching the expected size. Subsequently, the nude mice were administered with KD, and the results

showed that KD administration after radiotherapy did not affect the efficacy of tumor radiotherapy.

The HSCs are the main cells that produce the ECM in the damaged liver. Protein α-SMA acts as an important marker for the activation of the HSCs, and FN is an important ECM regulatory component in the fibrosis process related to the HSCs activation (Rygiel et al., 2008; Zollinger and Smith 2017; Klingberg et al., 2018). The activated HSCs migrate and accumulate in the tissue repairing site, then secrete a large amount of ECM and regulate ECM degradation (Chen et al., 2020). In addition, during the chronic liver injury, liver parenchymal cells are damaged, along with increasing of the activated HSCs and inflammatory cells (Weiskirchen and Tacke 2016). We found that the HSCs, the main effector cells of liver fibrosis, were activated by radiation and proliferated actively after 6Gy of radiation, and the expression of the fibrosis-related proteins significantly increased. The administration of KD effectively inhibited the activation and proliferation of the HSCs, and promoted a significant reduction in the expression of the fibrosis-related proteins.

CTGF is a kind of matrix protein that is commonly up-regulated in the liver fibrosis, which plays a key role in liver fibrosis (Weiskirchen, 2016; Wu et al., 2018b; Makino et al., 2018). Studies have shown that hepatocytes, bile duct cells, HSCs and many other cells express and secrete CTGF protein in the fibrotic liver (Williams et al., 2014; Ding et al., 2016; Ramazani et al., 2018). As reported, CTGF is significantly upregulated and plays a key role in the liver fibrosis (Xu et al., 2015; Tomei et al., 2016). Furthermore, CTGF is a downstream regulator of TGF-β1, which is the final link leading to the accumulation of ECM (Wu et al., 2018b). Various activating factors can promote the latent TGF-β1 turning into activated TGF-β1, and the latter binds to the corresponding receptor on the effector cells (Hinck et al., 2016). Growing evidence have shown that activated and overexpressed TGF-β1 eventually lead to the depletion of parenchymal cells and excessive tissue fibrosis (Moses et al., 2016; Liu et al., 2019; Wang et al., 2019). In this study, we screened the key target gene regulated by KD through high-throughput sequencing of the transcriptome, and CTGF was found to be a key molecule in the RILF. The signaling pathway enrichment suggested the importance of TGF-β signaling pathway in regulating the RILF, and the IHC staining of liver tissue showed the reduced expression of TGF-β1 in the IR + KD group. Our data showed that the irradiation activated and upregulated TGF-β1, which stimulated the HSCs, resulting in the increased expression of the fibrosis-related proteins. Furthermore, treatment with KD reduced the activated TGF-β1 after radiotherapy. Taken together, we figured out that KD alleviated the RILF via inhibition of the TGF-β1/Smad/CTGF axis.

This study has several limitations. Firstly, we lacked continuous monitoring at different time points before

24 weeks. Secondly, we failed to use the imaging methods to assess the degree of liver fibrosis in this study. In the follow-up researches, the imaging detection will be used to further verify the experimental results. Thirdly, the intermolecular interaction in the signaling pathway needs to be detailed.

In summary, this study discovered that KD could ameliorate the RILF through the regulation of the key molecule CTGF and TGF-β1/Smad/CTGF pathway in the animal model and the cell-level experiments. Additionally, KD showed no adverse effects on the tumor radiotherapy. These results have provided supporting evidence for the clinical application of KD as an innovative drug for the treatment of the RILF, and provided a basis for the use of reagents targeting the TGF-β1 pathway and CTGF molecule to prevent and treat the RILF.

AUTHOR CONTRIBUTIONS

XN, YZ, HH, and XY designed the study. XN, QY, LL, MY, and HH performed the experiments and analyzed the data; YZ and XY provided the reagents and expertise; XN, YZ, HH, and XY discussed the results; XN, QY, BW, and YH wrote the manuscript; HH and XY revised the manuscript; All authors have read and corrected the manuscript.

ACKNOWLEDGMENTS

We thank the School of Pharmacy from Tongji Medical College, Huazhong University of Science and Technology for generation of the KD powder.

REFERENCES

Alatas, F. S., Matsuura, T., Pudjiadi, A. H., Wijaya, S., and Taguchi, T. (2020). Peroxisome Proliferator-Activated Receptor Gamma Agonist Attenuates Liver Fibrosis by Several Fibrogenic Pathways in an Animal Model of Cholestatic Fibrosis. *Pediatr. Gastroenterol. Hepatol. Nutr.* 23, 346–355. doi:10.5223/pghn.2020.23.4.346

Atta, H. M. (2015). Reversibility and Heritability of Liver Fibrosis: Implications for Research and Therapy. *World J. Gastroenterol.* 21, 5138–5148. doi:10.3748/wjg.v21.i17.5138

Aydın, M. M., and Akçalı, K. C. (2018). Liver Fibrosis. *Turk J. Gastroenterol.* 29, 14–21. doi:10.5152/tjg.2018.17330

Bedossa, P., and Poynard, T. (1996). An Algorithm for the Grading of Activity in Chronic Hepatitis C. The METAVIR Cooperative Study Group. *Hepatology* 24, 289–293. doi:10.1002/hep.510240201

Chen, Y., Yuan, B., Chen, G., Zhang, L., Zhuang, Y., Niu, H., et al. (2020). Circular RNA RSF1 Promotes Inflammatory and Fibrotic Phenotypes of Irradiated Hepatic Stellate Cell by Modulating miR-146a-5p. *J. Cel Physiol* 235, 8270–8282. doi:10.1002/jcp.29483

Chen, Y., Yuan, B., Wu, Z., Dong, Y., Zhang, L., and Zeng, Z. (2017). Microarray Profiling of Circular RNAs and the Potential Regulatory Role of Hsa_circ_0071410 in the Activated Human Hepatic Stellate Cell Induced by Irradiation. *Gene* 629, 35–42. doi:10.1016/j.gene.2017.07.078

Chen, Y. X., Zeng, Z. C., Sun, J., Zeng, H. Y., Huang, Y., and Zhang, Z. Y. (2015). Mesenchymal Stem Cell-Conditioned Medium Prevents Radiation-Induced Liver Injury by Inhibiting Inflammation and Protecting Sinusoidal Endothelial Cells. *J. Radiat. Res.* 56, 700–708. doi:10.1093/jrr/rrv026

Cheng, W., Xiao, L., Ainiwaer, A., Wang, Y., Wu, G., Mao, R., et al. (2015). Molecular Responses of Radiation-Induced Liver Damage in Rats. *Mol. Med. Rep.* 11, 2592–2600. doi:10.3892/mmr.2014.3051

Derynck, R., and Budi, E. H. (2019). Specificity, Versatility, and Control of TGF-β Family Signaling. *Sci. Signal.* 12. doi:10.1126/scisignal.aav5183

Dewidar, B., Meyer, C., Dooley, S., and Meindl-Beinker, A. N. (2019a). TGF-β in Hepatic Stellate Cell Activation and Liver Fibrogenesis-Updated 2019. *Cells* 8, 1419. doi:10.3390/cells8111419

Dewidar, B., Meyer, C., Dooley, S., and Meindl-Beinker, N. (2019b). TGF-β in Hepatic Stellate Cell Activation and Liver Fibrogenesis-Updated 2019. *Cells* 8, 1419. doi:10.3390/cells8111419

Ding, Z. Y., Jin, G. N., Wang, W., Sun, Y. M., Chen, W. X., Chen, L., et al. (2016). Activin A-Smad Signaling Mediates Connective Tissue Growth Factor Synthesis in Liver Progenitor Cells. *Int. J. Mol. Sci.* 17, 408. doi:10.3390/ijms17030408

Dituri, F., Mancarella, S., Cigliano, A., Chieti, A., and Giannelli, G. (2019). TGF-β as Multifaceted Orchestrator in HCC Progression: Signaling, EMT, Immune Microenvironment, and Novel Therapeutic Perspectives. *Semin. Liver Dis.* 39, 53–69. doi:10.1055/s-0038-1676121

Du, S. S., Qiang, M., Zeng, Z. C., Zhou, J., Tan, Y. S., Zhang, Z. Y., et al. (2010). Radiation-induced Liver Fibrosis Is Mitigated by Gene Therapy Inhibiting Transforming Growth Factor-β Signaling in the Rat. *Int. J. Radiat. Oncol. Biol. Phys.* 78, 1513–1523. doi:10.1016/j.ijrobp.2010.06.046

Feng, Z., Hai-ning, Y., Xiao-man, C., Zun-chen, W., Sheng-rong, S., and Das, U. N. (2014). Effect of Yellow Capsicum Extract on Proliferation and Differentiation of 3T3-L1 Preadipocytes. *Nutrition* 30, 319–325. doi:10.1016/j.nut.2013.08.003

Guha, C., and Kavanagh, B. D. (2011). Hepatic Radiation Toxicity: Avoidance and Amelioration. *Semin. Radiat. Oncol.* 21, 256–263. doi:10.1016/j.semradonc.2011.05.003

Han, N. K., Jung, M. G., Jeong, Y. J., Son, Y., Han, S. C., Park, S., et al. (2019). Plasma Fibrinogen-like 1 as a Potential Biomarker for Radiation-Induced Liver Injury. *Cells* 8, 1042. doi:10.3390/cells8091042

Hasan, H. F., Abdel-Rafei, M. K., and Galal, S. M. (2017). Diosmin Attenuates Radiation-Induced Hepatic Fibrosis by Boosting PPAR-γ Expression and Hampering miR-17-5p-Activated Canonical Wnt-β-Catenin Signaling. *Biochem. Cel Biol* 95, 400–414. doi:10.1139/bcb-2016-0142

Hinck, A. P., Mueller, T. D., and Springer, T. A. (2016). Structural Biology and Evolution of the TGF-β Family. *Cold Spring Harb Perspect. Biol.* 8. doi:10.1101/cshperspect.a022103

Hu, Z., Qin, F., Gao, S., Zhen, Y., Huang, D., and Dong, L. (2018). Paeoniflorin Exerts Protective Effect on Radiation-Induced Hepatic Fibrosis in Rats via TGF-β1/Smads Signaling Pathway. *Am. J. Transl Res.* 10, 1012–1021.

Jung, J., Yoon, S. M., Kim, S. Y., Cho, B., Park, J. H., Kim, S. S., et al. (2013). Radiation-induced Liver Disease after Stereotactic Body Radiotherapy for Small Hepatocellular Carcinoma: Clinical and Dose-Volumetric Parameters. *Radiat. Oncol.* 8, 249. doi:10.1186/1748-717x-8-249

Katsuno, Y., Meyer, D. S., Zhang, Z., Shokat, K. M., Akhurst, R. J., Miyazono, K., et al. (2019). Chronic TGF-β Exposure Drives Stabilized EMT, Tumor Stemness, and Cancer Drug Resistance with Vulnerability to Bitopic mTOR Inhibition. *Sci. Signal.* 12. doi:10.1126/scisignal.aau8544

Kim, J., and Jung, Y. (2017). Radiation-induced Liver Disease: Current Understanding and Future Perspectives. *Exp. Mol. Med.* 49, e359. doi:10.1038/emm.2017.85

Kim, Y., Ratziu, V., Choi, S. G., Lalazar, A., Theiss, G., Dang, Q., et al. (1998). Transcriptional Activation of Transforming Growth Factor Beta1 and its Receptors by the Kruppel-like Factor Zf9/core Promoter-Binding Protein and Sp1. Potential Mechanisms for Autocrine Fibrogenesis in Response to Injury. *J. Biol. Chem.* 273, 33750–33758. doi:10.1074/jbc.273.50.33750

Kisseleva, T., and Brenner, D. (2021). Molecular and Cellular Mechanisms of Liver Fibrosis and its Regression. *Nat. Rev. Gastroenterol. Hepatol.* 18, 151–166. doi:10.1038/s41575-020-00372-7

Klingberg, F., Chau, G., Walraven, M., Boo, S., Koehler, A., Chow, M. L., et al. (2018). The Fibronectin ED-A Domain Enhances Recruitment of Latent TGF-β-Binding Protein-1 to the Fibroblast Matrix. *J. Cel Sci* 131. doi:10.1242/jcs.201293

Lee, U. E., and Friedman, S. L. (2011). Mechanisms of Hepatic Fibrogenesis. *Best Pract. Res. Clin. Gastroenterol.* 25, 195–206. doi:10.1016/j.bpg.2011.02.005

Liang, J., Song, X., Xiao, Z., Chen, H., Shi, C., and Luo, L. (2018). Using IVIM-MRI and R2 Mapping to Differentiate Early Stage Liver Fibrosis in a Rat Model of Radiation-Induced Liver Fibrosis. *Biomed. Res. Int.* 2018, 4673814. doi:10.1155/2018/4673814

Liu, M., Xu, Y., Han, X., Yin, L., Xu, L., Qi, Y., et al. (2015). Dioscin Alleviates Alcoholic Liver Fibrosis by Attenuating Hepatic Stellate Cell Activation via the TLR4/MyD88/NF-Kb Signaling Pathway. *Sci. Rep.* 5, 18038. doi:10.1038/srep18038

Liu, N., Feng, J., Lu, X., Yao, Z., Liu, Q., Lv, Y., et al. (2019). Isorhamnetin Inhibits Liver Fibrosis by Reducing Autophagy and Inhibiting Extracellular Matrix Formation via the TGF-β1/Smad3 and TGF-B1/p38 MAPK Pathways. *Mediators Inflamm.* 2019, 6175091. doi:10.1155/2019/6175091

Makino, Y., Hikita, H., Kodama, T., Shigekawa, M., Yamada, R., Sakamori, R., et al. (2018). CTGF Mediates Tumor-Stroma Interactions between Hepatoma Cells and Hepatic Stellate Cells to Accelerate HCC Progression. *Cancer Res.* 78, 4902–4914. doi:10.1158/0008-5472.can-17-3844

Ming, J., Xu, Q., Gao, L., Deng, Y., Yin, J., Zhou, Q., et al. (2021). Kinsenoside Alleviates 17α-Ethinylestradiol-Induced Cholestatic Liver Injury in Rats by Inhibiting Inflammatory Responses and Regulating FXR-Mediated Bile Acid Homeostasis. *Pharmaceuticals (Basel)* 14. doi:10.3390/ph14050452

Moses, H. L., Roberts, A. B., and Derynck, R. (2016). The Discovery and Early Days of TGF-β: A Historical Perspective. *Cold Spring Harb Perspect. Biol.* 8. doi:10.1101/cshperspect.a021865

Mu, M., Zuo, S., Wu, R. M., Deng, K. S., Lu, S., Zhu, J. J., et al. (2018). Ferulic Acid Attenuates Liver Fibrosis and Hepatic Stellate Cell Activation via Inhibition of TGF-β/Smad Signaling Pathway. *Drug Des. Devel Ther.* 12, 4107–4115. doi:10.2147/dddt.s186726

Munoz-Schuffenegger, P., Ng, S., and Dawson, L. A. (2017). Radiation-Induced Liver Toxicity. *Semin. Radiat. Oncol.* 27, 350–357. doi:10.1016/j.semradonc.2017.04.002

Natarajan, V., Harris, E. N., and Kidambi, S. (2017). SECs (Sinusoidal Endothelial Cells), Liver Microenvironment, and Fibrosis. *Biomed. Res. Int.* 2017, 4097205. doi:10.1155/2017/4097205

Ni, Y., Li, J. M., Liu, M. K., Zhang, T. T., Wang, D. P., Zhou, W. H., et al. (2017). Pathological Process of Liver Sinusoidal Endothelial Cells in Liver Diseases. *World J. Gastroenterol.* 23, 7666–7677. doi:10.3748/wjg.v23.i43.7666

Oakley, F., Meso, M., Iredale, J. P., Green, K., Marek, C. J., Zhou, X., et al. (2005). Inhibition of Inhibitor of kappaB Kinases Stimulates Hepatic Stellate Cell Apoptosis and Accelerated Recovery from Rat Liver Fibrosis. *Gastroenterology* 128, 108–120. doi:10.1053/j.gastro.2004.10.003

Qi, C. X., Zhou, Q., Yuan, Z., Luo, Z. W., Dai, C., Zhu, H. C., et al. (2018). Kinsenoside: A Promising Bioactive Compound from Anoectochilus Species. *Curr. Med. Sci.* 38, 11–18. doi:10.1007/s11596-018-1841-1

Ramazani, Y., Knops, N., Elmonem, M. A., Nguyen, T. Q., Arcolino, F. O., Van Den Heuvel, L., et al. (2018). Connective Tissue Growth Factor (CTGF) from Basics to Clinics. *Matrix Biol.* 68-69, 44–66. doi:10.1016/j.matbio.2018.03.007

Roehlen, N., Crouchet, E., and Baumert, T. F. (2020). Liver Fibrosis: Mechanistic Concepts and Therapeutic Perspectives. *Cells* 9, 875. doi:10.3390/cells9040875

Rosenbloom, J., Macarak, E., Piera-Velazquez, S., and Jimenez, S. A. (2017). Human Fibrotic Diseases: Current Challenges in Fibrosis Research. *Methods Mol. Biol.* 1627, 1–23. doi:10.1007/978-1-4939-7113-8_1

Rygiel, K. A., Robertson, H., Marshall, H. L., Pekalski, M., Zhao, L., Booth, T. A., et al. (2008). Epithelial-mesenchymal Transition Contributes to portal Tract Fibrogenesis during Human Chronic Liver Disease. *Lab. Invest.* 88, 112–123. doi:10.1038/labinvest.3700704

Tomei, P., Masola, V., Granata, S., Bellin, G., Carratù, P., Ficial, M., et al. (2016). Everolimus-induced Epithelial to Mesenchymal Transition (EMT) in Bronchial/pulmonary Cells: when the Dosage Does Matter in Transplantation. *J. Nephrol.* 29, 881–891. doi:10.1007/s40620-016-0295-4

Tullius, S. G., Biefer, H. R., Li, S., Trachtenberg, A. J., Edtinger, K., Quante, M., et al. (2014). NAD+ Protects against EAE by Regulating CD4+ T-Cell Differentiation. *Nat. Commun.* 5, 5101. doi:10.1038/ncomms6101

Wan, Y., Meng, F., Wu, N., Zhou, T., Venter, J., Francis, H., et al. (2017). Substance P Increases Liver Fibrosis by Differential Changes in Senescence of Cholangiocytes and Hepatic Stellate Cells. *Hepatology* 66, 528–541. doi:10.1002/hep.29138

Wang, K., Fang, S., Liu, Q., Gao, J., Wang, X., Zhu, H., et al. (2019). TGF-β1/p65/MAT2A Pathway Regulates Liver Fibrogenesis via Intracellular SAM. *EBioMedicine* 42, 458–469. doi:10.1016/j.ebiom.2019.03.058

Wang, S., Lee, Y., Kim, J., Hyun, J., Lee, K., Kim, Y., et al. (2013). Potential Role of Hedgehog Pathway in Liver Response to Radiation. *PLoS One* 8, e74141. doi:10.1371/journal.pone.0074141

Wei, J., Feng, L., Li, Z., Xu, G., and Fan, X. (2013). MicroRNA-21 Activates Hepatic Stellate Cells via PTEN/Akt Signaling. *Biomed. Pharmacother.* 67, 387–392. doi:10.1016/j.biopha.2013.03.014

Weiskirchen, R. (2016). Hepatoprotective and Anti-fibrotic Agents: It's Time to Take the Next Step. *Front. Pharmacol.* 6, 303. doi:10.3389/fphar.2015.00303

Weiskirchen, R., and Tacke, F. (2016). Liver Fibrosis: From Pathogenesis to Novel Therapies. *Dig. Dis.* 34, 410–422. doi:10.1159/000444556

Williams, M. J., Clouston, A. D., and Forbes, S. J. (2014). Links between Hepatic Fibrosis, Ductular Reaction, and Progenitor Cell Expansion. *Gastroenterology* 146, 349–356. doi:10.1053/j.gastro.2013.11.034

Wu, X., Zhi, F., Lun, W., Deng, Q., and Zhang, W. (2018a). Baicalin Inhibits PDGF-BB-Induced Hepatic Stellate Cell Proliferation, Apoptosis, Invasion, Migration and Activation via the miR-3595/ACSL4 axis. *Int. J. Mol. Med.* 41, 1992–2002. doi:10.3892/ijmm.2018.3427

Wu, Y., Wang, W., Peng, X. M., He, Y., Xiong, Y. X., Liang, H. F., et al. (2018b). Rapamycin Upregulates Connective Tissue Growth Factor Expression in Hepatic Progenitor Cells through TGF-β-Smad2 Dependent Signaling. *Front. Pharmacol.* 9, 877. doi:10.3389/fphar.2018.00877

Xiang, M., Liu, T., Tan, W., Ren, H., Li, H., Liu, J., et al. (2016a). Effects of Kinsenoside, a Potential Immunosuppressive Drug for Autoimmune Hepatitis, on Dendritic cells/CD8+ T Cells Communication in Mice. *Hepatology* 64, 2135–2150. doi:10.1002/hep.28825

Xiang, M., Liu, T., Tan, W., Ren, H., Li, H., Liu, J., et al. (2016b). Effects of Kinsenoside, a Potential Immunosuppressive Drug for Autoimmune Hepatitis, on Dendritic cells/CD8+ T Cells Communication in Mice. *Hepatology* 64, 2135–2150. doi:10.1002/hep.28825

Xu, F., Liu, C., Zhou, D., and Zhang, L. (2016). TGF-β/SMAD Pathway and its Regulation in Hepatic Fibrosis. *J. Histochem. Cytochem.* 64, 157–167. doi:10.1369/0022155415627681

Xu, X., Dai, H., Geng, J., Wan, X., Huang, X., Li, F., et al. (2015). Rapamycin Increases CCN2 Expression of Lung Fibroblasts via Phosphoinositide 3-kinase. *Lab. Invest.* 95, 846–859. doi:10.1038/labinvest.2015.68

Ye, S., Shao, Q., and Zhang, A. (2017). Anoectochilus Roxburghii: A Review of its Phytochemistry, Pharmacology, and Clinical Applications. *J. Ethnopharmacol* 209, 184–202. doi:10.1016/j.jep.2017.07.032

Yuan, B., Chen, Y., Wu, Z., Zhang, L., Zhuang, Y., Zhao, X., et al. (2019a). Proteomic Profiling of Human Hepatic Stellate Cell Line LX2 Responses to Irradiation and TGF-B1. *J. Proteome Res.* 18, 508–521. doi:10.1021/acs.jproteome.8b00814

Yuan, B. Y., Chen, Y. H., Wu, Z. F., Zhuang, Y., Chen, G. W., Zhang, L., et al. (2019b). MicroRNA-146a-5p Attenuates Fibrosis-Related Molecules in Irradiated and TGF-Beta1-Treated Human Hepatic Stellate Cells by Regulating PTPRA-SRC Signaling. *Radiat. Res.* 192, 621–629. doi:10.1667/rr15401.1

Zarzycka, M., Kotwicka, M., Jendraszak, M., Skibinska, I., Kotula-Balak, M., and Bilinska, B. (2014). Hydroxyflutamide Alters the Characteristics of Live Boar Spermatozoa. *Theriogenology* 82, 988–996. doi:10.1016/j.theriogenology.2014.07.013

Zollinger, A. J., and Smith, M. L. (2017). Fibronectin, the Extracellular Glue. *Matrix Biol.* 60-61, 27–37. doi:10.1016/j.matbio.2016.07.011

11

Circulating Collagen Metabolites and the Enhanced Liver Fibrosis (ELF) Score as Fibrosis Markers in Systemic Sclerosis

Chen Chen [1,2], Lingbiao Wang [1,2], Jinfeng Wu [3], Meijuan Lu [4], Sen Yang [1,2], Wenjing Ye [1,2], Ming Guan [4], Minrui Liang [1,2]* and Hejian Zou [1,2]*

[1]Department of Rheumatology, Huashan Hospital, Fudan University, Shanghai, China, [2]Institute of Rheumatology, Immunology and Allergy, Fudan University, Shanghai, China, [3]Department of Dermatology, Huashan Hospital, Fudan University, Shanghai, China, [4]Department of Laboratory Medicine, Huashan Hospital, Fudan University, Shanghai, China

*Correspondence:
Minrui Liang
mliang10@fudan.edu.cn
Hejian Zou
hjzou@fudan.edu.cn

Background: Serum fibrosis markers for systemic sclerosis (SSc) remain limited. The Enhanced Liver Fibrosis (ELF) score is a collagen marker set consisting of procollagen type III amino terminal propeptide (PIIINP), tissue inhibitor of metalloproteinases 1 (TIMP-1), and hyaluronic acid (HA). This longitudinal study aimed to examine the performance of the ELF score and its single analytes as surrogate outcome measures of fibrosis in SSc.

Methods: Eighty-five SSc patients fulfilling the 2013 ACR/EULAR criteria with the absence of chronic liver diseases were enrolled. Serum PIIINP, TIMP-1, HA, and the ELF score were measured and correlated with clinical variables including the modified Rodnan skin score (mRSS) and interstitial lung disease (ILD). Twenty SSc patients underwent a follow-up serological testing and mRSS evaluation during treatment with immunosuppressants and/or anti-fibrotic drugs.

Results: Serum PIIINP, TIMP-1, and ELF score were significantly higher in patients with SSc than in healthy controls [PIIINP: 10.31 (7.83–14.10) vs. 5.61 (4.69–6.30), $p < .001$; TIMP-1: 110.73 (66.21–192.45) vs. 61.81 (48.86–85.24), $p < .001$; ELF: 10.34 (9.91–10.86) vs. 9.68 (9.38–9.99), $p < .001$]. Even higher levels of PIIINP, TIMP-1, and ELF score were found in patients with diffuse cutaneous SSc than those with limited cutaneous SSc. At baseline, both PIIINP and ELF score showed good correlation with mRSS (PIIINP: $r = .586$, $p < .001$; ELF: $r = .482$, $p < .001$). Longitudinal analysis showed that change in PIIINP positively correlated with change in mRSS ($r = 0.701$, $p = .001$), while change in ELF score were not related, in a statistical context, to the change in mRSS (ELF: $r = .140$, $p = .555$). Serum TIMP-1 was significantly higher in SSc patients with ILD,

---

Abbreviations: ACA, anti-centromere antibody; ARA, anti-RNA polymerase III antibody; ATA, anti-topoisomerase I antibody; dcSSc, diffuse cutaneous systemic sclerosis; DU, digital ulcer; ECM, extracellular matrix; ELF, Enhanced Liver Fibrosis; ELISA, enzyme-linked immunosorbent assay; HA, hyaluronic acid; HC, healthy control; HRCT, high-resolution computed tomography; ILD, interstitial lung disease; lcSSc, limited cutaneous systemic sclerosis; MaxFIB, maximum fibrosis score; MPCLIA, chemiluminescence immunoassay combined with the magnetic particles; mRSS, modified Rodnan skin score; PAH, pulmonary arterial hypertension; PIIINP, procollagen type III amino terminal propeptide; RP, Raynaud's phenomenon; SSc: systemic sclerosis; TIMP-1, tissue inhibitor of metalloproteinases 1.

compared to the matched group of patients without ILD [109.45 (93.05–200.09) vs. 65.50 (40.57–110.73), p = 0.007].

Conclusion: In patients with SSc, the ELF score well correlates with the extent of skin fibrosis, while serum PIIINP is a sensitive marker for longitudinal changes of skin fibrosis. In the future, circulating collagen metabolites may potentially be used to evaluate therapeutic effects of anti-fibrotic treatments in the disease.

Keywords: enhanced liver fibrosis (ELF) score, hyaluronic acid, modified rodnan skin score (mRSS), procollagen type iii aminoterminal propeptide, systemic sclerosis (SSc), tissue inhibitor for metalloproteinase (TIMP)

INTRODUCTION

Systemic sclerosis (SSc) is a multisystemic connective tissue disease characterized by progressive fibrosis in the skin, lung and other internal organs. Pathological hallmarks of the disease include autoimmune response, collagen accumulation in affected tissues, and obliterative vasculopathy of the peripheral and visceral vasculature (Allanore et al., 2015).

There is an urgent clinical need to identify serum fibrosis markers in SSc. Ideally, the markers should be able to reflect the extent of fibrosis, run parallel with disease progression or regression, and respond to therapeutic interventions. Prior evidence has shown increased collagen synthesis and decreased collagenase activity in SSc derived fibroblasts (LeRoy, 1974; Stone et al., 1995). Consequently, a number of circulating collagen metabolites have been evaluated as candidate biomarkers for SSc over the past decades. However, at the moment, still no validated ones can be reliably used as surrogate outcome measures in clinical trials or routine medical care.

The Enhanced Liver Fibrosis (ELF) score is a serum marker panel consisting of three collagen metabolites, namely procollagen type III amino terminal propeptide (PIIINP), tissue inhibitor of metalloproteinases 1 (TIMP-1) and hyaluronic acid (HA). The composite index was originally derived from patients with chronic liver disease and shown to be predictive of liver fibrosis (Rosenberg et al., 2004; Parkes et al., 2010; Parkes et al., 2011). PIIINP is the amino terminal peptide released during the synthesis and deposition of type III collagen (Lapiere et al., 1971). TIMP-1 is a specific inhibitor of extracellular matrix (ECM) degradation enzymes (Kikuchi et al., 1997). HA is a large glycosaminoglycan involved in the formation of ECM and maintenance of myofibroblast phenotype (Webber et al., 2009). Serum levels of PIIINP, HA, or TIMP-1 were found to be increased in patients with SSc compared with healthy controls (Scheja et al., 1992; Freitas et al., 1996; Young-Min et al., 2001). The clinical implication of those markers further lied in their correlation with SSc disease activity and organ involvement (Kikuchi et al., 1995; Scheja et al., 2000; Yoshizaki et al., 2008). High levels of PIIINP and HA were also demonstrated as unfavorable predictors for survival in SSc (Scheja et al., 1992; Nagy and Czirják, 2005). More recently, the composite index ELF score was found to be superior to its individual components in reflecting overall fibrotic activity in two independent SSc cohorts (Abignano et al., 2014; Abignano et al., 2018). Besides, a pilot study on IgG4-related disease,

another immune-mediated fibrotic disease, revealed that the ELF score could also be an useful indicator of treatment response (Della-Torre et al., 2015). However, evidence on SSc is still in limited amounts and longitudinal data are lacking.

This longitudinal study aimed to examine the performance of the ELF score and its single analytes as surrogate outcome measures of fibrosis in SSc.

MATERIALS AND METHODS
Study Subjects
A total of 85 SSc patients were enrolled in this single-center retrospective study. All patients fulfilled the 2013 ACR/EULAR classification criteria for SSc. Exclusion criteria were 1) chronic hepatitis B and C virus infection; 2) alcoholic liver disease; 3) non-alcoholic fatty liver disease; 4) primary biliary cirrhosis; 5) autoimmune hepatitis; 6) primary sclerosing cholangitis; 7) acute liver injury. Eighty-five age- and gender-matched healthy volunteers were recruited as controls. All SSc patients and controls had normal liver function with no signs of liver cirrhosis on ultrasound assessment. The study was approved by the local ethics committee and informed consent was obtained from all participants.

For patients with SSc, disease duration was calculated from the onset of both Raynaud's phenomenon (RP) and the first non-RP symptom. Modified Rodnan skin score (mRSS) assessment was performed by a same experienced rheumatologist, blinded to the serological testing. Digital ulcer (DU) and pulmonary arterial hypertension (PAH) were identified based on previous literature (Plastiras et al., 2007; Baron et al., 2014). All patients underwent chest high-resolution computed tomography (HRCT) scan. Interstitial lung disease (ILD) was defined as typical radiologic changes affecting more than 5% of the lung parenchyma; the changes include ground-glass attenuation, reticular opacities, and honeycombing, with or without traction bronchiolectasis or bronchiectasis. Two visual semiquantitative HRCT scores were assessed. The overall HRCT score, based on the method describe by Ichikado and colleagues (Ichikado et al., 2006), was graded according to the types and extent (to the nearest 5%) of parenchymal abnormalities in six lung zones. The maximum fibrosis score (MaxFIB) was exclusively calculated from the zone of maximal lung involvement on a scale of 0–4 based on the percentage of area affected (Goldin et al., 2008). Two independent observers evaluated the images and the results were averaged to get the final HRCT scores.

Serum levels of PIIINP, TIMP-1, and HA were measured and clinical evaluations (including mRSS assessment and HRCT scan) were conducted in all the enrolled patients at baseline. Twenty SSc patients underwent a follow-up serological testing and mRSS evaluation during treatment with immunosuppressants and/or anti-fibrotic drugs. Serum was separated and stored at −80°C. The mRSS assessment and HRCT scan were performed within 3 days of the collection of blood samples.

Biochemical Measurements

The ELF score is an algorithm based on quantitative serum measurements of PIIINP, HA, and TIMP-1. Serum concentrations of PIIINP and HA were measured using the chemiluminescence immunoassay combined with the magnetic particles (MPCLIA) (Autobio Diagnostics, Zhengzhou, China). The MPCLIA combines the competitive enzyme immunoassay with the chemiluminescence technique. In this two-step assay, antigens (PIIINP or HA derivatives) are first pre-coated onto microtiter wells, then reference standards, specimens, and solution containing anti-PIIINP antibody or HA binding proteins are added, respectively. Then the plate is incubated. During incubation, PIIINP or HA presents in specimens or reference standards compete with precoated antigens for combining with PIIINP antibodies or HA binding proteins. When this step is fully completed, wash the microtiter plate to remove unbound materials. Add enzyme conjugate reagent, which combines with anti-PIIINP antibody or HA binding proteins attached on microtiter wells in the previous step. After a second incubation, remove unbound enzyme conjugates by washing. Add chemiluminescent substrates, measure the relative light unit (RLU) value for each well, construct calibration curves with values obtained from reference standards, calculate the serum concentrations of PIIINP and HA in each specimen through the calibration curves. PIIINP and HA concentrations in specimens are inversely proportional to relative light unit (RLU) values. Serum concentrations of TIMP-1 were determined by the sandwich enzyme-linked immunosorbent assay (ELISA) (Sangon Biotech and Bio Basic, Shanghai, China). The procedures are as follow. Add standard and sample to the microplate that have been pre-coated with anti-TIMP-1 antibody. After incubation, add biotin-conjugated anti-TIMP-1 antibody. It is then combined with horseradish peroxidase-conjugated streptavidin to form an immune complex, then incubated and washed to remove unbound enzyme, and then added to the chromogenic substrate TMB (3,3′,5,5′-Tetramethylbenzidine) to produce a blue color and converted to the final yellow under the action of acid. Finally, the absorbance (OD) value was measured at 450 nm. The concentration of TIMP-1 in the sample was proportional to the absorbance (OD) value and can be calculated by drawing a standard curve. The ELF score was calculated using the Siemens algorithm (Vali et al., 2020):

TABLE 1 | Demographic and clinical characteristics of 85 SSc patients.

Characteristics	N = 85
Gender (female/male)	68/17 (80.0%/20.0%)
Age, years	53 (38–62)
Subtype (dcSSc/lcSSc)	47/38 (55.3%/44.7%)
Disease duration from RP, years	3.0 (1.0–9.0)
Disease duration from first non-RP, years	2.0 (1.0–5.0)
mRSS	8.0 (3.5–17.5)
Raynaud's phenomenon	79 (92.9%)
Puffy fingers	58 (68.2%)
Telangiectasia	46 (54.1%)
Digital ulcer	28 (32.9%)
Interstitial lung disease	49 (57.6%)
Pulmonary arterial hypertension	4 (4.7%)
ESR, mm/h	21.0 (12.0–37.0)
Disease specific autoantibodies	
ATA positive	47 (55.3%)
ACA positive	19 (22.4%)
ARA positive	4 (4.7%)

ACA, anti-centromere antibody; ARA, anti-RNA polymerase III antibody; ATA, anti-topoisomerase I antibody; dcSSc, diffuse cutaneous SSc; ESR, erythrocyte sedimentation rate; lcSSc, limited cutaneous SSc; mRSS, modified Rodnan skin score; RP, Raynaud's phenomenon; SSc, systemic sclerosis.

$$ELF\ score = 2.494 + 0.846\ln(C_{HA}) + 0.735\ln(C_{PIIINP})$$
$$+ 0.391\ln(C_{TIMP-1})$$

Statistical Analysis

Statistical analysis was performed using SPSS Statistics (version 28.0), and graphs were constructed using R statistical package (version 4.1.2). Continuous variables were expressed as median (interquartile range) and categorical data as number and percentage. Welch's t test was used to compare continuous variables between two groups and Mann-Whitney U test was applied as an alternative when the parametric assumptions were not met. Chi-square test and when indicated, Fisher's exact test were used to compare the distribution of categorical variables between groups. Spearman's rank correlation tests were employed to search for possible relationships between variables and post-hoc power analysis was conducted using Fisher's asymptotic method. Multiple linear regression was used to evaluate independent predictors of the ELF score. Propensity score matching was used to generate comparable study groups. Propensity scores were estimated by logistic regression and matching was done at 1:1 ratio with a match tolerance of 0.05, based on the maximize execution performance analysis. p values of less than .05 (two-sided) were considered statistically significant.

RESULTS

A total of 85 SSc patients were enrolled, 47 with diffuse cutaneous SSc (dcSSc) and 38 with limited cutaneous SSc (lcSSc). Patient demographic and clinical features are summarized in **Table 1**. Medium age was 53 (38–62) years, and medium disease duration

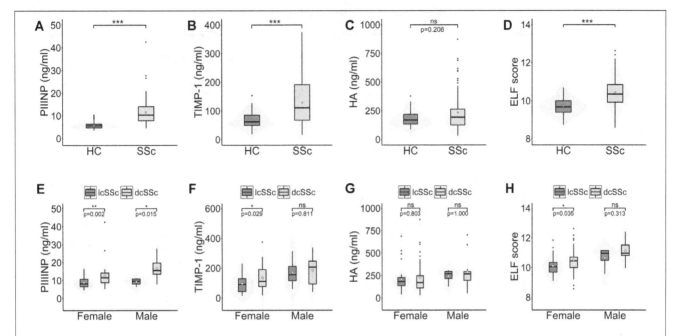

FIGURE 1 | Serum PIIINP, TIMP-1, HA levels and ELF score in patients with SSc. **(A–D)** Serum PIIINP, TIMP-1, HA levels and ELF score in patients with SSc compared with healthy controls. **(E–H)** Serum PIIINP, TIMP-1, HA levels and ELF score in patients with diffuse cutaneous SSc compared with limited cutaneous SSc in males and females. A violin plot includes a fat line showing the median of the data, a box representing the interquartile range, upper and lower bars indicating the 5th and 95th centiles, and a shadow presenting the kernel probability density of the data at different values. The black dots stand for outliers and the white diamonds stand for mean values. HC, healthy controls; dcSSc, diffuse cutaneous SSc; lcSSc, limited cutaneous SSc; ns, not significant. ***p < .001, **p < .01, *p < .05.

from the first non-RP symptom was 2.0 (1.0–5.0) years. Patient mRSS ranged from 0 to 41 with a medium of 8 (interquartile range: 3.5–17.5). Patients with DU, ILD, and PAH accounted for 32.9% (28), 57.6% (49), and 4.7% (4) of the study population, respectively. Positive anti-topoisomerase I antibody (ATA), anti-centromere antibody (ACA), and anti-RNA polymerase III antibody (ARA) were present in 47 (55.3%), 19 (22.4%), and 4 (4.7%) patients, respectively.

Elevated Collagen Metabolites in Patients With SSc

Serum PIIINP, TIMP-1, and ELF score were significantly higher in patients with SSc than in healthy controls [PIIINP: 10.31 (7.83–14.10) vs. 5.61 (4.69–6.30), p < .001; TIMP-1: 110.73 (66.21–192.45) vs. 61.81 (48.86–85.24), p < .001; ELF: 10.34 (9.91–10.86) vs. 9.68 (9.38–9.99), p < .001], while no statistically significant difference was observed in serum HA between SSc patients and healthy controls [192.00 (124.17–265.07) vs. 168.16 (132.57–219.11) p = .206; **Figures 1A–D**]. Among patients, males showed remarkably higher PIIINP, TIMP-1, HA, and ELF score than females (p = .003, p = .008, p = .020, p = .001, respectively; **Table 2**), whereas no such gender dependency could be observed in healthy controls (p = .525, p = .160, p = .273, p = .257, respectively). Even higher levels of PIIINP, TIMP-1, and ELF score were found in dcSSc compared with lcSSc (p < .001, p = .017, p = .003, respectively; **Table 2**). Since there was a higher percentage of males in the dcSSc group than in the lcSSc group (27.7% vs. 10.5%, p = .050), a subgroup

analysis by gender was further conducted to eliminate possible confounding. The results demonstrated still higher levels of PIIINP, TIMP-1, and ELF score in dcSSc in the female subgroup (p = .002, p = .029, p = 0.035, respectively; **Figures 1E–H**).

As shown in **Table 3**, serum PIIINP, HA, and ELF score negatively correlated with disease duration from RP (PIIINP: r = −.348, p = .001, HA: r = −.320, p = .003; ELF: r = −.400, p < .001). Serum HA and ELF score positively correlated with age (HA: r = .456, p < .001, ELF: r = .353, p = .001). A similar age-related trend was also found in healthy controls (HA: r = .364, p = .001, ELF: r = .284, p = .012).

Collagen Metabolites as Indicators of Skin Fibrosis

At baseline, both PIIINP and ELF score showed strong correlation with mRSS, while only moderate correlations were observed for TIMP-1 or HA (PIIINP: r = .586, p < .001, power = .999; TIMP-1: .240, p = .035, HA: r = .237, p = .038; ELF: r = .482, p < .001; **Table 3** and **Figures 2A,B**). Multiple linear regression analysis was performed and all the variables that were significantly correlated with those serum collagen metabolites in the univariate analysis were included as covariates. In multiple linear regression models, mRSS maintained to be a strong predictor for serum PIIINP, HA, and ELF score (p<.001, p = .012, p<.001, respectively).

The follow-up mRSS evaluation and serological testing were made at a medium of 3.4 (interquartile range: 2.1–9.6) months after the baseline assessment in 20 SSc patients. The clinical

TABLE 2 | Serum PIIINP, TIMP-1, HA levels and ELF score in patients with SSc stratified by main clinical characteristics.

Characteristics	PIIINP (ng/ml)	TIMP-1 (ng/ml)	HA (ng/ml)	ELF score
Total	10.31 (7.83–14.10)	110.73 (66.21–192.45)	192.00 (124.17–265.07)	10.34 (9.91–10.86)
Gender				
female	9.50 (7.14–13.22)	104.90 (63.88–166.75)	178.33 (117.40–243.53)	10.23 (9.79–10.64)
male	14.05 (9.80–19.50)	197.73 (90.94–256.83)	266.97 (166.52–299.14)	10.96 (10.79–11.47)
p Value	0.003	0.008	0.020	0.001
Subtype				
dcSSc	13.34 (8.99–15.46)	116.00 (85.18–214.77)	195.88 (121.84–275.86)	10.60 (10.11–11.20)
lcSSc	8.39 (6.55–10.91)	98.32 (48.50–141.75)	188.50 (133.90–246.52)	10.10 (9.65–10.53)
p Value	<0.001	0.017	0.691	0.003
DU				
with DU	10.91 (8.62–14.18)	118.35 (70.89–199.50)	171.58 (124.17–302.18)	10.38 (9.98–11.10)
w/o DU	9.65 (7.23–14.10)	107.12 (53.06–185.34)	202.09 (121.87–255.24)	10.31 (9.84–10.81)
p Value	0.282	0.175	0.874	0.364
ILD				
with ILD	10.90 (7.99–14.06)	120.70 (80.00–206.49)	202.82 (113.63–273.63)	10.37 (9.95–11.05)
w/o ILD	9.61 (7.51–14.90)	95.83 (51.76–166.75)	179.83 (133.87–253.16)	10.24 (9.82–10.83)
p Value	0.715	0.054	0.803	0.600
PAH				
with PAH	10.99 (9.07–14.56)	92.81 (31.70–212.59)	172.34 (132.98–370.11)	10.24 (10.04–11.08)
w/o PAH	10.44 (7.83–14.13)	110.73 (66.93–193.66)	195.88 (123.77–266.97)	10.40 (9.91–10.88)
p Value	0.659	0.674	0.926	1.000
ATA				
ATA+	10.97 (7.97–14.42)	120.70 (85.18–205.80)	202.09 (121.84–266.97)	10.32 (9.91–11.01)
ATA-	9.61 (7.72–13.56)	99.76 (62.59–170.03)	178.33 (126.30–267.29)	10.39 (9.89–10.84)
p Value	0.331	0.110	0.757	0.965
ACA				
ACA+	8.59 (7.41–10.97)	65.50 (34.99–120.94)	178.26 (123.77–228.01)	10.20 (9.79–10.56)
ACA-	10.94 (7.93–14.27)	118.35 (82.58–202.52)	199.26 (123.89–273.50)	10.40 (9.94–11.13)
p Value	0.143	0.003	0.776	0.187

ACA, anti-centromere antibody; ARA, anti-RNA polymerase III antibody; ATA, anti-topoisomerase I antibody; dcSSc, diffuse cutaneous SSc; DU, digital ulcer; ELF, enhanced liver fibrosis; HA, hyaluronic acid; ILD, interstitial lung disease; lcSSc, limited cutaneous SSc; PAH, pulmonary arterial hypertension; PIIINP, procollagen type III amino terminal propeptide; SSc, systemic sclerosis; TIMP-1, tissue inhibitor of metalloproteinases 1; w/o, without.

TABLE 3 | Correlation coefficient (r) between PIIINP, TIMP-1, HA, ELF score and continuous clinical variables in patients with SSc.

Characteristics	PIIINP	TIMP-1	HA	ELF score
Age	−0.001	0.001	0.456***	0.353**
Disease duration from RP	−0.348**	−0.175	−0.320**	−0.400***
Disease duration from first non-RP	−0.226*	−0.134	−0.197	−0.264*
mRSS	0.586***	0.240*	0.237*	0.482***
Overall HRCT score[a]	−0.152	0.100	0.280	0.255
MaxFIB HRCT score[a]	−0.095	−0.001	0.189	0.158
ESR, mm/h	0.263*	0.105	0.086	0.215

ELF, enhanced liver fibrosis; ESR, erythrocyte sedimentation rate; HA, hyaluronic acid; HRCT, high resolution computed tomography; MaxFIB, maximum fibrosis score; mRSS, modified Rodnan skin score; PIIINP, procollagen type III amino terminal propeptide; RP, Raynaud's phenomenon; SSc, systemic sclerosis; TIMP-1, tissue inhibitor of metalloproteinases 1.
[a]Only patients with interstitial lung disease (N = 49) were included in the analysis.
***p < .001.
**p < .01.
*p < .05.

features and ongoing medications are summarized in **Table 4**. Specifically, immunosuppressants (including cyclophosphamide, mycophenolate mofetil, and methotrexate) and anti-fibrotic drugs (including nintedanib and pirfenidone) were used in 10 (50%) and 9 (45%) patients, respectively. In a longitudinal view, changes in PIIINP positively correlated with changes in mRSS (r = .701, p = .001, power = .895); in most cases, decrease in serum PIIINP levels was in parallel with improvement in skin fibrosis (**Figure 2C**). No significant correlations were observed between

changes in TIMP-1, HA, or ELF and changes in mRSS (TIMP-1: r = −.170, p = .474; HA: r = −.126, p = .596, ELF: r = .140, p = .555; **Figure 2D**).

Collagen Metabolites as Markers of Lung Fibrosis

Neither ELF nor its single components showed statistically significant differences between patients with or without ILD,

TABLE 4 | Clinical features and ongoing medications of the 20 SSc patients with longitudinal follow-ups.

Characteristics	N = 20
Follow-up time, months	3.4 (2.1–9.6)
Gender (female/male)	14/6 (70%/30%)
Age, years	56 (50–62)
Subtype (dcSSc/lcSSc)	14/6 (70%/30%)
Disease duration from RP, years	1.7 (0.5–6.0)
Disease duration from first non-RP, years	1.7 (0.6–3.0)
mRSS	9.5 (7.0–21.8)
Interstitial lung disease	14 (70%)
ESR, mm/h	27.0 (19.0–37.0)
Disease specific autoantibodies	
ATA positive	17 (85%)
ACA positive	1 (5%)
ARA positive	1 (5%)
Treatment	
Immunosuppressants[a]	10 (50%)
Anti-fibrotic drugs[b]	9 (45%)

ACA, anti-centromere antibody; ARA, anti-RNA polymerase III antibody; ATA, anti-topoisomerase I antibody; dcSSc, diffuse cutaneous SSc; ESR, erythrocyte sedimentation rate; lcSSc, limited cutaneous SSc; mRSS, modified Rodnan skin score; RP, Raynaud's phenomenon.
[a]Immunosuppressants include cyclophosphamide, mycophenolate mofetil, and methotrexate.
[b]Anti-fibrotic drugs include nintedanib and pirfenidone.

although trends toward higher serum levels of collagen metabolites in patients with ILD were observed (**Table 2**). No linear correlation between collagen markers and semi-quantitative HRCT scores could be established either (**Table 3**).

To balance the distribution of demographic and clinical features, SSc patients with and without ILD were matched for age, gender, disease subtype, disease duration from RP onset and mRSS using propensity score matching. After matching, 30 patients remained (15 in each group) and two groups were well balanced in terms of the matched variables (**Table 5**). Serum TIMP-1 was significantly higher in patients with ILD, compared to the matched group of patients without ILD [109.45 (93.05–200.09) vs. 65.50 (40.57–110.73), *p* = .007], while no

statistical difference was found in PIIINP, HA, and ELF score (*p* = .412, *p* = .285, *p* = .215, respectively; **Table 5**).

DISCUSSION

The present study illustrates longitudinal changes of serum collagen metabolites in SSc. A novel finding is the strong positive correlation between changes of PIIINP and changes of mRSS over time, which reveals that PIIINP could serve as a potent biomarker for monitoring skin sclerosis and active fibrosis in SSc.

Previous reports have documented a remarkable decrease in serum PIIINP after plasma exchange or immunosuppressive therapy in patients with SSc (Behr et al., 1995; Heickendorff et al., 1995; Cozzi et al., 2001). However, the clinical relevance of the serological changes remains elusive. In order to address this issue, we concurrently assess the serum collagen metabolites and the clinical parameter mRSS. Our data suggested that serum PIIINP could be a surrogate outcome measure in SSc, in parallel with the skin score. However, it should be noted that changes in serum PIIINP could not be linked to any specific treatment regimen in our study, since patients received various types of therapy, including immunosuppressants and anti-fibrotic drugs, either alone or in combination. Future studies are needed to investigate the potential of those collagen markers in monitoring therapeutic efficacy in different treatment subgroups of SSc patients.

Interestingly, longitudinal change in PIIINP exhibited strong correlation with longitudinal change in mRSS, probably superior to the ELF score in reflecting skin progression in patients with SSc. This may result from the multiparametric nature of the ELF algorithm, where every single marker reflects a different aspect of the fibrotic process. Indeed, PIIINP and TIMP-1 respectively represent increased collagen formation and decreased collagen degradation. HA was superior in identification of advanced fibrosis but much weaker than PIIINP or TIMP-1 in discriminating early fibrosis (Lichtinghagen et al., 2013). Considering the short disease duration and moderate mRSS of our study population, current data revealed that PIIINP could be a sensitive surrogate marker of fibrotic burden and disease

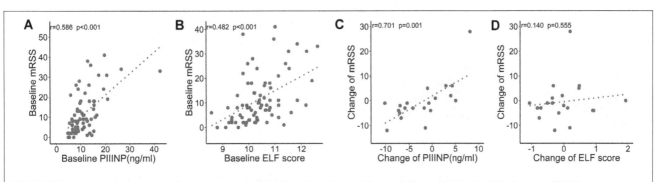

FIGURE 2 | Correlations between serum collagen markers and mRSS at baseline and during follow-up. **(A)** Serum PIIINP and mRSS at baseline. **(B)** ELF score and mRSS at baseline. **(C)** Change in PIIINP and change in mRSS over time. **(D)** Change in ELF score and change in mRSS over time.

TABLE 5 | Clinical and serological parameters of SSc patients with and without ILD matched by propensity score matching.

Characteristics	With ILD (n = 15)	Without ILD (n = 15)	SMD	p Value
Age, years	54 (41–62)	56 (44–64)	0.149	0.686
Gender (female/male)	12/3 (80%/20%)	14/1 (93.3%/6.7%)	0.400	0.598
Subtype (dcSSc/lcSSc)	10/5 (67%/33%)	10/5 (67%/33%)	<0.001	1.000
Disease duration from RP, years	3.0 (1.7–10.0)	4.0 (1.5–10.0)	0.126	0.967
mRSS	11.0 (6.0–24.0)	10 (3.0–14.0)	0.392	0.367
Overall HRCT score	145 (125–159)	—	—	—
MaxFIB HRCT score	3 (2–3)	—	—	—
PIIINP, ng/ml	9.66 (6.59–12.02)	12.29 (7.83–15.23)	0.318	0.412
TIMP-1, ng/ml	109.45 (93.05–200.09)	65.50 (40.57–110.73)	0.908	0.007
HA, ng/ml	228.14 (125.37–273.37)	178.26 (92.93–231.85)	0.090	0.285
ELF score	10.20 (9.89–10.68)	10.40 (10.15–11.13)	0.463	0.215

ELF, enhanced liver fibrosis; HA, hyaluronic acid; HRCT, high resolution computed tomography; ILD, interstitial lung disease; MaxFIB, maximum fibrosis score; mRSS, modified Rodnan skin score; PIIINP, procollagen type III amino terminal propeptide; RP, Raynaud's phenomenon; SMD, standardized mean difference; TIMP-1, tissue inhibitor of metalloproteinases 1.

progression in patients with early SSc. It should also be highlighted that the ELF score was initially derived from a chronic liver disease cohort. The algorithm and reference ranges, specially tailored to assess liver fibrosis and predict liver-related events, may not be readily applicable to SSc. Our results reaffirmed the necessity to develop a disease-specific algorithm based on the clinical implication and analytical performance of individual markers in SSc.

It should also be highlighted that every single marker is differentially affected by confounding factors, which can further complicate the results of the composite score ELF. In the present study as well as previous reports, age is established as a putative confounder for serum HA in both healthy controls and SSc patients (Lichtinghagen et al., 2013; Dellavance et al., 2016). Besides, the diet-related intraday variation of serum HA was reported to be as high as 70% (Lichtinghagen et al., 2013). Disease duration is another influencing factor to be reckoned with. Patients with shorter SSc disease course tended to have higher levels of collagen metabolites, which can be attributed to the active ECM turnover in early phase of the disease (Scheja et al., 2000), and is also in agree with the spontaneous regression of skin fibrosis in some SSc patients (Allanore et al., 2015). Hence, we believe that those serum collagen markers are more valuable when used for within-individual comparisons during follow-ups, while between-individual comparisons should be avoided to prevent misinterpretation of the results.

Recently, Dobrota and colleagues reported that high serum levels of PRO-C3 (the PIIINP neo-epitope) significantly predicted skin progression in SSc, after adjustment for mRSS, sex, and age (Dobrota et al., 2021). PRO-C3 is identified as a more dynamic marker of fibrogenesis than PIIINP, since the antibody applied in PRO-C3 assay only recognized the epitope on PIIINP where the propeptide is cleaved from the intact type III collagen (Nielsen et al., 2013). However, considering that previous investigations in healthy controls found no significant correlation between serum levels of PRO-C3 and PIIINP (Nielsen et al., 2013), the clinical implications of those two serum biomarkers still require further comparing and exploring in SSc cohorts. In the current study, an attempted has also been made to evaluate the predictive effects of serum collagen markers on

longitudinal change in mRSS. However, the results were inconclusive due to the small sample size and larger samples are required before valid conclusions can be drawn.

In regard to lung involvement, Abignano and colleagues demonstrated that the ELF score was significantly higher in patients with ILD compared to those without (Abignano et al., 2014), while in the present study, only TIMP-1 showed difference between the two groups of patients. The conflicting results may be explained by the fact that the ELF score is more of a marker for overall fibrotic activity in SSc, rather than a marker for specific organ involvement (Abignano et al., 2018). Though propensity score matching was used to balance the distribution of several demographic and clinical features in our study, multisystem fibrotic conditions could still complicate the results. Indeed, it is no easy job to evaluate ILD using serological markers alone, and a combined clinical and collagen marker algorithm to predict lung function decline in SSc is currently under development (Hutchinson et al., 2021).

This study is limited by the sample size and retrospective design. Serial measurements are warranted to determine the sensitivity of serum collagen markers to fibrotic changes over a longer period of time. Second, the minimal clinically important difference of serum biomarkers was not estimated in the study, making it hard to evaluate the effect of a given therapy through the serological measurements. Third, potential serum markers for progression of ILD are also well worthy to be explored in patients with SSc. However, due to the retrospective nature of the study, sequential pulmonary function tests were only performed in less than half of the patients and no conclusion can be drawn from this extremely small cohort at the moment. In addition, there is a technical detail to be mentioned that serum PIIINP, TIMP-1, and HA were analyzed using commercial reagents, rather than the integrated platform for ELF in the current study. Considering the inevitable manufacturer-based variation, cross-study comparisons of data from the present study and previous literature have to be made with care.

In conclusion, our study shed new light on the validity of serum collagen metabolites as reliable markers of fibrosis in SSc. We unveil for the first time that changes in PIIINP correlate well with changes in clinical outcome. In the future, collagen markers

In conclusion, our study shed new light on the validity of serum collagen metabolites as reliable markers of fibrosis in SSc. We unveil for the first time that changes in PIIINP correlate well with changes in clinical outcome. In the future, collagen markers could potentially be used to evaluate therapeutic effects of anti-fibrotic treatments in SSc. Research is also needed to establish a disease-specific collagen index to better reflect the fibrotic process in SSc.

AUTHOR CONTRIBUTIONS

CC: Data analysis, Writing—original draft. LW: Specimen collection. JW: Resources. ML: Biochemical measurements. SY and WY: Data collection. MG: Methodology, Validation. ML: Conceptualization, Investigation, Writing—Review and Editing, Funding acquisition. HZ: Conceptualization, Supervision, Funding acquisition.

REFERENCES

Abignano, G., Cuomo, G., Buch, M. H., Rosenberg, W. M., Valentini, G., Emery, P., et al. (2014). The Enhanced Liver Fibrosis Test: a Clinical Grade, Validated Serum Test, Biomarker of Overall Fibrosis in Systemic Sclerosis. *Ann. Rheum. Dis.* 73, 420–427. doi:10.1136/annrheumdis-2012-202843

Abignano, G., Blagojevic, J., Bissell, L.-A., Dumitru, R. B., Eng, S., Allanore, Y., et al. (2018). European Multicentre Study Validates Enhanced Liver Fibrosis Test as Biomarker of Fibrosis in Systemic Sclerosis. *Rheumatology* 58, 254. doi:10.1093/rheumatology/key271

Allanore, Y., Simms, R., Distler, O., Trojanowska, M., Pope, J., Denton, C. P., et al. (2015). Systemic Sclerosis. *Nat. Rev. Dis. Primers* 1, 15002. doi:10.1038/nrdp.2015.2

Baron, M., Chung, L., Gyger, G., Hummers, L., Khanna, D., Mayes, M. D., et al. (2014). Consensus Opinion of a North American Working Group Regarding the Classification of Digital Ulcers in Systemic Sclerosis. *Clin. Rheumatol.* 33, 207–214. doi:10.1007/s10067-013-2460-7

Behr, J., Adelmann-Grill, B. C., Hein, R., Beinert, T., Schwaiblmair, M., Krombach, F., et al. (1995). Pathogenetic and Clinical Significance of Fibroblast Activation in Scleroderma Lung Disease. *Respiration* 62, 209–216. doi:10.1159/000196449

Cozzi, F., Marson, P., Rosada, M., De Silvestro, G., Bullo, A., Punzi, L., et al. (2001). Long-term Therapy with Plasma Exchange in Systemic Sclerosis: Effects on Laboratory Markers Reflecting Disease Activity. *Transfus. Apher. Sci.* 25, 25–31. doi:10.1016/s1473-0502(01)00078-7

Della-Torre, E., Feeney, E., Deshpande, V., Mattoo, H., Mahajan, V., Kulikova, M., et al. (2015). B-cell Depletion Attenuates Serological Biomarkers of Fibrosis and Myofibroblast Activation in IgG4-Related Disease. *Ann. Rheum. Dis.* 74, 2236–2243. doi:10.1136/annrheumdis-2014-205799

Dellavance, A., Fernandes, F., Shimabokuro, N., Latini, F., Baldo, D., Barreto, J. A., et al. (2016). Enhanced Liver Fibrosis (ELF) Score: Analytical Performance and Distribution Range in a Large Cohort of Blood Donors. *Clin. Chim. Acta* 461, 151–155. doi:10.1016/j.cca.2016.08.006

Dobrota, R., Jordan, S., Juhl, P., Maurer, B., Wildi, L., Bay-Jensen, A.-C., et al. (2021). Circulating Collagen Neo-Epitopes and Their Role in the Prediction of Fibrosis in Patients with Systemic Sclerosis: a Multicentre Cohort Study. *Lancet Rheumatol.* 3, e175–e184. doi:10.1016/S2665-9913(20)30385-4

Freitas, J. P., Filipe, P., Emerit, I., Meunier, P., Manso, C. F., and Guerra Rodrigo, F. (1996). Hyaluronic Acid in Progressive Systemic Sclerosis. *Dermatology* 192, 46–49. doi:10.1159/000246314

Goldin, J. G., Lynch, D. A., Strollo, D. C., Suh, R. D., Schraufnagel, D. E., Clements, P. J., et al. (2008). High-Resolution CT Scan Findings in Patients with Symptomatic Scleroderma-Related Interstitial Lung Disease. *Chest* 134, 358–367. doi:10.1378/chest.07-2444

Heickendorff, L., Zachariae, H., Bjerring, P., Halkier-Sørensen, L., and Søndergaard, K. (1995). The Use of Serologic Markers for Collagen Synthesis and Degradation in Systemic Sclerosis. *J. Am. Acad. Dermatol.* 32, 584–588. doi:10.1016/0190-9622(95)90341-0

Hutchinson, M., Abignano, G., Blagojevic, J., Bosello, S. L., Allanore, Y., Denton, C., et al. (2021). Op0269 A Combined Clinical and Biomarker Algorithm to Predict Fvc Decline in Systemic Sclerosis Associated Interstitial Lung Disease: Results from an International Multicentre Observational Cohort. *Ann. Rheum. Dis.* 80, 2–164. doi:10.1136/annrheumdis-2021-eular.1861

Ichikado, K., Suga, M., Muranaka, H., Gushima, Y., Miyakawa, H., Tsubamoto, M., et al. (2006). Prediction of Prognosis for Acute Respiratory Distress Syndrome

with Thin-Section CT: Validation in 44 Cases. *Radiology* 238, 321–329. doi:10.1148/radiol.2373041515

Kikuchi, K., Kubo, M., Sato, S., Fujimoto, M., and Tamaki, K. (1995). Serum Tissue Inhibitor of Metalloproteinases in Patients with Systemic Sclerosis. *J. Am. Acad. Dermatol.* 33, 973–978. doi:10.1016/0190-9622(95)90289-9

Kikuchi, K., Kadono, T., Furue, M., and Tamaki, K. (1997). Tissue Inhibitor of Metalloproteinase 1 (TIMP-1) May Be an Autocrine Growth Factor in Scleroderma Fibroblasts. *J. Invest. Dermatol.* 108, 281–284. doi:10.1111/1523-1747.ep12286457

Lapière, C. M., Lenaers, A., and Kohn, L. D. (1971). Procollagen Peptidase: An Enzyme Excising the Coordination Peptides of Procollagen. *Proc. Natl. Acad. Sci. U S A.* 68, 3054–3058. doi:10.1073/pnas.68.12.3054

LeRoy, E. C. (1974). Increased Collagen Synthesis by Scleroderma Skin Fibroblasts *In Vitro*: a Possible Defect in the Regulation or Activation of the Scleroderma Fibroblast. *J. Clin. Invest.* 54, 880–889. doi:10.1172/JCI107827

Lichtinghagen, R., Pietsch, D., Bantel, H., Manns, M. P., Brand, K., and Bahr, M. J. (2013). The Enhanced Liver Fibrosis (ELF) Score: Normal Values, Influence Factors and Proposed Cut-Off Values. *J. Hepatol.* 59, 236–242. doi:10.1016/j.jhep.2013.03.016

Nagy, Z., and Czirják, L. (2005). Increased Levels of Amino Terminal Propeptide of Type III Procollagen Are an Unfavourable Predictor of Survival in Systemic Sclerosis. *Clin. Exp. Rheumatol.* 23, 165–172.

Nielsen, M. J., Nedergaard, A. F., Sun, S., Veidal, S. S., Larsen, L., Zheng, Q., et al. (2013). The Neo-Epitope Specific PRO-C3 ELISA Measures True Formation of Type III Collagen Associated with Liver and Muscle Parameters. *Am. J. Transl. Res.* 5, 303–315.

Parkes, J., Roderick, P., Harris, S., Day, C., Mutimer, D., Collier, J., et al. (2010). Enhanced Liver Fibrosis Test Can Predict Clinical Outcomes in Patients with Chronic Liver Disease. *Gut* 59, 1245–1251. doi:10.1136/gut.2009.203166

Parkes, J., Guha, I. N., Roderick, P., Harris, S., Cross, R., Manos, M. M., et al. (2011). Enhanced Liver Fibrosis (ELF) Test Accurately Identifies Liver Fibrosis in Patients with Chronic Hepatitis C. *J. Viral Hepat.* 18, 23–31. doi:10.1111/j.1365-2893.2009.01263.x

Plastiras, S. C., Karadimitrakis, S. P., Kampolis, C., Moutsopoulos, H. M., and Tzelepis, G. E. (2007). Determinants of Pulmonary Arterial Hypertension in Scleroderma. *Semin. Arthritis Rheum.* 36, 392–396. doi:10.1016/j.semarthrit.2006.10.004

Rosenberg, W. M., Voelker, M., Thiel, R., Becka, M., Burt, A., Schuppan, D., et al. (2004). Serum Markers Detect the Presence of Liver Fibrosis: A Cohort Study. *Gastroenterology* 127, 1704–1713. doi:10.1053/j.gastro.2004.08.052

Scheja, A., Akesson, A., and Hørslev-Petersen, K. (1992). Serum Levels of Aminoterminal Type III Procollagen Peptide and Hyaluronan Predict Mortality in Systemic Sclerosis. *Scand. J. Rheumatol.* 21, 5–9. doi:10.3109/03009749209095054

Scheja, A., Wildt, M., Wollheim, F. A., Akesson, A., and Saxne, T. (2000). Circulating Collagen Metabolites in Systemic Sclerosis. Differences between Limited and Diffuse Form and Relationship with Pulmonary Involvement. *Rheumatology (Oxford)* 39, 1110–1113. doi:10.1093/rheumatology/39.10.1110

Stone, P. J., Korn, J. H., North, H., Lally, E. V., Miller, L. C., Tucker, L. B., et al. (1995). Cross-linked Elastin and Collagen Degradation Products in the Urine of Patients with Scleroderma. *Arthritis Rheum.* 38, 517–524. doi:10.1002/art.1780380409

Vali, Y., Lee, J., Boursier, J., Spijker, R., Löffler, J., Verheij, J., et al. (2020). Enhanced Liver Fibrosis Test for the Non-invasive Diagnosis of Fibrosis in Patients with NAFLD: A Systematic Review and Meta-Analysis. *J. Hepatol.* 73, 252–262. doi:10.1016/j.jhep.2020.03.036

Webber, J., Meran, S., Steadman, R., and Phillips, A. (2009). Hyaluronan Orchestrates Transforming Growth Factor-beta1-dependent Maintenance of Myofibroblast Phenotype. *J. Biol. Chem.* 284, 9083–9092. doi:10.1074/jbc.M806989200

Yoshizaki, A., Iwata, Y., Komura, K., Hara, T., Ogawa, F., Muroi, E., et al. (2008). Clinical Significance of Serum Hyaluronan Levels in Systemic Sclerosis: Association with Disease Severity. *J. Rheumatol.* 35, 1825–1829.

Young-Min, S. A., Beeton, C., Laughton, R., Plumpton, T., Bartram, S., Murphy, G., et al. (2001). Serum TIMP-1, TIMP-2, and MMP-1 in Patients with Systemic Sclerosis, Primary Raynaud's Phenomenon, and in normal Controls. *Ann. Rheum. Dis.* 60, 846–851.

12

TMEM88 Modulates Lipid Synthesis and Metabolism Cytokine by Regulating Wnt/β-Catenin Signaling Pathway in Non-Alcoholic Fatty Liver Disease

Huan Zhou [1,2,3*†], Xingyu Zhu [1,2†], Yan Yao [4†], Yue Su [1,3], Jing Xie [1], Minhui Zhu [1,2], Cuixia He [1,2], Jiaxiang Ding [1,3], Yuanyuan Xu [1,2], Rongfang Shan [1,2], Ying Wang [1,2], Xiangdi Zhao [1,2], Yuzhou Ding [1], Bingyan Liu [1], Zhonghuan Shao [1], Yuanyuan Liu [1], Tao Xu [4*] and Yunqiu Xie [1*]

[1]National Drug Clinical Trial Center, The First Affiliated Hospital of Bengbu Medical College, Bengbu, China, [2]School of Pharmacy, Bengbu Medical College, Bengbu, China, [3]School of Public Foundation, Bengbu Medical University, Bengbu, China, [4]Inflammation and Immune Mediated Diseases Laboratory of Anhui Province, Anhui Institute of Innovative Drugs, School of Pharmacy, Anhui Medical University, Hefei, China

*Correspondence:
Huan Zhou
zhouhuan@bbmc.edu.cn
Tao Xu
xutao@ahmu.edu.cn
Yunqiu Xie
xieyunqiuu@126.com

†These authors have contributed equally to this work

Objective: To clarify the molecular mechanism of TMEM88 regulating lipid synthesis and metabolism cytokine in NAFLD.

Methods: *In vivo*, NAFLD model mice were fed by a Methionine and Choline-Deficient (MCD) diet. H&E staining and immunohistochemistry experiments were used to analyze the mice liver tissue. RT-qPCR and Western blotting were used to detect the lipid synthesis and metabolism cytokine. *In vitro*, pEGFP-C1-TMEM88 and TMEM88 siRNA were transfected respectively in free fat acid (FFA) induced AML-12 cells, and the expression level of SREBP-1c, PPAR-α, FASN, and ACOX-1 were evaluated by RT-qPCR and Western blotting.

Results: The study found that the secretion of PPAR-α and its downstream target ACOX-1 were upregulated, and the secretion of SREBP-1c and its downstream target FASN were downregulated after transfecting with pEGFP-C1-TMEM88. But when TMEM88 was inhibited, the experimental results were opposite to the aforementioned conclusions. The data suggested that it may be related to the occurrence, development, and end of NAFLD. Additionally, the study proved that TMEM88 can inhibit Wnt/β-catenin signaling pathway. Meanwhile, TMEM88 can accelerate the apoptotic rate of FFA-induced AML-12 cells.

Conclusion: Overall, the study proved that TMEM88 takes part in regulating the secretion of lipid synthesis and metabolism cytokine through the Wnt/β-catenin signaling pathway in AML-12 cells. Therefore, TMEM88 may be involved in the progress of NAFLD. Further research will bring new ideas for the study of NAFLD.

Keywords: lipid metabolism, AML-12 cells, Wnt/β-catenin, FFA, TMEM88

INTRODUCTION

Non-alcoholic fatty liver disease (NAFLD) is a disorder of liver lipid metabolism under non-alcoholic stimulation and excessive precipitation of liver cell fat, leading to fatty liver, non-alcoholic steatohepatitis (NASH), and other related diseases (Maurice and Manousou 2018; Geh et al., 2021). With the global obesity epidemic, the incidence of NAFLD continues to increase, and it has become the most common chronic liver disease on a global scale (Younossi 2019). The incidence of NAFLD in adults is about 17–33%, and the incidence in obese people is as high as 75%. Among them, the incidence of cirrhosis in NAFLD for 10 years is 25% (Borrelli et al., 2018; Maurice and Manousou 2018). Although there are many theories and hypotheses about the pathogenesis of NAFLD, they fail to cover the whole process of occurrence and development. A lot of evidence showed that it was related to the imbalance of lipid homeostasis caused by abnormal regulation of lipid metabolism (Buzzetti et al., 2016). The accumulation of triglycerides in liver parenchymal cells is the main feature of NAFLD. The main mechanism of hepatocyte fat deposition is the imbalance of triglyceride synthesis and output in the liver (Mashek 2021). Most of the sterol regulatory elements of transcription cytokine are also downstream target genes of the binding protein such as fatty acid synthase (FAS). They have also been involved in the synthesis of carbohydrate reactive element–binding protein (ChREBP) in the liver (Barbaro et al.). According to relevant experimental reports, the Wnt/β-catenin signaling pathway can regulate liver lipid anabolism by regulating other regulatory cytokines, such as SREBP-1c, FAS, and PPAR family (Xu et al., 2014; Seo et al., 2016).

Additionally, TMEM88 is a potential type 2 transmembrane protein generated by transcription and translation on chromosome 17p13.1. However, as far as the current research was concerned, the research on the related expression mechanism of this protein was still limited, and its potential application value is gradually receiving attention. Recent studies showed that β-catenin located in the cytoplasm was recognized by the phosphorylation site of GSK3β and phosphorylated and degraded, thereby inhibiting the classic Wnt/β-catenin signaling pathway. Research on TMEM88 indicated that TMEM88 had an inhibitory effect on the Wnt/β-catenin signaling pathway in HEK293 cells, and this impact can also mediate the development of human embryonic stem cells to cardiomyocytes. In addition, an experiment found that TMEM88 has a protective function on alcoholic liver fibrosis (Li et al., 2020). It proved that TMEM88 can play a certain regulatory role in the happening and progress of liver diseases. Therefore, this experiment further speculated that TMEM88 may mediate the Wnt/β-catenin signaling pathway to maintain lipid homeostasis and protect liver cells.

This research was devised to probe the metabolic function and molecular mechanisms of TMEM88 in NAFLD. In vivo study, the MCD-fed mice were used to study the mechanism of TMEM88 in NAFLD. FFA-induced AML-12 cells were used to observe the regulatory mechanism of TMEM88 in vitro. The results showed that TMEM88 can regulate lipid metabolism cytokine which provided a strategy for the diagnosis and treatment for NAFLD-related diseases.

MATERIALS AND METHODS

Materials

Dulbecco's modified Eagle medium was purchased from HyClone (Beijing, China). Lipofectamine™ 2000 and TRIzol were purchased from Invitrogen (Carlsbad, CA, United States). An ECL-Chemiluminescence kit was purchased from ThermoFisher Scientific (NYC, United States). An FITC Annexin V Apoptosis Detection Kit I was purchased from BestBio (Shanghai, China). Fetal bovine serum (FBS) and Opti-MEM were purchased from Gibco (Grand Island, NY, United States). The primers of TMEM88, SREBP-1c, PPAR-α, FASN, and ACOX-1 were produced by Sheng gong Biotechnology Company (Shanghai, China). TBST was purchased from Boster (Boster, China). Extraction buffer, PMSF, and RIPA lysis buffer were purchased from Beyotime (Hangzhou, China). β-catenin inhibitor FH535 (HY-15721) was purchased from MCE (Shanghai, China). Methionine- and choline-deficient diet (MCD) (TP 3006) and methionine- and choline-supplement diet (MCS) (TP 3006S) were purchased from Trophic (Nantong, China). Palmitoleic acid (P860713) and oleic acid (O815202) were purchased from Macklin (Shanghai, China). TMEM88 (sc135525) monoclonal antibody was purchased from Santa Cruz Biotechnology (CA, United States). Anti-β-actin (Cat: TA-09) monoclonal antibody was purchased from Santa Cruz Biotechnology (CA, United States). c-myc (2278T), cyclin D1 (2978T) monoclonal antibodies were purchased from Cell Signaling Technology (MA, United States). PPAR-α(DF6073) and SREBP-1c (AF6283) monoclonal antibodies were purchased from Affinity (Cincinnati, United States). FASN (ab128870) and ACOX-1 (ab32072) were purchased from Abcam (Cambridge, United Kingdom). Goat anti-mouse immunoglobulin (IgG) (ZB-2305) and goat anti-rabbit immunoglobulin (IgG) (ZB-2301) secondary antibodies were purchased from ZSGBBIO (Beijing, China).

Construction of Non-Alcoholic Fatty Liver Disease Model

The mice used to construct the NAFLD model were 8-weeks-old male C57BL/6J mice. The animal trial procedure was approved by the Ethics Committee of Bengbu Medical College. All male mice were randomly divided into two groups ($n = 10$). Normal group mice were fed with MCS feed, experimental group mice were fed with MCD. After 8 weeks of continuous feeding, the mice were anesthetized and killed in the early morning of the last day. Blood and liver tissue were collected for further analysis.

Cell Culture

AML-12 cells were nourished in DME/F12 medium containing 10% FBS and nurtured in a 37°C moist incubator and 5% CO_2. Different times and concentrations of FFA were used to stimulate AML-12 cells.

Oil Red

The AML-12 cells were divided into two groups. The experimental group was induced by FFA for 24 h, then ORO Fixative was used to fix AML-12 cells for 15–25 min, 60% isopropyl alcohol was used to wash the cells for 5 min, and the ORO Stain was used to stain the AML-12 cells, then stained for 10–15 min by airtight, and water was used to remove the staining solution. Then Mayer hematoxylin staining solution was used to counter-stain the cell nucleus for 1~2 min, then discard the staining solution and wash with water 3 times, then microscope was used to observe the stain.

Edu Staining

4% fixative was used to fixate the fresh liver tissues for 24 h, then the tissues were dehydrated with ethanol from high concentration to low concentration, and put in xylene. The treated tissues were embedded in paraffin and sectioned, and then xylene and gradient alcohol were used to dewax and dehydrate. Then HE was used to dye, gradient alcohol was used to dehydrate. After permeation with xylene for 5 min, the tissues were observed by microscope.

siRNA and Plasmid Transfection

The AML-12 cells were seeded into 6-well plates and transfected according to previous research methods (Barbaro, Romito, and Alisi). After 6 h of transfection, the cells were cultured in DMF/F12 medium for 24 h, and the siRNA sequence used for transfection is as follows: F:5′-UCAUGUUAGGCUUCGGCUUTT-3′; R:5′-AAGCCGAAGCCUAACAUGATT -3′; negative control: F: 5′-UUCUCCGAACGUGUCACGUTT-3′, R:5′-ACGUG ACACUG GCGGAGAATT-3′.

Cell Viability Assays

Cell proliferation was analyzed by using CCK-8 assay. Cells were transferred into 96-well plates with a volume of 100 ul per well, with a cell density of 1×10^4 cells, and placed in the incubator until they adhere to the wall. Different concentrations of FFA were used to induce cells for 24 h. Then 10 ul of CCK8 solution was added to each well and incubated for 3 h in the incubator. Then a microplate reader was used to measure the optical density (OD) at a wavelength of 490 nm, and the percent viability was calculated. The experimental data were repeated three times.

Flow Cytometry

After transfection and FFA stimulation, AML-12 cells were lysed with trypsin for 2 min and then gently pipetted into a 1.5-ml EP tube for centrifugation. The supernatant was discarded, and cold PBS was added for washing and centrifugation, and the previous operation was repeated three times. Annexin V working solution was added to resuspend the cells and then PI staining was performed, and the solution was incubated for 10 min in the dark.

RNA Isolation and RT-qPCR

TRIzol reagent and chloroform were used to extract RNA from AML-12 cells, then RNA was transferred in the water phase to another RNase-free centrifuge tube and isopropanol was added to precipitate, and the resulting RNA was dissolved in enzyme-free water. The first-strand cDNA synthesis kit was used for RNA reversing. GAPDH was used as an internal reference for detection in an RT-qPCR instrument. The primers used for PCR are shown in **Table 1**.

Western Blotting

A new RIPA lysis buffer containing 1% PMSF was used to extract proteins from liver tissue and AML-12 cells. The BCA protein detection kit measured the protein concentration. The same amount of protein was resolved by SDS-PAGE then the PVDF membrane was used to transfer. After blocking in blocking buffer, the membrane was washed three times in TBS-Tween buffer. The membrane with the specific primary antibody was incubated in the primary antibody dilution buffer in a 4°C refrigerator for 12 h. Meanwhile, β-actin was used by mouse secondary antibody. TMEM88, SREBP-1c, PPAR-α, FASN, ACOX-1, and β-catenin were used by rabbit secondary antibody. After washing three times with TBST, the ECL chemiluminescence kit was used to detect the protein.

Immunohistochemistry

Before dewaxing, the liver slices were placed in a constant temperature oven at 60°C for 1 h. The tissue slices were soaked in xylene and ethanol of different concentrations for hydration, and then the slices were immersed in a sodium citrate buffer. Then the antigen was repaired by high pressure. After cooling to room temperature, 3% H_2O_2 was added and allowed to stand for 15 min for inhibiting endogenous peroxidase activity and then 2% bovine serum albumin (BSA), TMEM88 (1:100) was added. And α-SMA (1: 100), the primary antibody was incubated at 4°C for 16 h. The expression was identified by using DAB color-developing solution. The sections were subsequently counterstained with hematoxylin for 5 min and then dehydrated in

TABLE 1 | Primer sequences for quantitative real-time reverse transcription polymerase chain reaction.

Gene	Primer pair	
TMEM88	F:5′-GCGCTAGCATGGCGGATGGCCCCAGG -3′	R:5′-GCGCGGCCGCTTAGGCTTCATTTGTCTTTTCTTCAG-3′
SREBP-1c	F:5′-GCAGCAACGGGACCATTCT -3′	R:5′- CCCCATGACTAAGTCCTTCAACT -3′
PPAR-α	F:5′- AACATCGAGTGTCGAATATGTGG -3′	R:5′- CCGAATAGTTCGCCGAAAGAA -3′
FASN	F:5′- GGAGGTGGTGATAGCCGGTAT -3′	R:5′- TGGGTAATCCATAGAGCCCAG -3′
ACOX-1	F:5′- TAACTTCCTCACTCGAAGCCA -3′	F:5′- AGTTCCATGACCCATCTCTGTC -3′
β-actin	F:5′-GCCAACACAGTGCTGTCTGG-3′	R:5′-CTCAGGAGGAGCAATGATCTTG-3′

reduced concentration ethanol, dried, photographed, mounted, and stored.

Statistical Analysis

All experimental data were repeated in triplicate. The difference between groups was analyzed by t-tests or one-way ANOVA and processed by SPSS 18.0 software. The data were presented as mean ± standard deviation (SD). If a p-value was less than 0.05, the data were considered statistically significant. If a p-value was less than 0.01, the data were considered statistically significant.

RESULTS

TMEM88 was Downregulated in Liver Tissue of Non-Alcoholic Fatty Liver Disease Mice

To observe the pathological changes of NAFLD *in vivo*. In this experiment, all MCD-fed mice which developed fatty liver and injury caused by the imbalance of lipid metabolism. The H&E staining results proved that the the NAFLD liver of the MCD-fed group exhibited fatty vacuoles and inflammatory infiltration, the gap between cells was enlarged, and the liver cord was disordered (**Figure 1A**). Immunohistochemistry results indicated that the expression level of TMEM88 was reduced in the MCD-fed group (**Figure 1B**). In addition, the blood collected from the corner of the eye was used to test the serum. The result indicated that the expression level of ALT and AST was upregulated in the MCD-fed group (**Figure 1C**). The expression level of TMEM88 in NAFLD mice liver was tested to make sure that whether TMEM88 was involved in NAFLD. RT-qPCR and Western blotting results indicated that the expression level of TMEM88 was reduced in the MCD-fed group (**Figures 1D,E**).

SREBP-1c, PPAR-α, FASN, and ACOX-1 are representative lipid metabolism cytokines. The results suggested that expression of levels of PPAR-α and ACOX-1 were reduced, while SREBP-1c and FASN were upregulated in liver samples (**Figures 2A,B**).

TMEM88 was Reduced in Free Fat Acid–Induced AML-12 Cells

To observe the pathological changes of NAFLD *in vitro* and the expression level of TMEM88 in FFA-induced AML-12 cells. AML-12 cells were stimulated by different concentrations of FFA and at different times. First, the oil red staining results demonstrated that compared with the normal group, it can be seen that the FFA-induced group was successfully constructed (**Figure 3A**). Second, different concentrations of FFA were used to induce AML-12 cells for 24 h. It indicated a dose-dependent decrease in cell viability (**Figure 3B**). Third, the experimental results indicated that the expression level of TMEM88 continued to decrease with the increasing concentration of FFA stimulation in the experiment and reached a bottom protein level after 24 h of inducing by 2 mM FFA (**Figure 3C**). Fourth, the AML-12 cells were induced by 2 mM FFA in different hours to observe the

expression level of TMEM88. Western blotting results proved that the TMEM88 protein level reached a valley when AML-12 cells were stimulated by FFA for 24 h (**Figure 3D**). Last, AML-12 cells were transfected with TMEM88siRNA and pEGFP-C1-TMEM88, respectively. The results showed that the TMEM88siRNA or pEGFP-C1-TMEM88, has been successfully transfected in AML-12 cells (**Figures 3E,F**).

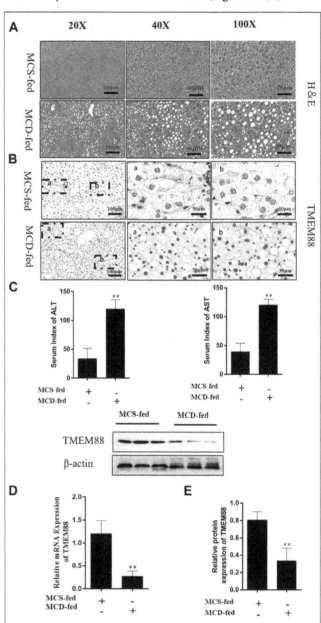

FIGURE 1 | TMEM88 expression was suppressed in NAFLD model. **(A)** The H&E stain in liver tissues. Fat vacuoles and intercellular spaces dilatation were appeared in NAFLD liver tissues, while the normal liver tissues indicated that normal lobular architecture. **(B)** Immunohistochemistry indicated that the expression of TMEM88 was reduced in MCD-fed mice liver tissues of **(C)**. The serum levels of ALT and AST in the MCD-fed group were increased. **(D,E)** RNA and protein results showed that compared with the normal group, TMEM88 was inhibited in MCD-fed mice. (Data are represented by at least three independent mean ± SD, $*p < 0.05$, $**p < 0.01$ vs normal group).

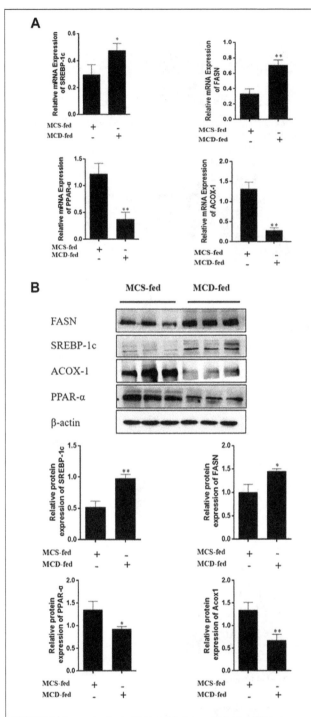

FIGURE 2 | Expression level of lipid metabolism cytokine in MCD-fed mice. (A,B) The mRNA and protein expression levels of FASN and SERBP-1C were increased. PPAR-α and ACOX-1 expression were decreased in NAFLD liver tissues. (Data are represented by at least three independent mean ± SD, *p < 0.05, **p < 0.01 vs normal group).

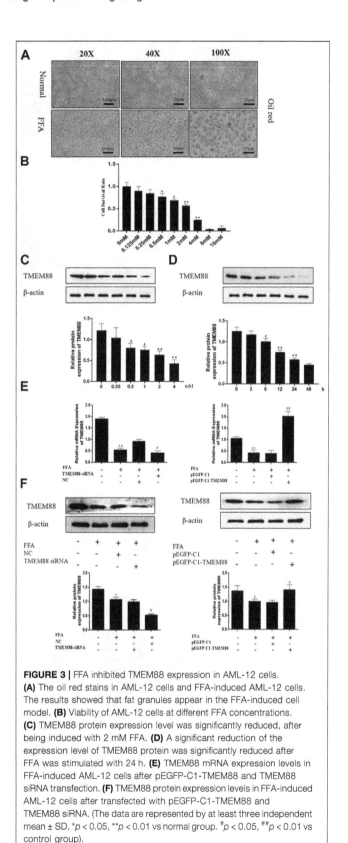

FIGURE 3 | FFA inhibited TMEM88 expression in AML-12 cells. (A) The oil red stains in AML-12 cells and FFA-induced AML-12 cells. The results showed that fat granules appear in the FFA-induced cell model. (B) Viability of AML-12 cells at different FFA concentrations. (C) TMEM88 protein expression level was significantly reduced, after being induced with 2 mM FFA. (D) A significant reduction of the expression level of TMEM88 protein was significantly reduced after FFA was stimulated with 24 h. (E) TMEM88 mRNA expression levels in FFA-induced AML-12 cells after pEGFP-C1-TMEM88 and TMEM88 siRNA transfection. (F) TMEM88 protein expression levels in FFA-induced AML-12 cells after transfected with pEGFP-C1-TMEM88 and TMEM88 siRNA. (The data are represented by at least three independent mean ± SD, *p < 0.05, **p < 0.01 vs normal group. #p < 0.05, ##p < 0.01 vs control group).

TMEM88 Promoted Lipid Metabolism in Free Fat Acid–Induced AML-12 Cells

To analyze the regulation mechanism of TMEM88 on lipid synthesis and metabolism cytokines, AML-12 cells were transfected with the TMEM88siRNA or pEGFP-C1-TMEM88. The results indicated that upregulation of TMEM88 inhibited the expression levels of SREBP-1c and FASN and upregulated PPAR-

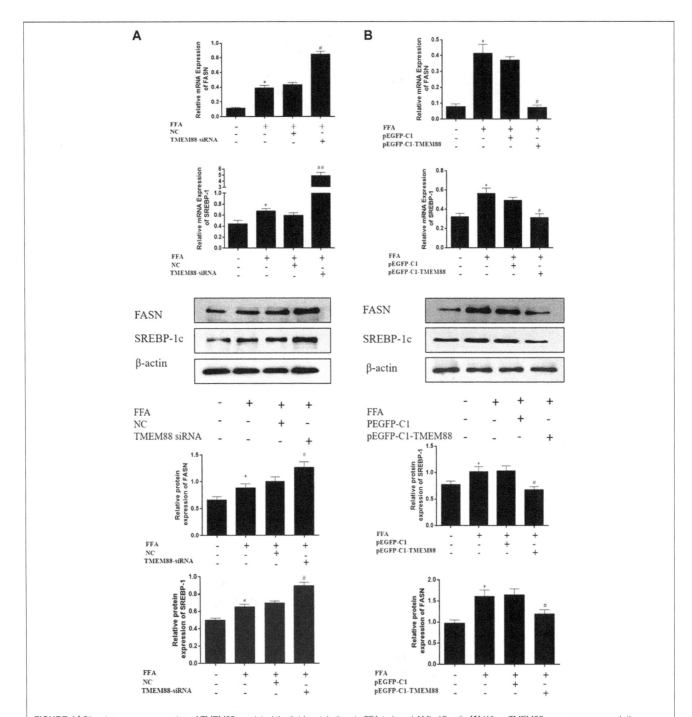

FIGURE 4 | Silencing or overexpression of TMEM88 regulated the lipid metabolism in FFA-induced AML-12 cells **(A)** When TMEM88 was overexpressed, the expression levels of FASN and SREBP-1c decreased. In contrast, **(B)** When TMEM88 was silenced, the expression levels of FASN and SREBP-1c were upregulated. (Data are represented by at least three independent mean ± SD, *$p < 0.05$ vs normal group, #$p < 0.05$, ##$p < 0.01$ vs control group).

α and ACOX-1 in FFA-induced AML-12 cells (**Figure 4A**, **Figure 5A**). Meanwhile, the expression level of lipid synthesis and metabolism cytokines was opposite when TMEM88 was knocked out (**Figure 4B**, **Figure 5B**). All in all, these results indicated that the secretion of PPAR-α and ACOX-1 was positively regulated by TMEM88, while SREBP-1c and FASN were negatively regulated.

TMEM88 Inhibited Cell Proliferation in Free Fat Acid–Induced AML-12 Cells

To explore the effect of TMEM88 on cell proliferation in FFA-induced AML-12 cells. Edu staining was used to detect proliferation. Cell reproduction was represented by the image of AML-12 cells stained with EDU (red), while the nucleus was

TMEM88 Modulates Lipid Synthesis and Metabolism Cytokine by Regulating Wnt/β-Catenin Signaling...

143

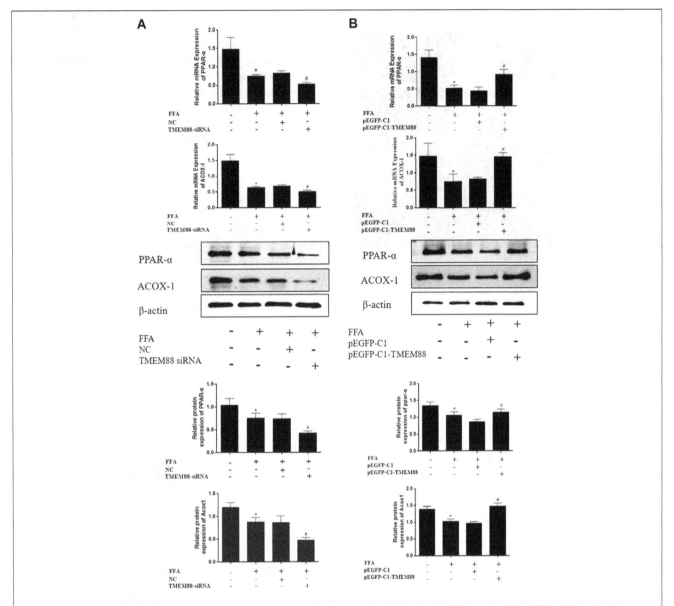

FIGURE 5 | Silencing or overexpression of TMEM88 regulated the lipid metabolism in FFA-induced AML-12 cells. **(A)** The results of RT-qPCR and Western blotting showed that transfection of TMEM88 siRNA downregulated the expression levels of PPAR-α and ACOX-1. Conversely, **(B)** pEGFP-C1-TMEM88 upregulated the expression levels of PPAR-α and ACOX-1. (The data are represented by at least three independent mean ± SD, *p < 0.05 vs normal group, #p < 0.05 vs control group).

marked with Hochest (blue). The results showed that TMEM88 siRNA can significantly promote the proliferation of activated AML-12 cells. On the contrary, the image indicated that the cell proliferation was inhibited after transfecting with pEGFP-C1-TMEM88 in FFA-induced AML-12 cells (**Figure 6A**).

TMEM88 Promoted Cell Apoptosis in Free Fat Acid–Induced AML-12 Cells

To research the function of TMEM88 on the cell apoptotic rate. Annexin V-FITC/PI double staining flow cytometry was used to process apoptosis. The result showed that the apoptosis of AML-12 cells was significantly inhibited when TMEM88 was knocked

out. On the other hand, the overexpression of TMEM88 induced a higher apoptotic rate (**Figures 7A,B**). Above all, TMEM88 can regulate the apoptosis of AML-12 cells.

TMEM88-Mediated Wnt/β-Catenin Signaling Pathway in Free Fat Acid–Induced AML-12 Cells

To detect the regulated mechanism of Wnt/β-catenin in NAFLD, this study found that the expression of the Wnt/β-catenin signaling pathway was increased in FFA-induced AML-12 cells. In addition, the Western blotting results suggested that the expression of β-catenin, c-myc, and cyclin D1 was greatly

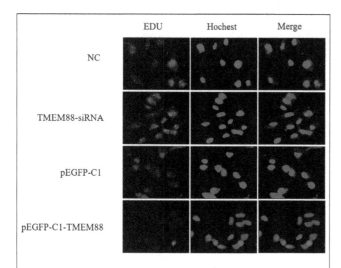

FIGURE 6 | TMEM88 inhibited the proliferation of AML-12 cells stimulated by FFA. **(A)** Edu staining detected the effect of TMEM88 on the proliferation of AML-12 cells stimulated by FFA. The image of AML-12 cells stained by Edu (red) represents cell proliferation, and Hochest (blue) was used to mark the cell nucleus.

increased when knocking out TMEM88 (**Figure 8A**). On the other hand, β-catenin, c-myc, and cyclin D1 signaling pathways were significantly downregulated when TMEM88 was overexpressed in AML-12 cells (**Figure 8B**). Furthermore, the β-catenin inhibitor FH535 was used to inhibit the β-catenin signaling pathway. The result showed that the downregulation of β-catenin can promote lipid metabolism (**Figure 8C**). Briefly, these results showed that the Wnt/β-catenin signaling pathway may regulate the lipid metabolism of TMEM88 in AML-12 cells.

DISCUSSION

There is currently no effective treatment for NAFLD. Its pathogenesis is generally difficult to detect at the beginning. Its process includes fat accumulation, inflammatory infiltration, cell damage, fibrosis, oxidative stress, and cancerous, similar to alcoholic fatty liver (Cobbina and Akhlaghi 2017; Baselli and Valenti 2019; Hu et al., 2019). It is the main life-threatening reason for liver disease. The main feature is the accumulation of fat in the liver caused by lipid anabolism (Tian et al., 2016; Barbaro

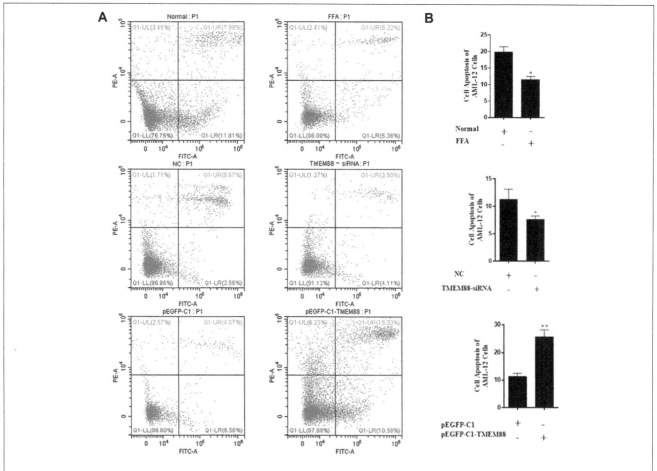

FIGURE 7 | Apoptosis of AML-12 cells induced was inhibited by FFA. **(A,B)** Flow cytometer results indicated that the expression of TMEM88 was positively correlated with AML-12 cell apoptosis. (The data are represented by at least three independent mean ± SD, *$p < 0.05$, **$p < 0.01$ vs control group).

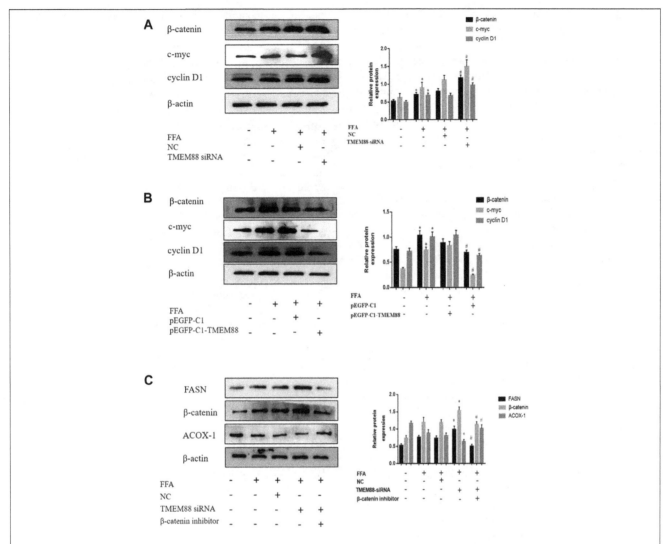

FIGURE 8 | Expression of β-catenin and related signaling pathways in FFA-induced AML-12 cells. **(A,B)** The Wnt/β-catenin, c-myc, and cyclin D1 signaling pathways were elevated in FFA-induced AML-12 cells. **(C)** The downregulated of β-catenin can promote lipid metabolism. (The data are represented by at least three independent mean ± SD, $^*p < 0.05$ vs control group, $^#p < 0.05$ vs siRNA+β-catenin inhibitor group).

et al., 2018; Del Campo et al., 2018). Moreover, as the living environment changes, the incidence of non-alcoholic fatty liver disease (NAFLD) is increasing globally (Younossi et al., 2016; Zhou et al., 2019; Ray 2021). The prevalence of NAFLD worldwide is approximately 25% (Younossi et al., 2016), the lowest incidence in Africa is 13% (26707365 (Younossi et al., 2016), and the incidence in Southeast Asia is as high as 42% (Li et al., 2019). It is estimated that the prevalence of NASH in western Europe, the United States, Japan, and China will show an increase by 56% in the next 10 years (Huang et al., 2021). Furthermore, TMEM88 can inhibit the Wnt/β-catenin–mediated in inflammatory and cancer (Ma et al., 2017; Xu et al., 2018). This experiment explores whether the Wnt/β-catenin signaling pathway can be mediated by TMEM88 and then regulated lipid metabolism in NAFLD models.

Currently, the underlying molecular mechanism of lipid metabolism imbalance in liver cells is still not fully understood. In addition, the experiment indicated that TMEM88 also mediated

the secretion of inflammatory cytokines, which showed that TMEM88 played a role in inflammatory diseases (Li et al., 2020). Moreover, the results of our past research showed that TMEM88 was reduced in HCC tissues and can be used to regulate HCC (Zhang et al., 2017). While TMEM88 in NAFLD has not been studied. The current research clarified the regulatory effect of TMEM88 in the fatty liver and its internal mechanism. First of all, protein and RNA results proved that the expression of TMEM88 was significantly reduced, compared with the normal group. The results demonstrated that TMEM88 may play an indispensable role in FFA-induced AML-12 cells. Furthermore, our research showed that in FFA-induced AML-12 cells and MCD-fed mice, the expression levels of SREBP-1c and FASN are higher in NAFLD, and ACOX-1 and PPAR-α expression levels were lower. Therefore, the experimental results demonstrated that the secretion of lipid metabolism cytokine SREBP-1c, PPAR-α, FASN, and ACOX-1 was regulated by TMEM88 *in vivo*. Moreover, this study also proved that the FASN and SREBP-1c were downregulated, while PPAR-α and ACOX-1 were increased by transfecting FFA-induced AML-12 cells with pEGFP-C1-TMEM88. Additionally, compared with the pEGFP-C1 transfection group, the FFA stimulation group and pEGFP-C1 transfection group were not statistically significant. In addition, the experiment proved that FASN and SREBP-1c were overexpressed, while the expression of PPAR-α and ACOX-1 was reduced by FFA-induced intracellular transfection with TMEM88 siRNA. Therefore, this experiment can infer that the baseline level of TMEM88 was essential for the expression of cell lipid metabolism cytokine genes. It can increase the level of lipid oxidation cytokines in AML-12 cells and negatively regulate lipid synthesis.

The classic Wnt/β-catenin signaling pathway is the best characterized Wnt pathway that participates in the development of animal embryos, and its dysfunction is closely related to a variety of other malignant tumors (Baselli and Valenti 2019). The β-catenin signaling pathway was phosphorylated and degraded by GSK3β when the Wnt signaling pathway was inhibited (Lee et al., 2021). In addition, the Wnt/β-catenin signaling pathway is the main target of the Hippo signaling pathway (Heallen et al., 2011). It also has the function of mediating liver fibrosis (Bhalla et al., 2012), liver regeneration (Cai et al., 2021), and HCC (Baselli and Valenti), and it can also influence the cell cycle (Barbaro, Romito, and Alisi). Studies showed that the Wnt/β-catenin signaling pathway can mediate tissue growth, development, homeostasis, and repair in a variety of ways (Majidinia et al., 2018; Fan et al., 2020). The Wnt/β-catenin signaling pathway was mediated by TMEM88 and then regulated the secretion of lipid metabolism cytokines. However, the molecular mechanism of the Wnt/β-catenin signaling pathway is still unclear in NAFLD HCC. There was no relevant research on the regulation effect of TMEM88 on the Wnt/β-catenin signaling pathway. Furthermore, hepatic steatosis needed further research. The previous research reports showed that liver fibrosis can be reduced by reversing the activation of HSCs and accelerating

hepatocyte apoptosis by blocking the Wnt/β-catenin signaling pathway (Chen et al., 2020; Huang et al., 2021; Jing et al., 2021). However, the relationship between the Wnt/β-catenin signaling pathway and NAFLD has not been reported yet. Therefore, this study deduced the key pathway of TMEM88 regulation mechanism *in vivo*. Moreover, the study result proved that the expression of the Wnt/β-catenin signaling pathway was decreased after FFA-induced AML-12 cells transfected with the TMEM88 overexpression plasmid. In conclusion, research results showed that the influence of intracellular lipid metabolism cytokines by Wnt/β-catenin, cyclin D1, and c-myc were inseparable from the mediation of TMEM88 in FFA-induced AML-12 cells.

In summary, this study showed that in FFA-induced AML-12 cells, the TMEM88 transmembrane protein and the Wnt/β-catenin signaling pathway can mutually regulate the secretion of cell lipid metabolism cytokines. In the next experiment, transcriptome sequencing will be performed on FFA-stimulated AML cells to find upstream regulatory cytokines of TMEM88, such as RNA or DNA. It is a great task to master the principle of these lipid metabolism regulators, but we must explore these regulators as a breakthrough point in the treatment of NAFLD-related diseases. Furthermore, with the continuous in-depth research on NAFLD and the development of science and technology, it is believed that the pathogenesis of NAFLD can be better clarified in the near future, a target for the treatment of NAFLD can be explored, and more patients can be cured.

AUTHOR CONTRIBUTIONS

HZ and XZ performed the design and conception. TX, YY, and YS contributed to the date data analysis and drafted. JX, CH, MZ, JD, and YX participated in data collection and animal feeding. RS, YW, DX-Z, and YD contributed to sample collection and cell culture. BL, ZS, YL, and YX contributed to the discussion.

REFERENCES

Barbaro, B., Romito, I., and Alisi, A. (2018). Commentary: The Histone Demethylase Phf2 Acts as a Molecular Checkpoint to Prevent NAFLD Progression during Obesity. *Front. Genet.* 9, 443. doi:10.3389/fgene.2018.00443

Baselli, G., and Valenti, L. (2019). Beyond Fat Accumulation, NAFLD Genetics Converges on Lipid Droplet Biology. *J. Lipid Res.* 60, 7–8. doi:10.1194/jlr.C091116

Bhalla, K., Hwang, B. J., Dewi, R. E., Twaddel, W., Goloubeva, O. G., Wong, K. K., et al. (2012). Metformin Prevents Liver Tumorigenesis by Inhibiting Pathways Driving Hepatic Lipogenesis. *Cancer Prev. Res. (Phila)* 5, 544–552. doi:10.1158/1940-6207.CAPR-11-0228

Borrelli, A., Bonelli, P., Tuccillo, F. M., Goldfine, I. D., Evans, J. L., Buonaguro, F. M., et al. (2018). Role of Gut Microbiota and Oxidative Stress in the Progression of Non-alcoholic Fatty Liver Disease to Hepatocarcinoma: Current and Innovative Therapeutic Approaches. *Redox Biol.* 15, 467–479. doi:10.1016/j.redox.2018.01.009

Buzzetti, E., Pinzani, M., and Tsochatzis, E. A. (2016). The Multiple-Hit Pathogenesis of Non-alcoholic Fatty Liver Disease (NAFLD). *Metabolism* 65, 1038–1048. doi:10.1016/j.metabol.2015.12.012

Cai, D., Li, Y., Zhang, K., Zhou, B., Guo, F., Holm, L., et al. (2021). Co-option of PPARα in the Regulation of Lipogenesis and Fatty Acid Oxidation in CLA-induced Hepatic Steatosis. *J. Cel Physiol* 236, 4387–4402. doi:10.1002/jcp.30157

Chen, Y., Chen, X., Ji, Y. R., Zhu, S., Bu, F. T., Du, X. S., et al. (2020). PLK1 Regulates Hepatic Stellate Cell Activation and Liver Fibrosis through Wnt/β-Catenin Signalling Pathway. *J. Cel Mol Med* 24, 7405–7416. doi:10.1111/jcmm.15356

Cobbina, E., and Akhlaghi, F. (2017). Non-alcoholic Fatty Liver Disease (NAFLD) - Pathogenesis, Classification, and Effect on Drug Metabolizing Enzymes and Transporters. *Drug Metab. Rev.* 49, 197–211. doi:10.1080/03602532.2017.1293683

Del Campo, J. A., Gallego-Durán, R., Gallego, P., and Grande, L. (2018). Genetic and Epigenetic Regulation in Nonalcoholic Fatty Liver Disease (NAFLD). *Int. J. Mol. Sci.* 19, 19. doi:10.3390/ijms19030911

Fan, R., Kim, Y. S., Wu, J., Chen, R., Zeuschner, D., Mildner, K., et al. (2020). Wnt/Beta-catenin/Esrrb Signalling Controls the Tissue-Scale Reorganization and Maintenance of the Pluripotent Lineage during Murine Embryonic Diapause. *Nat. Commun.* 11, 5499. doi:10.1038/s41467-020-19353-0

Geh, D., Anstee, Q. M., and Reeves, H. L. (2021). NAFLD-associated HCC: Progress and Opportunities. *J. Hepatocell Carcinoma* 8, 223–239. doi:10.2147/JHC.S272213

Heallen, T., Zhang, M., Wang, J., Bonilla-Claudio, M., Klysik, E., Johnson, R. L., et al. (2011). Hippo Pathway Inhibits Wnt Signaling to Restrain Cardiomyocyte Proliferation and Heart Size. *Science* 332, 458–461. doi:10.1126/science.1199010

Hu, S., Li, S. W., Yan, Q., Hu, X. P., Li, L. Y., Zhou, H., et al. (2019). Natural Products, Extracts and Formulations Comprehensive Therapy for the Improvement of Motor Function in Alcoholic Liver Disease. *Pharmacol. Res.* 150, 104501. doi:10.1016/j.phrs.2019.104501

Huang, D. Q., El-Serag, H. B., and Loomba, R. (2021). Global Epidemiology of NAFLD-Related HCC: Trends, Predictions, Risk Factors and Prevention. *Nat. Rev. Gastroenterol. Hepatol.* 18, 223–238. doi:10.1038/s41575-020-00381-6

Jing, C. Y., Fu, Y. P., Zhou, C., Zhang, M. X., Yi, Y., Huang, J. L., et al. (2021). Hepatic Stellate Cells Promote Intrahepatic Cholangiocarcinoma Progression via NR4A2/osteopontin/Wnt Signaling axis. *Oncogene* 40, 2910–2922. doi:10.1038/s41388-021-01705-9

Lee, I. H., Im, E., Lee, H. J., Sim, D. Y., Lee, J. H., Jung, J. H., et al. (2021). Apoptotic and Antihepatofibrotic Effect of Honokiol via Activation ofGSK3βand Suppression of Wnt/β-catenin Pathway in Hepatic Stellate Cells. *Phytotherapy Res.* 35, 452–462. doi:10.1002/ptr.6824

Li, J., Zou, B., Yeo, Y. H., Feng, Y., Xie, X., Lee, D. H., et al. (2019). Prevalence, Incidence, and Outcome of Non-alcoholic Fatty Liver Disease in Asia, 1999-2019: a Systematic Review and Meta-Analysis. *Lancet Gastroenterol. Hepatol.* 4, 389–398. doi:10.1016/S2468-1253(19)30039-1

Li, L. Y., Yang, C. C., Li, S. W., Liu, Y. M., Li, H. D., Hu, S., et al. (2020). TMEM88 Modulates the Secretion of Inflammatory Factors by Regulating YAP Signaling Pathway in Alcoholic Liver Disease. *Inflamm. Res.* 69, 789–800. doi:10.1007/s00011-020-01360-y

Ma, R., Feng, N., Yu, X., Lin, H., Zhang, X., Shi, O., et al. (2017). Promoter Methylation of Wnt/β-Catenin Signal Inhibitor TMEM88 Is Associated with Unfavorable Prognosis of Non-small Cell Lung Cancer. *Cancer Biol. Med. Nov* 14, 377–386. doi:10.20892/j.issn.2095-3941.2017.0061

Majidinia, M., Aghazadeh, J., Jahanban-Esfahlani, R., and Yousefi, B. (2018). The Roles of Wnt/β-Catenin Pathway in Tissue Development and Regenerative Medicine. *J. Cel Physiol* 233, 5598–5612. doi:10.1002/jcp.26265

Mashek, D. G. (2021). Hepatic Lipid Droplets: A Balancing Act between Energy Storage and Metabolic Dysfunction in NAFLD. *Mol. Metab.* 50, 101115. doi:10.1016/j.molmet.2020.101115

Maurice, J., and Manousou, P. (2018). Non-alcoholic Fatty Liver Disease. *Clin. Med. (Lond)* 18, 245–250. doi:10.7861/clinmedicine.18-3-245

Ray, K. (2021). Examining the Prevalence of NAFLD and NASH in a US Cohort. *Nat. Rev. Gastroenterol. Hepatol.* 18, 286. doi:10.1038/s41575-021-00446-0

Seo, M. H., Lee, J., Hong, S. W., Rhee, E. J., Park, S. E., Park, C. Y., et al. (2016). Exendin-4 Inhibits Hepatic Lipogenesis by Increasing β-Catenin Signaling. *PLoS One* 11, e0166913. doi:10.1371/journal.pone.0166913

Tian, Y., Mok, M. T., Yang, P., and Cheng, A. S. (2016). Epigenetic Activation of Wnt/β-Catenin Signaling in NAFLD-Associated Hepatocarcinogenesis. *Cancers (Basel)* 8, 8. doi:10.3390/cancers8080076

Xu, H., Wang, J., Chang, Y., Xu, J., Wang, Y., Long, T., et al. (2014). Fucoidan from the Sea Cucumber Acaudina Molpadioides Exhibits Anti-adipogenic Activity by Modulating the Wnt/β-Catenin Pathway and Down-Regulating the SREBP-1c Expression. *Food Funct.* 5 (5), 1547–1555. doi:10.1039/c3fo60716j

Xu, T., Pan, L. X., Ge, Y. X., Li, P., Meng, X. M., Huang, C., et al. (2018). TMEM88 Mediates Inflammatory Cytokines Secretion by Regulating JNK/P38 and Canonical Wnt/β-Catenin Signaling Pathway in LX-2 Cells. *Inflammopharmacology* 26, 1339–1348. doi:10.1007/s10787-017-0419-z

Younossi, Z. M., Koenig, A. B., Abdelatif, D., Fazel, Y., Henry, L., and Wymer, M. (2016). Global Epidemiology of Nonalcoholic Fatty Liver Disease-Meta-Analytic Assessment of Prevalence, Incidence, and Outcomes. *Hepatology* 64 (Jul), 73–84. doi:10.1002/hep.28431

Younossi, Z. M. (2019). Non-alcoholic Fatty Liver Disease - A Global Public Health Perspective. *J. Hepatol.* 70, 531–544. doi:10.1016/j.jhep.2018.10.033

Zhang, X., Wan, J. X., Ke, Z. P., Wang, F., Chai, H. X., and Liu, J. Q. (2017). TMEM88, CCL14 and CLEC3B as Prognostic Biomarkers for Prognosis and Palindromia of Human Hepatocellular Carcinoma. *Tumour Biol.* 39, 1010428317708900. doi:10.1177/1010428317708900

Zhou, F., Zhou, J., Wang, W., Zhang, X. J., Ji, Y. X., Zhang, P., et al. (2019). Unexpected Rapid Increase in the Burden of NAFLD in China from 2008 to 2018: A Systematic Review and Meta-Analysis. *Hepatology* 70, 1119–1133. doi:10.1002/hep.30702

13

Milk Fat Globule-EGF Factor 8 Alleviates Pancreatic Fibrosis by Inhibiting ER Stress-Induced Chaperone-Mediated Autophagy in Mice

Yifan Ren[1,2†], Qing Cui[3†], Jia Zhang[1,4], Wuming Liu[1,4], Meng Xu[2], Yi Lv[1,4], Zheng Wu[4], Yuanyuan Zhang[5]* and Rongqian Wu[1]*

[1]National Local Joint Engineering Research Center for Precision Surgery and Regenerative Medicine, Shaanxi Provincial Center for Regenerative Medicine and Surgical Engineering, First Affiliated Hospital of Xi'an Jiaotong University, Xi'an, China, [2]Department of General Surgery, The Second Affiliated Hospital of Xi'an Jiaotong University, Xi'an, China, [3]Department of Cardiology, Xi'an Central Hospital, Xi'an, China, [4]Department of Hepatobiliary Surgery, First Affiliated Hospital of Xi'an Jiaotong University, Xi'an, China, [5]Department of Department of Pediatrics, First Affiliated Hospital of Xi'an Jiaotong University, Xi'an, China

*Correspondence:
Rongqian Wu
rwu001@mail.xjtu.edu.cn
Yuanyuan Zhang
yuanyuanzhang@xjtu.edu.cn

[†]These authors have contributed equally to this work

Pancreatic fibrosis is an important pathophysiological feature of chronic pancreatitis (CP). Our recent study has shown that milk fat globule-EGF factor 8 (MFG-E8) is beneficial in acute pancreatitis. However, its role in CP remained unknown. To study this, CP was induced in male adult *Mfge8*-knockout (*Mfge8*-KO) mice and wild type (WT) mice by six intraperitoneal injections of cerulein (50 µg/kg/body weight) twice a week for 10 weeks. The results showed that knockout of *mfge8* gene aggravated pancreatic fibrosis after repeated cerulein injection. In WT mice, pancreatic levels of MFG-E8 were reduced after induction of CP and administration of recombinant MFG-E8 alleviated cerulein-induced pancreatic fibrosis. The protective effect of MFG-E8 in CP was associated with reduced autophagy and oxidative stress. In human pancreatic stellate cells (PSCs), MFG-E8 inhibited TGF-β1-induced ER stress and autophagy. MFG-E8 downregulated the expression of lysosomal associated membrane protein 2A (LAMP2A), a key factor in ER stress-induced chaperone-mediated autophagy (CMA). QX77, an activator of CMA, eliminated the effects of MFG-E8 on TGF-β1-induced PSC activation. In conclusion, MFG-E8 appears to mitigate pancreatic fibrosis *via* inhibiting ER stress-induced chaperone-mediated autophagy. Recombinant MFG-E8 may be developed as a novel treatment for pancreatic fibrosis in CP.

Keywords: chronic pancreatitis, MFG-E8, fibrosis, pancreatic stellate cell, chaperone-mediated autophagy, LAMP2A

INTRODUCTION

Pancreatic fibrosis is an important pathophysiological feature of chronic pancreatitis (CP). Its management remains a serious clinical challenge (Kleeff et al., 2017; Gardner et al., 2020). Activation of the pancreatic stellate cell (PSC) is a key step in the development of pancreatic fibrosis (Ren et al., 2020). In normal pancreas, PSCs surround acinar cells in a resting state. When the pancreas is challenged by inflammation or mechanical stimulation, PSCs' phenotype changes from a resting to

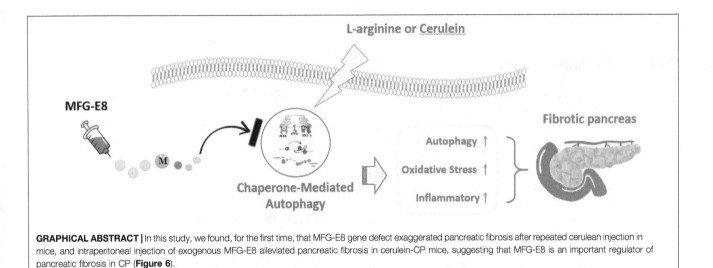

GRAPHICAL ABSTRACT | In this study, we found, for the first time, that MFG-E8 gene defect exaggerated pancreatic fibrosis after repeated cerulean injection in mice, and intraperitoneal injection of exogenous MFG-E8 alleviated pancreatic fibrosis in cerulein-CP mice, suggesting that MFG-E8 is an important regulator of pancreatic fibrosis in CP (**Figure 6**).

an active state (Bynigeri et al., 2017). The production of α-SMA is a hallmark of PSC activation, and is accompanied by the production of large amounts of collagen I and III (Xue et al., 2018), which together form the pathological process of pancreatic fibrosis in CP. However, the molecular mechanism of PSC activation during the development of CP is still obscure.

Autophagy is involved in the activation of PSCs (Endo et al., 2017; Ren et al., 2020). Suppressing autophagy has been shown to inhibit the activation of PSCs and reduce the development of pancreatic fibrosis (Xue et al., 2019). Chaperone-mediated autophagy (CMA) is a process in which lysosomal degradation occurs when cytoplasmic proteins with special modules are recognized by molecular chaperones and bind to lysosomal-associated membrane protein 2A (LAMP2A) (Kaushik and Cuervo, 2018). LAMP2A, a special receptor on the lysosomal membrane, is believed to be a key regulator of CMA (Pajares et al., 2018). Endoplasmic reticulum (ER) stress is an important trigger of CMA (Li et al., 2017). Our previous study has shown that activation of PSCs is associated with oxidative and ER stress (Ren et al., 2020). However, the specific role of CMA in pancreatic fibrosis during CP remains largely unknown.

Milk fat globule epidermal growth factor (EGF) factor 8 (MFG-E8), also known as lactadherin, is a lipophilic glycoprotein. It is expressed and secreted by a variety of cells and tissues including the pancreas (D'Haese et al., 2013). MFG-E8 contains an RGD motif and can interact with integrins (Franchi et al., 2011; Aziz et al., 2015). Through binding to integrin receptors, MFG-E8 exhibits versatile functions and is involved in a variety of cellular processes, such as maintenance and repair of intestinal epithelial cells, angiogenesis, and clearance of apoptotic cells (Kranich et al., 2010; Deng et al., 2017; Gao et al., 2018). Previous studies have indicated that MFG-E8 inhibited the activation of fibroblasts induced by TGF-β1, and recombinant MFG-E8 alleviated the development of fibrosis in the skin, heart, kidney and liver in mice (An et al., 2017; Fujiwara et al., 2019; Shi et al., 2020; Wang et al., 2020). Our recent study has shown that MFG-E8 restores mitochondrial function in acute

pancreatitis (Ren et al., 2021). However, whether MFG-E8 plays any role in the development of pancreatic fibrosis has not been studied. The main purpose of the current study is to investigate the role of MFG-E8 in ER stress, CMA, PSC activation and pancreatic fibrosis in CP.

MATERIALS AND METHODS

Experimental Animal

C57BL/6J adult mice were purchased from Animal Experimental Center of Xi'an Jiaotong University Health Science Center, and *Mfge8*-knockout (*Mfge8*-KO) mice were purchased from Nanfang Biotech Technology Co., Ltd (Shanghai, China). *Mfge8*-KO mice were obtained by knocking out 2–6 exons of *mfge8* gene using CRISPR/Cas9 gene editing technology. All experimental animals are housed in a temperature-controlled room on a 12-h light/dark cycle with *ad libitum* access to food and water. The mice were fasted for 12 h before collecting samples. The study protocol was approved by the Institutional Animal Care and Use Committee of the Ethics Committee of Xi'an Jiaotong University Health Science Center.

Mouse Model of Chronic Pancreatitis and Administration of MFG-E8

Chronic pancreatitis was induced in male adult mice by six intraperitoneal injections of cerulein (50 μg/kg/body weight, C6660, Solarbio, Beijing, China) twice a week for 10 weeks, as described by Sendler M. et al. (Sendler et al., 2015) and used by us recently (Ren et al., 2020). During the last 5 weeks, 1 hour after cerulein injection, normal saline (vehicle) or 20 μg/kg recombinant murine MFG-E8 (RD System, Inc. Minnesota, United States) was administered through intraperitoneal injection. The animals were sacrificed 2 days after the last injection of cerulein. The doses of MFG-E8 used in this study were chosen on the basis of our previous publications in acute pancreatitis (Ren et al., 2021). Blood and tissue samples were collected.

Cell Culture and Treatment

Human pancreatic stellate cells (PSCs) were purchased from FengHui Biotechnology (FHHUM-CELL-0124, China) and cultured in Ham's F-12K medium (PM150910C, Procell, Wuhan, China) with 20% fetal bovine serum (164210-100, Procell, Wuhan, China) in a humidified incubator at 37°C with 5% CO_2. HPSCs (1×10^6/well) were planted into 6-well plates for 24 h. The cells appeared to be in quiescent state. Then, the cells were treated with 5 ng/mL TGF-β1 (5154LC, Cell Signaling Technology, United States) with 10 ng/ml or 20 ng/mL recombinant human MFG-E8 or equal volume of PBS for 24 h. In additional groups of cells, QX77 (5 ng/ml, S6797, SELLEK, United States), a LAMP2A-specific activator (Zhang et al., 2017), was added simultaneously with 20 ng/mL MFG-E8 in TGF-β1-treated HPSCs. 24 h later, the cells were collected for various measurements.

Histologic Evaluation

Pancreatic tissue sections were stained with H&E. The pathological staining scoring system introduced by Schmidt et al. (Schmidt et al., 1992) was used to evaluate the pancreatic tissue damage.

Immunohistochemical Staining

Immunohistochemical staining was performed as we described before (Bi et al., 2020). Paraffin sections of mouse pancreatic tissue were prepared, and Sirius red and Masson-Goldner staining were used to indicate the degree of tissue fibrosis. α-smooth muscle actin (α-SMA) staining (A5228, mouse monoclonal clone, Sigma-Aldrich, United States) and Collagen I (ab34710, rabbit polyclonal, Abcam, United States) staining were used to mark the deposition of extracellular matrix. MPO (ab45977, rabbit polyclonal, Abcam, United States) was used to mark the infiltration of neutrophils. Gr1 (LY6G) (ab25377, antibody, Abcam, United States), CD11b (ab216445, rabbit polyclonal, Abcam, United States) and F4/80 (ab240946, rabbit polyclonal, Abcam, United States) were used to demonstrate macrophage infiltration, LC3B (ab48394, rabbit polyclonal, Abcam, United States) were used to demonstrate autophagy levels. The immunohistochemical staining was photographed with a light microscope. Three fields were randomly selected for each image, and the images were quantitatively and statistically analyzed with ImageJ Pro Plus 6.0 software.

Immunofluorescence Staining

The expression of Collagen I, α-SMA and DHE were assessed by immunofluorescence staining as described by us previous (Ren et al., 2020). Quantitative determination of fluorescence intensity was perfumed by Image Pro Plus 6.0 software.

Enzyme-Linked Immunosorbent Assay

The mouse IL-6 ELISA kit (SEA079Mu, Cloud-Clone Corp USCN Life Science, Wuhan, CN), tumor necrosis factor-α (TNF-α) ELISA kit (SEA133Mu, Cloud-Clone Corp USCN Life Science, Wuhan, CN), IL-10 ELISA kit (SEA056Mu, Cloud-Clone Corp USCN Life Science, Wuhan, CN) and MFG-E8 ELISA kit (SEB286Mu, Cloud-Clone Corp USCN Life Science, Wuhan, CN) were used for the detection of IL-6, TNF-α, IL-10 and MFG-E8 according to the manufacturer's instructions.

Detection of SOD, FRAP GSH and MDA Levels

Pancreatic tissue and HPSCs homogenate was obtained and superoxide dismutase (SOD), total antioxidant capacity assay kit with FRAP method (FRAP value), glutathione (GSH) and malonaldehyde (MDA) were measured as we described before (Ren et al., 2019a; Ren et al., 2019b; Ren et al., 2020).

Western Blot Analysis

Pancreatic tissues were lysed in cold RIPA (P0013B, Beyotime, Beijing, China). The protein concentration was evaluated with the BCA Protein Assay Kit (P0012S, Beyotime, Beijing, China). After gel electrophoresis, the protein was transferred to PVDF membrane and incubation in blocking solution (3% BSA or 5% skimmed milk) at room temperature. Then the membranes were incubated overnight at 4°C with the primary antibodies (**Supplementary Table S1**). Primary antibodies were diluted in Primary Antibody Dilution Buffer for Western Blot (P0256, Beyotime, Beijing, China). Membranes were washed and then incubated with specific HRP-conjugated secondary antibodies (**Supplementary Table S1**) for 1.5 h at room temperature. Bands were developed using Digital gel image analysis system (Bio-Rad, California, United States) and quantitative of protein level were calculated by ImageJ2x software. Information about the antibodies used in this study are listed in **Supplementary Table S1**.

Statistical Analysis

All measurement data are expressed as the mean ± standard error (SEM). The t-test or one-way ANOVA with the Tukey-Kramer test was used to analyze the differences between groups. All analyses were conducted with data statistics software GraphPad Prism version 8.0 (GraphPad Software, Inc., San Diego, CA, United States). $p < 0.05$ represented a significant difference.

RESULTS

MFG-E8 Deficiency Exaggerates Repeated Cerulein Injection-Induced CP *in Vivo*

To evaluate the pathophysiological role of MFG-E8 in CP, we induced CP in *Mfge8*-KO mice (The efficacy of MFG-E8 knockout was confirmed by Western blotting, **Supplementary Figure S1**) by repeated intraperitoneal injection of cerulein. H&E staining showed that MFG-E8 deficiency did not result in any significant changes in pancreatic histomorphology in sham mice (**Figure 1A**). However, repeated cerulein injection caused much more severe pancreatic damage in *Mfge8*-KO mice than their WT littermates (**Figures 1A,B**). *Mfge8*-KO mice also had larger area of necrosis than WT mice after repeated cerulein injection (**Figures 1A,C**). Masson and Sirius red staining showed more severe fibrosis in the pancreatic tissue of *Mfge8*-KO mice than that of WT mice (**Figures 1A,D**). Consistently, α-SMA and

Milk Fat Globule-EGF Factor 8 Alleviates Pancreatic Fibrosis by Inhibiting ER Stress-Induced...

151

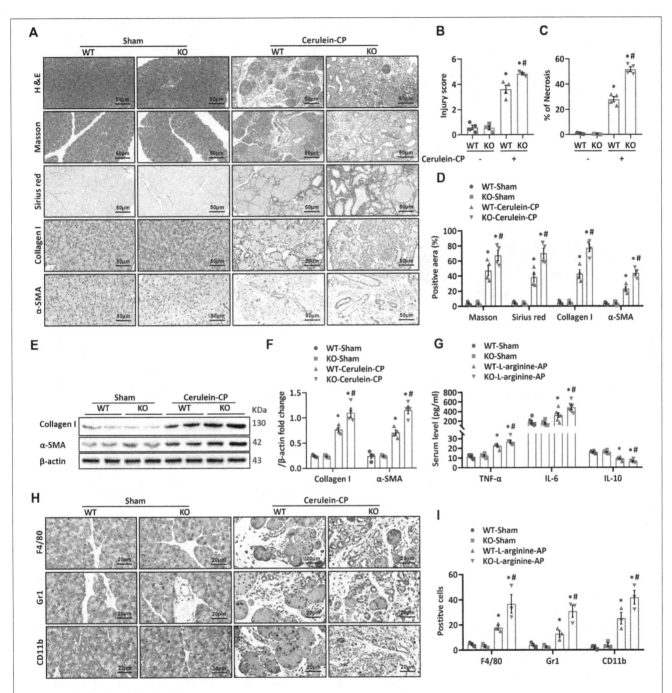

FIGURE 1 | MFG-E8 Deficiency Potentiates Cerulein-Induced CP *in Vivo*. Cerulein-CP was induced by six IP injections of cerulein (50 µg/kg/body weight) twice a week for 10 weeks. During the last 5 weeks, 1 h after cerulein injection, normal saline (vehicle) or 20 µg/kg MFG-E8 was administered through intraperitoneal injection. The control group received the same frequency and time of intraperitoneal injection of normal saline (Sham). The animals were sacrificed at 2 days after the last injection of cerulein or normal saline. Blood and tissue samples were collected. **(A)** Representative photos of H&E, Sirius red, Masson, Collagen I and α-SMA staining; **(B)** Quantitative analysis of H&E staining (one-way ANOVA with the Tukey-Kramer test); **(C)** Percentages of necrotic areas (one-way ANOVA with the Tukey-Kramer test); **(D)** Quantitative analysis of Sirius red Masson, Collagen I and α-SMA staining (one-way ANOVA with the Tukey-Kramer test); **(E,F)** Western blot analysis of the expression of α-SMA and collagen I in the pancreas (one-way ANOVA with the Tukey-Kramer test); **(G)** Serum levels of IL-6, IL-10 and TNF-α (one-way ANOVA with the Tukey-Kramer test); **(H,I)** Representative photos and quantitative analysis of F4/80, Gr1 and CD11b staining (one-way ANOVA with the Tukey-Kramer test). $n = 4$–6, mean ± SEM; $*p < 0.05$ versus Sham group; $\#p < 0.05$ versus Vehicle group. CP, chronic pancreatitis; H&E, hematoxylin and eosin; α-SMA, alpha-smooth muscle actin; WT, wild type; KO, knock out.

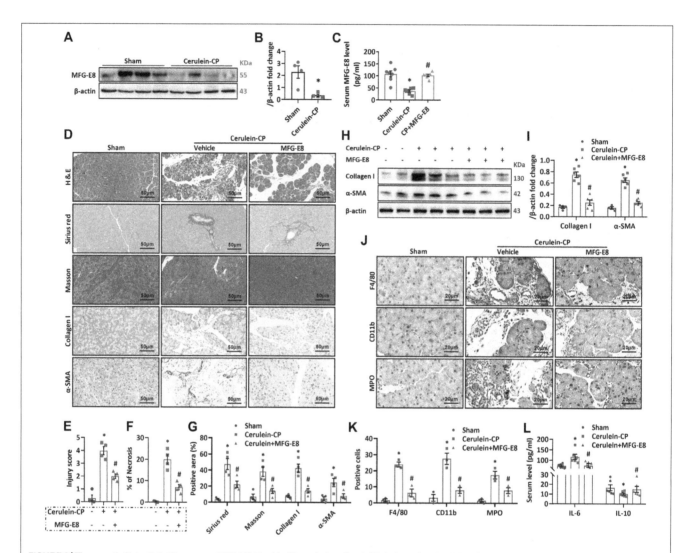

FIGURE 2 | Therapeutic Potential of Exogenous MFG-E8. Cerulein-CP was induced by six IP injections of cerulein (50 µg/kg/body weight) twice a week for 10 weeks. During the last 5 weeks, 1 h after cerulein injection, normal saline (vehicle) or 20 µg/kg MFG-E8 was administered through intraperitoneal injection. The control group received the same frequency and time of intraperitoneal injection of normal saline (Sham). The animals were sacrificed at 2 days after the last injection of cerulein or normal saline. Blood and tissue samples were collected. **(A,B)** Western blot analysis of the expression of MFG-E8 in the pancreas (t-test); **(C)** Serum MFG-E8 levels (one-way ANOVA with the Tukey-Kramer test); **(D)** Representative photos of H&E, Sirius red, Masson, Collagen I and α-SMA staining; **(E)** Quantitative analysis of H&E staining (one-way ANOVA with the Tukey-Kramer test); **(F)** Percentages of necrotic areas (one-way ANOVA with the Tukey-Kramer test); **(G)** Quantitative analysis of Sirius red Masson, Collagen I and α-SMA staining (one-way ANOVA with the Tukey-Kramer test); **(H,I)** Western blot analysis of the expression of α-SMA and collagen I in the pancreas (one-way ANOVA with the Tukey-Kramer test); **(J)** Representative photos of F4/80, MPO and CD11b staining; **(K)** Quantitative analysis of F4/80, MPO and CD11b staining (one-way ANOVA with the Tukey-Kramer test); **(L)** Serum levels of IL-6 and IL-10 (one-way ANOVA with the Tukey-Kramer test). n = 4–6, mean ± SEM; * p < 0.05 versus Sham group; #p < 0.05 versus Vehicle group. CP, chronic pancreatitis; MFG-E8, Milk Fat Globule-EGF Factor 8; H&E, hematoxylin and eosin; MPO, myeloperoxidase; α-SMA, alpha-smooth muscle actin.

Collagen I staining showed that repeated cerulein injection caused extracellular matrix deposition in the interstitial space of *Mfge8*-KO mice than that of WT mice (**Figures 1A,D**). These findings were confirmed by western blot analysis of α-SMA and Collagen I protein expression in the pancreatic tissues (**Figures 1E,F**). MFG-E8 Deficiency also potentiated inflammatory responses in CP. As shown in **Figure 1G**, serum proinflammatory cytokines TNF-α and IL-6 were further increased, while anti-inflammatory cytokine IL-10 was further decreased in *Mfge8*-KO mice than WT mice after repeated cerulein injection. Inflammatory cell infiltration in the pancreas was measured by F4/80, CD11b, and Gr1 staining.

As shown in **Figures 1H,I**, repeated cerulein injection also resulted in more inflammatory cell infiltration in the pancreas of *Mfge8*-KO mice than that of WT mice.

MFG-E8 Levels Are Decreased in the Pancreas of CP Mice and Exogenous MFG-E8 Treatment Is Beneficial in Experimental CP

To further investigate the role of MFG-E8 in CP, we measured MFG-E8 protein expression in the pancreas after repeated cerulein injection by western blot analysis. As shown in

Milk Fat Globule-EGF Factor 8 Alleviates Pancreatic Fibrosis by Inhibiting ER Stress-Induced...

153

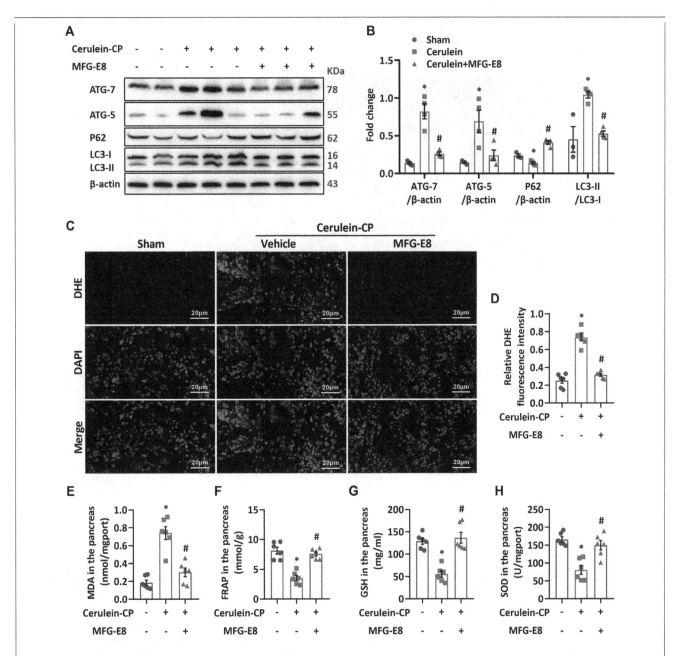

FIGURE 3 | Exogenous MFG-E8 Alleviates Autophagy and Oxidative Stress in Cerulein-CP. Cerulein-CP was induced by six IP injections of cerulein (50 μg/kg/body weight) twice a week for 10 weeks. During the last 5 weeks, 1 h after cerulein injection, normal saline (vehicle) or 20 μg/kg MFG-E8 was administered through intraperitoneal injection. The control group received the same frequency and time of intraperitoneal injection of normal saline (Sham). The animals were sacrificed at 2 days after the last injection of cerulein or normal saline. Blood and tissue samples were collected. **(A,B)** Western blot analysis of the expression of ATG7, ATG5, P62 and LC3B in the pancreas (one-way ANOVA with the Tukey-Kramer test); **(C,D)** Representative images and quantitative analysis of immunofluorescence staining of DHE in the pancreas (one-way ANOVA with the Tukey-Kramer test); **(E)** FRAP level in the pancreas (one-way ANOVA with the Tukey-Kramer test); **(F)** GSH level in the pancreas (one-way ANOVA with the Tukey-Kramer test); **(G)** MDA level in the pancreas (one-way ANOVA with the Tukey-Kramer test); **(H)** SOD level in the pancreas (one-way ANOVA with the Tukey-Kramer test). $n = 3$–6, mean ± SEM; * $p < 0.05$ versus Sham group; # $p < 0.05$ versus Vehicle group. CP, chronic pancreatitis; MFG-E8, Milk Fat Globule-EGF Factor 8; MDA, malondialdehyde; SOD, superoxide dismutase; FRAP, Ferric ion reducing antioxidant power; DHE, Dihydroethidium; GSH, glutathione.

Figures 2A,B, repeated intraperitoneal injection of cerulein significantly decreased MFG-E8 protein levels in the pancreas of WT mice. Because MFG-E8 is a secreted protein, we also measured the serum MFG-E8 levels in mice. As shown in

Figure 2C, serum MFG-E8 levels in cerulein-treated mice were significantly lower than those in the control group, while repeated intraperitoneal injection of exogenous MFG-E8 effectively maintained serum MFG-E8 levels ($p < 0.05$).

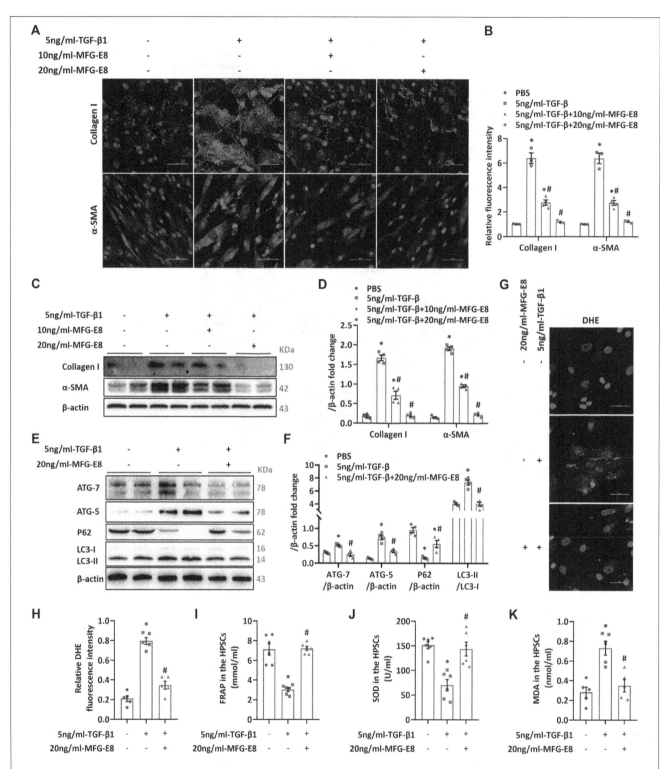

FIGURE 4 | Exogenous MFG-E8 Blocks TGF-β1–induced activation of HPSCs. Human pancreatic stellate cells (1×10⁶/well) were treated with 5 ng/ml TGF-β1 with or without 10 ng/ml or 20 ng/ml MFG-E8 for 24 h, the same volume of PBS was added to another group of HPSCs as a control group. **(A,B)** Representative images and quantitative analysis of immunofluorescence staining of α-SMA and collagen I in the HPSCs (one-way ANOVA with the Tukey-Kramer test); **(C,D)** Western blot analysis of the expression of α-SMA and collagen I in the HPSCs (one-way ANOVA with the Tukey-Kramer test); **(E,F)** Western blot analysis of the expression of ATG7, ATG5, P62 and LC3B in the HPSCs (one-way ANOVA with the Tukey-Kramer test); **(G,H)** Representative images and quantitative analysis of immunofluorescence staining of DHE in the HPSCs (one-way ANOVA with the Tukey-Kramer test); **(I)** FRAP level in the HPSCs (one-way ANOVA with the Tukey-Kramer test); **(J)** SOD level in the HPSCs (one-way ANOVA with the Tukey-Kramer test); **(K)** MDA level in the HPSCs (one-way ANOVA with the Tukey-Kramer test). $n = 3$–6, mean ± SEM; ∗ $p < 0.05$ versus Sham group; #$p < 0.05$ versus Vehicle group. α-SMA, alpha-smooth muscle actin; TGF-β1, transforming growth factor-β1; HPSCs, human pancreatic stellate cells; MDA, malondialdehyde; SOD, superoxide dismutase; MFG-E8, Milk Fat Globule-EGF Factor 8; FRAP, Ferric ion reducing antioxidant power; DHE, Dihydroethidium.

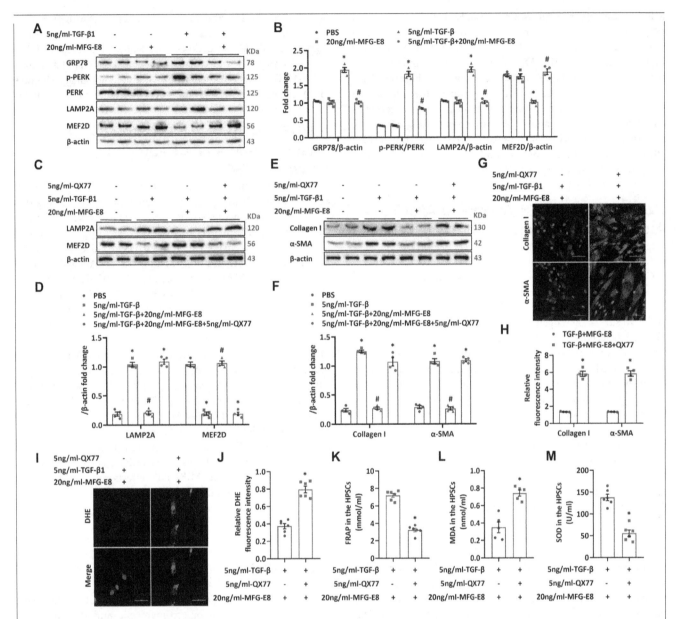

FIGURE 5 | ER Stress Induced CMA Mediate the Activation of HPSCs. Human pancreatic stellate cells (1×10⁶/well) were treated with 5 ng/ml TGF-β1 with or without 20 ng/ml MFG-E8 for 24 h, the same volume of PBS was added to another group of HPSCs as a control group. To determine the role of ER stress-mediated CMA activation in exogenous MFG-E8's effect in HPSCs, QX77, a LAMP2A-specific activator, was added simultaneously with 20 ng/mL-MFG-E8 in TGF-β1-treated HPSCs. **(A,B)** Western blot analysis of the expression of GRP78, p-PERK, PERK, LAMP2A and MEF2D in the HPSCs (one-way ANOVA with the Tukey-Kramer test); **(C,D)** Western blot analysis of the expression of LAMP2A and MEF2D in the HPSCs (one-way ANOVA with the Tukey-Kramer test); **(E,F)** Western blot analysis of the expression of α-SMA and Collagen I in the HPSCs (one-way ANOVA with the Tukey-Kramer test); **(G,H)** Representative images and quantitative analysis of immunofluorescence staining of α-SMA and collagen I in the HPSCs (t-test); **(I,J)** Representative images and quantitative analysis of immunofluorescence staining of DHE in the HPSCs (t-test); **(K)** FRAP level in the HPSCs (t-test); **(L)** MDA level in the HPSCs (t-test); **(M)** SOD level in the HPSCs (t-test). n = 4–6, mean ± SEM; *p < 0.05 versus Sham group; #p < 0.05 versus Vehicle group. α-SMA, alpha-smooth muscle actin; TGF-β1, transforming growth factor-β1; HPSCs, human pancreatic stellate cells, MFG-E8, Milk Fat Globule-EGF Factor 8; DHE, Dihydroethidium; LAMP2A, Lysosomal associated membrane proteins 2a; MDA, malondialdehyde; SOD, superoxide dismutase; FRAP, Ferric ion reducing antioxidant power.

Administration of recombinant MFG-E8 significantly reduced pancreatic injury (**Figures 2D,E**) and necrosis (**Figure 2F**) in cerulein-CP mice. Pancreatic fibrosis was evaluated by Sirius red, Masson, α-SMA and Collagen I staining. As shown in **Figures 2D,G**, exogenous MFG-E8 treatment reduced the positive staining of the above fibrosis-related indicators in the pancreatic tissue of cerulein-CP mice by 55.2, 59.5, 68.7, and 54.6%, respectively (p < 0.05). Western blot analysis also confirmed that α-SMA and Collagen I protein expression in pancreatic tissue of cerulein-CP mice was downregulated by

MFG-E8 treatment (**Figures 2H,I**). Similar beneficial effects of exogenous MFG-E8 treatment was observed in repeated L-arginine injection-induced CP in mice (**Supplementary Figures 2A–F**). MFG-E8 also inhibited inflammatory responses in cerulein-CP mice. As shown in **Figures 2J,K**, administration of exogenous MFG-E8 reduced the numbers of F4/80, CD11b and MPO positive cells in the pancreas of cerulein-CP mice by 82.6, 72.5 and 47.9%, respectively ($p < 0.05$). The abnormal serum levels of inflammatory mediators (IL-6 and IL-10) in cerulein-CP mice were restored to almost sham levels by exogenous MFG-E8 treatment (**Figure 2L**).

Exogenous MFG-E8 Treatment Alleviates Autophagy and Oxidative Stress in CP Mice

Impaired autophagy and oxidative stress activate PSCs and promote their release of large amounts of extracellular matrix (ECM), which, along with collagen deposition, initiates and accelerates the progression of pancreatic fibrosis (Bhardwaj and Yadav, 2013; Ryu et al., 2013; Diakopoulos et al., 2015; Li et al., 2018a). To investigate the mechanism responsible for MFG-E8's beneficial effects in CP, we measured indicators of autophagy and oxidative stress. We have confirmed that deleting the exons 4 to 6 of the MFG-E8 gene (*mfge8*-knockout) has no significant effect on the antioxidant capacity (Ren et al., 2021) and autophagy (**Supplementary Figure S3**) in the mouse pancreatic tissue. In this study, we further explored the effects of exogenous MFG-E8 on the levels of oxidative stress and autophagy in the pancreas of cerulein-treated CP mice. As shown in **Figures 3A,B**, pancreatic levels of ATG7, ATG5 and LC3 II/LC3 I increased, while P62 decreased significantly after repeated cerulein injection, indicating activated autophagy process in CP. Exogenous MFG-E8 treatment reversed these changes in cerulein-CP mice, suggesting MFG-E8 suppresses autophagy in CP. The enhancement of autophagy could induce the disorder of oxygen free radical regulation, resulting in oxidative stress (Li et al., 2021). Our results also indicated that repeated cerulein injection induced oxidative stress in the pancreas. As shown in **Figures 3C,D**, DHE staining in the pancreas increased dramatically after repeated cerulein injection. Consistently, pancreatic tissues levels of MDA (**Figure 3E**) were also significantly elevated in cerulein-CP. In the meantime, anti-oxidative indicators including FRAP (**Figure 3F**), GSH (**Figure 3G**) and SOD (**Figure 3H**) decreased after repeated cerulein injection. Exogenous MFG-E8 treatment decreased DHE, MDA, and increased FRAP, GSH, and SOD in the pancreas of cerulein-CP mice, suggesting MFG-E8 reduces oxidative stress in CP.

MFG-E8 Blocks TGF-β1-Induced PSC Activation, Autophagy and Oxidative Stress *in Vitro*

PSCs activation plays a fundamental role in the development of pancreatic fibrosis. Activated PSCs have upregulated α-SMA expression and release a large amount of extracellular matrix proteins such as collagen I. To determine the effects of MFG-E8

on PSCs activation *in vitro*, we treated human PSCs with TGF-β1 in the presence of various concentrations of MFG-E8. As shown in **Figures 4A–D**, MFG-E8 dose-dependently suppressed TGF-β1-induced collagen I and α-SMA production in cultured human PSCs. MFG-E8 also blocked TGF-β1-induced autophagy (**Figures 4E,F**) and oxidative stress (**Figures 4G–K**) in cultured human PSCs.

MFG-E8 Suppresses ER Stress and Chaperone-Mediated Autophagy in Activated PSCs

TGF-β1 treatment increased ER stress-related protein GRP78 expression and PERK phosphorylation in human PSCs (**Figures 5A,B**), suggesting activated ER stress. MFG-E8 decreased TGF-β1-induced GRP78 expression and PERK phosphorylation in human PSCs. ER stress can lead to CMA (Li et al., 2018b). LAMP2A is the rate-limiting receptor for CMA substrate flux. And increased CMA activity leads to MEF2D degradation (Li et al., 2017). As shown in **Figures 5A,B**, TGF-β1 also increased LAMP2A expression and decreased MEF2D expression in human PSCs, suggesting increased CMA activity. MFG-E8 decreased TGF-β1-induced LAMP2A express, while increased MEF2D expression in the meantime. Exogenous MFG-E8 also reduced ER stress and CMA in cerulein-treated CP mice ($p < 0.05$, **Supplementary Figures S4A,B**). QX77 is a specific CMA activator. It can upregulate LAMP2A expression (Zhang et al., 2017). As shown in **Figures 5C,D**, QX77 reversed MFG-E8's effects on LAMP2A and MEF2D expression. To explore the role of CMA in MFG-E8's effects on PSC activation, the expression of collagen I and α-SMA was measured. As shown in **Figures 5E–H**, QX77 eliminated MFG-E8's effects on collagen I and α-SMA expression. Similarly, the suppressive effect of MFG-E8 on oxidative stress in activated PSCs was also mitigated by the addition of QX77 (**Figures 5I–M**).

DISCUSSION

Pancreatic fibrosis, a characteristic feature of CP, is the result of abnormal activation of stromal cells and deposition of extracellular matrix (ECM) proteins. The development of fibrosis leads to the gradual loss of exocrine and endocrine functions of the pancreas. Currently, there is no specific treatment for pancreatic fibrosis. Clinical management of CP patients mainly relies on supportive therapies to alleviate pain and prevent complications. As such, identifying key factors in pancreatic fibrosis would greatly contribute to the development of effective treatment for CP. In this study, we found, for the first time, that MFG-E8 gene defect exaggerated pancreatic fibrosis after repeated cerulein injection in mice, and intraperitoneal injection of exogenous MFG-E8 alleviated pancreatic fibrosis in cerulein-CP mice, suggesting that MFG-E8 is an important regulator of pancreatic fibrosis in CP.

MFG-E8 was first identified in the lactation mammary gland (Hanayama and Nagata, 2005). Subsequent studies have demonstrated that MFG-E8 promotes the removal of apoptotic cells and inhibits inflammatory responses (Miksa et al., 2008; Kranich et al., 2010; Wu et al., 2010; Cheyuo et al., 2012; Shah et al., 2012). MFG-E8 deficiency has been linked to the development of autoimmune diseases such as rheumatoid arthritis and inflammatory bowel disease (Nagata, 2007; Albus et al., 2016; He et al., 2016). Our recent study has shown that MFG-E8 restores mitochondrial function *via* integrin-medicated activation of the FAK-STAT3 signaling pathway in acute pancreatitis (Ren et al., 2021). It is well known that repeated episodes of acute pancreatitis lead to the development of CP. To extend our investigation of MFG-E8 in pancreatitis, we evaluated the role of MFG-E8 in pancreatic fibrosis in the current study. The results suggest that MFG-E8 has an anti-fibrotic property in the pancreas. This is consistent with the reported function of MFG-E8 in hepatic fibrosis, renal fibrosis and skin fibrosis (Fujiwara et al., 2019; Shi et al., 2020; Wang et al., 2020). Thus, MFG-E8 may be a promising option for the treatment of pancreatic fibrosis.

Activation of PSCs plays a critical role in the development of pancreatic fibrosis in CP (Ramakrishnan et al., 2020). Activated stellate cells cause the deposition of extracellular matrix by releasing a series of collagen fibers including α-SMA, collagen I and III. Pathological changes were manifested as the loss of a large number of functional cells such as pancreatic acinus cells and pancreatic-beta cells, and replaced by a large number of proliferation of non-functional extracellular matrix (Masamune et al., 2009). Autophagy is necessary for the activation of PSCs (Endo et al., 2017). The increase of intracellular oxygen free radicals induced by autophagy aggravates oxidative stress and further stimulates the release of α-SMA by activated PSCs (Xue et al., 2019). Using two different mouse models of CP, we showed that intraperitoneal injection of exogenous MFG-E8 inhibited pancreatic fibrosis and inflammatory responses. Moreover, in our *in vitro* study, we found that exogenous MFG-E8 alleviated TGF-β1-induced activation of human PSCs, which is associated with reduced autophagy and oxidative stress, indicating that MFG-E8 might inhibit the activation of PSCs by suppressing autophagy.

Our previous study has found that TGF-β1-induced activation of HPSCs results in ER stress and aggravates cellular oxidative stress (Ren et al., 2020). ER stress leads to the activation of chaperone-mediated autophagy (CMA) (Abokyi et al., 2020). CMA is a unique form of autophagy, which was only found in mammalian cells. It requires the participation of lysosomal-associated membrane protein 2A (LAMP2A), which facilitates the translocation of cytosolic proteins containing a KFERQ-like peptide motif across the lysosomal membrane and subsequent MEF2D degradation (Pajares et al., 2018; Wang et al., 2018). As a rate-limiting molecule of CMA, the abnormal expression or function of LAMP2A is of great pathophysiological significance. In the current study, we found that TGF-β1 treatment led to the elevated expression of LAMP2A and the reduced level of MEF2D. MFG-E8, on the other hand, decreased LAMP2A expression and increased MEF2D expression in TGF-β1-treat human PSCs, suggesting MFG-E8 can suppress the CMA pathway. QX77, a specific CMA activator, not only

reversed MFG-E8's effects on LAMP2A and MEF2D expression, but also eliminated MFG-E8's effects on collagen I and α-SMA expression. These results, taken together, indicated that MFG-E8 mitigates pancreatic fibrosis by inhibiting the ER stress-induced CMA pathway. However, it is also possible that MFG-E8 directly inhibits ER stress. A recent study by Song M et al. has shown that activation of p-STAT3 alleviates ER-stress in splenocytes during chronic stress (Song et al., 2020). Our previous study has suggested that MFG-E8 can activate p-STAT3 (Ren et al., 2021). In this regard, the direct effect of MFG-E8 on ER-stress in pancreatitis warrants further investigation.

The impact of MFG-E8 in CP, however, remains controversial. D'Haese JG et al. found that compared with normal pancreatic tissue samples obtained from healthy organ donors, pancreatic tissues collected from chronic pancreatitis patients had significantly higher levels of MFG-E8 (D'Haese et al., 2013). How the normal pancreatic tissue samples were obtained and preserved, however, were not described in the paper. Pancreatic tissues obtained from organ donors might undergo ischemia reperfusion injury, machine perfusion and static cold storage. All these factors could alter the expression of MFG-E8. More importantly, the authors did not provide any direct evidence showing MFG-E8 plays a pathogenic role in chronic pancreatitis. In the current study, we found that administration of recombinant MFG-E8 alleviated pancreatic fibrosis in mouse models of CP and MFG-E8 inhibited TGF-β1-induced ER stress and chaperone-mediated autophagy in cultured human PSCs. In addition, knockout of *mfge8* gene exaggerated pancreatic fibrosis after repeated cerulein injection in mice. These results were consistent with several other studies, which also showed that MFG-E8 has anti-fibrotic effects (Brissette et al., 2016; Fujiwara et al., 2019; Shi et al., 2020; Kim et al., 2021).

There are some limitations of the study. First of all, due to the lack of clinical samples, we were unable to verify our findings in CP patients. The clinical significance of this study warrants further investigation. And alcohol consumption is the most common cause of CP in Western societies (Singh et al., 2019). Although we evaluated the anti-fibrotic effect of MFG-E8 in two different CP models, whether it has any effect on alcohol-induced CP remains unknown. The major biological effects of MFG-E8 are mediated through binding to αvβ3/5 integrins. Our previous study has shown that administration of cilengitide, a specific αvβ3/5 integrin inhibitor, abolished MFG-E8's beneficial effects in acute pancreatitis (Ren et al., 2021). Whether the recombinant MFG-E8 has any off-target effects in CP, however, remains to be determined. Furthermore, this study showed that MFG-E8 downregulated LAMP2A expression. However, the detailed molecular mechanism is still unknown.

CONCLUSION

MFG-E8 alleviates pancreatic fibrosis *via* inhibiting ER stress-induced chaperone-mediated autophagy in experimental CP. Recombinant MFG-E8 may be developed as a novel treatment for pancreatic fibrosis in CP.

AUTHOR CONTRIBUTIONS

YR acquired and analyzed the data, wrote the paper. QC, WL, JZ, and MX participated in data acquirement. ZW and YL interpreted the data. YZ interpreted the data and revised the paper. RW designed and supervised the study and revised the paper. All authors have read and agreed with the final manuscript.

ACKNOWLEDGMENTS

We appreciate the administrative support provided by Juan Zhao and Hui Yang during data collection.

REFERENCES

Abokyi, S., Shan, S. W., To, C. H., Chan, H. H., and Tse, D. Y. (2020). Autophagy Upregulation by the TFEB Inducer Trehalose Protects against Oxidative Damage and Cell Death Associated with NRF2 Inhibition in Human RPE Cells. *Oxid Med. Cel Longev* 2020, 5296341. doi:10.1155/2020/5296341

Albus, E., Sinningen, K., Winzer, M., Thiele, S., Baschant, U., Hannemann, A., et al. (2016). Milk Fat Globule-Epidermal Growth Factor 8 (MFG-E8) Is a Novel Anti-inflammatory Factor in Rheumatoid Arthritis in Mice and Humans. *J. Bone Miner Res.* 31, 596–605. doi:10.1002/jbmr.2721

An, S. Y., Jang, Y. J., Lim, H.-J., Han, J., Lee, J., Lee, G., et al. (2017). Milk Fat Globule-EGF Factor 8, Secreted by Mesenchymal Stem Cells, Protects against Liver Fibrosis in Mice. *Gastroenterology* 152, 1174–1186. doi:10.1053/j.gastro.2016.12.003

Aziz, M., Yang, W.-L., Corbo, L. M., Chaung, W. W., Matsuo, S., and Wang, P. (2015). MFG-E8 Inhibits Neutrophil Migration through αvβ3-integrin-dependent MAP Kinase Activation. *Int. J. Mol. Med.* 36, 18–28. doi:10.3892/ijmm.2015.2196

Bhardwaj, P., and Yadav, R. K. (2013). Chronic Pancreatitis: Role of Oxidative Stress and Antioxidants. *Free Radic. Res.* 47, 941–949. doi:10.3109/10715762.2013.804624

Bi, J., Zhang, J., Ren, Y., Du, Z., Zhang, Y., Liu, C., et al. (2020). Exercise Hormone Irisin Mitigates Endothelial Barrier Dysfunction and Microvascular Leakage-Related Diseases. *JCI Insight* 5. doi:10.1172/jci.insight.136277

Brissette, M.-J., Laplante, P., Qi, S., Latour, M., and Cailhier, J.-F. (2016). Milk Fat Globule Epidermal Growth Factor-8 Limits Tissue Damage through Inflammasome Modulation during Renal Injury. *J. Leukoc. Biol.* 100, 1135–1146. doi:10.1189/jlb.3a0515-213rr

Bynigeri, R. R., Jakkampudi, A., Jangala, R., Subramanyam, C., Sasikala, M., Rao, G. V., et al. (2017). Pancreatic Stellate Cell: Pandora's Box for Pancreatic Disease Biology. *Wjg* 23, 382–405. doi:10.3748/wjg.v23.i3.382

Cheyuo, C., Jacob, A., Wu, R., Zhou, M., Qi, L., Dong, W., et al. (2012). Recombinant Human MFG-E8 Attenuates Cerebral Ischemic Injury: its Role in Anti-inflammation and Anti-apoptosis. *Neuropharmacology* 62, 890–900. doi:10.1016/j.neuropharm.2011.09.018

D'Haese, J. G., Demir, I. E., Kehl, T., Winckler, J., Giese, N. A., Bergmann, F., et al. (2013). The Impact of MFG-E8 in Chronic Pancreatitis: Potential for Future Immunotherapy?. *BMC Gastroenterol.* 13, 14. doi:10.1186/1471-230X-13-14

Deng, K.-Q., Li, J., She, Z.-G., Gong, J., Cheng, W.-L., Gong, F.-H., et al. (2017). Restoration of Circulating MFGE8 (Milk Fat Globule-EGF Factor 8) Attenuates Cardiac Hypertrophy through Inhibition of Akt Pathway. *Hypertension* 70, 770–779. doi:10.1161/hypertensionaha.117.09465

Diakopoulos, K. N., Lesina, M., Wörmann, S., Song, L., Aichler, M., Schild, L., et al. (2015). Impaired Autophagy Induces Chronic Atrophic Pancreatitis in Mice via Sex- and Nutrition-dependent Processes. *Gastroenterology* 148, 626–638. doi:10.1053/j.gastro.2014.12.003

Endo, S., Nakata, K., Ohuchida, K., Takesue, S., Nakayama, H., Abe, T., et al. (2017). Autophagy Is Required for Activation of Pancreatic Stellate Cells, Associated with Pancreatic Cancer Progression and Promotes Growth of Pancreatic Tumors in Mice. *Gastroenterology* 152, 1492–1506. doi:10.1053/j.gastro.2017.01.010

Franchi, A., Bocca, S., Anderson, S., Riggs, R., and Oehninger, S. (2011). Expression of Milk Fat Globule EGF-Factor 8 (MFG-E8) mRNA and Protein in the Human Endometrium and its Regulation by Prolactin. *Mol. Hum. Reprod.* 17, 360–371. doi:10.1093/molehr/gaq102

Fujiwara, C., Uehara, A., Sekiguchi, A., Uchiyama, A., Yamazaki, S., Ogino, S., et al. (2019). Suppressive Regulation by MFG-E8 of Latent Transforming Growth Factor β-Induced Fibrosis via Binding to αv Integrin: Significance in the Pathogenesis of Fibrosis in Systemic Sclerosis. *Arthritis Rheumatol.* 71, 302–314. doi:10.1002/art.40701

Gao, Y. Y., Zhang, Z. H., Zhuang, Z., Lu, Y., Wu, L. Y., Ye, Z. N., et al. (2018). Recombinant Milk Fat Globule-EGF Factor-8 Reduces Apoptosis via Integrin beta3/FAK/PI3K/AKT Signaling Pathway in Rats after Traumatic Brain Injury. *Cell Death Dis.* 9, 845. doi:10.1038/s41419-018-0939-5

Gardner, T. B., Adler, D. G., Forsmark, C. E., Sauer, B. G., Taylor, J. R., and Whitcomb, D. C. (2020). ACG Clinical Guideline: Chronic Pancreatitis. *Am. J. Gastroenterol.* 115, 322–339. doi:10.14309/ajg.0000000000000535

Hanayama, R., and Nagata, S. (2005). Impaired Involution of Mammary Glands in the Absence of Milk Fat Globule EGF Factor 8. *Proc. Natl. Acad. Sci.* 102, 16886–16891. doi:10.1073/pnas.0508599102

He, Z., Si, Y., Jiang, T., Ma, R., Zhang, Y., Cao, M., et al. (2016). Phosphotidylserine Exposure and Neutrophil Extracellular Traps Enhance Procoagulant Activity in Patients with Inflammatory Bowel Disease. *Thromb. Haemost.* 115, 738–751. doi:10.1160/TH15-09-0710

Kaushik, S., and Cuervo, A. M. (2018). The Coming of Age of Chaperone-Mediated Autophagy. *Nat. Rev. Mol. Cel Biol.* 19, 365–381. doi:10.1038/s41580-018-0001-6

Kim, J. H., An, G. H., Kim, J. Y., Rasaei, R., Kim, W. J., Jin, X., et al. (2021). Human Pluripotent Stem-Cell-Derived Alveolar Organoids for Modeling Pulmonary Fibrosis and Drug Testing. *Cell Death Discov.* 7, 48. doi:10.1038/s41420-021-00439-7

Kleeff, J., Whitcomb, D. C., Shimosegawa, T., Esposito, I., Lerch, M. M., Gress, T., et al. (2017). Chronic Pancreatitis. *Nat. Rev. Dis. Primers* 3, 17060. doi:10.1038/nrdp.2017.60

Kranich, J., Krautler, N. J., Falsig, J., Ballmer, B., Li, S., Hutter, G., et al. (2010). Engulfment of Cerebral Apoptotic Bodies Controls the Course of Prion Disease in a Mouse Strain-dependent Manner. *J. Exp. Med.* 207, 2271–2281. doi:10.1084/jem.20092401

Li, C.-X., Cui, L.-H., Zhuo, Y.-Z., Hu, J.-G., Cui, N.-q., and Zhang, S.-K. (2018). Inhibiting Autophagy Promotes Collagen Degradation by Regulating Matrix Metalloproteinases in Pancreatic Stellate Cells. *Life Sci.* 208, 276–283. doi:10.1016/j.lfs.2018.07.049

Li, H., Gao, L., Min, J., Yang, Y., and Zhang, R. (2021). Neferine Suppresses Autophagy-Induced Inflammation, Oxidative Stress and Adipocyte Differentiation in Graves' Orbitopathy. *J. Cel Mol Med.* 25 (4), 1949–1957. doi:10.1111/jcmm.15931

Li, W., Yang, Q., and Mao, Z. (2018). Signaling and Induction of Chaperone-Mediated Autophagy by the Endoplasmic Reticulum under Stress Conditions. *Autophagy* 14, 1094–1096. doi:10.1080/15548627.2018.1444314

Li, W., Zhu, J., Dou, J., She, H., Tao, K., Xu, H., et al. (2017). Phosphorylation of LAMP2A by P38 MAPK Couples ER Stress to Chaperone-Mediated Autophagy. *Nat. Commun.* 8, 1763. doi:10.1038/s41467-017-01609-x

Masamune, A., Watanabe, T., Kikuta, K., and Shimosegawa, T. (2009). Roles of Pancreatic Stellate Cells in Pancreatic Inflammation and Fibrosis. *Clin. Gastroenterol. Hepatol.* 7, S48–S54. doi:10.1016/j.cgh.2009.07.038

Miksa, M., Amin, D., Wu, R., Jacob, A., Zhou, M., Dong, W., et al. (2008). Maturation-induced Down-Regulation of MFG-E8 Impairs Apoptotic Cell Clearance and Enhances Endotoxin Response. *Int. J. Mol. Med.* 22, 743–748. doi:10.3892/ijmm_00000080

Nagata, S. (2007). Autoimmune Diseases Caused by Defects in Clearing Dead Cells and Nuclei Expelled from Erythroid Precursors. *Immunol. Rev.* 220, 237–250. doi:10.1111/j.1600-065x.2007.00571.x

Pajares, M., Rojo, A. I., Arias, E., Díaz-Carretero, A., Cuervo, A. M., and Cuadrado, A. (2018). Transcription Factor NFE2L2/NRF2 Modulates Chaperone-Mediated Autophagy through the Regulation of LAMP2A. *Autophagy* 14, 1310–1322. doi:10.1080/15548627.2018.1474992

Ramakrishnan, P., Loh, W. M., Gopinath, S. C. B., Bonam, S. R., Fareez, I. M., Mac Guad, R., et al. (2020). Selective Phytochemicals Targeting Pancreatic Stellate Cells as New Anti-fibrotic Agents for Chronic Pancreatitis and Pancreatic Cancer. *Acta Pharmaceutica Sinica B* 10, 399–413. doi:10.1016/j.apsb.2019.11.008

Ren, Y., Qiu, M., Zhang, J., Bi, J., Wang, M., Hu, L., et al. (2019). Low Serum Irisin Concentration Is Associated with Poor Outcomes in Patients with Acute Pancreatitis and Irisin Administration Protects against Experimental Acute Pancreatitis. *Antioxid. Redox Signal.* 31 (11), 771–785. doi:10.1089/ars.2019.7731

Ren, Y.-F., Wang, M.-Z., Bi, J.-B., Zhang, J., Zhang, L., Liu, W.-M., et al. (2019). Irisin Attenuates Intestinal Injury, Oxidative and Endoplasmic Reticulum Stress in Mice with L-Arginine-Induced Acute Pancreatitis. *Wjg* 25, 6653–6667. doi:10.3748/wjg.v25.i45.6653

Ren, Y., Liu, W., Zhang, L., Zhang, J., Bi, J., Wang, T., et al. (2021). Milk Fat Globule EGF Factor 8 Restores Mitochondrial Function via Integrin-medicated Activation of the FAK-STAT3 Signaling Pathway in Acute Pancreatitis. *Clin. Translational Med.* 11, e295. doi:10.1002/ctm2.295

Ren, Y., Zhang, J., Wang, M., Bi, J., Wang, T., Qiu, M., et al. (2020). Identification of Irisin as a Therapeutic Agent that Inhibits Oxidative Stress and Fibrosis in a Murine Model of Chronic Pancreatitis. *Biomed. Pharmacother.* 126, 110101. doi:10.1016/j.biopha.2020.110101

Ryu, G. R., Lee, E., Chun, H.-J., Yoon, K.-H., Ko, S.-H., Ahn, Y.-B., et al. (2013). Oxidative Stress Plays a Role in High Glucose-Induced Activation of Pancreatic Stellate Cells. *Biochem. Biophysical Res. Commun.* 439, 258–263. doi:10.1016/j.bbrc.2013.08.046

Schmidt, J., Rattner, D. W., Lewandrowski, K., Compton, C. C., Mandavilli, U., Knoefel, W. T., et al. (1992). A Better Model of Acute Pancreatitis for Evaluating Therapy. *Ann. Surg.* 215, 44–56. doi:10.1097/00000658-199201000-00007

Sendler, M., Beyer, G., Mahajan, U. M., Kauschke, V., Maertin, S., Schurmann, C., et al. (2015). Complement Component 5 Mediates Development of Fibrosis, via Activation of Stellate Cells, in 2 Mouse Models of Chronic Pancreatitis. *Gastroenterology* 149, 765–776.e10. doi:10.1053/j.gastro.2015.05.012

Shah, K. G., Wu, R., Jacob, A., Molmenti, E. P., Nicastro, J., Coppa, G. F., et al. (2012). Recombinant Human Milk Fat Globule-EGF Factor 8 Produces Dose-dependent Benefits in Sepsis. *Intensive Care Med.* 38, 128–136. doi:10.1007/s00134-011-2353-7

Shi, Z., Wang, Q., Zhang, Y., and Jiang, D. (2020). Extracellular Vesicles Produced by Bone Marrow Mesenchymal Stem Cells Attenuate Renal Fibrosis, in Part by Inhibiting the RhoA/ROCK Pathway, in a UUO Rat Model. *Stem Cel Res Ther.* 11, 253. doi:10.1186/s13287-020-01767-8

Singh, V. K., Yadav, D., and Garg, P. K. (2019). Diagnosis and Management of Chronic Pancreatitis. *JAMA* 322, 2422–2434. doi:10.1001/jama.2019.19411

Song, M., Wang, C., Yang, H., Chen, Y., Feng, X., Li, B., et al. (2020). P-STAT3 Inhibition Activates Endoplasmic Reticulum Stress-Induced Splenocyte Apoptosis in Chronic Stress. *Front. Physiol.* 11, 680. doi:10.3389/fphys.2020.00680

Wang, B., Ge, Z., Wu, Y., Zha, Y., Zhang, X., Yan, Y., et al. (2020). MFGE8 Is Down-regulated in Cardiac Fibrosis and Attenuates Endothelial-mesenchymal Transition through Smad2/3-Snail Signalling Pathway. *J. Cel. Mol. Med.* 24, 12799–12812. doi:10.1111/jcmm.15871

Wang, C., Wang, H., Zhang, D., Luo, W., Liu, R., Xu, D., et al. (2018). Phosphorylation of ULK1 Affects Autophagosome Fusion and Links Chaperone-Mediated Autophagy to Macroautophagy. *Nat. Commun.* 9, 3492. doi:10.1038/s41467-018-05449-1

Wu, R., Chaung, W. W., Zhou, M., Ji, Y., Dong, W., Wang, Z., et al. (2010). Milk Fat Globule EGF Factor 8 Attenuates Sepsis-Induced Apoptosis and Organ Injury in Alcohol-Intoxicated Rats. *Alcohol. Clin. Exp. Res.* 34, 1625–1633. doi:10.1111/j.1530-0277.2010.01248.x

Xue, R., Jia, K., Wang, J., Yang, L., Wang, Y., Gao, L., et al. (2018). A Rising Star in Pancreatic Diseases: Pancreatic Stellate Cells. *Front. Physiol.* 9, 754. doi:10.3389/fphys.2018.00754

Xue, R., Wang, J., Yang, L., Liu, X., Gao, Y., Pang, Y., et al. (2019). Coenzyme Q10 Ameliorates Pancreatic Fibrosis via the ROS-Triggered mTOR Signaling Pathway. *Oxid Med. Cel Longev* 2019, 8039694. doi:10.1155/2019/8039694

Zhang, J., Johnson, J. L., He, J., Napolitano, G., Ramadass, M., Rocca, C., et al. (2017). Cystinosin, the Small GTPase Rab11, and the Rab7 Effector RILP Regulate Intracellular Trafficking of the Chaperone-Mediated Autophagy Receptor LAMP2A. *J. Biol. Chem.* 292, 10328–10346. doi:10.1074/jbc.m116.764076

14

Germacrone Attenuates Hepatic Stellate Cells Activation and Liver Fibrosis via Regulating Multiple Signaling Pathways

Zhiyong Li [1,2†], Zhilei Wang [3†], Fang Dong [4†], Wei Shi [2], Wenzhang Dai [2], Jing Zhao [2], Qiang Li [2], Zhi-e Fang [2], Lutong Ren [2], Tingting Liu [2], Ziying Wei [2], Wenqing Mou [2], Li Lin [2], Yan Yang [2], Xiaohe Xiao [2,5*], Li Ma [6*] and Zhaofang Bai [2,5*]

[1]School of Pharmacy, Chengdu University of Traditional Chinese Medicine, Chengdu, China, [2]Department of Hepatology, Fifth Medical Center of Chinese PLA General Hospital, Beijing, China, [3]TCM Regulating Metabolic Diseases Key Laboratory of Sichuan Province, Hospital of Chengdu University of Traditional Chinese Medicine, Chengdu, China, [4]School of Public Health and Health Management, Shandong First Medical University and Shandong Academy of Medical Sciences, Shandong, China, [5]China Military Institute of Chinese Materia, Fifth Medical Center of Chinese PLA General Hospital, Beijing, China, [6]School of Traditional Chinese Medicine, Capital Medical University, Beijing, China

*Correspondence:
Xiaohe Xiao
pharmacy_302@126.com
Li Ma
marytcm@ccmu.edu.cn
Zhaofang Bai
baizf2008@hotmail.com
†These authors have contributed equally to this work

Liver fibrosis is an abnormal proliferation of connective tissue in the liver caused by various pathogenic factors. Chronic liver injury leads to release of inflammatory cytokines and reactive oxygen species (ROS) from damaged hepatocytes, which activates hepatic stellate cells (HSCs) to secrete extracellular matrix proteins, thereby leading to fibrosis. Thus, inhibition of hepatocyte injury and HSC activation, and promotion of apoptosis of activated HSCs are important strategies for prevention of liver fibrosis. In this study, we showed that the germacrone (GER), the main component in the volatile oil of zedoary turmeric, inhibited hepatic fibrosis by regulating multiple signaling pathways. First, GER improved the cell survival rate by inhibiting the production of ROS after hepatocyte injury caused by acetaminophen (APAP). In addition, GER inhibited the activation of HSCs and expression of collagen I by blocking TGF-β/Smad pathway in LX-2 cells. However, when the concentration of GER was higher than 60 µM, it specifically induced HSCs apoptosis by promoting the expression and activation of apoptosis-related proteins, but it had no effect on hepatocytes. Importantly, GER significantly attenuated the methionine- and choline-deficient (MCD) diet-induced liver fibrosis by inhibiting liver injury and the activation of HSCs in vivo. In summary, GER can not only protect hepatocytes by reducing ROS release to avoid the liver injury-induced HSC activation, but also directly inhibit the activation and survival of HSCs by regulating TGF-β/Smad and apoptosis pathways. These results demonstrate that GER can be used as a potential therapeutic drug for the treatment of liver fibrosis.

Keywords: ROS: reactive oxygen species, HSCs: hepatic stellate cells, germacrone, TGF-β/Smad pathway, apoptosis

INTRODUCTION

In recent years, liver fibrosis has become a hot spot in liver disease research, and the complex mechanism of liver fibrosis formation has been revealed from many aspects (Parola and Pinzani, 2019). In the process of liver fibrosis, the dead and dying parenchymal cells release the danger signals, including inflammatory factors, damage associated molecular patterns (DAMPs), and reactive oxygen species (ROS), which can contribute to the activation of the hepatic stellate cells (HSCs) (Pellicoro et al., 2014). The ROS-generating enzymes, NADPH oxidase 1 (NOX1), NOX2, or NOX4, can induce liver fibrosis by activating HSCs (Lan et al., 2015). Importantly, HSCs are the most direct and relevant cell type for the formation of liver fibrosis. They are nonparenchymal cells of the liver, located in the space between liver sinusoidal endothelial cells (LSECs) and hepatocytes, and account for about 10% of the intrinsic cells of the liver (Higashi et al., 2017). Under the physiological conditions, the main function of HSCs is to metabolize and store retinol in lipid droplets in the cytoplasm; HSCs exhibit a nonproliferating quiescent phenotype, quite different from other cell morphologies. When the liver is damaged, the quiescent HSCs are activated and they differentiate into myofibroblasts, which secrete collagen and other components of the extracellular matrix (ECM). This transformation is an important step in the occurrence of liver fibrosis (Tsuchida and Friedman, 2017). The activated HSCs transform the main components of the ECM from type IV collagen, heparan sulfate proteoglycan (HSPG), and laminin (LN) to type I and III collagen, resulting in an increase in the density and hardness of the ECM (Cordero-Espinoza and Huch, 2018).

The activation of HSCs is related to the cytokines such as connective tissue growth factor (CTGF), transforming growth factor (TGF), platelet-derived growth factor (PDGF) and vascular endothelial growth factor (VEGF) released by liver parenchymal cells (Yang et al., 2014; Dewidar et al., 2019). TGF-β/Smad signaling is known as the classic HSC activation pathway. Under the stimulation by TGF-β1, the principal transforming growth factor isoform, the overexpressed TGF-β1 binds to HSC surface receptors and mediates the activation of HSCs. Then, the Smad2 and Smad3 are recruited to the TGF-β receptor and finally activated through phosphorylation. The activated Smad complex simultaneously recruits transcription co-activation molecules (such as P300/CBP and MSG1) and co-inhibitory molecules (TGIF and Ski/Sno N). Subsequently, phosphorylated Smad2/3 and Smad4 form a complex and then translocate into the nucleus to regulate the transcription of downstream pro-fibrosis genes, leading to liver fibrosis (Greenwel et al., 1997; Ghosh et al., 2000; Hata and Chen, 2016; Yoshida et al., 2018). In contrast, in the process of feedback regulation, Smad7 acts as a negative regulator (Bian et al., 2014). In addition, TGF-β1 can also activate the mitogen-activated protein kinase (MAPK) signaling pathway to promote HSC activation. TGF-β1 can regulate the activated MAPK signaling pathway, including extracellular signal-regulated kinase (ERK), P38 MAPK, and c-Jun N-terminal kinase (JNK), thereby promoting HSC activation (Engel et al., 1999; Hanafusa et al., 1999; Hernandez-Aquino and Muriel,

2018). Therefore, blocking HSC activation and promoting HSC apoptosis may be the strategies to prevent liver fibrosis.

The Liuweiwuling tablet, a traditional Chinese medicine preparation, has a significant effect on the treatment of liver fibrosis (Liu et al., 2018). Zedoary turmeric oil, the main medicinal material of Liuweiwuling prescriptions, has a significant antifibrotic effect (Jiang et al., 2005). In this study, we found that germarcone (GER), one of the main components of the volatile oil of zedoary turmeric, inhibited hepatic fibrosis by regulating multiple signaling pathways. We demonstrated that GER ameliorates liver fibrosis by inhibit the survival and activation of HSCs through apoptosis and TGF-β/Smad pathway *in vitro*. We further found that GER is able to reduce the release of ROS caused by APAP in L02, which plays an important role in protecting hepatocytes. Finally, GER also improves liver injury and prevents liver fibrosis through TGF-β/Smad pathway caused by methionine- and choline-deficient (MCD) diet.

MATERIALS AND METHODS

Reagents and Antibodies

Reagents: germacrone (TOPSCIENCE, T2945), acetaminophen (APAP, MCE, HY-66005), N-acetyl-L-cysteine (NAC, MCE, HY-B0215), hydrogen peroxide solution (H_2O_2, Sigma, 323381), Dulbecco's modified Eagle medium (DMEM, Macgene, CM10013), fetal bovine serum (FBS, Biological Industries, 04-001-1ACS), 1% penicillin–streptomycin (Macgene, CC004), 0.25% trypsin-EDTA (Macgene, CC012.100), 0.05% trypsin-EDTA (Macgene, C01712), TGF-β1 (PeproTech, AF-100-21C), Cell Counting Kit-8 (CCK-8, Dojindo, CK04), PE Annexin V Apoptosis Detection Kit I (BD Pharmingen™, 559763), MitoSOX™ red mitochondrial superoxide indicator (Invitrogen™, M36008), Carboxymethyl Cellulose-Na(CMC-Na, SCR, 9004-32-4), and methionine- and choline-sufficient, methionine- and choline-deficient (MCS/MCD, Dyets, MCDAA).

Antibodies: COL1A1 (R&D, AF6220), α-SMA (CST, 19245), P-Smad3 (CST, 9520), Smad3 (CST, 9523), PARP (CST, 9542S), cleaved PARP (CST, 5625S), caspase-3 (CST, 9665S), cleaved caspase-3 (CST, 96615), Bcl-2 (Abcam, ab32124), Bax (Abcam, ab32503), and GAPDH (GeneTex, GTX100118).

Cell Culture and Treatment

LX-2 human HSCs were purchased from Shanghai YuBo Biotechnology Co., Ltd. (YB-H3614), whereas human hepatocyte LO2 cells were kindly provided by Dr. Tao Li from National Center of Biomedical Analysis (Beijing, China). All the cells were cultured in 5% CO_2 incubator at 37°C using DMEM containing 10% FBS and 1% penicillin–streptomycin.

Cell viability test: LX-2 at 2.5×10^4 cells/well and LO2 at 2×10^4 cells/well were seeded in 96-well plates overnight. Then, the cells were incubated with different concentrations of GER (0–200 μM) for 24 h, and the cell viability was detected by CCK-8.

Drug effect detect: LX-2 at 7.5×10^4 cells/well were seeded in 24-well plates overnight. The LX-2 cells were starved with serum-free medium for 18 h. Then, the cells were pretreated with 10, 20, and 40 µM GER for 1 h. After stimulation with TGF-β1 (10 ng/ml) for 24 h, the cell lysate was collected for western blot and RT-qPCR analysis.

LX-2 cells at 7.5×10^4 cells/well were cultured in 24-well plates overnight. The cells were treated with 40–120 µM GER for 24 h, and the cell lysate was collected for western blot analysis. Alternatively, after the same treatment, the cells were collected and stained in line with the PE Annexin V Apoptosis Detection Kit I instructions, and the apoptotic cells were detected by flow cytometry.

LO2 cells at 6×10^4 cells/well were seeded in a 24-well plate overnight. The cells were pretreated with 10, 20, and 40 µM GER for 12 h, and then incubated with 20 mM APAP for 12 h. All the cells were collected and stained with MitoSOX red mitochondrial superoxide indicator. Finally, the mitochondrial ROS was detected by flow cytometry.

Mouse Model of Liver Fibrosis

Male C57BL/6 mice (6–7 weeks old) were purchased from SPF Biotechnology Co., Ltd. (Beijing, China). They were placed in the animal experiment center of the Fifth Medical Center of Chinese PLA General Hospital, Beijing 100039, China. This study was reviewed and approved by the animal ethics committee of the Fifth Medical Centre, Chinese PLA General Hospital (Beijing, China). All animals were fed adaptively under controlled temperature (25 ± 3°C) and 12-h dark/light cycle, during which sufficient food and water were provided. GER for the in vivo study was prepared with PBS containing 1% DMSO and 0.5% CMC-Na.

The animal model of liver fibrosis was developed using the MCS/MCD diet. All the mice were divided into five groups (n = 8). The control group was fed MCS diet and four experimental groups were fed MCD diet. Two weeks before the development of the model, all of the groups were fed MCS diet for transition, and then the experimental group gradually increased MCD diet. Two weeks later, the experimental groups were fed only MCD diet and began to receive drug treatment at the same time. The control group and the model group were given vehicle solvent, the positive drug group was given 0.2 mg/ml colchicine (COL), and the two treatment groups were given 25 or 50 mg/kg GER. The dosage of administration was 0.2 ml for per mouse through intragastric gavage (ig) every day for 6 weeks, and they were weighed twice a week. After the last administration, the mice fasted for 12 h and were killed by neck dislocation. The serum and liver were collected for detection and analysis.

Liver Function Parameter Tests

The levels of aspartate aminotransferase (AST) and alanine aminotransferase (ALT) in serum were detected in line with the instructions of AST (Nanjing JianChen Bioengineering Institute, C010-2-1) and ALT (Nanjing JianChen Bioengineering Institute, C009-2-1) kits.

TABLE 1 | Human primers for quantitative real-time PCR analysis.

Name		Sequence (5′ 3′)
ACTA2	Forward primer	CAGGGCTGTTTTCCCATCCAT
	Reverse primer	GCCATGTTCTATCGGGTACTTC
COL1A1	Forward primer	GTCGAGGGCCAAGACGAAG
	Reverse primer	CAGATCACGTCATCGCACAAC
Smad3	Forward primer	CCATCTCCTACTACGAGCTGAA
	Reverse primer	CACTGCTGCATTCCTGTTGAC
MMP-2	Forward primer	GTGAAGTATGGGAACGCCG
	Reverse primer	GCCGTACTTGCCATCCTTCT
GAPDH	Forward primer	AGCCACATCGCTCAGACAC
	Reverse primer	GCCCAATACGACCAAATCC

Liver Fibrosis Parameter Tests

The levels of hydroxyproline (Hyp) and PIIINP (procollagen type III N-terminal propeptide) were detected in line with instructions of ELISA Kit for hydroxyproline (Cloud-Clone Corp, CEA621Ge) and mouse procollagen type III N-terminal propeptide ELISA Kit (Novus Biologicals, NBP2-81204).

Histological and Immunohistochemical Assays

The liver tissue was fixed with 10% formalin solution, embedded in paraffin, cut into 7-mm-thick sections, and stained with hematoxylin-eosin (HE) and Masson. For immunohistochemical staining, the paraffin-embedded sections were incubated with the primary antibodies α-SMA and COL1A1, followed by incubation with the HRP-linked secondary antibodies. Finally, the quantitative analysis of α-SMA and COL1A1 were performed using K-Viewer software (K-Viewer V1, 1.5.3.1, KFBIO).

Western Blot Analysis

The collected total cellular proteins were separated by 10% SDS-PAGE gel electrophoresis and transferred to the polyvinylidene fluoride (PVDF) membrane, which was blocked with 5% skimmed milk for 1 h. Then, the membrane was incubated with the following antibodies: COL1A1, α-SMA, P-Smad3, Smad3, caspase-3, cleaved caspase-3, PARP, cleaved PARP, Bcl-2, and Bax. The GAPDH was used as a loading control. After incubating the linked-HRP secondary antibody, the bands were visualized using an ECL detection reagent and then develop it with the film.

We added 50 mg of liver tissue to 1 ml of RIPA lysate (including protease inhibitor) and homogenized at the frequency of 100 Hz for 90 s. The tissue lysate was placed on ice for 30 min and the supernatant was absorbed. The protein level was quantified by the cellular western blot method, and the following antibodies were incubated: α-SMA, Smad3, and P-Smad3. The β-actin was used as the loading control. After incubating the linked-HRP secondary antibody, the bands were visualized using an ECL detection reagent and then develop it with the film.

TABLE 2 | Mouse primers for quantitative real-time PCR analysis.

Name		Sequence (5′ 3′)
ACTA2	Forward primer	TCAGCGCCTCCAGTTCCT
	Reverse primer	AAAAAAAACCACGAGTAACAAATCAA
COL1A1	Forward primer	ACGTCCTGGTGAAGTTGGTC
	Reverse primer	CAGGGAAGCCTCTTTCTCCT
Smad3	Forward primer	AGGGGCTCCCTCACGTTATC
	Reverse primer	CATGGCCCGTAATTCATGGTG
TGF-β1	Forward primer	AGACCACATCAGCATTGAGTG
	Reverse primer	GGTGGCAACGAATGTAGCTGT
GAPDH	Forward primer	AATGGATTTGGACGCATTGGT
	Reverse primer	TTTGCACTGGTACGTGTTGAT

Quantitative Real-Time Polymerase Chain Reaction

TRlzol (Sigma, 93289) was used to extract cell total RNA or tissue total RNA in line with the manufacturer's protocol. Then, we reversed the extracted RNA to cDNA by RT Master Mix for qPCR (MCE, HY-K0510). Real-time PCR was performed with an Applied Biosystems ViiA6 Real-time PCR system using the SYBR Green qPCR Master Mix (MCE, HY-K0501). The PCR primer sequences are shown in **Tables 1**, **2**. The expression of related genes was calculated by ΔΔCt relative to GAPDH.

Data and Statistical Analysis

The data were presented as the mean ± standard error of mean (SEM). GraphPad Prism 5.0 (GraphPad Software, San Diego RRID:SCR_002798) was used for statistical analysis. A two-tailed unpaired Student's t test for two groups or one-way ANOVA for multiple groups was conducted to evaluate the significant differences. A p-value < 0.05 was considered statistically significant.

RESULTS

Screening of Effective Components Inhibiting HSC Activity in Zedoary Turmeric Oil

We found that the Liuweiwuling tablet, a prescription of traditional Chinese medicine, inhibited hepatic fibrosis in rats treated with carbon tetrachloride, and it was reported that zedoary turmeric oil was the main antifibrotic ingredient (Wu et al., 2010). Therefore, we screened out the component in zedoary turmeric oil that affected the activity of HSC in TGF-β1-induced LX-2 (**Figure 1A**). The western blot results showed that both GER and curdione (CUR) had more obvious inhibitory effect on the expression of collagen I than the other components. And the curcumol was reported to have anti-fibrotic effect (Jia

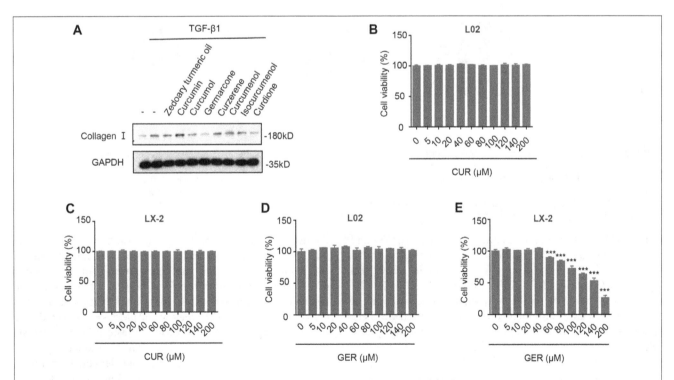

FIGURE 1 | Screening the effective components in zedoary turmeric oil which inhibit the activity of HSCs. **(A)** LX-2 cells were treated with Zedoary turmeric oil (0.2 μL/ml) and Curcumin, Curcumol, Germarcone (GER), Curzerene, Curcumenol, Isocurcumenol, and Curdione (CUR) (40 μM) for 25 h, and then were stimulated by TGF-β (10 ng/ml) for 24 h. The expression of collagen I was detected by western blot, and GAPDH was used as the loading control. **(B)** L02 cells were treated with CUR for 24 h, then the cell viability was detected by CCK-8 ($n = 3$). **(C)** LX-2 cells were treated with CUR for 24 h, then the cell viability was detected by CCK-8 ($n = 3$). **(D)** L02 cells were treated with GER for 24 h, then the cell viability was detected by CCK-8 ($n = 3$). **(E)** LX-2 cells were treated with GER for 24 h, then the cell viability was detected by CCK-8 ($n = 3$). All the results were compared with control group. All data are presented as means ± SEM. ***$p < 0.001$ vs. the control group.

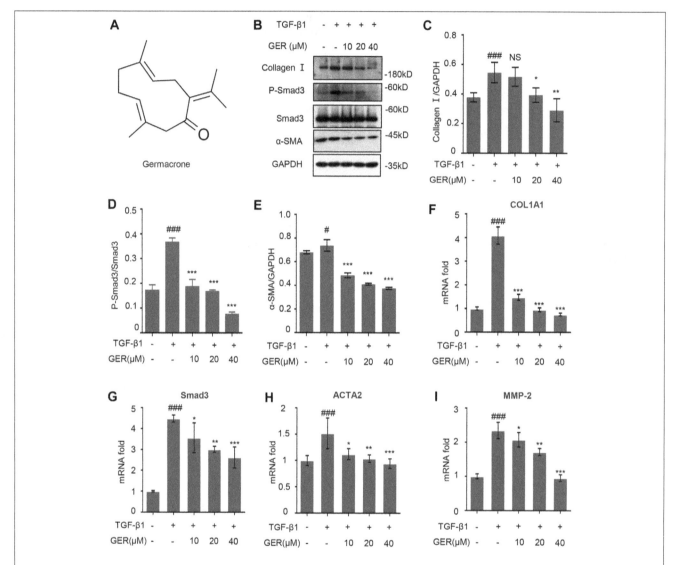

FIGURE 2 | GER suppresses TGF-β induced HSCs activation by inhibiting TGF-β/Smad signaling pathway. **(A)** The molecular structure of GER. **(B)** Western blot for collagen I, P-Smad3, Smad3, α-SMA protein level in LX-2, and GAPDH was used to as the loading control. **(C–E)** Quantitative analysis of collagen I, P-Smad3, Smad3, α-SMA, and GAPDH expression (n = 3). **(F-I)** Quantitative real-time PCR analysis of COL1A1, Smad3, ACTA2, and MMP-2 mRNA expression in LX-2. The $_{\Delta\Delta}C_t$ method was used to quantify relative changes (n = 3). All data are presented as means ± SEM. $^{\#}p < 0.05$, $^{\#\#\#}p < 0.001$ vs. the control group. $^{*}p < 0.05$, $^{**}p < 0.01$, $^{***}p < 0.001$ vs. the TGF-β group. NS, non-significant vs. the TGF-β group.

et al., 2018). Furthermore, we examined the effects of GER and CUR on the viability of L02 and LX-2 cells. The results showed that CUR (10–200 μM) did not affect the viability of L02 and LX-2 cells (**Figures 1B,C**). Although GER (10–200 μM) did not affect the viability of L02 cells, higher concentrations of GER (60–120 μM) inhibited the viability of LX-2 cells (**Figures 1D,E**); therefore, we continued to study the related effects of GER on LX-2 cells.

GER Inhibits the Activation of HSCs *in vitro* by Targeting the TGF-β/Smad Signaling Pathway

To explore whether GER could inhibit the activation of HSCs by blocking the TGF-β/Smad signaling pathway, we

conducted related experiments on LX-2 cells. First, the effect of GER on the viability of LX-2 cells was measured; the results showed that the concentration of GER below 60 μM had no cytotoxic effects on LX-2. To avoid the influence of cytotoxicity on the experimental results, the concentration of GER below 60 μM was selected for *in vitro* experimental research. Western blot analysis showed that GER reduced the TGF-β1–induced protein level of p-Smad3 and Smad3 in a dose-dependent manner, which directly regulating the expression of α-SMA and collagen I proteins in LX-2 (**Figures 2B–E**). furthermore, The RT-qPCR analysis revealed that GER significantly decreased the mRNA level of Smad3 and also reduced the mRNA level of its downstream genes ACTA2, MMP-2, and COL1A1 (**Figures 2F–I**). These results indicated that GER can

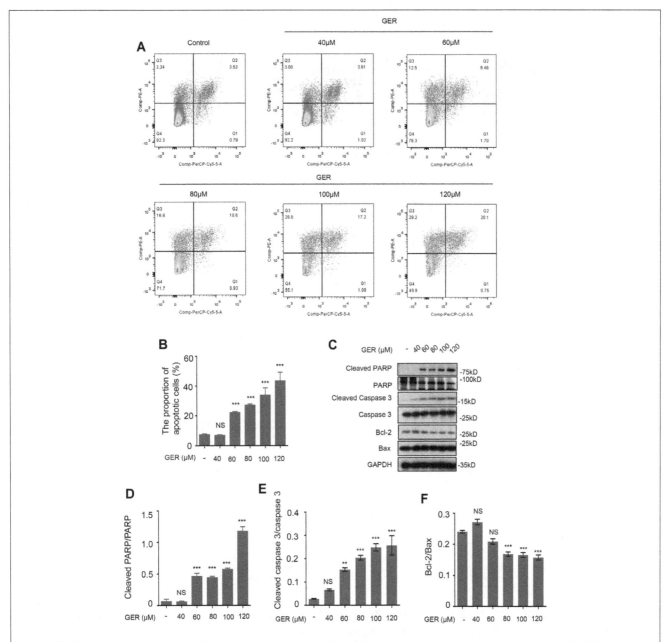

FIGURE 3 | GER promotes the apoptosis of HSCs. **(A)** Flow cytometric analysis of PI-stained apoptotic cells, and the cells in the upper right quadrant (Q2) were early apoptotic cells, and the cells in the upper left quadrant (Q3) were mid and late apoptotic cells. The apoptotic cells contained early, mid and late apoptotic cells. **(B)** Quantitative analysis of different group apoptotic cells after treatment with GER ($n = 3$). **(C)** Western blot for cleaved PARP, PARP, cleaved Caspase-3, Caspase-3, Bcl-2, Bax protein level in LX-2, and GAPDH was used as the loading control. **(D–F)** Quantitative analysis of cleaved PARP vs PARP, cleaved Caspase-3 vs. Caspase-3 and Bcl-2 vs Bax expression ($n = 3$). All data are presented as means ± SEM. *$p < 0.05$, **$p < 0.01$, ***$p < 0.001$ vs. the control group. NS, non-significant vs. the control group.

inhibit the activation of HSCs and the expression of ECMs through the TGF-β/Smad3 signaling pathway.

GER Inhibits the Survival of HSCs by Regulating Apoptotic Pathway *in vitro*

Previously, we observed that GER (10–40 µM) inhibited the activation of LX-2 cells; however, when the concentration of GER increased, it significantly inhibited the viability of LX-2

cells. Therefore, we explored the role of GER (40–120 µM) in apoptosis of LX-2 cells. First, flow cytometry was used to detect and analyze the proportion of apoptotic cells after GER treatment. The results showed that the proportion of early apoptotic cells (in the upper right quadrant, Q2) and the mid and late apoptotic cells (in the upper left quadrant, Q3) in the GER group were increased in a dose-dependent manner compared with those in the control group, indicating that apoptosis of LX-2 was promoted only by higher

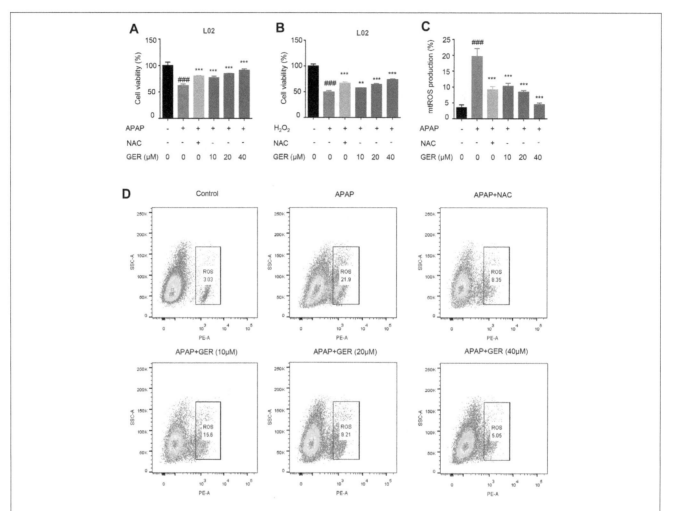

FIGURE 4 | GER protects the hepatocyte by inhibiting the release of mitochondrial ROS *in vitro*. **(A)** L02 cells were treated with APAP (20 mM) for 12 h, and then were treated with GER or NAC for 24 h, then the cell viability was detected by CCK-8 (*n* = 3). **(B)** L02 cells were treated with H_2O_2 (600 µM) for 12 h, and then were treated with GER or NAC for 24 h, then the cell viability was detected by CCK-8 (*n* = 3). **(C)** Quantitative analysis of different group mitochondrial ROS release (*n* = 3). **(D)** Flow cytometric analysis of the cell proportion of mitochondrial ROS in L02. The NAC was used as positive control, every group was treated with APAP except for control group. All data are presented as means ± SEM. $^{###}p < 0.001$ vs. the control group. $^{**}p < 0.01$, $^{***}p < 0.001$ vs. the APAP group.

concentrations of GER (60–120 µM) (**Figures 3A,B**). Furthermore, we detected the expression of relevant apoptotic proteins in LX-2 cells. Poly ADP-ribose polymerase (PARP), a DNA repair enzyme and the main cleavage substrate of caspase-3, is the core member of the apoptosis pathway; it plays an important role in DNA damage repair. Namely, the PARP substrate is cleaved by caspase-3 and becomes a form of cleaved PARP that loses its enzymatic activity (Morris et al., 2018). The increased cleaved PARP accelerates cell apoptosis. At the same time, Bax/Bcl-2 ratio is also important. Bax is a proapoptotic protein, which is antagonistic to Bcl-2 (Moldoveanu et al., 2020). In our study, western blot analysis was used to detect the expression of apoptotic proteins; we showed that GER (60, 80, 100, 120 µM) promoted the expression of cleaved PARP and cleaved caspase-3 proteins, and inhibited the expression of antiapoptotic protein Bcl-2 (**Figures 3C–F**). These results revealed that GER inhibited

the survival of HSCs by regulating the apoptotic pathway in a dose-dependent manner.

GER Protects Hepatocytes by Inhibiting the Production of Mitochondrial ROS *in vitro*

It has been reported that GER may protect hepatocytes (Hashem et al., 2021). In our study, we explored the hepatoprotective effects of GER in APAP cellular damage model. According to the results of preliminary experiments, the cells were treated with 20 mM APAP or 600 µM H_2O_2 to induce the hepatocyte damage model and then incubated with different concentrations (10, 20, and 40 µM) of GER. Cell viability was detected 24 h later. The results showed that GER increased the cell survival rate of L02 cells after APAP or H_2O_2 treatment in a dose-dependent manner, confirming the protective effect of GER on hepatocytes (**Figures 4A,B**). APAP mainly causes mitochondrial oxidative stress to

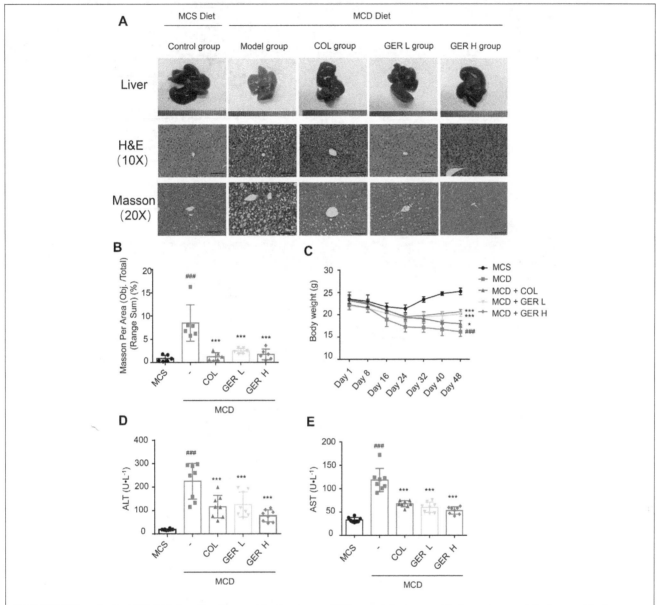

FIGURE 5 | GER ameliorates MCD diet-induced liver tissue and function damage. **(A)** Representative images of the liver and representative images of the liver sections stained with haematoxylin and eosin (H&E, scale bars, 50 µm) and masson (scale bars, 100 µm). Colchicine (COL) was used as positive control, GER L: the low dose (25 mg/kg) of GER group, GER H: the high dose (50 mg/kg) of GER group. **(B)** Quantification of masson changes in different treatment groups ($n = 6$). **(C)** The weight changes of mice in different group for per 7 days **(D,E)** Serum alanine transaminase (ALT) and aspartate transaminase (AST) levels ($n = 8$). All data are presented as means ± SEM. $^{###}p < 0.001$ vs. the MCS group. $^{***}p < 0.001$ vs. the model group.

produce ROS, which leads to mitochondrial damage and thus induces liver cell apoptosis. Therefore, we explored whether GER can inhibit the generation of ROS caused by APAP and protect hepatocytes. The MitoSOX red mitochondrial superoxide indicator (Ex/Em: 510/580 nm) was used to stain the cell mitochondrial ROS, followed by detection and analysis through flow cytometry. The flow cytometric results showed that APAP promoted the production of mitochondrial ROS, and the administration of GER was able to inhibit the production of mitochondrial ROS (**Figures 4C,D**),

demonstrating that GER protected hepatocytes from damage by inhibiting the production of mitochondrial ROS.

GER Ameliorates MCD Diet-Induced Liver Function and Tissue Damage

To explore the role of GER in the process of liver fibrosis, C57BL/ 6 mice were fed the MCD diet to induce liver fibrosis, and the MCS diet was used for comparison. As shown in **Figure 5**, compared with the MCS diet group, the liver surface in the

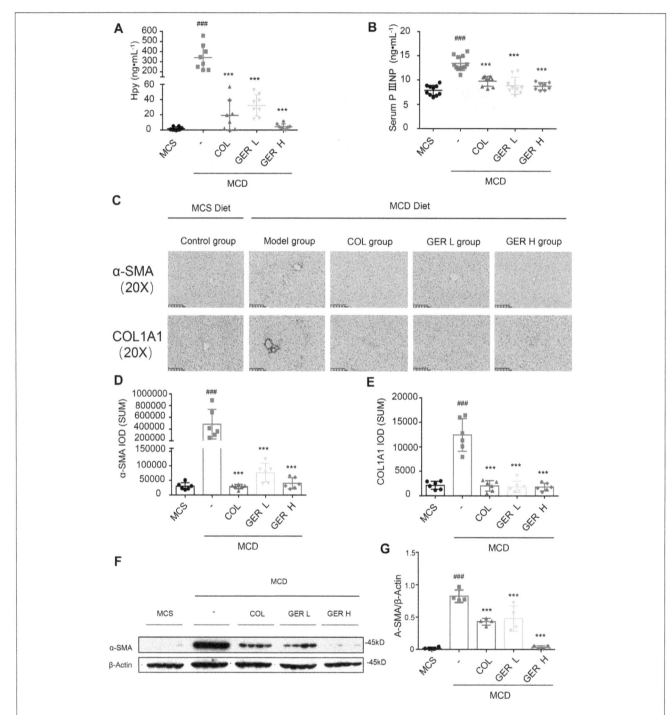

FIGURE 6 | GER inhibits the activation of HSCs via TGF-β/Smad signaling pathway *in* MCD diet-induced liver fibrosis model. **(A)** The content of hydroxyproline in liver tissue (*n* = 8). **(B)** The serum content of PIIINP (*n* = 8–11). **(C)** Immunohistochemistry for α-SMA and COL1A1 in liver sections (scale bars, 100 μm). **(D–E)** Quantification of α-SMA and COL1A1 expression in different treatment groups (*n* = 6). **(F)** Western blot for α-SMA and Smad3 protein levels in liver tissue, and β-actin was used as the loading control (*n* = 4). **(G)** Quantitative analysis of α-SMA and β-actin expression (*n* = 4). All data are presented as means ± SEM. $^{###}p < 0.001$ vs. the MCS group. $^{*}p < 0.05$, $^{***}p < 0.001$ vs. the model group.

MCD model group was rougher, with many nodular textures, and yellowish in color, which situations in GER treatment group were improved effectively (**Figure 5A**). Similarly, histopathological staining (H&E and Masson) revealed that the liver sections of the MCD diet model group were severely damaged, exhibiting

vesicular steatosis, ballooning degeneration of hepatocytes, and fibrosis around hepatocytes and sinuses in the liver; in contrast, the GER group had less liver damage, less steatosis, and less fibrosis (**Figures 5A,B**). In addition, the weight of the mice on the MCD diet, especially in the MCD model group, showed a

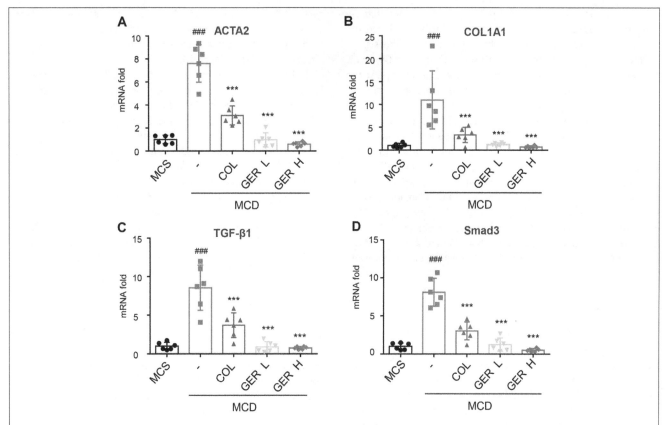

FIGURE 7 | GER inhibits the activation of HSCs via TGF-β/Smad signaling pathway *in* MCD diet-induced liver fibrosis model. **(A–D)** Quantitative real-time PCR analysis of ACTA2, COL1A1, TGF-β, and Smad3 mRNA expression in liver tissue (*n* = 6). All data are presented as means ± SEM. [###]*p* < 0.001 vs. the MCS group. *p < 0.05, ***p* < 0.001 vs. the model group.

downward trend compared with the MCS diet group. After treatment with GER in MCD diet, the weight first showed a tendency to decrease and then to increase, demonstrating that the body function of the mice in the MCD diet group was restored after the administration of GER (**Figure 5C**). The serum levels of ALT and AST in the MCD model group were significantly higher than those in the control group; in contrast, the levels of ALT and AST were significantly reduced after GER administration, indicating that GER ameliorated liver damage caused by the MCD diet (**Figures 5D,E**).

GER Inhibits the Activation of HSCs by Regulating TGF-β/Smad Signaling in MCD Diet-Induced Liver Fibrosis Model

Hydroxyproline is a characteristic biochemical marker that can be used to quantify the content of collagen in tissues, which is often used to indicate the degree of liver fibrosis (Lee et al., 2005; Gjaltema and Bank, 2017). PIIINP is a cleavage product of procollagen III, which can be detected in serum and used as a circulating biomarker of ECM remodeling in the process of liver fibrosis (Mosca et al., 2019). Therefore, we detected the content of hydroxyproline in the tissue and PIIINP in serum. The results showed that the levels of hydroxyproline and PIIINP in the MCD

model group were higher than those in the MCS group, whereas the concentration of hydroxyproline in the tissue and PIIINP in serum were significantly decreased in the GER group, indicating that GER had an antifibrotic effect (**Figure 6A,B**).

To further clarify the role of GER in the MCD diet-induced liver fibrosis model, immunohistochemical staining was used to analyze the expression of α-SMA and COL1A1 in liver tissues. We found a large amount of COL1A1 accumulation in the liver tissue of the MCD model group compared with the MCS group, while the distribution of COL1A1 was significantly reduced in the GER group, indicating that GER was able to reduce the expression of COL1A1 in liver fibrosis and reduce the deposition of collagen in fibrotic tissue (**Figures 6C–E**). We also detected the distribution of α-SMA, a marker of HSC activation, in the tissues. The results showed that compared with the MCD model group, the distribution of α-SMA in the liver tissues was reduced after the administration of GER (**Figures 6F–G**), demonstrating that GER was able to inhibit the expression of α-SMA and block HSC activation in mice with liver fibrosis. Furthermore, we extracted RNA from liver tissue and detected the expression of COL1A1 and ACTA2 genes by RT-qPCR. Consistent with the immunohistochemical results, the expression levels of COL1A1 and ACTA2 in the mice liver tissues of the GER group were lower than those of the MCD model group

(**Figures 7A,B**). Therefore, it was evident that GER inhibited the activation of HSCs in MCD diet-induced fibrosis, reduced the expression of COL1A1, and thereby improved liver fibrosis.

The TGF-β/Smad signaling pathway activation is the main pathway for HSC activation and ECM generation. To explore the cause of liver fibrosis in the MCD diet model and the mechanism of GER against liver fibrosis, we determined the content of TGF-β in serum and tissues. The results of RT-qPCR showed that the TGF-β levels in liver tissue in the MCD model group were significantly higher than those in the MCS group and the GER group (**Figure 7C**), indicating that the increase in the TGF-β level was the main cause of liver fibrosis induced by MCD diet. In addition, the GER group significantly reduced Smad3 protein expression compared with the MCD model group (**Figure 7D**). The above results demonstrated that GER was able to reduce the increase in TGF-β levels caused by MCD diet and to suppress the activation of HSCs through the TGF-β/Smad signaling pathway.

DISCUSSION

Fibrosis is a part of the wound healing response after catastrophic tissue damage, which maintains the integrity of organs, but can also lead to a variety of human pathological conditions, including cirrhosis (Bataller and Brenner, 2005; Lee et al., 2015). The reversal and treatment of liver fibrosis is an important means to reduce the severity of chronic liver disease; therefore, there is an urgent clinical need to develop an effective antifibrotic drug (Iredale, 2007; Roehlen et al., 2020). GER, which was screened out from zedoary turmeric oil in this study, is a kind of open double-ring sesquiterpene compound with ketone group in turmeric plants (An and Jang, 2020); it has numerous physiological activities and great medicinal potential, including anti-inflammatory, anti-virus, anti-tumor, and anti-oxidant effects (Aggarwal et al., 2013; An and Jang, 2020). In the last years, the mechanisms of antifibrotic effect were investigated. The results showed that the activation of HSCs into proliferative fibro/myo-fibroblasts has been found to be the central factor of liver fibrosis, and they found that the expression of α-SMA, a HSCs activation marker, and collagen I were increased after stimulating by TGF-β1 (Dewidar et al., 2019). However, few studies reported the effect of GER on liver fibrosis. In this study, GER inhibited the expression of α-SMA in TGF-β1-stimulated LX-2, indicating that the activation of HSCs might be prevented by GER.

TGF-β1, the most powerful fibrocytokine in the microenvironment of liver fibrosis (Hellerbrand et al., 1999), exerts its biological activity via the Smad signaling pathway. Smad signal transduction pathways mediated TGF-β1-induced collagen synthesis through the phosphorylating Smad2/3, which can translocate to the nucleus to regulate the target genes, and thus play a crucial role in the development of liver fibrosis (Roberts et al., 2006). To explore whether GER regulates liver fibrosis through TGF-β/Smad signaling pathway, the GER attenuated TGF-β1-induced LX-2 fibrosis was used. Ours results showed that both the protein level of phosphorylating Smad3 and Smad3 were decreased after GER treatment. Furthermore, the mRNA level of Smad3 and its downstream gene ACTA2, COL1A1, and MMP-2 were also downregulated. These results indicated that inhibiting of TGF-β/Smad signaling pathway may be a key mechanism to GER exerts its anti-fibrotic effect in TGF-β1-induced LX-2.

Inducing apoptosis of HSCs and inhibiting the survival of HSCs are also important mechanisms of anti-hepatic fibrosis. Various growth factors released by damaged hepatocytes are the main reasons for the rapid proliferation and activation of HSCs. On the one hand, the proliferation of HSCs is positively regulated by PDGF, on the other hand, it inhibits its apoptosis (Tsuchida and Friedman, 2017). Therefore, we can also inhibit the survival of HSCs by promoting the apoptosis of HSCs. It was reported that Gliotoxin promotes the apoptosis of HSCs by activating Caspase 3 and consuming ATP, thus improving liver fibrosis in rats (Dekel et al., 2003). Ours results showed that the dose of GER plays a regulatory effect on HSCs. At the low dose (lower than 40 μM), GER can inhibit the activation of HSCs through the TGF-β/Smad signaling pathway. However, when the concentration of GER is in the range of 60–120 μM, it can promote the apoptosis of HSCs by upregulating Cleaved-caspase 3 protein expression and inhibiting anti-apoptotic protein Bcl-2 expression as well as has no toxic effect on hepatocytes. These indicates that GER has a dual effect on HSCs, inhibiting the activity of HSCs in the therapeutic concentration range to exert an antifibrotic effect. When the concentration of GER increases, it can induce programmed apoptosis of HSCs, which can effectively inhibit the survival of HSCs in the process of fibrosis.

Liver injury contributes to liver fibrosis where hepatocytes change their gene expression and secretion profile in response to such injury, and the newly expressed fibrogenic factors including TGF-β and NADPH oxidase 4 (Lan et al., 2015; Wang et al., 2016). Nox4 mediates the synthesis of ROS that is also one of the reasons for the activation of HSCs (Novo et al., 2011). A large number of studies have shown that most of liver fibrosis *in vivo*, including CCl₄, alcohol, Thioacetamide (TAA) and nonalcoholic steatohepatitis (NASH), injured hepatocytes proposed to play a causative role in the induction of liver fibrosis (Ramos-Tovar and Muriel, 2020). Furthermore, it was found that HSCs cultured with ROS produced by stimulated neutrophils showed that an increased level of procollagen mRNA and protein (Casini et al., 1997). Therefore, ROS is also the one of the accomplices in liver fibrosis. In this study, APAP was used to produce ROS in L02, and we found that GER can protect hepatocytes and reduce the release of ROS from injured hepatocytes *in vitro*. And *in vivo* experiment showed that GER significantly improved the state of liver injury in mice with lower serum aminotransferase subjected level to MCD-diet group; through observing the pathological sections, we found that the hepatocytes with fatty degeneration and fat vacuoles of steatosis in the GER group were significantly less common. All these findings indicate that GER may not only directly prevent the damage of parenchymal cells, but also inhibit the activity of stellate cells by inhibiting the release of damage substances and ROS to attenuate liver fibrosis.

So according to *in vitro* study, We found that the effect of GER on attenuating liver fibrosis can be explained from two aspects. On the one hand, its direct effect is to inhibit the activation and survival of HSCs. In terms of what they have in common, they all act directly on HSCs to inhibit liver fibrosis, but the difference is that the concentration of GER effect is different, and the mechanism is also different. On the other hand, GER can indirectly prevent liver fibrosis by protecting hepatocytes. At the same time, the two effects of GER inducing HSCs apoptosis and GER protecting hepatocytes are synergistic in preventing liver fibrosis.

MCD-diet mice is a well-established nutritional model of liver fibrosis with serum aminotransferase elevation, and liver histological changes similar to human Non-alcoholic steatohepatitis (Li et al., 2018). To explore the effect of GER on hepatic fibrosis, a MCD-diet model of liver fibrosis was investigated. According to related research, MCD-diet can lead to abnormal liver metabolism, massive fat accumulation and weight loss (Li et al., 2020). But in our study, the mice weight showed that GER could prevent MCD-diet induced weight loss, and we detected lower level of ALT and AST in GER group, in addition, histopathological analysis showed that there was less vesicular steatosis, ballooning degeneration of hepatocytes, and fibrosis around hepatocytes and sinuses in the liver of the GER group. Consistent with *in vitro* data, GER could protect liver through reducing the release of ROS produced by damaged hepatocytes. These results indicated that GER may reduce liver injury, balance the level of oxidative stress in the liver, and then improve the liver function to play the anti-fibrotic effect.

Levels of hydroxyproline and PIIINP in liver are the important indicators reflecting the degree of liver fibrosis. In our study, MCD-diet mice showed increased levels of hydroxyproline and PIIINP in liver, which were significantly decreased after GER administration. Therefore, we further explored the anti-fibrotic mechanism of GER *in vivo*. Immunohistochemical analysis showed that there were a large number of α-SMA and COL1A1 proteins distributed in MCD-diet mice liver, but both of them were decreased after GER treatment. This phenomenon was consistent with the results of our *in vitro* experiments, which further confirmed that GER inhibited the activity of HSCs. RT-qPCR analysis showed that the gene level of TGF-β was upregulated in MCD-diet mice liver, at the same time, its transduction signal pathway Smad 3 and its downstream genes ACTA2 and COL1A1 were also upregulated, which indicating

that TGF-β/Smad signaling pathway was a important mechanism in MCD-diet induced liver fibrosis. However, GER could reduce the expression of TGF-β, Smad 3, ACTA2 ,and COL1A1 genes, so that inhibited TGF-β/Smad signaling pathway. The same results had been confirmed on LX-2.

In conclusion, we found GER could attenuate liver fibrosis through regulating multiple signaling pathways, the first was to inhibit the activity of HSCs through TGF-β/Smad signaling pathway, the second was to protect the liver, reduce hepatocytes injury and liver oxidative stress, and avoid ROS-induced the activation of HSCs. Finally, the survival of HSCs was inhibited through apoptosis pathway. To a certain extent, GER may be used in the treatment of clinical chronic hepatic fibrosis.

AUTHOR CONTRIBUTIONS

ZL: Investigation, Validation, Visualization, Formal analysis, Software, Writing-Original draft preparation. ZW: Investigation, Validation, Visualization, Formal analysis, Writing-Original draft preparation. FD: Investigation, Validation, Visualization, Formal analysis. WS, WD, JZ, and QL: Visualization, Software. ZF, LR, TL, ZW, WM, LL, and YY: Investigation. XX: Conceptualization, Visualization, Funding acquisition. LM: Investigation, Validation, Resources, Formal analysis, Data curation, Supervision, Writing-Reviewing and Editing. ZB: Conceptualization, Methodology, Investigation, Validation, Resources, Formal analysis, Data curation, Visualization, Supervision, Project administration, Writing-Reviewing and Editing, Funding acquisition.

ACKNOWLEDGMENTS

We thank Tao Li (National Center of Biomedical Analysis) for providing L02 cells. This work was supported by Science and Technology Major Project "Key New Drug Creation and Manufacturing Program" (2017ZX09301022), National Natural Science Foundation of China (81930110).

REFERENCES

Aggarwal, B. B., Yuan, W., Li, S., and Gupta, S. C. (2013). Curcumin-free Turmeric Exhibits Anti-inflammatory and Anticancer Activities: Identification of Novel Components of Turmeric. *Mol. Nutr. Food Res.* 57, 1529–1542. doi:10.1002/mnfr.201200838

An, S., and Jang, E. (2020). Preclinical Evidence of Curcuma Longa and its Noncurcuminoid Constituents against Hepatobiliary Diseases. *A Rev.* 2020, 8761435. doi:10.1155/2020/8761435

Bataller, R., and Brenner, D. A. (2005). Liver Fibrosis. *J. Clin. Invest.* 115, 209–218. doi:10.1172/JCI24282

Bian, E. B., Huang, C., Wang, H., Chen, X. X., Zhang, L., Lv, X. W., et al. (2014). Repression of Smad7 Mediated by DNMT1 Determines Hepatic Stellate Cell Activation and Liver Fibrosis in Rats. *Toxicol. Lett.* 224, 175–185. doi:10.1016/j.toxlet.2013.10.038

Casini, A., Ceni, E., Salzano, R., Biondi, P., Parola, M., Galli, A., et al. (1997). Neutrophil-derived Superoxide Anion Induces Lipid Peroxidation and Stimulates Collagen Synthesis in Human Hepatic Stellate Cells: Role of

Nitric Oxide. *Hepatology* 25, 361–367. doi:10.1053/jhep.1997.v25.pm0009021948

Cordero-Espinoza, L., and Huch, M. (2018). The Balancing Act of the Liver: Tissue Regeneration versus Fibrosis. *J. Clin. Invest.* 128, 85–96. doi:10.1172/JCI93562

Dekel, R., Zvibel, I., Brill, S., Brazovsky, E., Halpern, Z., and Oren, R. (2003). Gliotoxin Ameliorates Development of Fibrosis and Cirrhosis in a Thioacetamide Rat Model. *Dig. Dis. Sci.* 48, 1642–1647. doi:10.1023/a:1024792529601

Dewidar, B., Meyer, C., Dooley, S., and Meindl-Beinker, A. N. (2019). TGF-β in Hepatic Stellate Cell Activation and Liver Fibrogenesis-Updated. *Cells* 2019 (8). doi:10.3390/cells8111419

Engel, M. E., McDonnell, M. A., Law, B. K., and Moses, H. L. (1999). Interdependent SMAD and JNK Signaling in Transforming Growth Factor-Beta-Mediated Transcription. *J. Biol. Chem.* 274, 37413–37420. doi:10.1074/jbc.274.52.37413

Ghosh, A. K., Yuan, W., Mori, Y., and Varga, J. (2000). Smad-dependent Stimulation of Type I Collagen Gene Expression in Human Skin Fibroblasts by TGF-Beta Involves Functional Cooperation with P300/CBP Transcriptional Coactivators. *Oncogene* 19, 3546–3555. doi:10.1038/sj.onc.1203693

Gjaltema, R. A., and Bank, R. A. (2017). Molecular Insights into Prolyl and Lysyl Hydroxylation of Fibrillar Collagens in Health and Disease. *Crit. Rev. Biochem. Mol. Biol.* 52, 74–95. doi:10.1080/10409238.2016.1269716

Greenwel, P., Inagaki, Y., Hu, W., Walsh, M., and Ramirez, F. (1997). Sp1 Is Required for the Early Response of alpha2(I) Collagen to Transforming Growth Factor-Beta1. *J. Biol. Chem.* 272, 19738–19745. doi:10.1074/jbc.272.32.19738

Hanafusa, H., Ninomiya-Tsuji, J., Masuyama, N., Nishita, M., Fujisawa, J., Shibuya, H., et al. (1999). Involvement of the P38 Mitogen-Activated Protein Kinase Pathway in Transforming Growth Factor-Beta-Induced Gene Expression. *J. Biol. Chem.* 274, 27161–27167. doi:10.1074/jbc.274.38.27161

Hashem, S., Nisar, S., Sageena, G., Macha, M. A., Yadav, S. K., Krishnankutty, R., et al. (2021). Therapeutic Effects of Curcumol in Several Diseases; an Overview. *Nutr. Cancer* 73, 181–195. doi:10.1080/01635581.2020.1749676

Hata, A., and Chen, Y. G. (2016). TGF-β Signaling from Receptors to Smads. *Cold Spring Harb Perspect. Biol.* 8. doi:10.1101/cshperspect.a022061

Hellerbrand, C., Stefanovic, B., Giordano, F., Burchardt, E. R., and Brenner, D. A. (1999). The Role of TGFbeta1 in Initiating Hepatic Stellate Cell Activation *In Vivo*. *J. Hepatol.* 30, 77–87. doi:10.1016/s0168-8278(99)80010-5

Hernández-Aquino, E., and Muriel, P. (2018). Beneficial Effects of Naringenin in Liver Diseases: Molecular Mechanisms. *World J. Gastroenterol.* 24, 1679–1707. doi:10.3748/wjg.v24.i16.1679

Higashi, T., Friedman, S. L., and Hoshida, Y. (2017). Hepatic Stellate Cells as Key Target in Liver Fibrosis. *Adv. Drug Deliv. Rev.* 121, 27–42. doi:10.1016/j.addr.2017.05.007

Iredale, J. P. (2007). Models of Liver Fibrosis: Exploring the Dynamic Nature of Inflammation and Repair in a Solid Organ. *J. Clin. Invest.* 117, 539–548. doi:10.1172/JCI30542

Jia, Y., Wang, F., Guo, Q., Li, M., Wang, L., Zhang, Z., et al. (2018). Curcumol Induces RIPK1/RIPK3 Complex-dependent Necroptosis via JNK1/2-ROS Signaling in Hepatic Stellate Cells. *Redox Biol.* 19, 375–387. doi:10.1016/j.redox.2018.09.007

Jiang, Y., Li, Z. S., Jiang, F. S., Deng, X., Yao, C. S., and Nie, G. (2005). Effects of Different Ingredients of Zedoary on Gene Expression of HSC-T6 Cells. *World J. Gastroenterol.* 11, 6780–6786. doi:10.3748/wjg.v11.i43.6780

Lan, T., Kisseleva, T., and Brenner, D. A. (2015). Deficiency of NOX1 or NOX4 Prevents Liver Inflammation and Fibrosis in Mice through Inhibition of Hepatic Stellate Cell Activation. *PLoS One* 10. e0129743. doi:10.1371/journal.pone.0129743

Lee, H. S., Shun, C. T., Chiou, L. L., Chen, C. H., Huang, G. T., and Sheu, J. C. (2005). Hydroxyproline Content of Needle Biopsies as an Objective Measure of Liver Fibrosis: Emphasis on Sampling Variability. *J. Gastroenterol. Hepatol.* 20, 1109–1114. doi:10.1111/j.1440-1746.2005.03901.x

Lee, Y. A., Wallace, M. C., and Friedman, S. L. (2015). Pathobiology of Liver Fibrosis: a Translational success story. *Gut* 64, 830–841. doi:10.1136/gutjnl-2014-306842

Li, R., Li, J., Huang, Y., Li, H., Yan, S., Lin, J., et al. (2018). Polydatin Attenuates Diet-Induced Nonalcoholic Steatohepatitis and Fibrosis in Mice. *Int. J. Biol. Sci.* 14, 1411–1425. doi:10.7150/ijbs.26086

Li, X., Wang, T. X., Huang, X., Li, Y., Sun, T., Zang, S., et al. (2020). Targeting Ferroptosis Alleviates Methionine-Choline Deficient (MCD)-diet Induced NASH by Suppressing Liver Lipotoxicity. *Liver Int.* 40, 1378–1394. doi:10.1111/liv.14428

Liu, H., Zhang, Z., Hu, H., Zhang, C., Niu, M., Li, R., et al. (2018). Protective Effects of Liuweiwuling Tablets on Carbon Tetrachloride-Induced Hepatic Fibrosis in Rats. *BMC Complement. Altern. Med.* 18, 212. doi:10.1186/s12906-018-2276-8

Moldoveanu, T., and Czabotar, P. E., (2020). BAX, BAK, and BOK: A Coming of Age for the BCL-2 Family Effector Proteins. *Cold Spring Harb Perspect. Biol.* 12. doi:10.1101/cshperspect.a036319

Morris, G., Walker, A. J., Berk, M., Maes, M., and Puri, B. K. (2018). Cell Death Pathways: a Novel Therapeutic Approach for Neuroscientists. *Mol. Neurobiol.* 55, 5767–5786. doi:10.1007/s12035-017-0793-y

Mosca, A., Comparcola, D., Romito, I., Mantovani, A., Nobili, V., Byrne, C. D., et al. (2019). Plasma N-Terminal Propeptide of Type III Procollagen Accurately Predicts Liver Fibrosis Severity in Children with Non-alcoholic Fatty Liver Disease. *Liver Int.* 39, 2317–2329. doi:10.1111/liv.14225

Novo, E., Busletta, C., Bonzo, L. V., Povero, D., Paternostro, C., Mareschi, K., et al. (2011). Intracellular Reactive Oxygen Species Are Required for Directional Migration of Resident and Bone Marrow-Derived Hepatic Pro-fibrogenic Cells. *J. Hepatol.* 54, 964–974. doi:10.1016/j.jhep.2010.09.022

Parola, M., and Pinzani, M. (2019). Liver Fibrosis: Pathophysiology, Pathogenetic Targets and Clinical Issues. *Mol. Aspects Med.* 65, 37–55. doi:10.1016/j.mam.2018.09.002

Pellicoro, A., Ramachandran, P., Iredale, J. P., and Fallowfield, J. A. (2014). Liver Fibrosis and Repair: Immune Regulation of Wound Healing in a Solid Organ. *Nat. Rev. Immunol.* 14, 181–194. doi:10.1038/nri3623

Ramos-Tovar, E., and Muriel, P. (2020). Molecular Mechanisms that Link Oxidative Stress, Inflammation, and Fibrosis in the Liver. *Antioxidants.* 9, 1–21. doi:10.3390/antiox9121279

Roberts, A. B., Tian, F., Byfield, S. D., Stuelten, C., Ooshima, A., Saika, S., et al. (2006). Smad3 Is Key to TGF-Beta-Mediated Epithelial-To-Mesenchymal Transition, Fibrosis, Tumor Suppression and Metastasis. *Cytokine Growth Factor. Rev.* 17, 19–27. doi:10.1016/j.cytogfr.2005.09.008

Roehlen, N., Crouchet, E., and Baumert, T. F. (2020). Liver Fibrosis: Mechanistic Concepts and Therapeutic Perspectives. *Cells* 9. doi:10.3390/cells9040875

Tsuchida, T., and Friedman, S. L. (2017). Mechanisms of Hepatic Stellate Cell Activation. *Nat. Rev. Gastroenterol. Hepatol.* 14, 397–411. doi:10.1038/nrgastro.2017.38

Wang, X., Zheng, Z., Caviglia, J. M., Corey, K. E., Herfel, T. M., Cai, B., et al. (2016). Hepatocyte TAZ/WWTR1 Promotes Inflammation and Fibrosis in Nonalcoholic Steatohepatitis. *Cell Metab* 24, 848–862. doi:10.1016/j.cmet.2016.09.016

Wu, S. J., Tam, K. W., Tsai, Y. H., Chang, C. C., and Chao, J. C. (2010). Curcumin and Saikosaponin a Inhibit Chemical-Induced Liver Inflammation and Fibrosis in Rats. *Am. J. Chin. Med.* 38, 99–111. doi:10.1142/S0192415X10007695

Yang, L., Kwon, J., Popov, Y., Gajdos, G. B., Ordog, T., Brekken, R. A., et al. (2014). Vascular Endothelial Growth Factor Promotes Fibrosis Resolution and Repair in Mice. *Gastroenterology* 146, 1339–1350. doi:10.1053/j.gastro.2014.01.061

Yoshida, K., Matsuzaki, K., Murata, M., Yamaguchi, T., Suwa, K., and Okazaki, K. (2018). Clinico-Pathological Importance of TGF-β/Phospho-Smad Signaling during Human Hepatic Fibrocarcinogenesis. *Cancers (Basel)* 10. doi:10.3390/cancers10060183

15

Nonlinear Relationship Between Macrocytic Anemia and Decompensated Hepatitis B Virus Associated Cirrhosis

Tian-Yu Zhao, Qing-Wei Cong, Fang Liu, Li-Ying Yao and Ying Zhu*

Liver Disease Center of Integrated Traditional Chinese and Western Medicine, The First Affiliated Hospital of Dalian Medical University, Dalian, China

*Correspondence:
Ying Zhu
zhuyingsh53@126.com

Background: Mean corpuscular volume (MCV) is major used as an indicator for the differential diagnosis of anemia. Macrocytic anemia in decompensated cirrhosis is common. However, the relationship between macrocytic anemia and decompensated hepatitis B virus (HBV) associated cirrhosis has not been fully addressed.

Methods: In this cross-sectional study, a total of 457 patients diagnosed decompensated HBV associated cirrhosis who met all inclusion criteria from 2011 to 2018 were analyzed. Association between macrocytic anemia and the liver damaged (Model for End Stage Liver Disease (MELD) score) were examined using multiple logistic regression analyses and identified using smooth curve fitting.

Results: Compared with normocytic anemia, MCV and MELD are significantly positively correlated in macrocytic anemia ($p < 0.001$). A non-linear relationship of MCV and MELD association was found though the piecewise linear spline models in patients with decompensated HBV associated cirrhosis. MCV positive correlated with MELD when the MCV was greater than 98.2 fl (regression coefficient = 0.008, 95% CI 0.1, 0.4).

Conclusion: Macrocytic anemia may be a reliable predictor for mortality because it is closely related to the degree of liver damage in patients with decompensated HBV associated cirrhosis.

Keywords: macrocytic anemia, decompensated HBV associated cirrhosis, MELD score, degree of liver damage, mean corpuscular volume

INTRODUCTION

Liver cirrhosis is a frequent end stage of liver disease, which itself results from a long-term process of fibrosis and sustained inflammation and leads to chronic liver disease (Schuppan and Afdhal, 2008). Hepatitis B virus (HBV) infection remains a very common liver disease (Nguyen et al., 2020), over 70% of infected cases are diagnosed as liver cirrhosis in China (Xiao et al., 2019). During the natural course of the disease, cirrhosis has transitioned from the compensation stage to the decompensation stage, through the developmental processes of one of the following serious complications: variceal hemorrhage, spontaneous bacterial peritonitis (SBP), encephalopathy, or jaundice. The 5-years liver related decompensated incidences in patients with compensated cirrhosis are 15–20%, 5-years survival rate for patients with compensated cirrhosis is approximately 84%, while for patients with decompensated cirrhosis, survival rate drops to 14–35% (Peng et al., 2012).

Anemia is now identified as an important predictor of adverse outcomes in liver cirrhosis patients, such as the development of acute-on-chronic liver failure (ACLF) in outpatients with cirrhosis and hepatocellular carcinoma mortality rates (Finkelmeier et al., 2014; Piano et al., 2017). Mean corpuscular volume (MCV) is defined as a measure of the average volume of a red blood cell, anemia is classified into three categories depending on the level of the patient's MCV: macrocytic anemia (>100 fl), normocytic anemia (80–100 fl) and microcytic anemia (<80 fl). A study has indicated that an increase MCV level was correlated with the prognosis of liver cancer (Yoon et al., 2016). However, the exact mechanisms behind the relationship between MCV and liver function damage degree in patients with decompensated hepatitis B virus-related cirrhosis is still unknown. The model for End Stage Liver Disease (MELD) score was a preferred tool to use to predict the short-term mortality of end-stage liver disease and measure cirrhosis severity (Kamath and Kim, 2007). It had been considered to be an important predictor of survival for end-stage liver disease caused by many etiologies and was considered an organ allocation strategy for liver transplantation more accurate than Child-Pugh score since its application in the United States in 2002 (Wiesner et al., 2003; Bambha et al., 2004). Analysis demonstrated that the greater MELD scores (≥15), the greater risk of death from liver disease, as well as showed a significant survival benefit from liver transplantation compared to lower MELD scores (<15) (Merion et al., 2005). Thus, higher MELD score are expected to indicate worse liver function.

Previous a study showed that the relationship between MCV and MELD (Yang et al., 2018), however, this relationship has not been well studied. Therefore, we investigated whether MCV is independently associated with MELD in HBV-associated decompensated cirrhosis.

METHODS

Characteristics of the Participants
This is a retrospective study from the Big Data Platform of the First affiliated hospital of Dalian Medical university from May 2011 to April 2018, our data consists of 1732 patients with decompensated HBV associated decompensated cirrhosis. Our research used the International Classification of Diseases codes to identify decompensation cirrhosis with HBV hospitalized patients. Decompensated Cirrhosis in Patients with hepatitis B according to the China's Guidelines for the Prevention and Treatment of Chronic Hepatitis B (The guidelines of prevention and treatment for chronic hepatitis B (2019 version), 2019), 1) HBsAg carrier for study population≥6 months; 2) confirm the presence of cirrhosis according to biochemical, radiological, endoscopic and histological

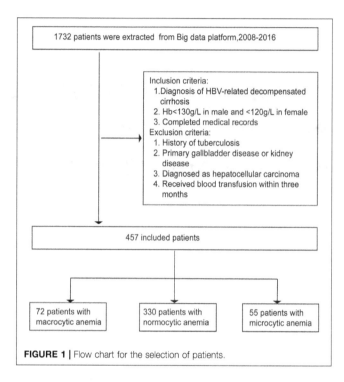

FIGURE 1 | Flow chart for the selection of patients.

criteria; 3) at least one episode of ascites, spontaneous bacterial peritonitis, hepatic encephalopathy, or variceal bleeding (Jang et al., 2015). The WHO defined anemia as a hemoglobin level <130 g/L in male and <120 g/L in female (McLean et al., 2009). Two investigators reviewed the charts of all patients, Any discrepancies between the two investigators will be adjudicated by a senior physician. 457 patients who met all inclusion criteria and none of the exclusion criteria were enrolled into the study. This cross-section hospital-based, observational study was conducted in a University Hospital (**Figure 1**).

The research protocol was reviewed and approved with a waiver of written informed consent by the Ethics Committee of the First affiliated hospital of Dalian Medical university, informed consent by telephone was obtained from each participant. All the methods were performed in accordance with relevant guidelines and regulations.

Data Collection
Demographic characteristics were obtained from face-to-face communication with patients or their families when the patient was admitted to our hospital. Blood samples were taken from the patients on an empty stomach for more than 10 h after the whole night and fast sent to the laboratory assessments. Having more than one cigarette per day is considered as smoking and alcohol intaking more than 20 g per day for at least a year is considered as drinking (Kim et al., 2013; Carter et al., 2015). Estimated GFR (eGFR) formula was derived from the modification of diet in renal disease (MDRD). Regrettably, due to missing data, HBV DNA data and body mass index (BMI) were excluded from this study (K/DOQI clinical practice guidelines for chronic kidney disease: evaluation, classification, and stratification, 2002; Ma et al., 2006).

MELD Score
Using the following formula to calculate the MELD score: 9.57 × loge (creatinine mg/dl) + 3.78 × loge (bilirubin mg/dl) + 11.2 ×

TABLE 1 | Baseline Characteristics of participants ($N = 457$).

Variable	Macrocytic anemia	Normocytic anemia	Microcytic anemia	p-value
No. of participants	72	330	55	
Mean corpuscular volume, fl	105.40 ± 4.49	91.14 ± 5.09	72.92 ± 5.16	<0.001
Age, years	66.29 ± 13.79	65.32 ± 12.65	65.78 ± 13.72	0.617
Sex				0.120
Male, n (%)	60 (83.33)	237 (71.82)	42 (76.36)	
Female, n (%)	12 (16.67)	93 (28.18)	13 (23.64)	
Smoke, n (%)	28 (41.18)	98 (31.11)	23 (43.40)	0.091
Alcohol, n (%)	25 (37.88)	88 (27.76)	19 (35.85)	0.171
Diabetes, n (%)	8 (11.11)	58 (17.58)	11 (20.00)	0.332
Hypertension, n (%)	9 (12.50)	55 (16.67)	12 (21.82)	0.376
Hemoglobin, g/L	102.48 ± 21.07	102.22 ± 18.98	73.15 ± 18.14	<0.001
Hemoglobin, categorical recoded, n (%)				<0.001
>90	57 (79.17)	245 (74.24)	9 (16.36)	
60–90	11 (15.28)	78 (23.64)	36 (65.45)	
<60	4 (5.56)	7 (2.12)	10 (18.18)	
Blood glucose, mmol/L	5.58 ± 2.00	6.19 ± 3.22	6.21 ± 2.57	0.588
SBP, mmHg	128.36 ± 17.88	128.86 ± 19.29	127.64 ± 19.71	0.715
DBP, mmHg	76.41 ± 10.40	77.56 ± 11.88	79.62 ± 12.71	0.378
Bilirubin,µmol/L	56.3 (25.6–120.2)	40.4 (25.1–75.0)	34.1 (19.2–71.6)	<0.001
Creatinine,µmol/L	63.5 (50.5–93.2)	62.0 (49.0–86.0)	66.0 (55.5–90.5)	0.209
INR	1.50 ± 0.69	1.27 ± 0.27	1.30 ± 0.22	<0.001
eGFR				
mL/min/1.73 m^2	110.0 (74.2–761.2)	112.3 (75.4–2,362.1)	121.5 (83.0–377.2)	0.091
ALB	31.31 ± 6.82	31.04 ± 6.06	33.04 ± 5.87	0.090
AST	60.5 (33.2–117.8)	59.0 (34.0–105.8)	47.0 (31.0–93.5)	0.518
ALT	37.5 (23.0–88.0)	42.0 (24.0–74.0)	37.0 (23.0–67.0)	0.864
ALP	121.0 (81.8–204.5)	123.5 (89.0–186.8)	138.0 (81.5–244.0)	0.924
GGT	80.5 (36.8–190.5)	94.0 (45.0–217.5)	107.0 (43.5–364.5)	0.663
MELD	17.02 ± 6.94	14.82 ± 4.20	15.16 ± 4.25	<0.001
Complications, n(%)				
UGB	10 (13.89)	50 (15.15)	2 (3.64)	0.069
SBP*	1 (1.39)	5 (1.52)	0 (0.00)	1.000
HE	0 (0.00)	12 (3.64)	0 (0.00)	0.093

Abbreviations: SBP, systolic blood pressure; DBP, diastolic blood pressure; MELD, model for end stage liver disease; UGB, upper gastrointestinal bleeding; SBP*, spontaneous bacterial peritonitis; HE, hepatic encephalopathy; INR, international normalized ratio; eGFR, estimated GFR; ALB, albumin; AST, aspartate aminotransferase; ALT, alanine aminotransferase; GGT, gamma-glutamyl transferase; ALP, alkaline phosphatase.

loge (INR) + 6.43, where INR is the international normalized ratio and 6.43 is the constant of the etiology of liver disease (Kamath and Kim, 2007).

Statistical Analysis

Categorical variables were described in counts (percentages) and continuous variables as means ± standard deviation (SD). Patients were distributed into 3 groups by mean corpuscular volume (MCV) classification. The variables were followed normal distribution and homogeneous in variance. The levels within 3 groups of the continuous variables were analyzed using one-way ANOVA. categorical variables were analyzed using Chi-square test. To evaluate the relationship between the MELD score and macrocytic anemia were analyzed using univariate and multivariate linear regression analyses. Only variables with a p-value < 0.05 in the univariate analyses were planned to be included in the multivariate model. The possible linear and nonlinear models were used to assess the relationship between MELD and MCV by multiple linear regression models and two-piece piecewise regression models adjusted for sex, age, smoking, drinking, SBP, DBP. We then performed stratified analyses in order to further explore potential modifier on the MELD-MCV association.

All data analysis and form generation were produced using the statistical package R (http://www.R-project.org, The R Foundation) and Empower (R) (www.empower stats.com; X&Y Solutions, Inc. Boston, MA). The results data were considered statistically significant When p-value was <0.05.

RESULTS

Characteristics of the Participants

The baseline characteristics of subjects with anemia were divided into three groups (**Table 1**). Among the 457 participants in this analysis, 330/457 patients (72.2%) of the anemic cases had normocytic anemia, with the remaining 127 (27.8%) having macrocytic ($n = 72$) and microcytic anemia ($n = 55$). The cohort was 74.2% male, had a mean age of 65.5 (SD = 12.9). In addition, we found significantly higher expression levels of serum bilirubin, international normalized ratio (INR) and MELD score in macrocytic anemia when compared to normocytic or microcytic anemia. However, no significant differences were found in age, gender, smoking, drinking, diabetes, hypertension, systolic blood pressure, diastolic blood pressure, creatinine, eGFR, albumin, alanine

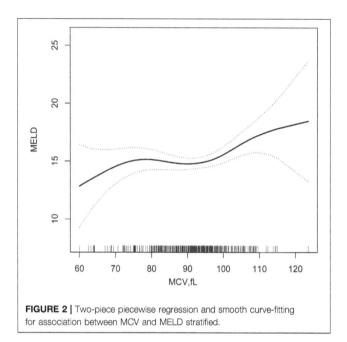

FIGURE 2 | Two-piece piecewise regression and smooth curve-fitting for association between MCV and MELD stratified.

TABLE 2 | Univariate analysis for MELD score.

	Statistics	β (95%CI)	p-value
Sex			
Female	118 (25.82%)	Ref	
Male	339 (74.18%)	−0.57 (−1.58, 0.43)	0.2627
Age	65.5 ± 12.9	−0.0 (−0.0, 0.0)	0.786
Smoking	149 (32.6%)	0.5 (−0.5, 1.4)	0.315
Drinking	132 (28.9%)	0.5 (−0.5, 1.4)	0.354
Diabetes	77 (16.8%)	−0.7 (−1.8, 0.5)	0.271
Hypertension	76 (16.6%)	−0.8 (−2.0, 0.4)	0.179
Hemoglobin, g/L			
>90	311 (68.1%)	Ref	
60–90	125 (27.4%)	0.6 (−0.4, 1.6)	0.248
<60	21 (4.6%)	1.9 (−0.2, 4.0)	0.074
Blood glucose	6.1 ± 3.0	−0.0 (−0.2, 0.1)	0.827
SBP	128.6 ± 19.1	−0.0 (−0.0, 0.0)	0.520
DBP	77.6 ± 11.8	0.0 (−0.0, 0.0)	0.988
MCV, fl	91.20 ± 9.86	0.04 (0.00, 0.09)	0.0485
Anemia classification			
Normocytic anemia	330 (72.21%)	Ref	
Macrocytic anemia	72 (15.75%)	2.20 (0.99, 3.41)	0.0004
Microcytic anemia	55 (12.04%)	0.34 (−1.01, 1.70)	0.6195

Abbreviations: MELD, model for end stage liver disease; β estimated coefficient; 95% CI 95% confidence interval; SBP, systolic blood pressure; DBP, diastolic blood pressure; MCV, mean corpuscular volume; fl.

aminotransferase (ALT), aspartate aminotransferase (AST), alkaline phosphatase (ALP), γ-glutamyltranspeptidase (γ-GT).

Association Between Macrocytic Anemia and MELD Score

In univariate regression analysis, we found that a significant correlation was present both macrocytic anemia and the MELD score (β = 2.20, 95% CI: 0.99–3.41, p < 0.001), normocytic group was used as a normalization control (**Table 2**). Moreover, this association persisted (β = 2.31, CI:1.09–3.52, p < 0.001) after adjustment for sex and age in Model I (β = 2.40, CI:1.06–3.74, p < 0.001) after adjustment for sex, age, smoking, drinking, SBP, DBP in Model II in multivariate analysis (**Table 3**).

Association Between MCV and MELD Score

The two-piece wise smooth curve for MCV-MELD association in decompensated HBV associated cirrhosis. MCV negatively correlated with MELD when the MCV was smaller or equal than 98.2 fl (regression coefficient = 0.793,95% CI—0.1, 0.1). There was a strong positive correlation if MCV greater than 98.2 fl (regression coefficient = 0.008,95% CI 0.1, 0.4) (**Figure 2**; **Table 4**).

DISCUSSION

In this study the analysis was done retrospectively, we suggested that macrocytic anemia (MCV >100 fl) related to the degree of liver damage in decompensated HBV associated cirrhosis patients. This variability persists even after adjusting for age, gender, smoking, drinking, SBP and DBP.

Positive association between MCV and MELD was found among HBV-associated decompensated cirrhosis. Our findings by the two-piece piece-wise regression model to display the relationship between MCV and MELD as non-linear relationship. Positive correlation was observed when the MCV was higher than 98.2 fl, while negative correlation occurred when the MCV was lower than 98.2 fl.

Macrocytosis, which is also known as MCV >100 fl, is not necessarily correlated with anemia. Moreover, in most of the cases it is unattached to anemia (Eisenga et al., 2019). We select anemia as an inclusion criteria in our model because 70% patients in our study have anemia. In patients with advanced chronic liver disease, a research reported that 66% of the population suffers from anemia of different etiologies, this result was consistent with our study (Scheiner et al., 2020). Furthermore, the cause of occurred anemia in patients with liver cirrhosis due to shortened erythrocyte survival, a lack of hematopoietic cytokine, gastrointestinal bleeding, bone marrow disorders. All these suggest serious impairment of liver function and a high risk of death.

The significance of macrocytosis remains an underestimated issue in the past. Only a small number of studies had relevant reports (Bourlon et al., 2016; Kloth et al., 2016; Lee et al., 2020). An article indicated that a high MCV was associated with increased risk of death from liver cancer in males (Yoon et al., 2016). One study with small sample size also found that the MCV was notably higher in chronic hepatic failure patients than in healthy individuals (Remková and Remko, 2009). A precious published finding also showed that macrocytic anemia was related to the degree of liver damage in patients with decompensated HBV associated cirrhosis (Yang et al., 2018). These results fit in with our study.

Macrocytosis is considered a structural and functional abnormality of the erythrocyte membrane. Several potential pathological mechanisms may explain our observations. First, irrespective of the etiology vitamin deficits is common in patients with cirrhosis, such as vitamin B12 and folate deficiency (Gupta et al., 2019; Ohfuji et al., 2021), macrocytic anemia usually occurs due to liver dysfunction, low intakes of dietary, low uptake and increased catabolism. Vitamin B12 and folate coenzymes deficiency are known to cause delayed in DNA

TABLE 3 | Relationship between MCV and MELD in different models.

Variable	Crude model		Model I		Model II	
	β (95%CI)	p-value	β (95%CI)	p-value	β (95%CI)	p-value
MCV, fl	0.04 (0.00, 0.09)	0.0485	0.05 (0.00, 0.09)	0.0428	0.05 (0.00, 0.10)	0.0367
Anemia classification						
Normocytic anemia	References		References		References	
Macrocytic anemia	2.20 (0.99, 3.41)	<0.001	2.31 (1.09, 3.52)	<0.001	2.40 (1.06, 3.74)	<0.001
Microcytic anemia	0.34 (−1.01, 1.70)	0.6195	0.39 (−0.97, 1.74)	0.5762	0.29 (−1.17, 1.76)	0.6958

Abbreviations: CI, confidence interval.
Model I adjusted for Sex and Age. Model II adjusted for Sex, Age, Smoking, Drinking, SBP, DBP.

TABLE 4 | Threshold Effect Analysis of MCV and MELD using Piece-wise Linear Regression.

Inflection point of MCV	Effect size(β)	95%CI	p Value
<98.2	0.0	−0.1 to 0.1	0.793
≥98.2	0.2	0.1 to 0.4	0.008

Effect: MELD Cause: MCV
adjusted :Sex, Age, Smoking, Drinking, SBP, DBP.

synthesis and eventually results in macrocytic anemia (Green and Dwyre, 2015; Lanier et al., 2018). Second, oxidative stress has been identified as an pivotal pathophysiological mechanism in chronic viral hepatitis B (Uchida et al., 2020). Because red blood cell is thought to be tightly related to whole-body antioxidant capacity (Tsantes et al., 2006). Oxidative stress decreases the RBC capacity to deform, reduces blood flow in microcirculation and compromises oxygen supply to certain tissues (Mohanty et al., 2014; Skjelbakken et al., 2014). Moreover, There are various factors that affect erythrocyte morphology in liver disease, such as etiology, severity of hepatic impairment, and use of drugs. There are many complicated mechanisms that affect the shape of red blood cells. These mechanisms may allow to perform effectively their independent or collaborative functions. Nevertheless, it's clear that macrocytic anemia has a positive correlation with the degree of liver damage in patients with decompensated HBV associated cirrhosis.

The MELD score is approved for assessing the degree of liver diseases. These variables include prothrombin time, INR, serum bilirubin and creatinine level. MELD score changes with variations in these variables. Higher MELD scores associate with increased risks of death and hepatic events in cirrhosis. In our study, among the parameters of MELD score, bilirubin and INR showed an increase on patients with macrocytic anemia. However, there was no remarkable difference with creatinine and

eGFR. Therefore, macrocytic anemia may not be relevant to renal injury in patients with decompensated HBV associated cirrhosis.

Several study limitations are noted. First, the main limitation of this study lies in its retrospective observational nature, the cross-sectional nature of our study does not permit the determination of causality between MCV and MELD. Second, this study included only Chinese participants, and therefore these findings may not be generalizable to other biogeographic ethnic groups. Third, we did not perform an analysis on the data of folate, serum vitamin B12 and reticulocyte count, which could provide a better understanding of macrocytic anemia in cirrhotic patients.

CONCLUSION

Macrocytic anemia was highly correlated with the degree of hepatic dysfunction and may be a reliable predictor for mortality in patients with decompensated HBV associated cirrhosis. We found a non-linear relationship between MCV and MELD. Moreover, further large-scale, well-designed and multicenter studies need to be conducted to confirm our conclusions, it is important to evaluate and investigate this association and to gain insight the underlying mechanisms.

AUTHOR CONTRIBUTIONS

T-YZ designed the study. Q-WC and FL interpreted the data. T-YZ and L-YY drafted the paper. YZ designed the experiments, improved the manuscript. All the authors have read and approved the final manuscript.

ACKNOWLEDGMENTS

We thank everyone who participated in the study.

REFERENCES

Bambha, K., Kim, W. R., Kremers, W. K., Therneau, T. M., Kamath, P. S., Wiesner, R., et al. (2004). Predicting Survival Among Patients Listed for Liver Transplantation: an Assessment of Serial MELD Measurements. *Am. J. Transpl.* 4 (11), 1798–1804. doi:10.1111/j.1600-6143.2004.00550.x

Bourlon, M. T., Gao, D., Trigero, S., Clemons, J. E., Breaker, K., Lam, E. T., et al. (2016). Clinical Significance of Sunitinib-Associated Macrocytosis in Metastatic Renal Cell Carcinoma. *Cancer Med.* 5 (12), 3386–3393. doi:10.1002/cam4.919

Carter, B. D., Abnet, C. C., Feskanich, D., Freedman, N. D., Hartge, P., Lewis, C. E., et al. (2015). Smoking and Mortality-Bbeyond Established Causes. *N. Engl. J. Med.* 372 (7), 631–640. doi:10.1056/NEJMsa1407211

Eisenga, M. F., Wouters, H. J. C. M., Kieneker, L. M., van der Klauw, M. M., van der Meer, P., Wolffenbuttel, B. H. R., et al. (2019). Active Smoking and Macrocytosis in the General Population: Two Population-Based Cohort Studies. *Am. J. Hematol.* 94 (2), E45–e48. doi:10.1002/ajh.25346

Finkelmeier, F., Bettinger, D., Köberle, V., Schultheiß, M., Zeuzem, S., Kronenberger, B., et al. (2014). Single Measurement of Hemoglobin Predicts Outcome of HCC Patients. *Med. Oncol.* 31 (1), 806. doi:10.1007/s12032-013-0806-2

Green, R., and Dwyre, D. M. (2015). Evaluation of Macrocytic Anemias. *Semin. Hematol.* 52 (4), 279–286. doi:10.1053/j.seminhematol.2015.06.001

Gupta, S., Read, S. A., Shackel, N. A., Hebbard, L., George, J., and Ahlenstiel, G. (2019). The Role of Micronutrients in the Infection and Subsequent Response to Hepatitis C Virus. *Cells* 8 (6), 8. doi:10.3390/cells8060603

Jang, J. W., Choi, J. Y., Kim, Y. S., Woo, H. Y., Choi, S. K., Lee, C. H., et al. (2015). Long-term Effect of Antiviral Therapy on Disease Course after Decompensation in Patients with Hepatitis B Virus-Related Cirrhosis. *Hepatology* 61 (6), 1809–1820. doi:10.1002/hep.27723

K/DOQI clinical practice guidelines for chronic kidney disease: evaluation, classification, and stratification (2002). K/DOQI Clinical Practice Guidelines for Chronic Kidney Disease: Evaluation, Classification, and Stratification. *Am. J. Kidney Dis.* 39 (2 Suppl. 1), S1–S266.

Kamath, P. S., and Kim, W. R. (2007). The Model for End-Stage Liver Disease (MELD). *Hepatology* 45 (3), 797–805. doi:10.1002/hep.21563

Kim, H. M., Kim, B. S., Cho, Y. K., Kim, B. I., Sohn, C. I., Jeon, W. K., et al. (2013). Elevated Red Cell Distribution Width Is Associated with Advanced Fibrosis in NAFLD. *Clin. Mol. Hepatol.* 19 (3), 258–265. doi:10.3350/cmh.2013.19.3.258

Kloth, J. S. L., Hamberg, P., Mendelaar, P. A. J., Dulfer, R. R., van der Holt, B., Eechoute, K., et al. (2016). Macrocytosis as a Potential Parameter Associated with Survival after Tyrosine Kinase Inhibitor Treatment. *Eur. J. Cancer* 56, 101–106. doi:10.1016/j.ejca.2015.12.019

Lanier, J. B., Park, J. J., and Callahan, R. C. (2018). Anemia in Older Adults. *Am. Fam. Physician* 98 (7), 437–442.

Lee, J. Y., Fagan, K. A., Zhou, C., Batten, L., Cohen, M. V., and Stevens, T. (2020). Biventricular Diastolic Dysfunction, Thrombocytopenia, and Red Blood Cell Macrocytosis in Experimental Pulmonary Arterial Hypertension. *Pulm. Circ.* 10 (2), 2045894020908787. doi:10.1177/2045894020908787

Ma, Y. C., Zuo, L., Chen, J. H., Luo, Q., Yu, X. Q., Li, Y., et al. (2006). Modified Glomerular Filtration Rate Estimating Equation for Chinese Patients with Chronic Kidney Disease. *J. Am. Soc. Nephrol.* 17 (10), 2937–2944. doi:10.1681/asn.2006040368

McLean, E., Cogswell, M., Egli, I., Wojdyla, D., and de Benoist, B. (2009). Worldwide Prevalence of Anaemia, WHO Vitamin and Mineral Nutrition Information System, 1993-2005. *Public Health Nutr.* 12 (4), 444–454. doi:10.1017/s1368980008002401

Merion, R. M., Schaubel, D. E., Dykstra, D. M., Freeman, R. B., Port, F. K., and Wolfe, R. A. (2005). The Survival Benefit of Liver Transplantation. *Am. J. Transpl.* 5 (2), 307–313. doi:10.1111/j.1600-6143.2004.00703.x

Mohanty, J. G., Nagababu, E., and Rifkind, J. M. (2014). Red Blood Cell Oxidative Stress Impairs Oxygen Delivery and Induces Red Blood Cell Aging. *Front. Physiol.* 5, 84. doi:10.3389/fphys.2014.00084

Nguyen, M. H., Wong, G., Gane, E., Kao, J. H., and Dusheiko, G. (2020). Hepatitis B Virus: Advances in Prevention, Diagnosis, and Therapy. *Clin. Microbiol. Rev.* 33 (2). doi:10.1128/cmr.00046-19

Ohfuji, S., Matsuura, T., Tamori, A., Kubo, S., Sasaki, S., Kondo, K., et al. (2021). Lifestyles Associated with Prognosis after Eradication of Hepatitis C Virus: A

Prospective Cohort Study in Japan. *Dig. Dis. Sci.* 66 (6), 2118–2128. doi:10.1007/s10620-020-06475-0

Peng, C. Y., Chien, R. N., and Liaw, Y. F. (2012). Hepatitis B Virus-Related Decompensated Liver Cirrhosis: Benefits of Antiviral Therapy. *J. Hepatol.* 57 (2), 442–450. doi:10.1016/j.jhep.2012.02.033

Piano, S., Tonon, M., Vettore, E., Stanco, M., Pilutti, C., Romano, A., et al. (2017). Incidence, Predictors and Outcomes of Acute-On-Chronic Liver Failure in Outpatients with Cirrhosis. *J. Hepatol.* 67 (6), 1177–1184. doi:10.1016/j.jhep.2017.07.008

Remková, A., and Remko, M. (2009). Homocysteine and Endothelial Markers Are Increased in Patients with Chronic Liver Diseases. *Eur. J. Intern. Med.* 20 (5), 482–486. doi:10.1016/j.ejim.2009.03.002

Scheiner, B., Semmler, G., Maurer, F., Schwabl, P., Bucsics, T. A., Paternostro, R., et al. (2020). Prevalence of and Risk Factors for Anaemia in Patients with Advanced Chronic Liver Disease. *Liver Int.* 40 (1), 194–204. doi:10.1111/liv.14229

Schuppan, D., and Afdhal, N. H. (2008). Liver Cirrhosis. *Lancet* 371 (9615), 838–851. doi:10.1016/s0140-6736(08)60383-9

Skjelbakken, T., Lappegård, J., Ellingsen, T. S., Barrett-Connor, E., Brox, J., Løchen, M. L., et al. (2014). Red Cell Distribution Width Is Associated with Incident Myocardial Infarction in a General Population: the Tromsø Study. *J. Am. Heart Assoc.* 3 (4). e001109. doi:10.1161/jaha.114.001109

The guidelines of prevention and treatment for chronic hepatitis B 2019 version (2019). The Guidelines of Prevention and Treatment for Chronic Hepatitis B (2019 Version). *Zhonghua Gan Zang Bing Za Zhi* 27 (12), 938–961. doi:10.3760/cma.j.issn.1007-3418.2019.12.007

Tsantes, A. E., Bonovas, S., Travlou, A., and Sitaras, N. M. (2006). Redox Imbalance, Macrocytosis, and RBC Homeostasis. *Antioxid. Redox Signal.* 8 (7-8), 1205–1216. doi:10.1089/ars.2006.8.1205

Uchida, D., Takaki, A., Oyama, A., Adachi, T., Wada, N., Onishi, H., et al. (2020). Oxidative Stress Management in Chronic Liver Diseases and Hepatocellular Carcinoma. *Nutrients* 12 (6). 1576. doi:10.3390/nu12061576

Wiesner, R., Edwards, E., Freeman, R., Harper, A., Kim, R., Kamath, P., et al. (2003). Model for End-Stage Liver Disease (MELD) and Allocation of Donor Livers. *Gastroenterology* 124 (1), 91–96. doi:10.1053/gast.2003.50016

Xiao, J., Wang, F., Wong, N. K., He, J., Zhang, R., Sun, R., et al. (2019). Global Liver Disease Burdens and Research Trends: Analysis from a Chinese Perspective. *J. Hepatol.* 71 (1), 212–321. doi:10.1016/j.jhep.2019.03.004

Yang, J., Yan, B., Yang, L., Li, H., Fan, Y., Zhu, F., et al. (2018). Macrocytic Anemia Is Associated with the Severity of Liver Impairment in Patients with Hepatitis B Virus-Related Decompensated Cirrhosis: a Retrospective Cross-Sectional Study. *BMC Gastroenterol.* 18 (1), 161. doi:10.1186/s12876-018-0893-9

Yoon, H. J., Kim, K., Nam, Y. S., Yun, J. M., and Park, M. (2016). Mean Corpuscular Volume Levels and All-Cause and Liver Cancer Mortality. *Clin. Chem. Lab. Med.* 54 (7), 1247–1257. doi:10.1515/cclm-2015-0786

16

The Roles and Mechanisms of lncRNAs in Liver Fibrosis

Zhifa Wang[1†], Xiaoke Yang[2†], Siyu Gui[3†], Fan Yang[4†], Zhuo Cao[4], Rong Cheng[5], Xiaowei Xia[5] and Chuanying Li[5]*

[1]Department of Rehabilitation Medicine, Chaohu Hospital of Anhui Medical University, Hefei Anhui, China, [2]Department of Rheumatology and Immunology, The First Affiliated Hospital of Anhui Medical University, Hefei, China, [3]Department of Ophthalmology, The Second Affiliated Hospital of Anhui Medical University, Hefei, China, [4]The First Clinical Medical College, Anhui Medical University, Hefei, China, [5]Department of Gastroenterology, Anhui Provincial Children's Hospital, Hefei, China

*Correspondence:
Chuanying Li
lcy056500@hotmail.com

[†]*These authors have contributed equally to this work*

Long non-coding RNAs (lncRNAs) can potentially regulate all aspects of cellular activity including differentiation and development, metabolism, proliferation, apoptosis, and activation, and benefited from advances in transcriptomic and genomic research techniques and database management technologies, its functions and mechanisms in physiological and pathological states have been widely reported. Liver fibrosis is typically characterized by a reversible wound healing response, often accompanied by an excessive accumulation of extracellular matrix. In recent years, a range of lncRNAs have been investigated and found to be involved in several cellular-level regulatory processes as competing endogenous RNAs (ceRNAs) that play an important role in the development of liver fibrosis. A variety of lncRNAs have also been shown to contribute to the altered cell cycle, proliferation profile associated with the accelerated development of liver fibrosis. This review aims to discuss the functions and mechanisms of lncRNAs in the development and regression of liver fibrosis, to explore the major lncRNAs involved in the signaling pathways regulating liver fibrosis, to elucidate the mechanisms mediated by lncRNA dysregulation and to provide new diagnostic and therapeutic strategies for liver fibrosis.

Keywords: lncRNAs, liver fibrosis, ceRNAs, HSCs, therapeutic strategies

INTRODUCTION

Overview of Liver Fibrosis

As a globally important public health problem, liver fibrosis is typically characterized by a reversible wound healing response and an accompanying imbalance between increased synthesis and deposition and decreased degradation of extracellular matrix (ECM), resulting in programmed overaccumulation of ECM components (Nudelman et al., 1998; Aydin and Akcali, 2018). Numerous epidemiological studies have revealed the etiological role of various chronic liver diseases and associated liver injury-healing reactions in liver fibrosis, such as hepatitis (non-alcoholic

---

Abbreviations: AMPK, AMP-activated protein kinase; ncRNAs, non-coding RNAs; lncRNAs, Long non-coding RNAs; ceRNAs, competing endogenous RNAs; miRNAs, micro RNAs; ECM, extracellular matrix; NASH, non-alcoholic steatohepatitis; HSCs, hepatic stellate cells; Xist X, chromosome inactivation specific transcript; HULC, hepatocellular carcinoma; NEAT1, Nuclear paraspeckle assembly transcript 1; SNHG7, small nucleolar RNA host gene 7; MALAT1, metastasis-associated lung adenocarcinoma transcript; HOTTIP, HOXA transcript at the distal tip; TUG1, taurine upregulated gene 1; MEG3, maternally expressed gene 3.

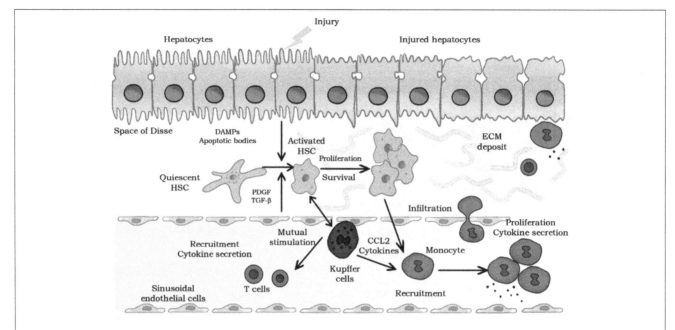

FIGURE 1 | Pathogenesis of liver fibrosis. The release of damage-related patterns (DAMPs). and apoptotic bodies can be induced by chronic hepatocyte injury, which activates hematopoietic stem cells and recruits immune cells. Moreover, the complex multidirectional interaction between activated hematopoietic stem cells and Kupffer cells and innate immune cells promotes transformation and differentiation into proliferation and ECM to generate myofibroblasts.

steatohepatitis (NASH), hepatitis B and C and so on) and biliary obstruction, which are closely associated with its progression (Parola and Pinzani, 2019). Mechanistic studies at the cellular level suggest that hepatic stellate cells (HSCs) located in the Disse space between hepatic sinusoidal endothelial cells and hepatic epithelial cells and maintaining a close interaction with both are the main sites for the production of ECM components (Geerts, 2001; Khomich et al., 2019), and furthermore, numerous studies have revealed that their intracellular lipid droplets, which are specific organelles for hepatic retinoic acid storage (Blaner et al., 2009; Elpek, 2014), could lead to liver disease disorders through efflux, depletion, and loss. undesirable progression (Yin et al., 2013; Ray, 2014; Krizhanovsky et al., 2008). Thus, studies on the activation mechanisms of hematopoietic stem cells are of great concern in proposing new therapies against hepatic fibrosis and in improving the original strategies (**Figure 1**).

Overview of LncRNAs

In recent years, numerous non-coding RNAs (ncRNAs) molecules have been identified benefiting from the application of RNA microarrays and next-generation transcriptome sequencing technologies, enabling humans to deepen their understanding of the pathophysiology of multiple diseases from a new perspective (Consortium et al., 2007). ncRNAs are well known for not encoding proteins at the RNA level but can perform as key regulators of multiple regulatory gene expression as well as cellular signaling pathways (Heo et al., 2019). NcRNAs are categorized according to their relative size into two types: small or short non-coding RNAs (miRNAs) of less than 200 nucleotides (nt) and long non-coding RNAs (lncRNAs) of greater than 200 nucleotides (Riaz and Li, 2019). The most prominently researched endogenous small ncRNAs,

known as miRNAs, mainly regulate the post-transcriptional levels of target genes by binding to the 3′ untranslated region (3′ UTR) of mRNAs, thus playing an important role in regulating the cell growth cycle as well as the expression of specific cell differentiation and cell death-related genes, lipid metabolism, and inflammatory responses. miRNAs have shown association with various liver diseases including liver fibrosis (Zhang CY. et al., 2016; Lan et al., 2018; Zhao et al., 2019).

As a novel ncRNAs, lncRNAs are predominantly transcribed by RNA polymerase II and exhibit multiple functions at the molecular level (**Figure 2**) (Ma et al., 2016b), the lncRNAs are classified according to their relative position on the chromosome to the coding gene as: 1. antisense lncRNAs, 2. intronic lncRNAs, 3. divergent lncRNAs, 4. intergenic lncRNAs, 5. promoter upstream lncRNAs, 6. promter-associated lncRNAs, 7. transcription start site-associated lncRNAs. LncRNAs regulate the expression of different genes based on their different cellular locations in multiple molecular mechanistic pathways including chromatin modification, transcriptional regulation, and post-transcriptional regulation (Zhang et al., 2014; Kopp and Mendell, 2018).

LncRNA Regulates DNA Methylation Modifications

Tsix inhibits Xist transcription by recruiting CTCF to the Xist promoter region, while JPx inhibits CTCF transcriptional repression of Xist by binding CTCC (CCCTC-binding factor); Khps1a participates in the T-DMR (tissue-dependent) region demethylation of Sphk1 by an unknown mechanism; Dum *cis*-recruits DNMT1, DNMT3A, DNMT3B, and etc. to the promoter region of the neighboring gene Dppa2. differentially methylated region) of Sphk1; Dum *cis*-recruits DNMT1, DNMT3A and

DNMT3B to the promoter region of the neighboring gene Dppa2 and causes silencing of methylation in this region, thereby suppressing Dppa2 expression and leading to differentiation of skeletal muscle myogenic cells into myoblasts (Guttman et al., 2011; Bian et al., 2019; He et al., 2020).

LncRNAs Are Involved in Pre-transcriptional Regulation

Xist (X chromosome inactivation specific transcript) and RepA (transcript of the adenine repeat region at the $5'$ end of the Xist gene) synergistically wrap the X chromosome and recruit PRC2 to establish H3K27me3 to cause X chromosome inactivation; Bxd (Bithoraxoid) binds to ubx-TRE (Ubx cis-regulatory trithorax response elements) and recruits ASH1 to activate Ubx transcription; HOTAIR regulates the expression of the HoxD gene cluster in trans by interacting with two histone modification complexes: catalytic PRC2 complex established by H3K27me3, and the LSD1-CoREST-REST complex catalyzing H3K4me2/3 erasure (lysine-specific demethylase1-RE1-Silencing Transcription factor corepressor 1-RE1 -Silencing Transcription factor complex); HOTTIP (HoxA transcript at the distal tip) recruits MLL (Mixed lineage) via WDR5 (WD repeat-containing protein 5) leukemia) to the $5'$ region of the HoxA gene cluster, which catalyzes the establishment of H3K4me3 and activates the expression of genes such as Hoxa11 and Hoxa13 in cis; Mira can form a DNA/RNA heterodimer with its locus and recruit MLL1, a member of the TrxG complex, which catalyzes the establishment of H3K4me3 and activates adjacent genes Hoxa6 and Hoxa7 expression, leading to differentiation of mES to the germline; Evf2 acts as a coactivator of DLX2 at high concentrations, enhancing Dlx5/6 enhancer activity and activating Dlx5 and Dlx6 transcription, while at low concentrations it can cis-suppress Dlx6 transcription through its Dlx6 antisense property, by recruiting MECP2, and thus HDAC Dlx5; asOct4-pg5 can recruit histone methyltransferases such as EZH2 and G9a to bind to the promoter regions of Oct4 and Oct4-pg5, establishing repressive chromatin modifications such as H3K27me3 and H3K9me3, which in turn repress transcription of Oct4 and Oct4-pg5, and when as Oct4-pg5 is combined with PURA (purine rich element binding protein A) and NCL (nucleolin), the ability to recruit EZH2 and G9a is lost and the repressive function is lost; the nascent ANRIL (antisense noncoding RNA in the INK4 locus) binds to CBX7 and ANRIL binds to CBX7 and promotes heterochromatin formation, while the formed ANRIL-CBX7 complex unbinds CBX7 to H3K27me3, leaving transcriptional repression in a dynamic state of flux. ANRIL recruits PRC2, allowing the INK4β/INK4α/ARF gene cluster to establish repressive modifications such as H3K27me3. ANRIL binds to SUZ12 and cis-represses INK4β transcription; DBE-T cis-recruits Ash1L to the 4q35 region, catalyzing the establishment of activating chromatin modifications such as H3K36me2, which activates gene transcription in the 4q35 region, ultimately leading to FSHD (facioscapulohumeral muscular dystrophy) disease (Guttman et al., 2011; Kopp and Mendell, 2018; Riaz and Li, 2019).

LncRNAs Are Involved in Transcriptional Regulation

Xite and DXPas34 regulate Tsix expression in cis with enhancer activity; transcription of SER3 gene biosynthesis-associated 3-phosphoglycerate dehydrogenase in the biosynthesis of serine is regulated by lncRNA SRG1 (SER3 regulatory gene 1); Pwr1 interferes with the transcription of Icr1; Icr1 interferes with the transcription of Fol11; DHFRtinc interferes with the transcription of DHFR; Airn interferes with the transcription of Igf2r; Gas5 inhibits the binding of activated GR to target genes (Zhang et al., 2014; Ma et al., 2016b).

LncRNAs Are Involved in Post-transcriptional Regulation

Malat1 regulates variable shear of Cat1 pre-mRNA; Zeb2-anti is involved in variable shear of Zed2; PTENpg1 asRNA β promotes PTENpg1 exit from the nucleus; Neat1 promotes retention of mRNA with IRAlus structure in the $3'$ UTR region within paraspeckles; BACE1-AS increases BACE1 stability; MDRL as ceRNA promotes pri-miR484 maturation (Bian et al., 2019; He et al., 2020).

It has been reported that lncRNAs are usually involved in the progression of human-related diseases by such ways as being deregulated (Guttman et al., 2011; He et al., 2020), and some studies have shown that lncRNAs are involved in the key process of liver fibrosis by acting as regulators of HSC activation (Wang et al., 2014; Bian et al., 2019). Even though we can observe an impressive amount of literature suggesting an important role of lncRNAs in the liver fibrosis process, it is undeniable that the detailed mechanisms of lncRNAs in liver fibrosis remain unclear until now. In this review, we aim to provide a review of the latest developments in lncRNAs research, elaborate on the interactions between lncRNAs and miRNAs, and further evaluate the potential of lncRNAs as new therapeutic targets in liver fibrosis.

THE REGULATORY ROLE OF LNCRNAS IN LIVER FIBROSIS

The distribution of lncRNAs in liver fibrosis has been detected by the latest high-throughput methods such as next-generation sequencing and microarrays (Zheng et al., 2015; Xiong et al., 2016), and the pleiotropic nature of lncRNAs has been demonstrated in the activation and apoptosis of HSCs and the progression of multiple liver fibrosis by interacting with molecules such as miRNAs, specific structural domains, and proteins to regulate key genes in liver fibrosis, thus exerting their potential (Bu et al., 2020). In this paper, we review the role of lncRNAs in liver fibrosis and their potential mechanisms in the development of liver fibrosis. **Table 1** provides a summary of the expression patterns, functional roles, and regulatory mechanisms of lncRNAs.

LncRNAs Involved in the Promotion of Liver Fibrosis
LncRNA HULC

Panzitt et al. identified for the first time the highly up-regulated hepatocellular carcinoma LncRNA (HULC) of approximately 500 nucleotides containing two exons located on chromosome

TABLE 1 | The expression of lncRNA in liver fibrosis.

lncRNAs	Expression	Role	Functional role	References
lncRNA NEAT1	Upregulated	Promotion of liver fibrosis	HSC activation, inflammatory response	Yu et al. (2017b); Ye et al. (2020)
lncRNA SNHG7	Upregulated	Promotion of liver fibrosis	HSC activation, autophagy and proliferation, survival, cell cycle	Yu et al. (2019); Xie et al. (2021)
lncRNA H19	Upregulated	Promotion of liver fibrosis	proliferation, activation, metabolism of lipid droplets, *trans*-differentiation	Song et al. (2017); Wang et al. (2020a)
lncRNA MALAT1	Upregulated	Promotion of liver fibrosis	HSC proliferation, cell cycle, and activation	Yu et al. (2015a); Wu et al. (2015)
lncRNA HOTTIP	Upregulated	Promotion of liver fibrosis	HSC cell proliferation and activation	Li et al. (2018a); Zheng et al. (2019)
lncRNA TUG1	Upregulated	Promotion of liver fibrosis	HSC activation	Han et al. (2018); Zhang et al. (2020a)
lncRNA HULC	Downregulated	Inhibition of liver fibrosis	Hepatic steatosis, inflammation, hepatocyte red lipid vesicles, HSC apoptosis	Shen et al. (2019a)
lincRNA-p21	Downregulated	Inhibition of liver fibrosis	HSC activation, proliferation, apoptosis	Yu et al. (2017c); Tu et al. (2017)
lncRNA MEG3	Downregulated	Inhibition of liver fibrosis	HSC activation, proliferation, EMT	Yu et al. (2018); Chen et al. (2019)
lncRNA GAS5	Downregulated	Inhibition of liver fibrosis	HSC activation, EMT	Yu et al. (2015b); Dong et al. (2019a)

6p24.3 as the most highly expressed lncRNA in human hepatocellular carcinoma, whose transcribed RNA does not have a considerable open reading frame nor does it produce any protein (Panzitt et al., 2007). The HULC promoter and its first exon are in a long terminal repeat sequence (LTR) retrotransposon-like sequence (Kapusta et al., 2013). The upregulation trend of HULC can be observed in all accessible studies on hepatocellular carcinoma (HCC) (Chen et al., 2017; Xin et al., 2018; Ghafouri-Fard et al., 2020b). Several literatures have reported that HULC is upregulated in cancer and is regulated as an oncogene lncRNA in tumorigenesis and progression (Kitagawa et al., 2013; Parasramka et al., 2016). Considering its high expression in HCC cells, previous studies have also shown the potential of HULC as a novel antitumor therapeutic agent (Klec et al., 2019). cAMP response element binding protein (CREB) is usually bound to and activated by the target promoter (Mayr and Montminy, 2001; Kong et al., 2016), and Wang et al. demonstrated the presence of CREB binding sites in the HULC promoter region and the ability to further activate the HULC promoter (Wang et al., 2010), which can affect the expression of HULC at the transcriptional level (Shen X. et al., 2019). Shen et al. revealed the role of lncRNA HULC in the progression of liver fibrosis in rats with nonalcoholic fatty liver disease (NFALD) and that inhibition of HULC suppressed steatosis. The degree of hepatic steatosis, inflammation, hepatocyte red lipid vesicles and apoptosis were also significantly reduced with the knockdown of HULC gene. Inhibition of HULC significantly reduced liver fibrosis scores and liver fibrosis indices (HA, LN, PC III, and IV-C) (Shen X. et al., 2019). Inhibition of HULC improved liver fibrosis and reduced hepatocyte apoptosis in NAFLD rats. In general, the above findings not only provide valuable candidate molecular markers for liver fibrosis and indicators of advanced liver fibrosis but also provide new insights into the role of lncRNA in the biology of cancer.

LncRNA Nuclear Paraspeckle Assembly Transcript 1

Nuclear paraspeckle assembly transcript 1 (NEAT1) was characterized as an unusual RNA polymerase II transcript that

lacks introns and accompanied by non-canonical processing of the non-polyadenylated 3′-end by RNase P (Ding et al., 2019). NEAT1 was found to be upregulated in gastric adenocarcinoma and human laryngeal squamous cell carcinoma (Ma et al., 2016a; Wang et al., 2016), which suggested that it promotes tumor development by promoting cell proliferation and survival as well as inhibiting apoptosis (Choudhry et al., 2015). A similar situation has been observed in hepatocellular carcinoma (Guo et al., 2015). Yu et al. examined NEAT1 expression in cCl4-induced mice. qRT-PCR analysis showed increased expression of NEAT1 in CCl4-treated livers compared to control livers, and a significant increase in NEAT1 expression in HSCs was also observed during different weeks of CCl4 treatment (Yu et al., 2017b), Huang et al. screened the aberrantly expressed microRNAs in the CCl4-induced mouse liver fibrosis model by analyzing the GSE77271 microRNA microarray based on the Agilent-046065 mouse miRNA V19.0 platform. Neat1 simultaneously targeted miR-148a-3p and miR-22-3p, and showed the most significant increase in liver fibrosis mice that displayed the most marked increase in expression upregulation, and its expression in the CCl4 group exceeded 2-fold that of the control group (Huang et al., 2021), and inhibition of NEAT1 was observed to reverse isotropic liver fibrosis with concomitant reduction in α-SMA and type I collagen content, which was further confirmed by NEAT1 knockdown assays and NEAT1 overexpression assays (Yu et al., 2017b). A similar situation was confirmed in the alcoholic steatohepatitis (ASH) assay by Ye et al. (Ye et al., 2020). Inhibition of NEAT1 suppressed ethanol-stimulated elevated lipid metabolism and inhibited inflammatory responses in AML-12 cells. More importantly, inhibition of NEAT1 upregulated ethanol-induced hepatic function in ASH mice and inhibited lipid, inflammatory responses, hepatocyte apoptosis, and hepatic fibrosis, demonstrating that knockdown of NEAT1 inhibited hepatic fibrosis in ASH mice and thus slowed down the development of ASH (Ye et al., 2020). Related mechanistic studies suggest that Kruppel-like factor 6 (KLF6), as an important pro-fibrotic gene, is involved in the regulation of liver fibrosis by NEAT1 (Yu et al., 2017b), and that NEAT1 overexpression induces KLF6 mRNA and protein expression. However, it is of interest that KLF6 knockdown experiments showed NEAT1-induced proliferation of HSC, while KLF6 siRNA blocked NEAT1-induced α-SMA and type I collagen production, suggesting that NEAT1 could mediate HSC activation through KLF6 (Yu et al., 2017b). Huang et al. suggested that NEAT1 knockdown could inhibit the process of liver fibrosis and HSCs activation by regulating the expression of a cellular adhesion element 3 (Cyth3) associated with allosteric insulin signaling in mammals (Jux et al., 2019; Huang et al., 2021). And Ye et al. further identified that downregulation of NEAT1 could limit the inflammatory response and liver fibrosis in ASH mice by reducing suppressor of cytokine signaling 2 (SOCS2) (Ye et al., 2020), which is a feedback inhibitor of the growth hormone/insulin-like growth factor axis (Monti-Rocha et al., 2018).

LncRNA Small Nucleolar RNA Host Gene 7

It was first reported by Chaudhry in 2013 that a new full-length 2,176 bp oncogenic lncRNA, known as lncRNA small nucleolar rna host gene 7 (SNHG7), expressed in lymphoblastoid cell lines TK6 and WTK1 (Chaudhry, 2013), which is located on chromosome 9q34.3. Recent studies have shown a significant increase in its expression in tumor cells of digestive system, breast, and prostate (Wu F. et al., 2020; Wu X. et al., 2020), and further studies have demonstrated that SNHG7 is widely involved in the proliferation, invasion and migration of various tumor cells (Xia et al., 2020), including its regulation in the progression of HCC and liver fibrosis (Cui et al., 2017). Just as Xie et al. found increased expression of SNHG7 in primary HSC mice as well liver fibrosis, suggesting its regulation of HSC activation (Xie et al., 2021), and SNHG7 knockdown experiments showed decreased expression levels of α-SMA and Col. I (Xie et al., 2021), similarly SNHG7 inhibition was associated with reduced survival and proliferation rates in liver fibrosis mice. Current studies have identified several types of high confidence indicators of autophagy, such as the cytoplasmic form of LC3, a key protein in autophagosome formation (LC3-I), the active membrane-bound form of LC3 (LC3-II), and Beclin1 (Wirawan et al., 2012; Alirezaei et al., 2015; Dodson et al., 2017; Feng et al., 2017). Xie et al. revealed that knockdown of SNHG7 could reduce the decrease the expression level of Beclin1, LC3-II and LC3-I ratio, demonstrating the inhibitory effect of SNHG7 knockdown on HSC autophagy (Xie et al., 2021). DNMT3A induces a DNMT-regulated DNA ab initio methylation process, and DNA methylation/hydroxy methylation, a key step in HSC activation and liver fibrosis development, can be inhibited by activation of DNMT3A expression in HSCs (Garzon et al., 2009; Page et al., 2016). Several recent mechanistic studies suggest that SNHG7 knockdown is significantly associated with low expression levels of DNMT3A. These results confirm the relationship between SNHG7 and DNMT3A, which are novel regulators of HSC activation, autophagy, and proliferation in liver fibrosis (Xie et al., 2021). Yu et al. identified a positive correlation between SNHG7 levels and type I collagen mRNA levels in patients with cirrhosis (Yu et al., 2017b). In addition, SNHG7 showed a significant association in regulating activated HSCs

proliferation and the cell cycle associated with increased G0/G1 phase cells and decreased S phase cells. SNHG7 knockdown experiments performed in activated HSCs inhibited type I collagen expression (Yu et al., 2017b), as well as collagen deposition and hydroxyproline due to carbon tetrachloride were similarly blocked by silencing of SNHG7 in vivo, suggesting that inhibition of liver fibrosis can be mediated by downregulation of SNHG7 (Yu et al., 2017b). Furthermore, Yu et al. demonstrated at the mechanistic level the role of SNHG7 in regulating the expression level of irregular fragment polarity protein 2 (DVL2) (Yu et al., 2017b; Nielsen et al., 2019), which was positively correlated with DVL2, the deletion of which also blocked its effect on HSCs activation (Yu et al., 2017b). In conclusion, all these data suggest that SNHG7 is an impressive possible therapeutic target and a potential diagnostic marker for liver fibrosis.

LncRNA H19

LncRNA H19 is expressed only by the maternal allele 11p15.5, which can encode 2.3 kb RNA and is transcribed by RNA polymerase II (Gabory et al., 2006), splicing and polyadenylation (Ghafouri-Fard et al., 2020a). It is exported from the nucleus to the cytoplasm, adjacent to the insulin-like growth factor 2 (IGF2) gene, and they are expressed from the maternal and paternal genetic chromosomes, respectively (Raveh et al., 2015; Wang J. et al., 2020). H19 RNA molecules have now been observed to be present in the cytoplasm at much higher levels than in the nucleus. H19 plays an essential role in biological processes such as apoptosis, angiogenesis, inflammation and cell death through regulatory RNA or ribosomal regulators (Yoshimura et al., 2018). This includes the regulation of proliferation, invasion, and metastasis processes in a variety of tumors of the digestive system (Zhou et al., 2017; Wei LQ. et al., 2019). Multiple complex mechanisms have been demonstrated in different cancers (Zhang D. M. et al., 2017; Zhou et al., 2017). Of interest is the upregulation of the level of intracellular transcripts (Zhu et al., 2019) and extracellular exosomes (Li X. et al., 2018), known as lncRNA-H19, observed in activated HSCs, which is thought to be associated with HSCs-activated metabolic processes like lipid (Liu et al., 2018) and cholesterol metabolism (Xiao et al., 2019). Previous research concluded that the level of fibrosis in the liver was positively correlated with the level of H19, and that H19 knockdown attenuated Bcl-2-induced liver injury (Zhang Y. et al., 2016), while conversely H19 overexpression significantly exacerbated the process of HSCs and EMT activation in hepatocytes (Zhu et al., 2019). Song et al. demonstrated the overexpression of H19 in bile duct ligation (BDL)-induced liver fibrosis with abnormal liver function parameters (Song et al., 2017), and identified a new downstream target gene of ZEB1, called EpCAM (Song et al., 2017), which promotes cholestatic liver fibrosis by interacting with the ZEB1 protein to prevent its binding to the EpCAM promoter and thus the inhibitory effect of ZEB1 (Song et al., 2017). Liu et al. reported that cholangiocyte-derived exosomal H19 promotes cholestatic liver injury in Mdr2$^{-/-}$ mice and promotes HSCs transdifferentiation and activation, along with upregulation of fibrotic gene expression in HSCs-derived fibroblasts (Liu et al.,

2019). Wang et al. discovered that H19 can promote RARα and RXRβ mRNA and protein synthesis (Wang ZM. et al., 2020), and its reduced expression reversed the extent of HSCs activation induced due to increased retinoic acid signaling. Meanwhile, it should be mentioned that H19 knockdown-mediated HSCs inactivation was inhibited by the activation of retinoic acid signaling. Furthermore, they demonstrated that H19 enhancement was positively associated with a synergistic increase in retinoic acid metabolism during HSCs activation (Wang ZM. et al., 2020). More significantly, they confirmed that inhibition of ethanol dehydrogenase III (ADH3) completely abolished the effect of H19-mediated retinoic acid signaling, and that dihydroartemisinin (DHA), a natural inhibitor of H19, reduced both H19 and ADH3 expression and thus inhibited HSC activation (Wang ZM. et al., 2020). Taken together, these results reveal some of the molecular mechanisms underlying the increase in retinoic acid signaling during HSCs activation and suggest that the lncRNA-H19/ADH3 pathway is a potential target for the treatment of liver fibrosis. Similarly, H19 expression levels were increased in CCl4-induced fibrotic liver thereby activating HSCs (Wang Z. et al., 2020). Further studies revealed the role of hypoxia-inducible factor-1α (HIF-1α) in promoting H19 expression by binding to the H19 promoter at two hypoxia response element (HRE) sites located at 492–499 and 515–522 bp (Wang Z. et al., 2020). H19 knockdown experiments also resulted in significant inhibition of HSC activation and attenuated liver fibrosis, suggesting that lncRNAH19 may be a potential target for antifibrotic therapeutic approaches. Moreover, the H19 silencing assay reduced the degree of lipid oxidation and the H19 knockdown assay restored the levels of lipid droplets, triglycerides, cholesteryl esters and retinyl esters in HSCs without changes in lipid uptake and synthesis (Wang Z. et al., 2020). In conclusion, as described above, the results highlight the role of H19 in the proliferation, activation and metabolism of lipid droplets in HSCs and reveal its feasibility as a new molecular target to attenuate liver fibrosis.

LncRNA Metastasis-Associated Lung Adenocarcinoma Transcript1

Ji et al. characterized a metastasis-associated lung adenocarcinoma transcript (MALAT1) transcribed by RNA polymerase II located on human chromosome 11q13 and mouse chromosome 19qA (Zhang et al., 2012; Wilusz, 2016), which is widely known for its properties in predicting early NSCLC metastasis and survival (Ji et al., 2003), the major transcript of MALAT1 is approximately mid-8 kb in humans and 6.7 kb in mice (Wilusz et al., 2008). MALAT1-associated small cytoplasmic RNA (mascRNA) is a larger fragment of approximately 6.7 kb and a smaller fragment of 61 nucleotides produced by the action of ribonuclease P and ribonuclease Z on MALAT1 (Brown et al., 2014), while the larger fragment or mature transcript is highly stable due to a unique triple-helix structure at the $3'$ end that protects it from nucleic acid exonucleases (Zhang et al., 2012). The highly conserved and widespread expression of MALAT1 in mammalian tissues and cancers implies its functional importance; MALAT-1 dysregulation in a variety of cancers has been extensively

studied. In most cases, it functions as a promoting role in the development of different types of tumors (Kim et al., 2018; Feng et al., 2019). MALAT1 upregulation is closely associated with the development of cancers such as lung (Wei S. et al., 2019), glioblastoma (Voce et al., 2019), esophageal squamous cell carcinoma (Chen M. et al., 2018), renal cell carcinoma (Zhang H. et al., 2019), colorectal cancer (Zhang H. et al., 2019; Xie et al., 2019), osteosarcoma (Chen Y. et al., 2018), multiple myeloma (Amodio et al., 2018), gastric cancer (Zhang YF. et al., 2020), gallbladder cancer (Lin et al., 2019), and other cancers (Tian and Xu, 2015), as well as other clinicopathological features including tumor location, tumor size, differentiation and tumor stage (Goyal et al., 2021). Numerous studies have shown that as a biomarker for tumor diagnosis and prognosis, the abnormal expression of MALAT1 in tumor tissues and/or body fluids is highly indicative (Leti et al., 2017; Peng et al., 2018). In a physical and functional interaction study with the liver fibrosis process, Yu et al. found that MALAT1 expression was significantly upregulated in fibrotic liver tissues and simultaneously activated HSCs (Yu et al., 2015a), while silencing MALAT1 suppressed the mRNA levels of α-SMA and Col.I and downregulated the protein levels of α-SMA and collagen type I in HSC respectively (Yu et al., 2015a). Sirius red staining of collagen in mouse liver tissue resulted in the observation that mice transduced by silencing MALAT1 showed a 54% downregulation of collagen accumulation compared to CCl4-treated mice (Yu et al., 2015a), reflecting the role of MALAT1 in accelerating the progression of liver fibrosis in vivo. Dai et al. used arsenite treatment of L-02 cells as well as co-culture of LX-2 cells and found that MALAT1 expression levels increased as well as co-culture promoting activation of LX-2 cells (Dai et al., 2019). They further discovered that MALAT1 levels were increased in exosomes of arsenite-treated L-02 cells and LX-2 cells exposed to exosomes from arsenite-treated L-02 cells (Dai et al., 2019), and these exosomes also promoted LX-2 cell activation; blocking MALAT1 expression simultaneously inhibited these changes, thus suggesting a mechanism by which MALAT1 induces LX-2 cell activation via exosomes. Silent information regulator 1 (SIRT1), as a member of the mammalian sirtuin family of proteins (SIRT1-SIRT7) (Dai et al., 2019), is homologous to the yeast Sir2 protein, and SIRT1 is involved in a variety of biological processes and exhibits multiple physiological functions through the deacetylation of many non-histone proteins (Houtkooper et al., 2012). Wu et al. verified the important role of SIRT1 in hepatic stellate cell activation and reversal and its overexpression countering TGF-β1-induced LX-2 cell activation (Wu et al., 2015), suggesting its potential as an alternative for the treatment of liver fibrosis. Further studies found that the evolutionarily highly conserved MALAT1 has a strong tendency to interact with SIRT1 (discriminatory power 100%) (Wu et al., 2015), which was verified in CCL4-treated mice and LX-2 cells exposed to TGF-β1, considering that the expression level of MALAT1 mRNA was significantly upregulated and accompanied by negative changes in SIRT1 protein (Wu et al., 2015). MALAT1 silencing assay yielded results that eliminated the TGF-β1-induced upregulation of myofibroblast markers and the downregulation of SIRT1 protein. These phenomena suggest a role for MALAT1 in mediating the expression as well as the function of SIRT1 in regulating liver fibrosis. In conclusion, these findings highlight the role of MALAT1 in liver fibrosis and suggest a mechanism for fibrosis development (Wu et al., 2015). However, future efforts should be devoted to elucidating other regulatory mechanisms and clinical implications of MALAT1 in liver fibrosis.

LncRNA HOXA Transcript at the Distal Tip

HOXA transcript at the distal tip (HOTTIP) is a functionally characterized lncRNA (Li et al., 2016). Wang et al. demonstrated that the HOTTIP gene is located at chromosomal locus 7p15.2 and encodes a 4665 bp transcript (Wang et al., 2011). Its function is to directly interact with the Trithorax protein WDR5 and induce open DNA chromatin conformation, target the WDR5/MLL complex and drive histone H3 lysine 4 trimethylation for transcriptional regulation of the 50-terminal HOXA locus gene (Wang et al., 2011). This suggests that HOTTIP is not only involved in developmental processes but also enhances the effect of this lncRNA as a cancer-associated lncRNA considering its role as a signaling transmitter from higher-order chromosome conformation to chromatin coding (Wang et al., 2011). Overall survival (OS), distant metastasis (DM), lymph node metastasis (LNM), and tumor staging of human tumors have been extensively studied and determined to be closely associated with HOTTIP expression, suggesting that HOTTIP expression may influence the prognosis and metastasis of several human cancers (Broerse and Crassini, 1984; Quagliata et al., 2014). The most representative case is the high HOTTIP expression in human HCC specimens (Quagliata et al., 2014) and its close correlation with clinical progression and disease outcome (Tsang et al., 2015). It is worth mentioning that HOTTIP has long been shown to be dysregulated in the early stages of hepatocellular carcinoma formation, and recent studies suggest a positive correlation between its expression and liver fibrosis progression (Yang et al., 2019; He et al., 2020). Zheng et al. verified the specific expression status of HOTTIP in liver fibrotic tissue and primary quiescent HSC (Zheng et al., 2019), and their qRT-PCR results showed a 22.6-fold increase in HOTTIP expression on day 10 compared to day 2 increased 22.6-fold, similar to the results from the group of oil-treated mice compared to the group of CCl$_4$-treated mice suggesting a significant upregulation of HOTTIP expression in HSCs however this phenomenon was not observed in hepatocytes (Zheng et al., 2019). Furthermore, the mRNA and protein levels of α-SMA and Col. I was also found to be reduced by hot-end silencing but Edu incorporation assay demonstrated that hot-end downregulation inhibited the proliferation of activated HSCs. The above results suggest that HOTTIP downregulation could inhibit HSCs activation and proliferation. Related mechanistic studies suggest that HOTTIP is a target of miR-150 and is also recruited to Ago2-associated miRNPs (Zheng et al., 2019), possibly acting through miR-150 association. In addition, bioinformatics analysis and luciferase analysis of a series of experiments also confirmed the role of serum response factor (SRF) as a target of miR-150. They further demonstrated that the inhibition of HSCs activation was caused by an increase in SRF

mRNA expression due to HOTTIP overexpression (Zheng et al., 2019). Li et al. revealed that HOTTIP expression was significantly upregulated in fibrotic and cirrhotic liver samples, with the highest in cirrhotic samples (Li Z. et al., 2018), and this was also found in liver fibrotic tissue, primary HSC and activated LX-2 cells. Inhibition of HOTTIP at the mRNA and protein levels was effective in reducing the expression of α- SMA and Col. I. They found that downregulation of HOTTIP attenuated CCl$_4$-induced liver fibrosis in mice. In contrast, the relative survival of HSC in LX-2 cells and the mRNA and protein levels of α-SMA and Col. I were significantly reduced by HOTTIP knockdown (Li Z. et al., 2018). Li et al. proposed a possible mechanism to promote HSC activation, i.e., negative regulation of HOTTIP mediated by miR-148a, considering that TGFBR1 and TGFBR2 were identified as miR-148a novel targets in HSCs. TGFBR1 and TGFBR2 levels were increased by high levels of HOTTIP, which led to the progression of liver fibrosis (Li Z. et al., 2018). These results highlight the potential of the HOTTIP/miR-148a/TGFBR1/TGFBR2 axis as a potential marker and target in patients with liver fibrosis. In conclusion, HOTTIP promotes HSCs cell proliferation and activation suggesting its possible role as a fibrogenic gene in liver fibrosis and plays a key role as a prognostic marker and novel therapeutic target. However, these still need to be investigated further.

LncRNA Taurine Upregulated Gene 1

The 7,598 nucleotide lncRNA sequence localized on chromosome 22q12.2, also known as taurine upregulated gene 1 (TUG1), was initially identified in a genomic screen of taurine-treated mouse retinal cells (Young et al., 2005; Zhang et al., 2013). Functional studies in mice further demonstrated that knockdown of TUG1 inhibits retinal developmental processes (Khalil et al., 2009). Khalil et al. demonstrated by whole genome RNA immunoprecipitation analysis that approximately 20% of lncRNAs (including TUG1) with methyltransferase activity promote demethylation and trimethylation of lysine residue 27 of histone 3 (H3K27me3) in the target gene and inhibit its expression by binding to polyclonal repressor complex 2 (PRC2), which inhibits its expression (van Kruijsbergen et al., 2015). Besides other PRC2-associated lncRNAs involved in tumorigenesis and progression, TUG1 regulates the biological behavior and molecular mechanisms of different cancer cells, including cell proliferation, invasion, apoptosis, differentiation, migration, drug resistance, radiation resistance, angiogenesis, mitochondrial bioenergetics, epithelial-mesenchymal transition (EMT), and regulation of blood-tumor barrier permeability among other different cancer cell (Niland et al., 2012; Katsushima et al., 2016; Cai et al., 2017; Chiu et al., 2018). TUG1 is closely associated with the mediation of radio resistance and angiogenesis in hepatoblastoma (Dong et al., 2016). TUG1 has also been extensively studied in liver diseases such as cirrhosis and liver fibrosis. Zhang et al. demonstrated that TUG1 is highly expressed in liver sinusoidal endothelial cells (LSEC), and the results of TUG1 knockdown experiments revealed inhibition of the extent of expression of autophagy and EMT-related genes (Zhang R. et al., 2020). In contrast, knockdown of TUG1 eliminated the most significant increase in autophagy-related genes in LPS-treated LSEC under starvation. The increase in ATG5 expression while inhibition of ATG5 attenuated autophagy and EMT (Zhang R. et al., 2020). Han et al. demonstrated that TUG1 was overexpressed in liver samples from patients with CCl4 and BDL-induced liver fibrosis *in vivo* as well as cirrhosis and activated HSCs while promoting a degree of expression of SMA, Col1a1, Mmp2/9/10, and Timp1. The possibility that TUG1 accelerates the progression of liver fibrosis by promoting the expression of these pro-fibrotic genes through downregulation of miR-29b is mechanistically argued (Han et al., 2018). Collectively, these studies revealed the mechanisms of TUG1 play a crucial role in liver fibrosis, suggesting its ability to monitor human liver fibrosis and its potential to be a candidate biomarker for new therapeutic strategies.

LncRNAs Involved in the Inhibition of Liver Fibrosis
Long Intergenic Non-Coding RNA p21

LincRNA-p21 (long intergenic non-coding RNA p21) localized at human chromosome 6p21.2 situated approximately 15 kb upstream of the cell cycle regulatory gene p21/Cdkn1a and approximately 3.0 kb in length has been described as an inducer of p53-dependent apoptosis in mouse embryonic fibroblasts (Huarte et al., 2010). lincRNA-p21 is available in two types both containing an exon and an Alu isoforms with a reverse repeat element (Yoon et al., 2012a; Yoon et al., 2012b; Wilusz and Wilusz, 2012). Coordinates the degree of autoregulation and expression of its target transcripts by interacting with RNA-binding proteins, miRNA, and mRNA targets (Yoon et al., 2012a). As a transcriptional target of p53 it is involved in the p53 pathway, downregulating many p53 target genes and triggering the apoptotic process by physically interacting with the p53 repressor complex (Fatica and Bozzoni, 2014). lincRNA-p21 has also been reported to regulate gene expression by directing protein binding partners in chromatin localization and thus directly binding to target mRNAs to act as a translational repressor and thus by activating p21 in cis participate in the regulation of the G1/S checkpoint (Dimitrova et al., 2014). It is also noteworthy that it can feedback regulate p53 activity by regulating the interaction of p53, p300, and MDM2 (Wu et al., 2014; Tang et al., 2015), thus participating in different tumorigenesis including hepatocellular carcinoma (Jia et al., 2016). In terms of tumor invasion lincRNA-p21 overexpression can be inhibited by Notch pathway (Wang et al., 2017). Besides it plays a key regulatory role in DNA damage response, apoptosis, and cell proliferation among other different processes (Ozgur et al., 2013). Zheng et al. observed in animal experiments that lincRNA-p21 expression was downregulated in liver fibrosis (Zheng et al., 2015). lincRNA-p21 was negatively correlated with disease progression and HSCs activation status, while *in vitro* and *in vivo* distribution inhibited HSCs activation and reduced liver fibrosis progression. Notably the reversibility of the inhibitory effect of lincRNA-p21 was confirmed by the removal of lincRNA-p21 leading to classical morphological changes associated with HSCs activation. lincRNA-p21 was

found by Zhang et al. to inhibit the cell cycle and proliferation of primary HSCs by enhancing p21 (Zheng et al., 2015), while Tu et al. found a significant increase in hepatocyte lincRNA-p21 expression during hepatic fibrosis (Tu et al., 2017). These suggest that lincRNA-p21 contributes to a positive role in hepatocyte apoptosis and inhibition of hepatocyte growth in fibrotic livers. Knockdown of hepatocyte lincRNA-p21 attenuated CCl4-induced hepatocyte apoptosis thereby reducing CCl4-induced inflammatory cell infiltration and secretion levels of pro-inflammatory and pro-fibrotic cytokines in the fibrotic liver. Mechanistic studies have shown that inhibition of miR-30 impairs the effect of lincRNA-p21 in the development of liver fibrosis (Tu et al., 2017). lincRNA-p21/miR-30 axis has been highlighted as a potential marker and target for patients with liver fibrosis. Yang et al. found that lincRNA-p21 overexpression promotes hepatocyte apoptosis, but its results can be blocked by thymosin β4 (Tβ4) blocked, and additionally Tβ4 reversed lincRNA-p21- induced cleavage of caspase-3 and caspase-9 levels (Tu et al., 2017). LincRNA-p21 overexpression increases the levels of fibrosis-associated proteins (type I collagen, α- SMA, and TIMP-1) and induces hydroxyproline and ALT production leading to pathological damage of liver tissue and progression of fibrosis. The potential utility of lincRNA-p21 in predicting cirrhosis is supported by the results of downregulation of serum lincRNA-p21 levels in cirrhotic patients (Yang L. et al., 2020). Yu et al. reported a decrease in serum lincRNA-p21 levels in patients with chronic hepatitis B that negatively correlated with the stage of liver fibrosis, thus revealing its diagnostic value (Yu et al., 2017c). There was also a negative correlation between serum lincRNA-p21 levels and markers of liver fibrosis (including α-SMA and Col. I) but not in markers of viral replication, liver inflammatory activity and liver function. The primary HSC culture results suggested that the deletion of lincRNA-p21 expression was associated with promoter methylation, and these conditions implied the potential of serum lincRNA-p21 as a potential biomarker of liver fibrosis in patients with chronic hepatitis B/cirrhosis. Promoter methylation may be involved in the downregulation of lincRNA-p21 in liver fibrosis (Yu et al., 2017c). Collectively, these findings demonstrate the ability of lincRNA-p21 to act as a mediator of HSCs activation and proliferation, suggesting its potential as a new therapeutic target for liver fibrosis.

LncRNA Maternally Expressed Gene 3

The maternally expressed gene 3 (MEG3), located within the human chromosome 14q32.3 DLK1-MEG3 locus (Wylie et al., 2000), is 35 kb in size consisting of 10 exons (Zhou et al., 2012) and encodes an approximately 1.6 kb long non-coding RNA as a contained 10 exons (Zhang et al., 2010). Selectively spliced transcripts of Gtl2 (gene trap site 2 (Gtl2) is the mouse homolog of human MEG3) extend to contain intron-encoded C/D box SNORNAs and miRNAs, suggesting that Gtl2 may function as a host gene for these small RNAs (Cavaille et al., 2002; Lin et al., 2003; Tierling et al., 2006). MEG3 can be observed in unimprinted embryonic cells to silence genes involved in neurogenesis by regulating the chromatin targeting of multicomb proteins and plays an important role in neuronal development (Mercer et al., 2008; Kaneko et al., 2014; Mondal et al., 2015). Recent studies have suggested that MEG3 may act as a tumor suppressor considering the extent to which its loss of expression in several cancers is associated with inhibition of cell proliferation (Ghafouri-Fard and Taheri, 2019). Yu et al. showed that the process of liver fibrosis is accompanied by a decrease in MEG3 *in vivo* and *in vitro* and that restoration of MEG3 expression inhibits liver fibrosis while reducing α-SMA and type I collagen production (Yu et al., 2018). MEG3 overexpression inhibits HSC activation through EMT and is associated with E-calcium activation. The Hedgehog (Hh) pathway is one of the pathways involved in HSC activation by MEG3 as an EMT process. Smoothing (SMO) plays an important role in the Hh pathway. Bioinformatics analysis, RNA immunoprecipitation and deletion mapping results suggest that the interaction between MEG3 and SMO is involved in EMT repression caused by MEG3 overexpression (Yu et al., 2018). Gene expression in the DLK1-MEG3 region is controlled by two differentially methylated regions (DMRs) consisting of multiple methylated CpG sites located approximately 13 kb upstream of the MEG3 transcription start site intergenic DMR (IG-DMR) and overlaps with a 1.5-kb upstream promoter in the post-fertilization-derived secondary (MEG3-DMR) (Murphy et al., 2003), indicating the important role that DNA methylation plays in silencing the MGE3 gene (Anwar et al., 2012). The most widely studied epigenetic modification, DNA methylation and its relevance to the pathogenesis of liver fibrosis have been well established experimentally (Benetatos et al., 2008; Li et al., 2010), and previous studies have suggested a role for DNA methylation in the deletion of MEG3 expression in tumors (Zhao et al., 2005; Benetatos et al., 2008). He et al. revealed that MEG3 levels were significantly reduced in CCl4-induced liver fibrosis in mice and humans, while MSP was significantly reduced in CCl4-treated mouse liver tissue and human liver fibrosis tissue and TGF-β1-treated LX-2 cells where MEG3 promoter methylation was observed (He et al., 2014). The effect of 5-azadC to block MEG3 methylation could be achieved by the methylation inhibitor 5-azadC significantly eliminating TGF-β1-induced aberrant MEG3 hypermethylation and restoring MEG3 in TGF-β1-treated LX-2 cells thereby inhibiting HSC activation and proliferation expression illustration (He et al., 2014). The inhibition of activation and the degree of proliferation of LX-2 cells and the reversal of methylation of the MEG3 promoter were both closely associated with the deletion of DNMT1 thereby restoring MEG3 expression. While 5-azadC treatment or knockdown of DNMT1 downregulated mRNA and protein production of α-SMA and Col. I in TGF-β1-treated LX-2 cells, overexpression of MEG3 was detected in TGF-β1-treated LX-2 cells (He et al., 2014), which significantly activated p53 protein levels and induced a Bax/Bcl-2 ratio accompanied by a significant increase in cytoplasmic cytochrome c significantly increased. These suggest that the p53-dependent mitochondrial apoptotic pathway is partially involved in the MEG3-induced apoptosis process (He et al., 2014). In conclusion, these findings demonstrate that MEG3 may play an important role in stellate cell activation and liver fibrosis

progression and presents as a new potential treatment target for liver fibrosis.

LncRNA GAS5

Situated at 1q25 and composed of 12 exons, GAS5 was originally identified from a subtractive cDNA library, named according to the increased level of expression found in mammalian cells at growth arrest (Sun et al., 2017). Its exons are selectively spliced to produce two possible mature lncRNAs: GAS5a and GAS5b (Li J. et al., 2018) and 11 introns responsible for encoding 10 cassettes of C/D small nucleolar RNA (snoRNA) (Ni et al., 2019). Sequence similarity to the hormone receptor element of the glucocorticoid receptor (GR) in terms of function inhibits the effect of GR on its target gene expression (Zhong et al., 2020). Considering other regions of sequence similarity suggests a role for this lncRNA in regulating the function of other hormones such as androgen, progesterone, and salt corticosteroid receptors (Dong P. et al., 2019; Yang X. et al., 2020). Additionally, plasma GAS5 is involved during diabetes and coronary heart disease. Yu et al. showed that GAS5 could directly bind to miR-222 in mouse, rat and human fibrotic liver samples as well as in activated HSC but its overexpression inhibited the activation of primary HSC *in vitro* while attenuating collagen accumulation levels in fibrotic liver tissues *in vivo*, but this was not observed in response to GAS5 is predominantly localized in the cytoplasm (Yu et al., 2015b) accompanied by a higher copy number than miR-222 and is noted to increase p27 protein levels by binding to miR-222, thereby acting as a suppressor in HSC activation and proliferation (Yu et al., 2015b). Han et al. revealed that GAS5 expression was strongly correlated with liver fibrosis in patients with nonalcoholic fatty liver disease (NAFLD) (Han et al., 2020), and plasma GAS5 expression was significantly higher in patients with advanced stages than in non-advanced stages (Han et al., 2020). The progression of fibrosis was linearly correlated with plasma GAS5 expression, which also suggests the potential of plasma GAS5 as a noninvasive marker of liver fibrosis in patients with NAFLD (Dong Z. et al., 2019). Dong et al. investigated CCl4-induced *in vivo* assays in model rats and TGF-β1-induced *in vitro* assays in HSC and found that miR-23a expression was significantly increased while compared with miR-23a Compared with the NC group (Dong Z. et al., 2019), miR-23a inhibitor did not affect the expression levels of E-calmodulin, α-SMA and type I collagen in normal rats while up-regulating the expression levels of E-calmodulin and down-regulating the expression levels of α-SMA and type I collagen in model rats, suggesting that miR-23a plays a critical regulatory role in the development of liver fibrosis (Dong Z. et al., 2019). Further co-transfection revealed that the relative luciferase activity of pGL3-GAS5-wt was inhibited by miR-23a mimics while the luciferase activity of miR-23a NC and pGL3- GAS5-mut was unchanged (Dong Z. et al., 2019). RNA pull-down analysis suggested that approximately 5% of GAS5 bound to miR-23a compared to 100% of GAS5 in total RNA, and these results suggest that miR-23a could pull down GAS5 in liver tissue and HSC. lncRNA GAS5 silencing resulted in increased expression levels of miR-23a while addition of exogenous miR-23a resulted in downregulation of lncRNA GAS5 expression levels, this evidence suggested the

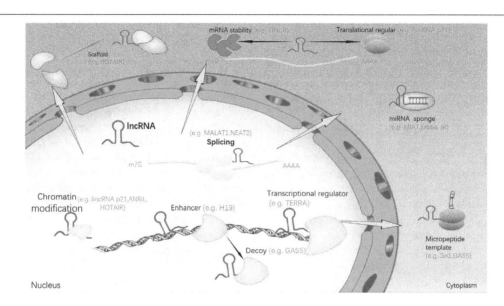

FIGURE 2 | The function and regulation mechanism of lncRNA. (1): In the nucleus, lncRNA could inhibit and/or activate gene expression by transferring chromatin modifiers and various transcriptional regulators into DNA. In addition, target gene activation could be further enhanced by lncRNA. They can also induce proteins to move away from specific DNA locations and pass as molecular decoys. (2): In the cytoplasm, lncRNA could bring two or more proteins into a complex by acting as a scaffold. In addition, they could regulate other transcripts or proteins by acting as sponges and protein templates, or regulating mRNA degradation and translation.

ability of lncRNA GAS5 to bind directly to miR-23a. Thus, the ability of lncRNA GAS5 to act as a sponge platform for miR-23a and competitively reduce the expression level of miR-23a to inhibit liver fibrosis can be confirmed. Additionally, it is essential to mention the fact that TCM has been selected as an alternative therapy for liver fibrosis in view of the ineffectiveness and frequent occurrence of adverse side effects of synthetic drugs currently used to treat liver diseases, including liver fibrosis (Lam et al., 2016). Dahuang Zhezhuo Pill (DHZCP) as a typical Chinese medicine can inhibit the proliferation of vascular smooth muscle cells or further development of liver fibrosis *in vivo* by inhibiting the MAPK pathway (Zhang et al., 2009; Cai et al., 2010). Gong et al. identified that the proliferation of HSC was significantly inhibited after overexpression of GAS5 and DHZCP reversed the relative mRNA expression of GAS5, which suggest that DHZCP can mitigate liver fibrosis by enhancing the GAS5 expression (Gong et al., 2018).

LncRNAs Functions as Competitive Endogenous RNAs in Liver Fibrosis

Competitive endogenous RNAs (ceRNAs) act as reciprocal regulators of transcripts at the post-transcriptional level through competing shared miRNAs (Salmena et al., 2011; Qi et al., 2015). ceRNA hypothesis suggests that it provides a pathway to predict the non-coding function of any non-featured RNA transcript by identifying putative miRNA binding sites and linking the function of protein-coding mRNAs to that of e.g., miRNA, lncRNA, and MiRNAs negatively regulate gene expression at the post-transcriptional level by direct base pairing with target sites within the untranslated region of messenger RNAs (Franco-

Zorrilla et al., 2007; Thomson and Dinger, 2016; Braga et al., 2020), considering that more than 60% of human protein-coding genes are under the selective pressure of MiRNAs and that any transcript containing miRNA response elements could theoretically function as ceRNAs the ability to function (Salmena et al., 2011; Li et al., 2014; Yang X. et al., 2020), which may typify a wide range of post-transcriptional forms of regulation of gene expression in physiology and pathology (Karreth et al., 2011; An et al., 2017; Wang L. X. et al., 2019). Many lncRNAs may have poor results on their effectiveness as ceRNAs under steady-state conditions due to low abundance and/or nuclear localization. Thousands of lncRNAs have cell type, tissue type, developmental stage, and disease-specific expression patterns and localization suggesting that in some cases individual lncRNAs may be effective natural miRNA sponges (Guttman and Rinn, 2012; Tay et al., 2014) (**Figure 3**). Preliminary experimental evidence has been given for ceRNA crosstalk results between the tumor suppressor gene PTEN and the pseudogene PTENP1 (Tay et al., 2011), and recent studies have focused on the ability of lncRNAs to act as ceRNAs to regulate miRNA concentrations and biological functions in hepatic fibrosis. using CCl4-induced mice (Zhang et al., 2018; He et al., 2020; Mahpour and Mullen, 2021). Zhu et al. explored that overexpression of H19 significantly exacerbated hepatocyte HSC and EMT activation (Zhu et al., 2019). Dual luciferase reporter analysis mechanistically revealed that miR-148a significantly inhibited the luciferase activity of pmirGLO-H19-WT and deregulated this inhibition by targeted mutation of the binding site. miR-148a inhibitor rescued H19 levels in LX-2 cells but miR-148a mimicked the down-regulated H19 levels in L-02 cells. Overexpression of H19 did not affect miR-148a levels in fibrotic livers but miR-148a could inhibit HSC and EMT activation by targeting ubiquitin-specific protease 4 (USP4) (Zhu et al., 2019). They demonstrated that the maintenance of USP4 levels could be mediated by H19 as ceRNA spongy miR-148a hair, and this evidence suggests that H19 may be a promising target for the treatment of liver fibrosis through the novel H19/miR-148a/USP4 axis that can promote liver fibrosis in HSC and hepatocytes (Zhu et al., 2019). Yu et al. found that liver fibrosis tissue and activation reduced levels of lincRNA-p21 expression in HSC, and overexpression of lincRNA-p21 played a key role in the inhibition of its activation by inducing a significant reduction in HSC expression of α-SMA and Col (Yu et al., 2016). Noticeably, these effects were blocked if in the absence of lincRNA-p21-induced PTEN enhancement, and these circumstances demonstrate the fact that lincRNAp21 inhibits liver fibrosis through PTEN. Further studies showed that miR-181b mimics inhibited the effect of lincRNA-p21 on PTEN expression and HSC activation. Combined with the above data lincRNA-p21 enhances PTEN expression levels by competitively binding miR-181b (Yu et al., 2016). Thus, these results reveal a novel lincRNA-p21-miR-181b-PTEN signaling cascade in liver fibrosis and its potential to suggest lincRNA-p21 as a molecular target for anti-fibrotic therapy. Yu et al. confirmed that lincRNA-p21 inhibits miR-17-5p levels, with this phenomenon missing in lincRNA-p21-miR-17-5p binding site could block miR-17-5p expression in the inhibition assay (Yu et al., 2017a). The function of miR-29b in mediating the downregulation of extracellular matrix genes involved in the TGF-β and NF-κB signaling pathways in HSC has long been reported (Roderburg et al., 2011). Han et al. suggested that TUG1 promotes the expression of these pro-fibrotic genes through the downregulation of miR-29b and thus plays a ceRNA role in accelerating the progression of liver fibrosis (Han et al., 2018). Xie et al. demonstrated that SNHG7 as a ceRNA can also bind to miR-29b in HSC and inhibit the expression level of miR-29b, which may affect the expression of DNMT3A (a downstream target gene of miR-29b) thus regulating the activation, autophagy, and proliferation of HSC (Xie et al., 2021). The downregulation of miR-378a-3p, a target of SNHG7, which is co-localized with SNHG7 in the cytoplasm, could block SNHG7 deletion and thus alleviate the outcome of HSC activation. Analogously, SNHG7-induced HSC activation was almost confirmed to be blocked by irregular fragment polarity protein 2 (DVL2) knockdown of the target site of miR-378a-3p (Yu et al., 2019). These discoveries suggest that lncRNA SNHG7 may interact with different miRNAs to play a critical role in the development of liver fibrosis. Zhou et al. investigated sperm-mediated primary HSC and found that lncRNA Gm5091 overexpressed and knocked downplayed important roles in negatively regulating cell migration, ROS content, IL-1β secretion and HSC activation, respectively (Zhou et al., 2018). lncRNA Gm5091 exhibited direct binding to miR-27b, miR-23b, and miR-24 and inhibited miR-27b, miR-23b, and miR-24 expression. All these suggest the potential of lncRNA Gm5091 to function as ceRNA and thus attenuate liver fibrosis through spongy miR-27b/23b/24 (Zhou et al., 2018). lncRNA ATB containing a common binding site for miR-200a was found to be upregulated in fibrotic liver tissue and simultaneously involved in LX-2 cell activation by Fu et al. in the same field. Knockdown experiments of lncRNA ATB upregulated

endogenous miR-200a while downregulating β-catenin expression while suppressing the activation state of LX-2 cells (Fu et al., 2017). Significant increase in lncRNA NEAT1 expression *in vitro* and *in vivo*, as well as the inhibitory effect of its deletion on liver fibrosis were observed (Yu et al., 2017b). lncRNA NEAT1 and miR-122 interacted directly in that lncRNA NEAT1 could regulate KLF6 expression in liver fibrosis by competitively binding to miR-122, thereby accelerating HSC activation and increased cell proliferation and collagen activation (Yu et al., 2017b). The lncRNA NEAT1, which is upregulated in NAFLD progression, binds to miR-506, and GLI3, and regulates GLI3 expression levels as well as fibrosis, inflammatory response and lipid metabolism in NAFLD by secreting miR-506 and miR-506/GLI3 axis, respectively (Jin et al., 2019). lncRNA NEAT1 was found to be elevated in ash by Ye et al. was elevated in ash and acted as a ceRNA sponge for miR-129-5p's ability to suppress SOCS2 expression. It is also important to note that inhibition of lncRNA NEAT1 inhibits the development of liver fibrosis and ASH by elevating miR-129-5p and inhibiting SOCS2 (Ye et al., 2020). These findings clarify that lncRNA NEAT1 may contribute to the development of liver fibrosis and provide new insights into the pathogenesis and potential therapeutic strategies for liver fibrosis. In conclusion these results suggest that lncRNA-miRNA interactions regulate target genes and play a role in liver fibrosis, and these evidence will provide the basis for a better understanding of this interaction to develop a new liver fibrosis treatment strategy (**Table 2**).

REGULATORY MECHANISM OF LNCRNAS IN LIVER FIBROSIS

Deep understanding of the disease is essential to improve patient survival and to identify effective biomarkers for the development of liver fibrosis. How to detect liver fibrosis early in disease progression and develop effective therapies is critical in reducing the risk of cirrhosis, subsequent decompensation or liver cancer and reducing cancer mortality (Chang et al., 2015; Tacke and Trautwein, 2015; Aydin and Akcali, 2018). We already know that multiple signaling pathways are involved in the pathogenesis of liver fibrosis (Yang et al., 2014; Roehlen et al., 2020; Zhu et al., 2021). We therefore summarize some of the regulatory mechanisms associated with hepatic fibrosis development and progression (**Figure 4**).

Notch Signaling Pathway

The importance of lncRNAs in mediating various signaling pathways has been recently highlighted in the direction of liver fibrosis onset and progression as well (Peng et al., 2018; Yang et al., 2019; Ganguly and Chakrabarti, 2021). The Notch signaling pathway, which induces developmental interactions and is a major player in liver biology and pathophysiology (Kovall et al., 2017; Nowell and Radtke, 2017; Meurette and Mehlen, 2018), is thought to be involved in cell proliferation, survival, apoptosis and differentiation events at various stages of development thereby controlling events such as organogenesis and morphogenesis (Zhang K. et al., 2019; Chen T. et al., 2020), as well as being significantly associated with HSC activation and

TABLE 2 | lncRNA as ceRNA in liver fibrosis.

lncRNAs	miRNA	Mechanism of interaction	Targets	References
lncRNA NEAT1	miR-122/miR-506/miR-129-5p	lncRNA NEAT1 act as sponge of miR-122/miR-506/miR-129-5p	KLF6/GLI3/SOCS2	Yu et al. (2017b); Jin et al. (2019); Ye et al. (2020)
lncRNA SNHG7	miR-29b/miR-378a-3p	lncRNA SNHG7 act as sponge of miR-29b/miR-378a-3p	DNMT3A/DVL2	32893175 Yu et al. (2019); Xie et al. (2021)
lncRNA H19	miR-148a	lncRNA H19 act as sponge of miR-148a	USP4	Zhu et al. (2019)
lncRNA Gm5091	miR-27b/23b/24	lncRNA Gm5091 act as sponge of miR-27b/23b/24	–	Zhou et al. (2018)
lncRNA TUG1	miR-29b	lncRNA TUG1 act as sponge of miR-29b	–	Han et al. (2018)
lincRNA-p21	miR-181b/miR-17-5p	lncRNA lincRNA-p21 act as sponge of miR-181b/miR-17-5p	PTEN/β-catenin	Yu et al. (2016); Yu et al. (2017a)
lncRNA ATB	miR-200a	lncRNA ATB act as sponge of miR-200a	β-catenin	Fu et al. (2017)

HCs EMT in liver fibrosis (Zhang K. et al., 2019). Chen et al. found that lncRNA Meg8, through the Notch pathway inhibited hepatic stellate cell activation and EMT in hepatocytes while its silencing assay exhibited a significant promotion of Notch2, Notch3 and Hes1 expression levels in primary HSC and LX-2 cells (Chen T. et al., 2020). lncRNAs Notch2, Notch3, and Hes1 expression could also be inhibited by knocking down lncRNAs in primary HCs and AML-12 cells Meg8 was significantly increased. Increased mRNA and protein levels of type I collagen and α-SMA were observed in LX-2 cells transfected with lncRNA Meg8 siRNA, while knockdown lncRNA Meg8 experiments showed that overexpression of type I collagen and α-SMA was eliminated by RO4929097, evidence suggesting that this signal may be involved in mediating the function of lncRNA Meg8 (Chen T. et al., 2020). The regulatory role of lncRNAs in liver fibrosis via the Notch signaling pathway was recently reported, and protein and mRNA levels of Notch signaling-related molecules and target genes Notch2, Notch3, and Hes1 were reduced in HSCs with lncRNA LFAR1 downregulation and increased in HSCs with lncRNA LFAR1 overexpression (Zhang K. et al., 2017). CCl4-and BDL-treated mice showed significantly increased expression of Notch2, Notch3, Hes1, and Hey2 compared to lenti NC infection. Lentivirus-mediated knockdown of lncRNA LFAR1 resulted in decreased expression of Notch2, Notch 3, Hes1, and Hey2 while suppressing CCl4-and BDL-induced upregulation of these genes, and this evidence suggests that lncRNA LFAR1 promotes processes such as liver fibrosis and HSC activation through activation of the Notch signaling pathway as well as acting as a Notch signaling pathway provides new insights to elucidate the molecular mechanisms of liver fibrosis (Zhang K. et al., 2017).

Wnt/β-Catenin Signaling Pathway

The Wnt/β-catenin signaling pathway, which is highly conserved among species and controls a variety of biological processes during animal development and life cycle (Zhou and Liu, 2015; Fu et al., 2018; Zuo et al., 2019), is essential in the regulation of EMT and can recur during the onset and progression of various diseases (Sebio et al., 2014; Schunk et al., 2021). Salvianolic acid B (Sal B), one of the water-soluble components extracted from Salvia miltiorrhiza, plays an important role in the treatment and inhibition of activated HSC, and increases the expression of lincRNA-p21 (Yu et al.,

2017a). Sal-B increased the expression of P-β-catenin and decreased the cytoplasmic and nuclear expression levels of β-catenin thus significantly reducing the pathway activity while this phenomenon could be restored by lincRNA-p21 knockdown. The deletion of lincRNA-p21 is involved in the inhibition of Sal-B-induced P-β-cateni and the restoration of reduced β-linked proteins in the cytoplasm and nucleus, suggesting that Sal-B may inhibit Wnt/β-linked protein pathway processes through lincRNA-p21 (Yu et al., 2017a). In conclusion, the Wnt/β-linked protein pathway inhibited by lincRNA-p21 is involved in the effect of Sal B on HSC activation and thus inhibits HSC activation and provides new evidence for the role of Wnt/β-linked protein signaling inhibited by lincRNA-p21 in the progression of liver fibrosis disease. proliferation, survival, differentiation, and invasion (Lee JJ. et al., 2015; Alzahrani, 2019; Corti et al., 2019).

PI3K/AKT/mTOR Signaling Pathway

lncRNAs silencing experiments can reduce the phosphorylation levels of ERK, Akt, and mTOR, while PI3K/AKT/mTOR signaling has also been reported to be closely associated with HSC proliferation, activation, and ECM synthesis, which is also significantly inhibited by pharmacological and genetic approaches through inhibition of PI3K signaling (Khemlina et al., 2017; Kong et al., 2020; Jung et al., 2021). Huang et al. revealed that increased expression of H19 could be inhibited by LY294002. These results suggest a role for lncRNA H19 in HSC activation as a downstream site regulated by the PI3K/AKT/mTOR pathway (Huang et al., 2019). Beyond this the pathway of lncRNA H19 promoting HSC activation through autophagy must be highlighted. It has also been reported that lncRNA H19 significantly decreased the expression of p-AKT and p-mTOR, and this effect was further enhanced by LY294002 and rapamycin (Huang et al., 2019). This suggests that lncRNA H19 can be involved in the PI3K/AKT/mTOR-promoted autophagy-activated HSC pathway 30735452. Dong et al. reported that silencing of lncRNA GAS5 increased the expression levels of p-PI3K, p-Akt, and p-mTOR thus revealing that activation of PI3K/Akt/mTOR signaling pathway in liver fibrosis can be mediated by the lncRNA GAS5 (Dong Z. et al., 2019). LOC102551149 knockdown assay promoted the expression of p-PI3K, p-Akt, and p-mTOR in activated HSC, while the overexpression of LOC102551149 in activated HSC 30735452 suppressed the expression levels of p-PI3K, *p*-Akt, and *p*-mTOR (Dong Z. et al., 2019). This evidence imply that lncRNAs can reduce the activation response of HSC by inhibiting the activation of PI3K/AKT/mTOR signaling pathway in liver fibrosis (Karin et al., 2002; De Simone et al., 2015).

NF-κB Signaling Pathway

The NF-κB signaling pathway, an important transcription factor for many inflammatory mediators and cytokines, remains a dormant molecule in the cytoplasm by binding tightly to IκB inhibitor proteins (Inoue et al., 1992; Yang et al., 2012), and phosphorylation of IκB by IκB kinase (IKK) upon stimulation separates IκB from NF-κB leading to translocation and activation of NF-κB, a process reported to be involved in the formation and progression of liver fibrosis (Luedde and Schwabe, 2011; Wang T. et al., 2019; Zhang K. et al., 2020; Zhao et al., 2020). Shi et al. found that LINC01093 31450097 knockdown assay confirmed the promotion of NF-κB p65 nuclear translocation and elevated levels of NF-kB p65 in the cytoplasm (Shi et al., 2019). On the contrary, overexpression of LINC01093 is involved in the inhibition of nuclear translocation of NF-κB p65 leading to an increase in the nuclear level of NF-κB p65 and a decrease in NF-κB p65 at the cytoplasmic level, and this evidence suggests that overexpression of LINC01093 could be involved in inhibiting hepatocyte apoptosis and attenuating the process of liver fibrosis by suppressing the NF-κB signaling pathway (Shi et al., 2019).

AMP-Activated Protein Kinase Signaling Pathway

The AMP-activated protein kinase (AMPK) signaling pathway, which plays an important role in regulating cellular energy homeostasis, could respond to changes in intracellular adenine nucleotide levels and is involved in the process of HSC activation (Shackelford and Shaw, 2009; Mihaylova and Shaw, 2011; Zhao et al., 2017). Yang et al. determined that the proliferation rate of HSC transfected with LncRNA- ANRIL siRNA was significantly higher than that of NC and vector-identified AMPK as a key gene in LncRNA-ANRIL-mediated HSC activation (Zhang T. et al., 2019; Kim MH. et al., 2020). Overexpression of LncRNA-ANRIL suppressed the level of phosphorylated AMPK in activated HSC while LncRNA-ANRIL-siRNA increased the level of phosphorylated AMPK in activated HSC, this evidence suggest that LncRNA-ANRIL deletion can trigger HSC activation through AMPK pathway (Yang JJ. et al., 2020). Wang et al. revealed that lncRNA- H19 regulates lipid droplet metabolism by mechanisms that rely on the AMPKα pathway acting as a sensor for maintaining energy homeostasis (Wang Z. et al., 2020). The upregulated lncRNA-H19 initiates the catabolic pathway by binding to AMPKα to maintain the necessary energy supply. In addition to acting as a scaffold between AMPKα and LKB1, lncRNA-H19 links AMPKα and LKB1 and plays a facilitating role in the phosphorylation of AMPKα by LKB1 (Wang Z. et al., 2020). lncRNA-H19/AMPKα pathway is thought to be involved in HSC activation-induced lipid droplet disappearance in liver fibrosis given that lncRNA-H19 can be observed to induce HSC

-formation of the AMPKα/LKB1 complex in LX2 cells and its potential as a novel target for liver fibrosis treatment (Wang Z. et al., 2020).

In conclusion, these findings highlight the possibility that there may be new therapeutic targets and biomarkers for liver fibrosis in the future from lncRNAs, **Figure 4** schematically demonstrates the potential mechanism of lncRNA on liver fibrosis.

POTENTIAL CLINICAL APPLICATION OF LNCRNAS IN HUMAN CANCERS

As a serious infectious disease caused by hepatitis B virus (HBV) infection, hepatitis B currently infects 350–400 million people worldwide (McMahon, 2009). Patients with chronic hepatitis B (CHB) are characterized by progressive liver fibrosis and inflammation (Guo et al., 2021) as the main pathological manifestations representing the ultimate common pathway for almost all types of CLD (Cai et al., 2020; Roehlen et al., 2020). However, it must be emphasized that liver fibrosis characterized by excessive accumulation of extracellular matrix (ECM) proteins also represents a manifestation of the liver's trauma healing response to various types of liver injury (e.g., HBV infection) (Lee Y. A. et al., 2015; Tacke and Trautwein, 2015). The application of liver biopsy as the gold standard for assessing the presence and staging of liver fibrosis is often limited by its invasive nature, possible complications, and potential sampling errors. Consequently, there is a need for effective early detection studies of liver fibrosis to control and treat the patient's liver fibrosis progression (Cadranel et al., 2000; Bravo et al., 2001; Rockey et al., 2009). lncRNAs are frequently deregulated in a variety of human diseases as well as in many important biological processes thereby generating abnormal lncRNAs involved in the development of various diseases 29330108 (Peng et al., 2017; Ma et al., 2018). It must be emphasized that lncRNAs are stable in the circulatory system and readily detectable in serum due to their inability to be degraded by nucleases (Faghihi et al., 2008; Gupta et al., 2010), a property that makes them highly diagnostic in different diseases including liver fibrosis (Zhang K. et al., 2017; Liu et al., 2019). They further demonstrated that reduced serum lincRNA-p21 levels in chronic hepatitis B patients correlated with fibrosis stage (Yu et al., 2017c). Subject operating characteristic curve (ROC) analysis suggested that serum lincRNA-p21 could differentiate chronic hepatitis B patients with liver fibrosis from healthy controls, specifically the area under the ROC curve (AUC) was 0.854 [0.805–0.894], with a sensitivity and specificity of 100 and 70%, respectively, at a critical value of 3.65. A sensitivity of 100% and specificity of 70% accompanied by an AUC of 0.760 (0.682–0.826) in differentiating chronic hepatitis B patients with low fibrosis scores from healthy controls; a sensitivity of 100% and specificity of 73.3% accompanied by an AUC of 0.856 in differentiating chronic hepatitis B patients with moderate fibrosis scores from healthy controls (0.801–0.901); 100% sensitivity and 77.5% specificity accompanied by an AUC of 0.935 (0.882–0.969) were observed in differentiating patients with chronic hepatitis B with high fibrosis

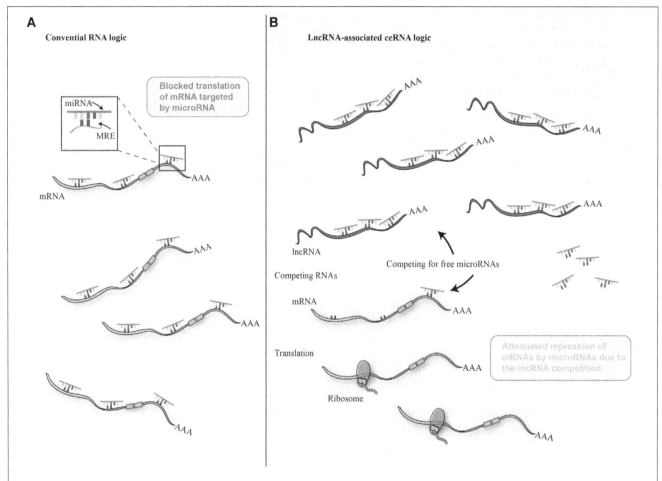

FIGURE 3 | The mechanism of ceRNA. **(A)** In the cytoplasm, miRNAs could regulate 3'- UTR of mRNAs through base pairing with partial complementarity in the conventional crosstalk of RNA transcripts, thus inhibiting mRNAs. **(B)** Under the ceRNA mechanism of cancer cells, miRNAs are isolated from each other by abnormally expressed lncrna and MREs, thus reducing the interaction between miRNA and mRNA, thereby weakening the inhibition of downstream mRNA.

score versus healthy controls (Yu et al., 2017c). Furthermore, the levels of lincRNA-p21 could be distinguished in chronic hepatitis B patients with different fibrosis scores, specifically: 70.9% sensitivity and 92.3% specificity (AUC 0.875, 0.800–0.930) for moderate fibrosis score and mild fibrosis score; 81.4% sensitivity and 96.1% specificity (AUC 0.954, 0.859–0.993) for high fibrosis score and low fibrosis score; and Yu et al. showed that serum lincRNA-p21 levels were associated with liver Fibrosis markers including α-SMA and Col1A1 were negatively correlated but markers of viral replication, liver inflammatory activity and liver function showed no correlation (Yu et al., 2017c). lncRNA SNHG7 was also found to be correlated with liver fibrosis progression by Yu et al. (Yu et al., 2019) and ROC curve analysis showed an area under the ROC curve (AUC) of 0.955 (95% confidence interval [CI], 0.868–0.990), where it is noteworthy that at a critical value of 1.0, its sensitivity is 90% and specificity is 100%, suggesting its potential as a potential diagnostic biomarker for liver fibrosis. lncRNA SNHG7 is higher in the cytoplasm of human LX-2 cells as well as primary HSC than in the nucleus (Yu et al., 2019), and this evidence indicates that the expression of lincRNA-p21 and lncRNA SNHG7 plays a

key role in the progression of liver fibrosis and its potential as a potential biomarker of liver fibrosis. Han et al. experimentally confirmed that plasma lncRNA GAS5 was significantly elevated in patients with advanced fibrosis compared to patients without progressive fibrosis, but this did not show any statistical difference in tissues, but lncRNA GAS5 tissue expression was positively correlated with the stage of fibrosis prior to the development of cirrhosis as well as significantly downregulating lncRNA in plasma of NAFLD patients with cirrhosis GAS5 expression (Han et al., 2020). However, significant differences in tissue levels of lncRNA GAS5 were not shown in patients with advanced fibrosis and cirrhosis, a phenomenon that emphasizes the accuracy of the association between plasma levels and fibrosis stage. The significance of serum lncRNA GAS5 in the diagnosis of liver fibrosis was proposed by Gou et al. through the detection of abnormalities in lncRNA GAS5 in the serum of patients with chronic hepatitis B, and although the significance of serum lncRNA GAS5 in the age and gender distribution subgroups were not statistically significant (Han et al., 2020). The results of qRT PCR analysis suggested lower serum lncRNA GAS5 levels in CHB patients, and

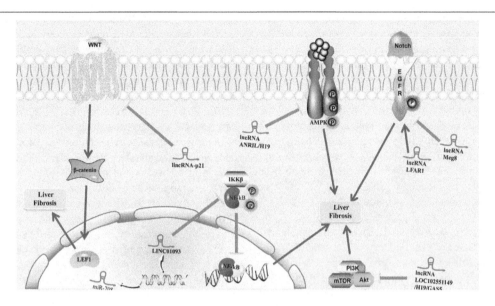

FIGURE 4 | The mechanism of lncRNA to liver fibrosis. Multiple stimuli such as chronic hepatitis B (CHB) damage hepatocytes to initiate wound healing responses, and LncRNAs play a role in promoting activation and apoptosis of hepatic stellate cells and inducing epithelial-mesenchymal transition (EMT) at multiple stages, leading to excessive accumulation of extracellular matrix (ECM) proteins in hepatocytes, resulting in liver fibrosis generation and progression.

the results of ROC curve analysis showed that serum lncRNA GAS5 could effectively differentiate between CHB liver fibrosis patients and healthy controls (AUC of 0.993, 0.972–0.992). Altogether, circulating elevated lncRNA GAS5 levels correlated with the progression of liver fibrosis prior to the development of cirrhosis can be used to serve as a valid non-invasive marker in patients with NAFLD and CHB with liver fibrosis (Han et al., 2020). Chen et al. contributed significantly to the promotion of lncRNA MEG3 as a serum bi-diagnostic marker for chronic hepatitis B and to improve early diagnosis and treatment outcomes (Chen et al., 2019). qRT PCR data showed a significant decrease in serum lncRNA MEG3 levels in patients with chronic hepatitis B. lncRNA MEG3 expression was negatively correlated with the degree of liver fibrosis (AUC of 0.8844 and the critical value was 5.112) in the low-level fibrosis group versus the control group (AUC and critical value were 0.5237 and 2.988, respectively) (Chen et al., 2019), in the moderate fibrosis group and the control group (AUC and critical value were 0.7085 and 3.812, respectively), and in the high fibrosis group and the control group (AUC and critical value were 0.9395 and 4.689, respectively). Finally, they focused on the possibility of lncRNA MEG3 levels as a differentiating marker in chronic hepatitis B types with different degrees of liver fibrosis (Chen et al., 2019). The AUC and critical values were found to be 0.8281 and 3.963 for the low and intermediate level fibrosis groups, respectively. 0.8857 and 4.818 for the high and low levels fibrosis groups, respectively, and conversely, 0.7861 and 5.312 for the high and intermediate level fibrosis groups, respectively. The results show the important diagnostic value of serum lncRNA MEG3 in patients with chronic hepatitis B combined with liver fibrosis. Yu et al. also concluded that lncRNA MEG3 was negatively correlated with the transcript level of α-

SMA and positively correlated with E-calmodulin mRNA expression. Moreover, the increase in fibrosis score was accompanied by a gradual increase in liver MEG3ΔCt value, which indicated that MEG3 expression was negatively correlated with fibrosis score (Yu et al., 2018). In conclusion, all the above results demonstrate that lncRNA MEG3 is a biomarker in the detection and prognosis of liver fibrosis.

Given the current delayed diagnosis and relapse as the biggest barriers to liver fibrosis treatment, ideal biomarkers are of great importance for clinical efforts such as improving early diagnosis rates. These results suggest a potential role of lncRNAs in the diagnosis and prognosis of liver fibrosis. Nevertheless, we must realize that the exact molecular mechanism of the role of lncRNAs in liver fibrosis is still unclear therefore the functional role of lncRNAs in liver fibrosis still needs further exploration and validation including clinical applications.

PROSPECTS

lncRNAs have been receiving increasing attention along with the rapid development of the field of molecular biology, and breakthroughs in new high-throughput sequencing technologies such as RNA-Seq, microarrays and deep sequencing have provided the basis for expanding our understanding of complex transcriptomic networks and enabling us to identify the dysregulated expression of various lncRNAs in liver fibrosis. Our review details the role of lncRNAs as important regulators in the development of liver fibrosis and the relationship between aberrant lncRNA expression and HSC activation (Yang et al., 2019; De Vincentis et al., 2020). In addition to this, given the increasing number of studies providing data on lncRNAs measured between normal and liver fibrotic tissues, it not only suggests that lncRNAs may be involved in the progression of liver fibrosis but also provides a solid theoretical basis for lncRNAs to become biomarkers for the clinical diagnosis of liver fibrosis (Jiang and Zhang, 2017; Unfried and Fortes, 2020). However, we still need to clarify the regulatory network of lncRNAs in liver fibrosis and the underlying molecular mechanisms are still complex and still inconclusive (Kim YA. et al., 2020; Ganguly and Chakrabarti, 2021). Therefore, the next work should focus on screening effective lncRNAs for the diagnosis and treatment of liver fibrosis and actively promote the development of effective lncRNAs that can be applied in the clinical setting.

On the other hand, a series of lipid bilayer membrane-bound organelles that are released by cells into the environment, which we call "EVs" (Xu et al., 2016), vary in size and could be released from almost all cells under appropriate physiological and pathological conditions (Walker et al., 2019; Mo et al., 2021). One of the hot topics of research is their cargo-carrying function given that their cargo can partially reflect the cellular properties of their origin, exosomes carry significantly different types of RNAs compared to parental cells (Abels and Breakefield, 2016; van Niel et al., 2018). Most importantly, ncRNAs can be shipped in a way that avoids the fate of unprotected ncRNAs that are readily degraded by RNA enzymes in the blood and can furthermore maintain their integrity and activity in circulation (Shen M. et al., 2019; Mori et al., 2019; Hu et al., 2020). Liu et al. found that hepatic lncRNA H19 expression levels correlated with serum exosomal lncRNA H19 levels and severity of liver fibrosis in a mouse model of cholestatic liver injury and in human patients with primary sclerosing cholangitis (PSC) and primary biliary cholangitis (PBC). In contrast, exogenous lncRNA H19 promotes liver fibrosis and enhances the activation and proliferation of HSC (Liu et al., 2019). Our review highlights the status of exogenous lncRNA H19 as a potential diagnostic marker and therapeutic target in the development of cholestatic liver fibrosis, and the potential of targeting these intercellular signaling mechanisms and mediators to increase sensitivity and improve response to conventional therapeutic agents used to treat liver fibrosis and to complement exogenous lncRNAs strategies in liver prevention, diagnosis and treatment. Finally, we must emphasize that gene editing is a technique for targeted modification of DNA nucleotide sequences characterized by the precise severing of targeted DNA fragments and insertion of new gene fragments (Jinek et al., 2012), and that CRISPR/Cas9, which has been successfully applied to the disruption of protein-coding24 sequences in various organisms (Sharma et al., 2021), is a very powerful gene editing tool, and that it also plays a key role in the progression and development of liver fibrosis (Barrangou et al., 2007; Strotskaya et al., 2017). For example, RSPO4-CRISPR applied in a rat model of liver fibrosis showed excellent performance in reducing liver injury and restoring the gut microbiota (Yu et al., 2021). HSC reprogramming via exon-mediated CRISPR/dCas9-VP64 delivery (Luo et al., 2021) has also been reported. Among them it is important to note that lncRNAs have been successfully edited/

regulated by the CRISPR/Cas9 system therefore no transgene needs to be introduced (Konermann et al., 2015; Chen B. et al., 2020). Due to its specificity, efficiency, simplicity, and versatility CRISPR/Cas9 has achieved many encouraging successes as a powerful genome engineering tool for the treatment of many diseases including cancer (Goyal et al., 2017; Esposito et al., 2019). For example, the fact that CRISPR/Cas9's specifically designed GRNA targeting suppresses the upregulated lncRNA UCA1 (uroepithelial carcinoma associated 1) in bladder cancer once again highlights the potential of the CRISPR/Cas9 system for regulating the expression of lncRNAs and for further use as a therapeutic approach in clinical cancer treatment (Yang et al., 2018; Shen M. et al., 2019). Therefore, it is reasonable to assume that CRISPR/Cas9 can regulate the expression of lncRNAs and thus achieve the treatment of liver fibrosis through relevant molecular mechanisms. Importantly, our review provides a summary of the stages by which this budding and maturing technology can be used in the future for drug discovery, cancer therapy, and treatment of other genetic diseases previously considered incurable.

CONCLUSION

Research on the involvement of lncRNAs in regulating the development of liver fibrosis are increasing year by year, and the results of *in vivo* and *ex vivo* experiments confirm the significant effect of overexpression and knockdown of lncRNAs in reducing or enhancing the extent of liver fibrosis, suggesting that lncRNAs are promising as new targets for liver fibrosis treatment. The expression of lncRNAs may be a suitable candidate in the issue of potential markers for the diagnosis and prognosis of liver fibrosis. lncRNAs regulate the proliferation, activation and apoptosis of HSC involved in the process of liver fibrosis. The regulation of lncRNAs expression mediated by miRNAs and the inverse regulation of miRNAs expression by lncRNAs are demonstrated. miRNAs are involved in the regulation of lncRNAs expression through sequence-specific binding between them. Multiple molecular mechanisms regulated by lncRNAs including NF-κB signaling pathway are involved in the pathological process of liver fibrosis, while examples of successful implementation of strategies applying regulation of lncRNA expression in preclinical models can already be observed. On the one hand, we can optimistically anticipate the promising clinical applications of therapeutic strategies based on the regulation of lncRNA expression, but on the other hand, we must realize that their safety and reliability still depend on the advancement of knowledge and sophisticated technologies.

AUTHOR CONTRIBUTIONS

ZW, XY, SG, and FY drafted the manuscript. CL revised the manuscript. ZC, RC, and XX reviewed and modified the manuscript. All authors agreed on the final version.

REFERENCES

Abels, E. R., and Breakefield, X. O. (2016). Introduction to Extracellular Vesicles: Biogenesis, RNA Cargo Selection, Content, Release, and Uptake. *Cell Mol Neurobiol* 36 (3), 301–312. doi:10.1007/s10571-016-0366-z

Alirezaei, M., Flynn, C. T., Wood, M. R., Harkins, S., and Whitton, J. L. (2015). Coxsackievirus Can Exploit LC3 in Both Autophagy-dependent and -independent Manners *In Vivo*. *Autophagy* 11 (8), 1389–1407. doi:10.1080/15548627.2015.1063769

Alzahrani, A. S. (2019). PI3K/Akt/mTOR Inhibitors in Cancer: At the Bench and Bedside. *Semin. Cancer Biol.* 59, 125–132. doi:10.1016/j.semcancer.2019.07.009

Amodio, N., Stamato, M. A., Juli, G., Morelli, E., Fulciniti, M., Manzoni, M., et al. (2018). Drugging the lncRNA MALAT1 via LNA gapmeR ASO Inhibits Gene Expression of Proteasome Subunits and Triggers Anti-multiple Myeloma Activity. *Leukemia* 32 (9), 1948–1957. doi:10.1038/s41375-018-0067-3

An, Y., Furber, K. L., and Ji, S. (2017). Pseudogenes Regulate Parental Gene Expression via ceRNA Network. *J. Cel Mol Med* 21 (1), 185–192. doi:10.1111/jcmm.12952

Anwar, S. L., Krech, T., Hasemeier, B., Schipper, E., Schweitzer, N., Vogel, A., et al. (2012). Loss of Imprinting and Allelic Switching at the DLK1-MEG3 Locus in Human Hepatocellular Carcinoma. *PLoS One* 7 (11), e49462. doi:10.1371/journal.pone.0049462

Aydin, M. M., and Akcali, K. C. (2018). Liver Fibrosis. *Turk J. Gastroenterol.* 29 (1), 14–21. doi:10.5152/tjg.2018.17330

Barrangou, R., Fremaux, C., Deveau, H., Richards, M., Boyaval, P., Moineau, S., et al. (2007). CRISPR Provides Acquired Resistance against Viruses in Prokaryotes. *Science* 315 (5819), 1709–1712. doi:10.1126/science.1138140

Benetatos, L., Dasoula, A., Hatzimichael, E., Georgiou, I., Syrrou, M., and Bourantas, K. L. (2008). Promoter Hypermethylation of the MEG3 (DLK1/MEG3) Imprinted Gene in Multiple Myeloma. *Clin. Lymphoma Myeloma* 8 (3), 171–175. doi:10.3816/CLM.2008.n.021

Bian, E. B., Xiong, Z. G., and Li, J. (2019). New Advances of lncRNAs in Liver Fibrosis, with Specific Focus on lncRNA-miRNA Interactions. *J. Cel Physiol* 234 (3), 2194–2203. doi:10.1002/jcp.27069

Blaner, W. S., O'Byrne, S. M., Wongsiriroj, N., Kluwe, J., D'Ambrosio, D. M., Jiang, H., et al. (2009). Hepatic Stellate Cell Lipid Droplets: a Specialized Lipid Droplet for Retinoid Storage. *Biochim. Biophys. Acta* 1791 (6), 467–473. doi:10.1016/j.bbalip.2008.11.001

Braga, E. A., Fridman, M. V., Moscovtsev, A. A., Filippova, E. A., Dmitriev, A. A., and Kushlinskii, N. E. (2020). LncRNAs in Ovarian Cancer Progression, Metastasis, and Main Pathways: ceRNA and Alternative Mechanisms. *Int. J. Mol. Sci.* 21 (22). doi:10.3390/ijms21228855

Bravo, A. A., Sheth, S. G., and Chopra, S. (2001). Liver Biopsy. *N. Engl. J. Med.* 344 (7), 495–500. doi:10.1056/NEJM200102153440706

Broerse, J., and Crassini, B. (1984). Investigations of Perception and Imagery Using CAEs: the Role of Experimental Design and Psychophysical Method. *Percept Psychophys* 35 (2), 155–164. doi:10.3758/bf03203895

Brown, J. A., Bulkley, D., Wang, J., Valenstein, M. L., Yario, T. A., Steitz, T. A., et al. (2014). Structural Insights into the Stabilization of MALAT1 Noncoding RNA by a Bipartite Triple helix. *Nat. Struct. Mol. Biol.* 21 (7), 633–640. doi:10.1038/nsmb.2844

Bu, F. T., Wang, A., Zhu, Y., You, H. M., Zhang, Y. F., Meng, X. M., et al. (2020). LncRNA NEAT1: Shedding Light on Mechanisms and Opportunities in Liver Diseases. *Liver Int.* 40 (11), 2612–2626. doi:10.1111/liv.14629

Cadranel, J. F., Rufat, P., and Degos, F. (2000). Practices of Liver Biopsy in France: Results of a Prospective Nationwide Survey. For the Group of Epidemiology of the French Association for the Study of the Liver (AFEF). *Hepatology* 32 (3), 477–481. doi:10.1053/jhep.2000.16602

Cai, B., Dongiovanni, P., Corey, K. E., Wang, X., Shmarakov, I. O., Zheng, Z., et al. (2020). Macrophage MerTK Promotes Liver Fibrosis in Nonalcoholic Steatohepatitis. *Cell Metab* 31 (2), 406–e7. e407. doi:10.1016/j.cmet.2019.11.013

Cai, H., Liu, X., Zheng, J., Xue, Y., Ma, J., Li, Z., et al. (2017). Long Non-coding RNA Taurine Upregulated 1 Enhances Tumor-Induced Angiogenesis through Inhibiting microRNA-299 in Human Glioblastoma. *Oncogene* 36 (3), 318–331. doi:10.1038/onc.2016.212

Cai, H. B., Sun, X. G., Liu, Z. F., Liu, Y. W., Tang, J., Liu, Q., et al. (2010). Effects of Dahuangzhechong Pills on Cytokines and Mitogen Activated Protein Kinase Activation in Rats with Hepatic Fibrosis. *J. Ethnopharmacol* 132 (1), 157–164. doi:10.1016/j.jep.2010.08.019

Cavaillé, J., Seitz, H., Paulsen, M., Ferguson-Smith, A. C., and Bachellerie, J. P. (2002). Identification of Tandemly-Repeated C/D snoRNA Genes at the Imprinted Human 14q32 Domain Reminiscent of Those at the Prader-Willi/Angelman Syndrome Region. *Hum. Mol. Genet.* 11 (13), 1527–1538. doi:10.1093/hmg/11.13.1527

Chang, J., Lan, T., Li, C., Ji, X., Zheng, L., Gou, H., et al. (2015). Activation of Slit2-Robo1 Signaling Promotes Liver Fibrosis. *J. Hepatol.* 63 (6), 1413–1420. doi:10.1016/j.jhep.2015.07.033

Chaudhry, M. A. (2013). Expression Pattern of Small Nucleolar RNA Host Genes and Long Non-coding RNA in X-Rays-Treated Lymphoblastoid Cells. *Int. J. Mol. Sci.* 14 (5), 9099–9110. doi:10.3390/ijms14059099

Chen, B., Deng, S., Ge, T., Ye, M., Yu, J., Lin, S., et al. (2020a). Live Cell Imaging and Proteomic Profiling of Endogenous NEAT1 lncRNA by CRISPR/Cas9-mediated Knock-In. *Protein Cell* 11 (9), 641–660. doi:10.1007/s13238-020-00706-w

Chen, M., Xia, Z., Chen, C., Hu, W., and Yuan, Y. (2018a). LncRNA MALAT1 Promotes Epithelial-To-Mesenchymal Transition of Esophageal Cancer through Ezh2-Notch1 Signaling Pathway. *Anticancer Drugs* 29 (8), 767–773. doi:10.1097/CAD.0000000000000645

Chen, M. J., Wang, X. G., Sun, Z. X., and Liu, X. C. (2019). Diagnostic Value of LncRNA-MEG3 as a Serum Biomarker in Patients with Hepatitis B Complicated with Liver Fibrosis. *Eur. Rev. Med. Pharmacol. Sci.* 23 (10), 4360–4367. doi:10.26355/eurrev_201905_17943

Chen, T., Lin, H., Chen, X., Li, G., Zhao, Y., Zheng, L., et al. (2020b). LncRNA Meg8 Suppresses Activation of Hepatic Stellate Cells and Epithelial-Mesenchymal Transition of Hepatocytes via the Notch Pathway. *Biochem. Biophys. Res. Commun.* 521 (4), 921–927. doi:10.1016/j.bbrc.2019.11.015

Chen, X., Lun, L., Hou, H., Tian, R., Zhang, H., and Zhang, Y. (2017). The Value of lncRNA HULC as a Prognostic Factor for Survival of Cancer Outcome: A Meta-Analysis. *Cell Physiol Biochem* 41 (4), 1424–1434. doi:10.1159/000468005

Chen, Y., Huang, W., Sun, W., Zheng, B., Wang, C., Luo, Z., et al. (2018b). LncRNA MALAT1 Promotes Cancer Metastasis in Osteosarcoma via Activation of the PI3K-Akt Signaling Pathway. *Cel Physiol Biochem* 51 (3), 1313–1326. doi:10.1159/000495550

Chiu, H. S., Somvanshi, S., Patel, E., Chen, T. W., Singh, V. P., Zorman, B., et al. (2018). Pan-Cancer Analysis of lncRNA Regulation Supports Their Targeting of Cancer Genes in Each Tumor Context. *Cell Rep* 23 (1), 297–e12. e212. doi:10.1016/j.celrep.2018.03.064

Choudhry, H., Albukhari, A., Morotti, M., Haider, S., Moralli, D., Smythies, J., et al. (2015). Tumor Hypoxia Induces Nuclear Paraspeckle Formation through HIF-2α Dependent Transcriptional Activation of NEAT1 Leading to Cancer Cell Survival. *Oncogene* 34 (34), 4482–4490. doi:10.1038/onc.2014.378

Consortium, E. P., Birney, E., Stamatoyannopoulos, J. A., Dutta, A., Guigó, R., Gingeras, T. R., et al. (2007). Identification and Analysis of Functional Elements in 1% of the Human Genome by the ENCODE Pilot Project. *Nature* 447 (7146), 799–816. doi:10.1038/nature05874

Corti, F., Nichetti, F., Raimondi, A., Niger, M., Prinzi, N., Torchio, M., et al. (2019). Targeting the PI3K/AKT/mTOR Pathway in Biliary Tract Cancers: A Review of Current Evidences and Future Perspectives. *Cancer Treat. Rev.* 72, 45–55. doi:10.1016/j.ctrv.2018.11.001

Cui, H., Zhang, Y., Zhang, Q., Chen, W., Zhao, H., and Liang, J. (2017). A Comprehensive Genome-wide Analysis of Long Noncoding RNA Expression Profile in Hepatocellular Carcinoma. *Cancer Med.* 6 (12), 2932–2941. doi:10.1002/cam4.1180

Dai, X., Chen, C., Xue, J., Xiao, T., Mostofa, G., Wang, D., et al. (2019). Exosomal MALAT1 Derived from Hepatic Cells Is Involved in the Activation of Hepatic Stellate Cells via miRNA-26b in Fibrosis Induced by Arsenite. *Toxicol. Lett.* 316, 73–84. doi:10.1016/j.toxlet.2019.09.008

De Simone, V., Franzè, E., Ronchetti, G., Colantoni, A., Fantini, M. C., Di Fusco, D., et al. (2015). Th17-type Cytokines, IL-6 and TNF-α Synergistically Activate STAT3 and NF-kB to Promote Colorectal Cancer Cell Growth. *Oncogene* 34 (27), 3493–3503. doi:10.1038/onc.2014.286

De Vincentis, A., Rahmani, Z., Muley, M., Vespasiani-Gentilucci, U., Ruggiero, S., Zamani, P., et al. (2020). Long Noncoding RNAs in Nonalcoholic Fatty Liver Disease and Liver Fibrosis: State-Of-The-Art and Perspectives in Diagnosis and Treatment. *Drug Discov. Today* 25 (7), 1277–1286. doi:10.1016/j.drudis.2020.05.009

Dimitrova, N., Zamudio, J. R., Jong, R. M., Soukup, D., Resnick, R., Sarma, K., et al. (2014). LincRNA-p21 Activates P21 in Cis to Promote Polycomb Target Gene Expression and to Enforce the G1/S Checkpoint. *Mol. Cel* 54 (5), 777–790. doi:10.1016/j.molcel.2014.04.025

Ding, F., Lai, J., Gao, Y., Wang, G., Shang, J., Zhang, D., et al. (2019). NEAT1/miR-23a-3p/KLF3: a Novel Regulatory axis in Melanoma Cancer Progression. *Cancer Cel Int* 19, 217. doi:10.1186/s12935-019-0927-6

Dodson, M., Wani, W. Y., Redmann, M., Benavides, G. A., Johnson, M. S., Ouyang, X., et al. (2017). Regulation of Autophagy, Mitochondrial Dynamics, and Cellular Bioenergetics by 4-hydroxynonenal in Primary Neurons. *Autophagy* 13 (11), 1828–1840. doi:10.1080/15548627.2017.1356948

Dong, P., Xiong, Y., Yue, J., J B Hanley, S., Kobayashi, N., Todo, Y., et al. (2019a). Exploring lncRNA-Mediated Regulatory Networks in Endometrial Cancer Cells and the Tumor Microenvironment: Advances and Challenges. *Cancers (Basel)* 11 (2), 234. doi:10.3390/cancers11020234

Dong, R., Liu, G. B., Liu, B. H., Chen, G., Li, K., Zheng, S., et al. (2016). Targeting Long Non-coding RNA-TUG1 Inhibits Tumor Growth and Angiogenesis in Hepatoblastoma. *Cell Death Dis* 7 (6), e2278. doi:10.1038/cddis.2016.143

Dong, Z., Li, S., Wang, X., Si, L., Ma, R., Bao, L., et al. (2019b). lncRNA GAS5 Restrains CCl4-Induced Hepatic Fibrosis by Targeting miR-23a through the PTEN/PI3K/Akt Signaling Pathway. *Am. J. Physiol. Gastrointest. Liver Physiol.* 316 (4), G539–G550. doi:10.1152/ajpgi.00249.2018

Elpek, G. Ö. (2014). Cellular and Molecular Mechanisms in the Pathogenesis of Liver Fibrosis: An Update. *World J. Gastroenterol.* 20 (23), 7260–7276. doi:10.3748/wjg.v20.i23.7260

Esposito, R., Bosch, N., Lanzós, A., Polidori, T., Pulido-Quetglas, C., and Johnson, R. (2019). Hacking the Cancer Genome: Profiling Therapeutically Actionable Long Non-coding RNAs Using CRISPR-Cas9 Screening. *Cancer Cell* 35 (4), 545–557. doi:10.1016/j.ccell.2019.01.019

Faghihi, M. A., Modarresi, F., Khalil, A. M., Wood, D. E., Sahagan, B. G., Morgan, T. E., et al. (2008). Expression of a Noncoding RNA Is Elevated in Alzheimer's Disease and Drives Rapid Feed-Forward Regulation of Beta-Secretase. *Nat. Med.* 14 (7), 723–730. doi:10.1038/nm1784

Fatica, A., and Bozzoni, I. (2014). Long Non-coding RNAs: New Players in Cell Differentiation and Development. *Nat. Rev. Genet.* 15 (1), 7–21. doi:10.1038/nrg3606

Feng, C., Zhao, Y., Li, Y., Zhang, T., Ma, Y., and Liu, Y. (2019). LncRNA MALAT1 Promotes Lung Cancer Proliferation and Gefitinib Resistance by Acting as a miR-200a Sponge. *Arch. Bronconeumol* 55 (12), 627–633. doi:10.1016/j.arbres.2019.03.026

Feng, L., Zhang, J., Zhu, N., Ding, Q., Zhang, X., Yu, J., et al. (2017). Ubiquitin Ligase SYVN1/HRD1 Facilitates Degradation of the SERPINA1 Z Variant/α-1-Antitrypsin Z Variant via SQSTM1/p62-dependent Selective Autophagy. *Autophagy* 13 (4), 686–702. doi:10.1080/15548627.2017.1280207

Franco-Zorrilla, J. M., Valli, A., Todesco, M., Mateos, I., Puga, M. I., Rubio-Somoza, I., et al. (2007). Target Mimicry Provides a New Mechanism for Regulation of microRNA Activity. *Nat. Genet.* 39 (8), 1033–1037. doi:10.1038/ng2079

Fu, N., Zhao, S. X., Kong, L. B., Du, J. H., Ren, W. G., Han, F., et al. (2017). LncRNA-ATB/microRNA-200a/β-catenin Regulatory axis Involved in the Progression of HCV-Related Hepatic Fibrosis. *Gene* 618, 1–7. doi:10.1016/j.gene.2017.03.008

Fu, X., Zhu, X., Qin, F., Zhang, Y., Lin, J., Ding, Y., et al. (2018). Linc00210 Drives Wnt/β-Catenin Signaling Activation and Liver Tumor Progression through CTNNBIP1-dependent Manner. *Mol. Cancer* 17 (1), 73. doi:10.1186/s12943-018-0783-3

Gabory, A., Ripoche, M. A., Yoshimizu, T., and Dandolo, L. (2006). The H19 Gene: Regulation and Function of a Non-coding RNA. *Cytogenet. Genome Res.* 113 (1-4), 188–193. doi:10.1159/000090831

Ganguly, N., and Chakrabarti, S. (2021). Role of Long Non-coding RNAs and R-elated E-pigenetic M-echanisms in L-iver F-ibrosis (Review). *Int. J. Mol. Med.* 47 (3). doi:10.3892/ijmm.2021.4856

Garzon, R., Liu, S., Fabbri, M., Liu, Z., Heaphy, C. E. A., Callegari, E., et al. (2009). MicroRNA-29b Induces Global DNA Hypomethylation and Tumor Suppressor Gene Reexpression in Acute Myeloid Leukemia by Targeting Directly DNMT3A and 3B and Indirectly DNMT1. *Blood* 113 (25), 6411–6418. doi:10.1182/blood-2008-07-170589

Geerts, A. (2001). History, Heterogeneity, Developmental Biology, and Functions of Quiescent Hepatic Stellate Cells. *Semin. Liver Dis.* 21 (3), 311–335. doi:10.1055/s-2001-17550

Ghafouri-Fard, S., Esmaeili, M., Taheri, M., and Samsami, M. (2020b). Highly Upregulated in Liver Cancer (HULC): An Update on its Role in Carcinogenesis. *J. Cel Physiol* 235 (12), 9071–9079. doi:10.1002/jcp.29765

Ghafouri-Fard, S., and Taheri, M. (2019). Maternally Expressed Gene 3 (MEG3): A Tumor Suppressor Long Non Coding RNA. *Biomed. Pharmacother.* 118, 109129. doi:10.1016/j.biopha.2019.109129

Ghafouri-Fard, S., Esmaeili, M., and Taheri, M. (2020a). H19 lncRNA: Roles in Tumorigenesis. *Biomed. Pharmacother.* 123, 109774. doi:10.1016/j.biopha.2019.109774

Gong, Z., Deng, C., Xiao, H., Peng, Y., Hu, G., Xiang, T., et al. (2018). Effect of Dahuang Zhechong Pills on Long Non-coding RNA Growth Arrest Specific 5 in Rat Models of Hepatic Fibrosis. *J. Tradit Chin. Med.* 38 (2), 190–196. doi:10.1016/j.jtcm.2018.04.007

Goyal, A., Myacheva, K., Gross, M., Klingenberg, M., Duran Arqué, B., and Diederichs, S. (2017). Challenges of CRISPR/Cas9 Applications for Long Non-coding RNA Genes. *Nucleic Acids Res.* 45 (3), e12. doi:10.1093/nar/gkw883

Goyal, B., Yadav, S. R. M., Awasthee, N., Gupta, S., Kunnumakkara, A. B., and Gupta, S. C. (2021). Diagnostic, Prognostic, and Therapeutic Significance of Long Non-coding RNA MALAT1 in Cancer. *Biochim. Biophys. Acta Rev. Cancer* 1875 (2), 188502. doi:10.1016/j.bbcan.2021.188502

Guo, S., Chen, W., Luo, Y., Ren, F., Zhong, T., Rong, M., et al. (2015). Clinical Implication of Long Non-coding RNA NEAT1 Expression in Hepatocellular Carcinoma Patients. *Int. J. Clin. Exp. Pathol.* 8 (5), 5395–5402.

Guo, Y., Li, C., Zhang, R., Zhan, Y., Yu, J., Tu, J., et al. (2021). Epigenetically-regulated Serum GAS5 as a Potential Biomarker for Patients with Chronic Hepatitis B Virus Infection. *Cbm* 32, 137–146. doi:10.3233/CBM-203169

Gupta, R. A., Shah, N., Wang, K. C., Kim, J., Horlings, H. M., Wong, D. J., et al. (2010). Long Non-coding RNA HOTAIR Reprograms Chromatin State to Promote Cancer Metastasis. *Nature* 464 (7291), 1071–1076. doi:10.1038/nature08975

Guttman, M., Donaghey, J., Carey, B. W., Garber, M., Grenier, J. K., Munson, G., et al. (2011). lincRNAs Act in the Circuitry Controlling Pluripotency and Differentiation. *Nature* 477 (7364), 295–300. doi:10.1038/nature10398

Guttman, M., and Rinn, J. L. (2012). Modular Regulatory Principles of Large Non-coding RNAs. *Nature* 482 (7385), 339–346. doi:10.1038/nature10887

Han, M. H., Lee, J. H., Kim, G., Lee, E., Lee, Y. R., Jang, S. Y., et al. (2020). Expression of the Long Noncoding RNA GAS5 Correlates with Liver Fibrosis in Patients with Nonalcoholic Fatty Liver Disease. *Genes (Basel)* 11 (5), 545. doi:10.3390/genes11050545

Han, X., Hong, Y., and Zhang, K. (2018). TUG1 Is Involved in Liver Fibrosis and Activation of HSCs by Regulating miR-29b. *Biochem. Biophys. Res. Commun.* 503 (3), 1394–1400. doi:10.1016/j.bbrc.2018.07.054

He, Y., Wu, Y. T., Huang, C., Meng, X. M., Ma, T. T., Wu, B. M., et al. (2014). Inhibitory Effects of Long Noncoding RNA MEG3 on Hepatic Stellate Cells Activation and Liver Fibrogenesis. *Biochim. Biophys. Acta* 1842 (11), 2204–2215. doi:10.1016/j.bbadis.2014.08.015

He, Z., Yang, D., Fan, X., Zhang, M., Li, Y., Gu, X., et al. (2020). The Roles and Mechanisms of lncRNAs in Liver Fibrosis. *Int. J. Mol. Sci.* 21 (4), 1482. doi:10.3390/ijms21041482

Heo, M. J., Yun, J., and Kim, S. G. (2019). Role of Non-coding RNAs in Liver Disease Progression to Hepatocellular Carcinoma. *Arch. Pharm. Res.* 42 (1), 48–62. doi:10.1007/s12272-018-01104-x

Houtkooper, R. H., Pirinen, E., and Auwerx, J. (2012). Sirtuins as Regulators of Metabolism and Healthspan. *Nat. Rev. Mol. Cel Biol* 13 (4), 225–238. doi:10.1038/nrm3293

Hu, W., Liu, C., Bi, Z. Y., Zhou, Q., Zhang, H., Li, L. L., et al. (2020). Comprehensive Landscape of Extracellular Vesicle-Derived RNAs in Cancer Initiation, Progression, Metastasis and Cancer Immunology. *Mol. Cancer* 19 (1), 102. doi:10.1186/s12943-020-01199-1

Huang, T. J., Ren, J. J., Zhang, Q. Q., Kong, Y. Y., Zhang, H. Y., Guo, X. H., et al. (2019). IGFBPrP1 Accelerates Autophagy and Activation of Hepatic Stellate

Cells via Mutual Regulation between H19 and PI3K/AKT/mTOR Pathway. *Biomed. Pharmacother.* 116, 109034. doi:10.1016/j.biopha.2019.109034

Huang, W., Huang, F., Zhang, R., and Luo, H. (2021). LncRNA Neat1 Expedites the Progression of Liver Fibrosis in Mice through Targeting miR-148a-3p and miR-22-3p to Upregulate Cyth3. *Cell Cycle* 20 (5-6), 490–507. doi:10.1080/15384101.2021.1875665

Huarte, M., Guttman, M., Feldser, D., Garber, M., Koziol, M. J., Kenzelmann-Broz, D., et al. (2010). A Large Intergenic Noncoding RNA Induced by P53 Mediates Global Gene Repression in the P53 Response. *Cell* 142 (3), 409–419. doi:10.1016/j.cell.2010.06.040

Inoue, J., Kerr, L. D., Kakizuka, A., and Verma, I. M. (1992). I Kappa B Gamma, a 70 Kd Protein Identical to the C-Terminal Half of P110 NF-Kappa B: a New Member of the I Kappa B Family. *Cell* 68 (6), 1109–1120. doi:10.1016/0092-8674(92)90082-n

Ji, P., Diederichs, S., Wang, W., Böing, S., Metzger, R., Schneider, P. M., et al. (2003). MALAT-1, a Novel Noncoding RNA, and Thymosin Beta4 Predict Metastasis and Survival in Early-Stage Non-small Cell Lung Cancer. *Oncogene* 22 (39), 8031–8041. doi:10.1038/sj.onc.1206928

Jia, M., Jiang, L., Wang, Y. D., Huang, J. Z., Yu, M., and Xue, H. Z. (2016). lincRNA-p21 Inhibits Invasion and Metastasis of Hepatocellular Carcinoma through Notch Signaling-Induced Epithelial-Mesenchymal Transition. *Hepatol. Res.* 46 (11), 1137–1144. doi:10.1111/hepr.12659

Jiang, X., and Zhang, F. (2017). Long Noncoding RNA: a New Contributor and Potential Therapeutic Target in Fibrosis. *Epigenomics* 9 (9), 1233–1241. doi:10.2217/epi-2017-0020

Jin, S. S., Lin, X. F., Zheng, J. Z., Wang, Q., and Guan, H. Q. (2019). lncRNA NEAT1 Regulates Fibrosis and Inflammatory Response Induced by Nonalcoholic Fatty Liver by Regulating miR-506/GLI3. *Eur. Cytokine Netw.* 30 (3), 98–106. doi:10.1684/ecn.2019.0432

Jinek, M., Chylinski, K., Fonfara, I., Hauer, M., Doudna, J. A., and Charpentier, E. (2012). A Programmable Dual-RNA-Guided DNA Endonuclease in Adaptive Bacterial Immunity. *Science* 337 (6096), 816–821. doi:10.1126/science.1225829

Jung, K., Kim, M., So, J., Lee, S. H., Ko, S., and Shin, D. (2021). Farnesoid X Receptor Activation Impairs Liver Progenitor Cell-Mediated Liver Regeneration via the PTEN-Pi3k-AKT-mTOR Axis in Zebrafish. *Hepatology* 74 (1), 397–410. doi:10.1002/hep.31679

Jux, B., Gosejacob, D., Tolksdorf, F., Mandel, C., Rieck, M., Namislo, A., et al. (2019). Cytohesin-3 Is Required for Full Insulin Receptor Signaling and Controls Body Weight via Lipid Excretion. *Sci. Rep.* 9 (1), 3442. doi:10.1038/s41598-019-40231-3

Kaneko, S., Bonasio, R., Saldaña-Meyer, R., Yoshida, T., Son, J., Nishino, K., et al. (2014). Interactions between JARID2 and Noncoding RNAs Regulate PRC2 Recruitment to Chromatin. *Mol. Cel* 53 (2), 290–300. doi:10.1016/j.molcel.2013.11.012

Kapusta, A., Kronenberg, Z., Lynch, V. J., Zhuo, X., Ramsay, L., Bourque, G., et al. (2013). Transposable Elements Are Major Contributors to the Origin, Diversification, and Regulation of Vertebrate Long Noncoding RNAs. *Plos Genet.* 9 (4), e1003470. doi:10.1371/journal.pgen.1003470

Karin, M., Cao, Y., Greten, F. R., and Li, Z. W. (2002). NF-kappaB in Cancer: from Innocent Bystander to Major Culprit. *Nat. Rev. Cancer* 2 (4), 301–310. doi:10.1038/nrc780

Karreth, F. A., Tay, Y., Perna, D., Ala, U., Tan, S. M., Rust, A. G., et al. (2011). In Vivo identification of Tumor- Suppressive PTEN ceRNAs in an Oncogenic BRAF-Induced Mouse Model of Melanoma. *Cell* 147 (2), 382–395. doi:10.1016/j.cell.2011.09.032

Katsushima, K., Natsume, A., Ohka, F., Shinjo, K., Hatanaka, A., Ichimura, N., et al. (2016). Targeting the Notch-Regulated Non-coding RNA TUG1 for Glioma Treatment. *Nat. Commun.* 7, 13616. doi:10.1038/ncomms13616

Khalil, A. M., Guttman, M., Huarte, M., Garber, M., Raj, A., Rivea Morales, D., et al. (2009). Many Human Large Intergenic Noncoding RNAs Associate with Chromatin-Modifying Complexes and Affect Gene Expression. *Proc. Natl. Acad. Sci. U S A.* 106 (28), 11667–11672. doi:10.1073/pnas.0904715106

Khemlina, G., Ikeda, S., and Kurzrock, R. (2017). The Biology of Hepatocellular Carcinoma: Implications for Genomic and Immune Therapies. *Mol. Cancer* 16 (1), 149. doi:10.1186/s12943-017-0712-x

Khomich, O., Ivanov, A. V., and Bartosch, B. (2019). Metabolic Hallmarks of Hepatic Stellate Cells in Liver Fibrosis. *Cells* 9 (1). doi:10.3390/cells9010024

Kim, J., Piao, H. L., Kim, B. J., Yao, F., Han, Z., Wang, Y., et al. (2018). Long Noncoding RNA MALAT1 Suppresses Breast Cancer Metastasis. *Nat. Genet.* 50 (12), 1705–1715. doi:10.1038/s41588-018-0252-3

Kim, M. H., Seong, J. B., Huh, J. W., Bae, Y. C., Lee, H. S., and Lee, D. S. (2020a). Peroxiredoxin 5 Ameliorates Obesity-Induced Non-alcoholic Fatty Liver Disease through the Regulation of Oxidative Stress and AMP-Activated Protein Kinase Signaling. *Redox Biol.* 28, 101315. doi:10.1016/j.redox.2019.101315

Kim, Y. A., Park, K. K., and Lee, S. J. (2020b). LncRNAs Act as a Link between Chronic Liver Disease and Hepatocellular Carcinoma. *Int. J. Mol. Sci.* 21 (8), 2883. doi:10.3390/ijms21082883

Kitagawa, M., Kitagawa, K., Kotake, Y., Niida, H., and Ohhata, T. (2013). Cell Cycle Regulation by Long Non-coding RNAs. *Cell Mol Life Sci* 70 (24), 4785–4794. doi:10.1007/s00018-013-1423-0

Klec, C., Gutschner, T., Panzitt, K., and Pichler, M. (2019). Involvement of Long Non-coding RNA HULC (Highly Up-Regulated in Liver Cancer) in Pathogenesis and Implications for Therapeutic Intervention. *Expert Opin. Ther. Targets* 23 (3), 177–186. doi:10.1080/14728222.2019.1570499

Konermann, S., Brigham, M. D., Trevino, A. E., Joung, J., Abudayyeh, O. O., Barcena, C., et al. (2015). Genome-scale Transcriptional Activation by an Engineered CRISPR-Cas9 Complex. *Nature* 517 (7536), 583–588. doi:10.1038/nature14136

Kong, D., Zhang, Z., Chen, L., Huang, W., Zhang, F., Wang, L., et al. (2020). Curcumin Blunts Epithelial-Mesenchymal Transition of Hepatocytes to Alleviate Hepatic Fibrosis through Regulating Oxidative Stress and Autophagy. *Redox Biol.* 36, 101600. doi:10.1016/j.redox.2020.101600

Kong, X., Qian, X., Duan, L., Liu, H., Zhu, Y., and Qi, J. (2016). microRNA-372 Suppresses Migration and Invasion by Targeting P65 in Human Prostate Cancer Cells. *DNA Cel Biol* 35 (12), 828–835. doi:10.1089/dna.2015.3186

Kopp, F., and Mendell, J. T. (2018). Functional Classification and Experimental Dissection of Long Noncoding RNAs. *Cell* 172 (3), 393–407. doi:10.1016/j.cell.2018.01.011

Kovall, R. A., Gebelein, B., Sprinzak, D., and Kopan, R. (2017). The Canonical Notch Signaling Pathway: Structural and Biochemical Insights into Shape, Sugar, and Force. *Dev. Cel* 41 (3), 228–241. doi:10.1016/j.devcel.2017.04.001

Krizhanovsky, V., Yon, M., Dickins, R. A., Hearn, S., Simon, J., Miething, C., et al. (2008). Senescence of Activated Stellate Cells Limits Liver Fibrosis. *Cell* 134 (4), 657–667. doi:10.1016/j.cell.2008.06.049

Lam, P., Cheung, F., Tan, H. Y., Wang, N., Yuen, M. F., and Feng, Y. (2016). Hepatoprotective Effects of Chinese Medicinal Herbs: A Focus on Anti-inflammatory and Anti-oxidative Activities. *Int. J. Mol. Sci.* 17 (4), 465. doi:10.3390/ijms17040465

Lan, T., Li, C., Yang, G., Sun, Y., Zhuang, L., Ou, Y., et al. (2018). Sphingosine Kinase 1 Promotes Liver Fibrosis by Preventing miR-19b-3p-Mediated Inhibition of CCR2. *Hepatology* 68 (3), 1070–1086. doi:10.1002/hep.29885

Lee, J. J., Loh, K., and Yap, Y. S. (2015a). PI3K/Akt/mTOR Inhibitors in Breast Cancer. *Cancer Biol. Med.* 12 (4), 342–354. doi:10.7497/j.issn.2095-3941.2015.0089

Lee, Y. A., Wallace, M. C., and Friedman, S. L. (2015b). Pathobiology of Liver Fibrosis: a Translational success story. *Gut* 64 (5), 830–841. doi:10.1136/gutjnl-2014-306842

Leti, F., Legendre, C., Still, C. D., Chu, X., Petrick, A., Gerhard, G. S., et al. (2017). Altered Expression of MALAT1 lncRNA in Nonalcoholic Steatohepatitis Fibrosis Regulates CXCL5 in Hepatic Stellate Cells. *Transl Res.* 190, 25–e21. doi:10.1016/j.trsl.2017.09.001

Li, J., Yang, C., Li, Y., Chen, A., Li, L., and You, Z. (2018a). LncRNA GAS5 Suppresses Ovarian Cancer by Inducing Inflammasome Formation. *Biosci. Rep.* 38 (2). doi:10.1042/BSR20171150

Li, J. H., Liu, S., Zhou, H., Qu, L. H., and Yang, J. H. (2014). starBase v2.0: Decoding miRNA-ceRNA, miRNA-ncRNA and Protein-RNA Interaction Networks from Large-Scale CLIP-Seq Data. *Nucleic Acids Res.* 42, D92–D97. Database issue. doi:10.1093/nar/gkt1248

Li, T., Mo, X., Fu, L., Xiao, B., and Guo, J. (2016). Molecular Mechanisms of Long Noncoding RNAs on Gastric Cancer. *Oncotarget* 7 (8), 8601–8612. doi:10.18632/oncotarget.6926

Li, X., Liu, R., Huang, Z., Gurley, E. C., Wang, X., Wang, J., et al. (2018b). Cholangiocyte-derived Exosomal Long Noncoding RNA H19 Promotes

Cholestatic Liver Injury in Mouse and Humans. *Hepatology* 68 (2), 599–615. doi:10.1002/hep.29838

Li, Y., Zhu, J., Tian, G., Li, N., Li, Q., Ye, M., et al. (2010). The DNA Methylome of Human Peripheral Blood Mononuclear Cells. *Plos Biol.* 8 (11), e1000533. doi:10.1371/journal.pbio.1000533

Li, Z., Wang, J., Zeng, Q., Hu, C., Zhang, J., Wang, H., et al. (2018c). Long Noncoding RNA HOTTIP Promotes Mouse Hepatic Stellate Cell Activation via Downregulating miR-148a. *Cel Physiol Biochem* 51 (6), 2814–2828. doi:10.1159/000496012

Lin, N., Yao, Z., Xu, M., Chen, J., Lu, Y., Yuan, L., et al. (2019). Long Noncoding RNA MALAT1 Potentiates Growth and Inhibits Senescence by Antagonizing ABI3BP in Gallbladder Cancer Cells. *J. Exp. Clin. Cancer Res.* 38 (1), 244. doi:10.1186/s13046-019-1237-5

Lin, S. P., Youngson, N., Takada, S., Seitz, H., Reik, W., Paulsen, M., et al. (2003). Asymmetric Regulation of Imprinting on the Maternal and Paternal Chromosomes at the Dlk1-Gtl2 Imprinted Cluster on Mouse Chromosome 12. *Nat. Genet.* 35 (1), 97–102. doi:10.1038/ng1233

Liu, C., Yang, Z., Wu, J., Zhang, L., Lee, S., Shin, D. J., et al. (2018). Long Noncoding RNA H19 Interacts with Polypyrimidine Tract-Binding Protein 1 to Reprogram Hepatic Lipid Homeostasis. *Hepatology* 67 (5), 1768–1783. doi:10.1002/hep.29654

Liu, R., Li, X., Zhu, W., Wang, Y., Zhao, D., Wang, X., et al. (2019). Cholangiocyte-Derived Exosomal Long Noncoding RNA H19 Promotes Hepatic Stellate Cell Activation and Cholestatic Liver Fibrosis. *Hepatology* 70 (4), 1317–1335. doi:10.1002/hep.30662

Luedde, T., and Schwabe, R. F. (2011). NF-kappaB in the Liver-Llinking Injury, Fibrosis, and Hepatocellular Carcinoma. *Nat. Rev. Gastroenterol. Hepatol.* 8 (2), 108–118. doi:10.1038/nrgastro.2010.213

Luo, N., Li, J., Chen, Y., Xu, Y., Wei, Y., Lu, J., et al. (2021). Hepatic Stellate Cell Reprogramming via Exosome-Mediated CRISPR/dCas9-VP64 Delivery. *Drug Deliv.* 28 (1), 10–18. doi:10.1080/10717544.2020.1850917

Ma, Y., Liu, L., Yan, F., Wei, W., Deng, J., and Sun, J. (2016a). Enhanced Expression of Long Non-coding RNA NEAT1 Is Associated with the Progression of Gastric Adenocarcinomas. *World J. Surg. Oncol.* 14 (1), 41. doi:10.1186/s12957-016-0799-3

Ma, Y., Yang, Y., Wang, F., Moyer, M. P., Wei, Q., Zhang, P., et al. (2016b). Long Non-coding RNA CCAL Regulates Colorectal Cancer Progression by Activating Wnt/β-Catenin Signalling Pathway via Suppression of Activator Protein 2α. *Gut* 65 (9), 1494–1504. doi:10.1136/gutjnl-2014-308392

Ma, Y., Zhang, J., Wen, L., and Lin, A. (2018). Membrane-lipid Associated lncRNA: A New Regulator in Cancer Signaling. *Cancer Lett.* 419, 27–29. doi:10.1016/j.canlet.2018.01.008

Mahpour, A., and Mullen, A. C. (2021). Our Emerging Understanding of the Roles of Long Non-coding RNAs in normal Liver Function, Disease, and Malignancy. *JHEP Rep.* 3 (1), 100177. doi:10.1016/j.jhepr.2020.100177

Mayr, B., and Montminy, M. (2001). Transcriptional Regulation by the Phosphorylation-dependent Factor CREB. *Nat. Rev. Mol. Cel Biol* 2 (8), 599–609. doi:10.1038/35085068

McMahon, B. J. (2009). The Natural History of Chronic Hepatitis B Virus Infection. *Hepatology* 49 (5 Suppl. l), S45–S55. doi:10.1002/hep.22898

Mercer, T. R., Dinger, M. E., Sunkin, S. M., Mehler, M. F., and Mattick, J. S. (2008). Specific Expression of Long Noncoding RNAs in the Mouse Brain. *Proc. Natl. Acad. Sci. U S A.* 105 (2), 716–721. doi:10.1073/pnas.0706729105

Meurette, O., and Mehlen, P. (2018). Notch Signaling in the Tumor Microenvironment. *Cancer Cell* 34 (4), 536–548. doi:10.1016/j.ccell.2018.07.009

Mihaylova, M. M., and Shaw, R. J. (2011). The AMPK Signalling Pathway Coordinates Cell Growth, Autophagy and Metabolism. *Nat. Cel Biol* 13 (9), 1016–1023. doi:10.1038/ncb2329

Mo, Z., Cheong, J. Y. A., Xiang, L., Le, M. T. N., Grimson, A., and Zhang, D. X. (2021). Extracellular Vesicle-Associated Organotropic Metastasis. *Cell Prolif* 54 (1), e12948. doi:10.1111/cpr.12948

Mondal, T., Subhash, S., Vaid, R., Enroth, S., Uday, S., Reinius, B., et al. (2015). MEG3 Long Noncoding RNA Regulates the TGF-β Pathway Genes through Formation of RNA-DNA Triplex Structures. *Nat. Commun.* 6, 7743. doi:10.1038/ncomms8743

Monti-Rocha, R., Cramer, A., Gaio Leite, P., Antunes, M. M., Pereira, R. V. S., Barroso, A., et al. (2018). SOCS2 Is Critical for the Balancing of Immune Response and Oxidate Stress Protecting against Acetaminophen-Induced Acute Liver Injury. *Front. Immunol.* 9, 3134. doi:10.3389/fimmu.2018.03134

Mori, M. A., Ludwig, R. G., Garcia-Martin, R., Brandão, B. B., and Kahn, C. R. (2019). Extracellular miRNAs: From Biomarkers to Mediators of Physiology and Disease. *Cel Metab* 30 (4), 656–673. doi:10.1016/j.cmet.2019.07.011

Murphy, S. K., Wylie, A. A., Coveler, K. J., Cotter, P. D., Papenhausen, P. R., Sutton, V. R., et al. (2003). Epigenetic Detection of Human Chromosome 14 Uniparental Disomy. *Hum. Mutat.* 22 (1), 92–97. doi:10.1002/humu.10237

Ni, W., Yao, S., Zhou, Y., Liu, Y., Huang, P., Zhou, A., et al. (2019). Long Noncoding RNA GAS5 Inhibits Progression of Colorectal Cancer by Interacting with and Triggering YAP Phosphorylation and Degradation and Is Negatively Regulated by the m6A Reader YTHDF3. *Mol. Cancer* 18 (1), 143. doi:10.1186/s12943-019-1079-y

Nielsen, C. P., Jernigan, K. K., Diggins, N. L., Webb, D. J., and MacGurn, J. A. (2019). USP9X Deubiquitylates DVL2 to Regulate WNT Pathway Specification. *Cel Rep* 28 (4), 1074–e5. e1075. doi:10.1016/j.celrep.2019.06.083

Niland, C. N., Merry, C. R., and Khalil, A. M. (2012). Emerging Roles for Long Non-coding RNAs in Cancer and Neurological Disorders. *Front. Genet.* 3, 25. doi:10.3389/fgene.2012.00025

Nowell, C. S., and Radtke, F. (2017). Notch as a Tumour Suppressor. *Nat. Rev. Cancer* 17 (3), 145–159. doi:10.1038/nrc.2016.145

Nudelman, R., Ardon, O., Hadar, Y., Chen, Y., Libman, J., and Shanzer, A. (1998). Modular Fluorescent-Labeled Siderophore Analogues. *J. Med. Chem.* 41 (10), 1671–1678. doi:10.1021/jm970581b

Özgür, E., Mert, U., Isin, M., Okutan, M., Dalay, N., and Gezer, U. (2013). Differential Expression of Long Non-coding RNAs during Genotoxic Stress-Induced Apoptosis in HeLa and MCF-7 Cells. *Clin. Exp. Med.* 13 (2), 119–126. doi:10.1007/s10238-012-0181-x

Page, A., Paoli, P., Moran Salvador, E., White, S., French, J., and Mann, J. (2016). Hepatic Stellate Cell Transdifferentiation Involves Genome-wide Remodeling of the DNA Methylation Landscape. *J. Hepatol.* 64 (3), 661–673. doi:10.1016/j.jhep.2015.11.024

Panzitt, K., Tschernatsch, M. M., Guelly, C., Moustafa, T., Stradner, M., Strohmaier, H. M., et al. (2007). Characterization of HULC, a Novel Gene with Striking Up-Regulation in Hepatocellular Carcinoma, as Noncoding RNA. *Gastroenterology* 132 (1), 330–342. doi:10.1053/j.gastro.2006.08.026

Parasramka, M. A., Maji, S., Matsuda, A., Yan, I. K., and Patel, T. (2016). Long Non-coding RNAs as Novel Targets for Therapy in Hepatocellular Carcinoma. *Pharmacol. Ther.* 161, 67–78. doi:10.1016/j.pharmthera.2016.03.004

Parola, M., and Pinzani, M. (2019). Liver Fibrosis: Pathophysiology, Pathogenetic Targets and Clinical Issues. *Mol. Aspects Med.* 65, 37–55. doi:10.1016/j.mam.2018.09.002

Peng, H., Wan, L. Y., Liang, J. J., Zhang, Y. Q., Ai, W. B., and Wu, J. F. (2018). The Roles of lncRNA in Hepatic Fibrosis. *Cell Biosci* 8, 63. doi:10.1186/s13578-018-0259-6

Peng, W. X., Koirala, P., and Mo, Y. Y. (2017). LncRNA-mediated Regulation of Cell Signaling in Cancer. *Oncogene* 36 (41), 5661–5667. doi:10.1038/onc.2017.184

Qi, X., Zhang, D. H., Wu, N., Xiao, J. H., Wang, X., and Ma, W. (2015). ceRNA in Cancer: Possible Functions and Clinical Implications. *J. Med. Genet.* 52 (10), 710–718. doi:10.1136/jmedgenet-2015-103334

Quagliata, L., Matter, M. S., Piscuoglio, S., Arabi, L., Ruiz, C., Procino, A., et al. (2014). Long Noncoding RNA HOTTIP/HOXA13 Expression Is Associated with Disease Progression and Predicts Outcome in Hepatocellular Carcinoma Patients. *Hepatology* 59 (3), 911–923. doi:10.1002/hep.26740

Raveh, E., Matouk, I. J., Gilon, M., and Hochberg, A. (2015). The H19 Long Non-coding RNA in Cancer Initiation, Progression and Metastasis - a Proposed Unifying Theory. *Mol. Cancer* 14, 184. doi:10.1186/s12943-015-0458-2

Ray, K. (2014). Liver: Hepatic Stellate Cells Hold the Key to Liver Fibrosis. *Nat. Rev. Gastroenterol. Hepatol.* 11 (2), 74. doi:10.1038/nrgastro.2013.244

Riaz, F., and Li, D. (2019). Non-coding RNA Associated Competitive Endogenous RNA Regulatory Network: Novel Therapeutic Approach in Liver Fibrosis. *Curr. Gene Ther.* 19 (5), 305–317. doi:10.2174/1566523219666191107113046

Rockey, D. C., Caldwell, S. H., Goodman, Z. D., Nelson, R. C., and Smith, A. D.American Association for the Study of Liver Diseases (2009). Liver Biopsy. *Hepatology* 49 (3), 1017–1044. doi:10.1002/hep.22742

Roderburg, C., Urban, G. W., Bettermann, K., Vucur, M., Zimmermann, H., Schmidt, S., et al. (2011). Micro-RNA Profiling Reveals a Role for miR-29 in

Human and Murine Liver Fibrosis. *Hepatology* 53 (1), 209–218. doi:10.1002/hep.23922

Roehlen, N., Crouchet, E., and Baumert, T. F. (2020). Liver Fibrosis: Mechanistic Concepts and Therapeutic Perspectives. *Cells* 9 (4), 875. doi:10.3390/cells9040875

Salmena, L., Poliseno, L., Tay, Y., Kats, L., and Pandolfi, P. P. (2011). A ceRNA Hypothesis: the Rosetta Stone of a Hidden RNA Language? *Cell* 146 (3), 353–358. doi:10.1016/j.cell.2011.07.014

Schunk, S. J., Floege, J., Fliser, D., and Speer, T. (2021). WNT-β-catenin Signalling - a Versatile Player in Kidney Injury and Repair. *Nat. Rev. Nephrol.* 17 (3), 172–184. doi:10.1038/s41581-020-00343-w

Sebio, A., Kahn, M., and Lenz, H. J. (2014). The Potential of Targeting Wnt/β-Catenin in colon Cancer. *Expert Opin. Ther. Targets* 18 (6), 611–615. doi:10.1517/14728222.2014.906580

Shackelford, D. B., and Shaw, R. J. (2009). The LKB1-AMPK Pathway: Metabolism and Growth Control in Tumour Suppression. *Nat. Rev. Cancer* 9 (8), 563–575. doi:10.1038/nrc2676

Sharma, G., Sharma, A. R., Bhattacharya, M., Lee, S. S., and Chakraborty, C. (2021). CRISPR-Cas9: A Preclinical and Clinical Perspective for the Treatment of Human Diseases. *Mol. Ther.* 29 (2), 571–586. doi:10.1016/j.ymthe.2020.09.028

Shen, M., Dong, C., Ruan, X., Yan, W., Cao, M., Pizzo, D., et al. (2019a). Chemotherapy-Induced Extracellular Vesicle MiRNAs Promote Breast Cancer Stemness by Targeting ONECUT2. *Cancer Res.* 79 (14), 3608–3621. doi:10.1158/0008-5472.CAN-18-4055

Shen, X., Guo, H., Xu, J., and Wang, J. (2019b). Inhibition of lncRNA HULC Improves Hepatic Fibrosis and Hepatocyte Apoptosis by Inhibiting the MAPK Signaling Pathway in Rats with Nonalcoholic Fatty Liver Disease. *J. Cel Physiol* 234 (10), 18169–18179. doi:10.1002/jcp.28450

Shi, X., Jiang, X., Yuan, B., Liu, T., Tang, Y., Che, Y., et al. (2019). LINC01093 Upregulation Protects against Alcoholic Hepatitis through Inhibition of NF-Kb Signaling Pathway. *Mol. Ther. Nucleic Acids* 17, 791–803. doi:10.1016/j.omtn.2019.06.018

Song, Y., Liu, C., Liu, X., Trottier, J., Beaudoin, M., Zhang, L., et al. (2017). H19 Promotes Cholestatic Liver Fibrosis by Preventing ZEB1-Mediated Inhibition of Epithelial Cell Adhesion Molecule. *Hepatology* 66 (4), 1183–1196. doi:10.1002/hep.29209

Strotskaya, A., Savitskaya, E., Metlitskaya, A., Morozova, N., Datsenko, K. A., Semenova, E., et al. (2017). The Action of *Escherichia coli* CRISPR-Cas System on Lytic Bacteriophages with Different Lifestyles and Development Strategies. *Nucleic Acids Res.* 45 (4), 1946–1957. doi:10.1093/nar/gkx042

Sun, D., Yu, Z., Fang, X., Liu, M., Pu, Y., Shao, Q., et al. (2017). LncRNA GAS5 Inhibits Microglial M2 Polarization and Exacerbates Demyelination. *EMBO Rep.* 18 (10), 1801–1816. doi:10.15252/embr.201643668

Tacke, F., and Trautwein, C. (2015). Mechanisms of Liver Fibrosis Resolution. *J. Hepatol.* 63 (4), 1038–1039. doi:10.1016/j.jhep.2015.03.039

Tang, S. S., Zheng, B. Y., and Xiong, X. D. (2015). LincRNA-p21: Implications in Human Diseases. *Int. J. Mol. Sci.* 16 (8), 18732–18740. doi:10.3390/ijms160818732

Tay, Y., Kats, L., Salmena, L., Weiss, D., Tan, S. M., Ala, U., et al. (2011). Coding-independent Regulation of the Tumor Suppressor PTEN by Competing Endogenous mRNAs. *Cell* 147 (2), 344–357. doi:10.1016/j.cell.2011.09.029

Tay, Y., Rinn, J., and Pandolfi, P. P. (2014). The Multilayered Complexity of ceRNA Crosstalk and Competition. *Nature* 505 (7483), 344–352. doi:10.1038/nature12986

Thomson, D. W., and Dinger, M. E. (2016). Endogenous microRNA Sponges: Evidence and Controversy. *Nat. Rev. Genet.* 17 (5), 272–283. doi:10.1038/nrg.2016.20

Tian, X., and Xu, G. (2015). Clinical Value of lncRNA MALAT1 as a Prognostic Marker in Human Cancer: Systematic Review and Meta-Analysis. *BMJ Open* 5 (9), e008653. doi:10.1136/bmjopen-2015-008653

Tierling, S., Dalbert, S., Schoppenhorst, S., Tsai, C. E., Oliger, S., Ferguson-Smith, A. C., et al. (2006). High-resolution Map and Imprinting Analysis of the Gtl2-Dnchc1 Domain on Mouse Chromosome 12. *Genomics* 87 (2), 225–235. doi:10.1016/j.ygeno.2005.09.018

Tsang, F. H., Au, S. L., Wei, L., Fan, D. N., Lee, J. M., Wong, C. C., et al. (2015). Long Non-coding RNA HOTTIP Is Frequently Up-Regulated in Hepatocellular

Carcinoma and Is Targeted by Tumour Suppressive miR-125b. *Liver Int.* 35 (5), 1597–1606. doi:10.1111/liv.12746

Tu, X., Zhang, Y., Zheng, X., Deng, J., Li, H., Kang, Z., et al. (2017). TGF-β-induced Hepatocyte lincRNA-P21 Contributes to Liver Fibrosis in Mice. *Sci. Rep.* 7 (1), 2957. doi:10.1038/s41598-017-03175-0

Unfried, J. P., and Fortes, P. (2020). LncRNAs in HCV Infection and HCV-Related Liver Disease. *Int. J. Mol. Sci.* 21 (6). doi:10.3390/ijms21062255

van Kruijsbergen, I., Hontelez, S., and Veenstra, G. J. (2015). Recruiting Polycomb to Chromatin. *Int. J. Biochem. Cel Biol* 67, 177–187. doi:10.1016/j.biocel.2015.05.006

van Niel, G., D'Angelo, G., and Raposo, G. (2018). Shedding Light on the Cell Biology of Extracellular Vesicles. *Nat. Rev. Mol. Cel Biol* 19 (4), 213–228. doi:10.1038/nrm.2017.125

Voce, D. J., Bernal, G. M., Wu, L., Crawley, C. D., Zhang, W., Mansour, N. M., et al. (2019). Temozolomide Treatment Induces lncRNA MALAT1 in an NF-Kb and P53 Codependent Manner in Glioblastoma. *Cancer Res.* 79 (10), 2536–2548. doi:10.1158/0008-5472.CAN-18-2170

Walker, S., Busatto, S., Pham, A., Tian, M., Suh, A., Carson, K., et al. (2019). Extracellular Vesicle-Based Drug Delivery Systems for Cancer Treatment. *Theranostics* 9 (26), 8001–8017. doi:10.7150/thno.37097

Wang, F., Yuan, J. H., Wang, S. B., Yang, F., Yuan, S. X., Ye, C., et al. (2014). Oncofetal Long Noncoding RNA PVT1 Promotes Proliferation and Stem Cell-like Property of Hepatocellular Carcinoma Cells by Stabilizing NOP2. *Hepatology* 60 (4), 1278–1290. doi:10.1002/hep.27239

Wang, J., Liu, X., Wu, H., Ni, P., Gu, Z., Qiao, Y., et al. (2010). CREB Up-Regulates Long Non-coding RNA, HULC Expression through Interaction with microRNA-372 in Liver Cancer. *Nucleic Acids Res.* 38 (16), 5366–5383. doi:10.1093/nar/gkq285

Wang, J., Sun, J., and Yang, F. (2020a). The Role of Long Non-coding RNA H19 in Breast Cancer. *Oncol. Lett.* 19 (1), 7–16. doi:10.3892/ol.2019.11093

Wang, K. C., Yang, Y. W., Liu, B., Sanyal, A., Corces-Zimmerman, R., Chen, Y., et al. (2011). A Long Noncoding RNA Maintains Active Chromatin to Coordinate Homeotic Gene Expression. *Nature* 472 (7341), 120–124. doi:10.1038/nature09819

Wang, L. X., Wan, C., Dong, Z. B., Wang, B. H., Liu, H. Y., and Li, Y. (2019a). Integrative Analysis of Long Noncoding RNA (lncRNA), microRNA (miRNA) and mRNA Expression and Construction of a Competing Endogenous RNA (ceRNA) Network in Metastatic Melanoma. *Med. Sci. Monit.* 25, 2896–2907. doi:10.12659/MSM.913881

Wang, P., Wu, T., Zhou, H., Jin, Q., He, G., Yu, H., et al. (2016). Long Noncoding RNA NEAT1 Promotes Laryngeal Squamous Cell Cancer through Regulating miR-107/CDK6 Pathway. *J. Exp. Clin. Cancer Res.* 35, 22. doi:10.1186/s13046-016-0297-z

Wang, T., Fu, X., Jin, T., Zhang, L., Liu, B., Wu, Y., et al. (2019b). Aspirin Targets P4HA2 through Inhibiting NF-Kb and LMCD1-AS1/let-7g to Inhibit Tumour Growth and Collagen Deposition in Hepatocellular Carcinoma. *EBioMedicine* 45, 168–180. doi:10.1016/j.ebiom.2019.06.048

Wang, X., Ruan, Y., Wang, X., Zhao, W., Jiang, Q., Jiang, C., et al. (2017). Long Intragenic Non-coding RNA lincRNA-P21 Suppresses Development of Human Prostate Cancer. *Cel Prolif* 50 (2). doi:10.1111/cpr.12318

Wang, Z., Yang, X., Kai, J., Wang, F., Wang, Z., Shao, J., et al. (2020b). HIF-1α-upregulated lncRNA-H19 Regulates Lipid Droplet Metabolism through the AMPKα Pathway in Hepatic Stellate Cells. *Life Sci.* 255, 117818. doi:10.1016/j.lfs.2020.117818

Wang, Z. M., Xia, S. W., Zhang, T., Wang, Z. Y., Yang, X., Kai, J., et al. (2020c). LncRNA-H19 Induces Hepatic Stellate Cell Activation via Upregulating Alcohol Dehydrogenase III-Mediated Retinoic Acid Signals. *Int. Immunopharmacol* 84, 106470. doi:10.1016/j.intimp.2020.106470

Wei, L. Q., Li, L., Lu, C., Liu, J., Chen, Y., and Wu, H. (2019a). Involvement of H19/miR-326 axis in Hepatocellular Carcinoma Development through Modulating TWIST1. *J. Cel Physiol* 234 (4), 5153–5162. doi:10.1002/jcp.27319

Wei, S., Wang, K., Huang, X., Zhao, Z., and Zhao, Z. (2019b). LncRNA MALAT1 Contributes to Non-small Cell Lung Cancer Progression via Modulating miR-200a-3p/programmed Death-Ligand 1 axis. *Int. J. Immunopathol Pharmacol.* 33, 2058738419859699. doi:10.1177/2058738419859699

Wilusz, C. J., and Wilusz, J. (2012). HuR and Translation-Tthe Missing Linc(RNA). *Mol. Cel* 47 (4), 495–496. doi:10.1016/j.molcel.2012.08.005

Wilusz, J. E., Freier, S. M., and Spector, D. L. (2008). 3' End Processing of a Long Nuclear-Retained Noncoding RNA Yields a tRNA-like Cytoplasmic RNA. *Cell* 135 (5), 919–932. doi:10.1016/j.cell.2008.10.012

Wilusz, J. E. (2016). Long Noncoding RNAs: Re-writing Dogmas of RNA Processing and Stability. *Biochim. Biophys. Acta* 1859 (1), 128–138. doi:10.1016/j.bbagrm.2015.06.003

Wirawan, E., Lippens, S., Vanden Berghe, T., Romagnoli, A., Fimia, G. M., Piacentini, M., et al. (2012). Beclin1: a Role in Membrane Dynamics and beyond. *Autophagy* 8 (1), 6–17. doi:10.4161/auto.8.1.16645

Wu, F., Sui, Y., Wang, Y., Xu, T., Fan, L., and Zhu, H. (2020a). Long Noncoding RNA SNHG7, a Molecular Sponge for microRNA-485, Promotes the Aggressive Behavior of Cervical Cancer by Regulating PAK4. *Onco Targets Ther.* 13, 685–699. doi:10.2147/OTT.S232542

Wu, G., Cai, J., Han, Y., Chen, J., Huang, Z. P., Chen, C., et al. (2014). LincRNA-p21 Regulates Neointima Formation, Vascular Smooth Muscle Cell Proliferation, Apoptosis, and Atherosclerosis by Enhancing P53 Activity. *Circulation* 130 (17), 1452–1465. doi:10.1161/CIRCULATIONAHA.114.011675

Wu, X., Yuan, Y., Ma, R., Xu, B., and Zhang, R. (2020b). lncRNA SNHG7 Affects Malignant Tumor Behaviors through Downregulation of EZH2 in Uveal Melanoma Cell Lines. *Oncol. Lett.* 19 (2), 1505–1515. doi:10.3892/ol.2019.11240

Wu, Y., Liu, X., Zhou, Q., Huang, C., Meng, X., Xu, F., et al. (2015). Silent Information Regulator 1 (SIRT1) Ameliorates Liver Fibrosis via Promoting Activated Stellate Cell Apoptosis and Reversion. *Toxicol. Appl. Pharmacol.* 289 (2), 163–176. doi:10.1016/j.taap.2015.09.028

Wylie, A. A., Murphy, S. K., Orton, T. C., and Jirtle, R. L. (2000). Novel Imprinted DLK1/GTL2 Domain on Human Chromosome 14 Contains Motifs that Mimic Those Implicated in IGF2/H19 Regulation. *Genome Res.* 10 (11), 1711–1718. doi:10.1101/gr.161600

Xia, Q., Li, J., Yang, Z., Zhang, D., Tian, J., and Gu, B. (2020). Long Non-coding RNA Small Nucleolar RNA Host Gene 7 Expression Level in Prostate Cancer Tissues Predicts the Prognosis of Patients with Prostate Cancer. *Medicine (Baltimore)* 99 (7), e18993. doi:10.1097/MD.0000000000018993

Xiao, Y., Liu, R., Li, X., Gurley, E. C., Hylemon, P. B., Lu, Y., et al. (2019). Long Noncoding RNA H19 Contributes to Cholangiocyte Proliferation and Cholestatic Liver Fibrosis in Biliary Atresia. *Hepatology* 70 (5), 1658–1673. doi:10.1002/hep.30698

Xie, J. J., Li, W. H., Li, X., Ye, W., and Shao, C. F. (2019). LncRNA MALAT1 Promotes Colorectal Cancer Development by Sponging miR-363-3p to Regulate EZH2 Expression. *J. Biol. Regul. Homeost Agents* 33 (2), 331–343.

Xie, Z., Wu, Y., Liu, S., Lai, Y., and Tang, S. (2021). LncRNA-SNHG7/miR-29b/ DNMT3A axis Affects Activation, Autophagy and Proliferation of Hepatic Stellate Cells in Liver Fibrosis. *Clin. Res. Hepatol. Gastroenterol.* 45 (2), 101469. doi:10.1016/j.clinre.2020.05.017

Xin, X., Wu, M., Meng, Q., Wang, C., Lu, Y., Yang, Y., et al. (2018). Long Noncoding RNA HULC Accelerates Liver Cancer by Inhibiting PTEN via Autophagy Cooperation to miR15a. *Mol. Cancer* 17 (1), 94. doi:10.1186/s12943-018-0843-8

Xiong, D., Sheng, Y., Ding, S., Chen, J., Tan, X., Zeng, T., et al. (2016). LINC00052 Regulates the Expression of NTRK3 by miR-128 and miR-485-3p to Strengthen HCC Cells Invasion and Migration. *Oncotarget* 7 (30), 47593–47608. doi:10.18632/oncotarget.10250

Xu, R., Greening, D. W., Zhu, H. J., Takahashi, N., and Simpson, R. J. (2016). Extracellular Vesicle Isolation and Characterization: toward Clinical Application. *J. Clin. Invest.* 126 (4), 1152–1162. doi:10.1172/JCI81129

Yang, J., Kantrow, S., Sai, J., Hawkins, O. E., Boothby, M., Ayers, G. D., et al. (2012). INK4a/ARF [corrected] Inactivation with Activation of the NF-κB/IL-6 Pathway Is Sufficient to Drive the Development and Growth of Angiosarcoma. *Cancer Res.* 72 (18), 4682–4695. doi:10.1158/0008-5472.CAN-12-0440

Yang, J., Meng, X., Pan, J., Jiang, N., Zhou, C., Wu, Z., et al. (2018). CRISPR/Cas9-mediated Noncoding RNA Editing in Human Cancers. *RNA Biol.* 15 (1), 35–43. doi:10.1080/15476286.2017.1391443

Yang, J. J., Tao, H., and Li, J. (2014). Hedgehog Signaling Pathway as Key Player in Liver Fibrosis: New Insights and Perspectives. *Expert Opin. Ther. Targets* 18 (9), 1011–1021. doi:10.1517/14728222.2014.927443

Yang, J. J., Yang, Y., Zhang, C., Li, J., and Yang, Y. (2020a). Epigenetic Silencing of LncRNA ANRIL Enhances Liver Fibrosis and HSC Activation through Activating AMPK Pathway. *J. Cel Mol Med* 24 (4), 2677–2687. doi:10.1111/jcmm.14987

Yang, L., Fu, W. L., Zhu, Y., and Wang, X. G. (2020b). Tβ4 Suppresses lincRNA-P21-Mediated Hepatic Apoptosis and Fibrosis by Inhibiting PI3K-AKT-NF-Kb Pathway. *Gene* 758, 144946. doi:10.1016/j.gene.2020.144946

Yang, X., Xie, Z., Lei, X., and Gan, R. (2020c). Long Non-coding RNA GAS5 in Human Cancer. *Oncol. Lett.* 20 (3), 2587–2594. doi:10.3892/ol.2020.11809

Yang, Z., Jiang, S., Shang, J., Jiang, Y., Dai, Y., Xu, B., et al. (2019). LncRNA: Shedding Light on Mechanisms and Opportunities in Fibrosis and Aging. *Ageing Res. Rev.* 52, 17–31. doi:10.1016/j.arr.2019.04.001

Ye, J., Lin, Y., Yu, Y., and Sun, D. (2020). LncRNA NEAT1/microRNA-129-5p/ SOCS2 axis Regulates Liver Fibrosis in Alcoholic Steatohepatitis. *J. Transl Med.* 18 (1), 445. doi:10.1186/s12967-020-02577-5

Yin, C., Evason, K. J., Asahina, K., and Stainier, D. Y. (2013). Hepatic Stellate Cells in Liver Development, Regeneration, and Cancer. *J. Clin. Invest.* 123 (5), 1902–1910. doi:10.1172/JCI66369

Yoon, J. H., Abdelmohsen, K., Srikantan, S., Yang, X., Martindale, J. L., De, S., et al. (2012a). LincRNA-p21 Suppresses Target mRNA Translation. *Mol. Cel* 47 (4), 648–655. doi:10.1016/j.molcel.2012.06.027

Yoon, J. H., Srikantan, S., and Gorospe, M. (2012b). MS2-TRAP (MS2-tagged RNA Affinity Purification): Tagging RNA to Identify Associated miRNAs. *Methods* 58 (2), 81–87. doi:10.1016/j.ymeth.2012.07.004

Yoshimura, H., Matsuda, Y., Yamamoto, M., Kamiya, S., and Ishiwata, T. (2018). Expression and Role of Long Non-coding RNA H19 in Carcinogenesis. *Front. Biosci. (Landmark Ed.* 23, 614–625. doi:10.2741/4608

Young, T. L., Matsuda, T., and Cepko, C. L. (2005). The Noncoding RNA Taurine Upregulated Gene 1 Is Required for Differentiation of the Murine Retina. *Curr. Biol.* 15 (6), 501–512. doi:10.1016/j.cub.2005.02.027

Yu, F., Dong, P., Mao, Y., Zhao, B., Huang, Z., and Zheng, J. (2019). Loss of lncRNA-SNHG7 Promotes the Suppression of Hepatic Stellate Cell Activation via miR-378a-3p and DVL2. *Mol. Ther. Nucleic Acids* 17, 235–244. doi:10.1016/j.omtn.2019.05.026

Yu, F., Geng, W., Dong, P., Huang, Z., and Zheng, J. (2018). LncRNA-MEG3 Inhibits Activation of Hepatic Stellate Cells through SMO Protein and miR-212. *Cel Death Dis* 9 (10), 1014. doi:10.1038/s41419-018-1068-x

Yu, F., Guo, Y., Chen, B., Shi, L., Dong, P., Zhou, M., et al. (2017a). LincRNA-p21 Inhibits the Wnt/β-Catenin Pathway in Activated Hepatic Stellate Cells via Sponging MicroRNA-17-5p. *Cel Physiol Biochem* 41 (5), 1970–1980. doi:10.1159/000472410

Yu, F., Jiang, Z., Chen, B., Dong, P., and Zheng, J. (2017b). NEAT1 Accelerates the Progression of Liver Fibrosis via Regulation of microRNA-122 and Kruppel-like Factor 6. *J. Mol. Med. (Berl)* 95 (11), 1191–1202. doi:10.1007/s00109-017-1586-5

Yu, F., Lu, Z., Cai, J., Huang, K., Chen, B., Li, G., et al. (2015a). MALAT1 Functions as a Competing Endogenous RNA to Mediate Rac1 Expression by Sequestering miR-101b in Liver Fibrosis. *Cell Cycle* 14 (24), 3885–3896. doi:10.1080/15384101.2015.1120917

Yu, F., Lu, Z., Chen, B., Dong, P., and Zheng, J. (2016). Identification of a Novel lincRNA-P21-miR-181b-PTEN Signaling Cascade in Liver Fibrosis. *Mediators Inflamm.* 2016, 9856538. doi:10.1155/2016/9856538

Yu, F., Zheng, J., Mao, Y., Dong, P., Lu, Z., Li, G., et al. (2015b). Long Non-coding RNA Growth Arrest-specific Transcript 5 (GAS5) Inhibits Liver Fibrogenesis through a Mechanism of Competing Endogenous RNA. *J. Biol. Chem.* 290 (47), 28286–28298. doi:10.1074/jbc.M115.683813

Yu, F., Zhou, G., Huang, K., Fan, X., Li, G., Chen, B., et al. (2017c). Serum lincRNA-P21 as a Potential Biomarker of Liver Fibrosis in Chronic Hepatitis B Patients. *J. Viral Hepat.* 24 (7), 580–588. doi:10.1111/jvh.12680

Yu, L., Wang, L., Wu, X., and Yi, H. (2021). RSPO4-CRISPR Alleviates Liver Injury and Restores Gut Microbiota in a Rat Model of Liver Fibrosis. *Commun. Biol.* 4 (1), 230. doi:10.1038/s42003-021-01747-5

Zhang, B., Arun, G., Mao, Y. S., Lazar, Z., Hung, G., Bhattacharjee, G., et al. (2012). The lncRNA Malat1 Is Dispensable for Mouse Development but its Transcription Plays a Cis-Regulatory Role in the Adult. *Cel Rep* 2 (1), 111–123. doi:10.1016/j.celrep.2012.06.003

Zhang, C. Y., Yuan, W. G., He, P., Lei, J. H., and Wang, C. X. (2016a). Liver Fibrosis and Hepatic Stellate Cells: Etiology, Pathological Hallmarks and

Therapeutic Targets. *World J. Gastroenterol.* 22 (48), 10512–10522. doi:10.3748/wjg.v22.i48.10512

Zhang, D. M., Lin, Z. Y., Yang, Z. H., Wang, Y. Y., Wan, D., Zhong, J. L., et al. (2017a). lncRNA H19 Promotes Tongue Squamous Cell Carcinoma Progression through Beta-catenin/GSK3beta/EMT Signaling via Association with EZH2. *Am. J. Transl Res.* 9 (7), 3474–3486.

Zhang, H., Li, W., Gu, W., Yan, Y., Yao, X., and Zheng, J. (2019a). MALAT1 Accelerates the Development and Progression of Renal Cell Carcinoma by Decreasing the Expression of miR-203 and Promoting the Expression of BIRC5. *Cel Prolif* 52 (5), e12640. doi:10.1111/cpr.12640

Zhang, K., Han, X., Zhang, Z., Zheng, L., Hu, Z., Yao, Q., et al. (2017b). The Liver-Enriched Lnc-LFAR1 Promotes Liver Fibrosis by Activating TGFβ and Notch Pathways. *Nat. Commun.* 8 (1), 144. doi:10.1038/s41467-017-00204-4

Zhang, K., Shi, Z., Zhang, M., Dong, X., Zheng, L., Li, G., et al. (2020a). Silencing lncRNA Lfar1 Alleviates the Classical Activation and Pyoptosis of Macrophage in Hepatic Fibrosis. *Cel Death Dis* 11 (2), 132. doi:10.1038/s41419-020-2323-5

Zhang, K., Shi, Z. M., Chang, Y. N., Hu, Z. M., Qi, H. X., and Hong, W. (2014). The Ways of Action of Long Non-coding RNAs in Cytoplasm and Nucleus. *Gene* 547 (1), 1–9. doi:10.1016/j.gene.2014.06.043

Zhang, K., Zhang, M., Yao, Q., Han, X., Zhao, Y., Zheng, L., et al. (2019b). The Hepatocyte-Specifically Expressed Lnc-HSER Alleviates Hepatic Fibrosis by Inhibiting Hepatocyte Apoptosis and Epithelial-Mesenchymal Transition. *Theranostics* 9 (25), 7566–7582. doi:10.7150/thno.36942

Zhang, Q., Geng, P. L., Yin, P., Wang, X. L., Jia, J. P., and Yao, J. (2013). Down-regulation of Long Non-coding RNA TUG1 Inhibits Osteosarcoma Cell Proliferation and Promotes Apoptosis. *Asian Pac. J. Cancer Prev.* 14 (4), 2311–2315. doi:10.7314/apjcp.2013.14.4.2311

Zhang, R., Huang, X. Q., Jiang, Y. Y., Li, N., Wang, J., and Chen, S. Y. (2020b). LncRNA TUG1 Regulates Autophagy-Mediated Endothelial-Mesenchymal Transition of Liver Sinusoidal Endothelial Cells by Sponging miR-142-3p. *Am. J. Transl Res.* 12 (3), 758–772.

Zhang, T., Hu, J., Wang, X., Zhao, X., Li, Z., Niu, J., et al. (2019c). MicroRNA-378 Promotes Hepatic Inflammation and Fibrosis via Modulation of the NF-Kb-Tnfα Pathway. *J. Hepatol.* 70 (1), 87–96. doi:10.1016/j.jhep.2018.08.026

Zhang, X., Rice, K., Wang, Y., Chen, W., Zhong, Y., Nakayama, Y., et al. (2010). Maternally Expressed Gene 3 (MEG3) Noncoding Ribonucleic Acid: Isoform Structure, Expression, and Functions. *Endocrinology* 151 (3), 939–947. doi:10.1210/en.2009-0657

Zhang, Y., Liu, C., Barbier, O., Smalling, R., Tsuchiya, H., Lee, S., et al. (2016b). Bcl2 Is a Critical Regulator of Bile Acid Homeostasis by Dictating Shp and lncRNA H19 Function. *Sci. Rep.* 6, 20559. doi:10.1038/srep20559

Zhang, Y. F., Li, C. S., Zhou, Y., and Lu, X. H. (2020c). Propofol facilitates cisplatin sensitivity via lncRNA MALAT1/miR-30e/ATG5 axis through suppressing autophagy in gastric cancer. *Life Sci.* 244, 117280. doi:10.1016/j.lfs.2020.117280

Zhang, Y. H., Liu, J. T., Wen, B. Y., and Liu, N. (2009). Mechanisms of Inhibiting Proliferation of Vascular Smooth Muscle Cells by Serum of Rats Treated with Dahuang Zhechong Pill. *J. Ethnopharmacol* 124 (1), 125–129. doi:10.1016/j.jep.2009.04.012

Zhang, Z., Qian, W., Wang, S., Ji, D., Wang, Q., Li, J., et al. (2018). Analysis of lncRNA-Associated ceRNA Network Reveals Potential lncRNA Biomarkers in Human Colon Adenocarcinoma. *Cel Physiol Biochem* 49 (5), 1778–1791. doi:10.1159/000493623

Zhao, J., Dahle, D., Zhou, Y., Zhang, X., and Klibanski, A. (2005). Hypermethylation of the Promoter Region Is Associated with the Loss of MEG3 Gene Expression in Human Pituitary Tumors. *J. Clin. Endocrinol. Metab.* 90 (4), 2179–2186. doi:10.1210/jc.2004-1848

Zhao, J., Han, M., Zhou, L., Liang, P., Wang, Y., Feng, S., et al. (2020). TAF and TDF Attenuate Liver Fibrosis through NS5ATP9, TGFβ1/Smad3, and NF-Kb/nlrp3 Inflammasome Signaling Pathways. *Hepatol. Int.* 14 (1), 145–160. doi:10.1007/s12072-019-09997-6

Zhao, Y., Hu, X., Liu, Y., Dong, S., Wen, Z., He, W., et al. (2017). ROS Signaling under Metabolic Stress: Cross-Talk between AMPK and AKT Pathway. *Mol. Cancer* 16 (1), 79. doi:10.1186/s12943-017-0648-1

Zhao, Z., Lin, C. Y., and Cheng, K. (2019). siRNA- and miRNA-Based Therapeutics for Liver Fibrosis. *Transl Res.* 214, 17–29. doi:10.1016/j.trsl.2019.07.007

Zheng, J., Dong, P., Mao, Y., Chen, S., Wu, X., Li, G., et al. (2015). lincRNA-p21 Inhibits Hepatic Stellate Cell Activation and Liver Fibrogenesis via P21. *FEBS J.* 282 (24), 4810–4821. doi:10.1111/febs.13544

Zheng, J., Mao, Y., Dong, P., Huang, Z., and Yu, F. (2019). Long Noncoding RNA HOTTIP Mediates SRF Expression through Sponging miR-150 in Hepatic Stellate Cells. *J. Cel Mol Med* 23 (2), 1572–1580. doi:10.1111/jcmm.14068

Zhong, Q., Wang, Z., Liao, X., Wu, R., and Guo, X. (2020). LncRNA GAS5/miR-4465 axis R-egulates the M-alignant P-otential of N-asopharyngeal C-arcinoma by T-argeting COX2. *Cell Cycle* 19 (22), 3004–3017. doi:10.1080/15384101.2020.1816280

Zhou, B., Yuan, W., and Li, X. (2018). LncRNA Gm5091 Alleviates Alcoholic Hepatic Fibrosis by Sponging miR-27b/23b/24 in Mice. *Cell Biol Int* 42 (10), 1330–1339. doi:10.1002/cbin.11021

Zhou, L., and Liu, Y. (2015). Wnt/β-catenin Signalling and Podocyte Dysfunction in Proteinuric Kidney Disease. *Nat. Rev. Nephrol.* 11 (9), 535–545. doi:10.1038/nrneph.2015.88

Zhou, W., Ye, X. L., Xu, J., Cao, M. G., Fang, Z. Y., Li, L. Y., et al. (2017). The lncRNA H19 Mediates Breast Cancer Cell Plasticity during EMT and MET Plasticity by Differentially Sponging miR-200b/c and Let-7b. *Sci. Signal.* 10 (483), eaak9557. doi:10.1126/scisignal.aak9557

Zhou, Y., Zhang, X., and Klibanski, A. (2012). MEG3 Noncoding RNA: a Tumor Suppressor. *J. Mol. Endocrinol.* 48 (3), R45–R53. doi:10.1530/JME-12-0008

Zhu, C., Tabas, I., Schwabe, R. F., and Pajvani, U. B. (2021). Maladaptive Regeneration - the Reawakening of Developmental Pathways in NASH and Fibrosis. *Nat. Rev. Gastroenterol. Hepatol.* 18 (2), 131–142. doi:10.1038/s41575-020-00365-6

Zhu, J., Luo, Z., Pan, Y., Zheng, W., Li, W., Zhang, Z., et al. (2019). H19/miR-148a/USP4 axis Facilitates Liver Fibrosis by Enhancing TGF-β Signaling in Both Hepatic Stellate Cells and Hepatocytes. *J. Cel Physiol* 234 (6), 9698–9710. doi:10.1002/jcp.27656

Zuo, X.-x., Yang, Y., Zhang, Y., Zhang, Z.-g., Wang, X.-f., and Shi, Y.-g. (2019). Platelets Promote Breast Cancer Cell MCF-7 Metastasis by Direct Interaction: Surface Integrin α2β1-contacting-mediated Activation of Wnt-β-Catenin Pathway. *Cell Commun Signal* 17 (1), 142. doi:10.1186/s12964-019-0464-x

17

Lipidomics Indicates the Hepatotoxicity Effects of EtOAc Extract of *Rhizoma Paridis*

Chaofeng Li[1†], Mingshuang Wang[1†], Tingting Fu[2], Zhiqi Li[1], Yang Chen[1], Tao He[2], Dan Feng[1], Zhaoyi Wang[1], Qiqi Fan[1], Meilin Chen[1], Honggui Zhang[2]*, Ruichao Lin[1]* and Chongjun Zhao[1]*

[1]Beijing Key Lab for Quality Evaluation of Chinese Materia Medica, School of Chinese Materia Medica, Beijing University of Chinese Medicine, Beijing, China, [2]School of Chinese Materia Medica, Beijing University of Chinese Medicine, Beijing, China

*Correspondence:
Honggui Zhang
zhanghg9@163.com
Ruichao Lin
linrch307@126.com
Chongjun Zhao
1014256537@qq.com

†These authors have contributed equally to this work

Rhizoma Paridis is a traditional Chinese medicine commonly used in the clinical treatment of gynecological diseases. Previous studies have shown that aqueous extracts of *Rhizoma Paridis* exhibit some hepatotoxicity to hepatocytes. Here, using lipidomics analysis, we investigated the potential hepatotoxicity of *Rhizoma Paridis* and its possible mechanism. The hepatic damaging of different solvent extracts of *Rhizoma Paridis* on zebrafish larvae were determined by a combination of mortality dose, biochemical, morphological, and functional tests. We found that ethyl acetate extracts (AcOEtE) were the most toxic fraction. Notably, lipidomic responsible for the pharmacological effects of AcOEtE were investigated by Q-Exactive HF-X mass spectrometer (Thermo Scientific high-resolution) coupled in tandem with a UHPLC system. Approximately 1958 unique spectral features were detected, of which 325 were identified as unique lipid species. Among these lipid species, phosphatidylethanolamine cardiolipin Ceramide (Cer), lysophosphatidylinositol sphingosine (Sph), etc., were significantly upregulated in the treated group. Pathway analysis indicates that *Rhizoma Paridis* may cause liver damage *via* interfering with the glycerophospholipid metabolism. Collectively, this study has revealed previously uncharacterized lipid metabolic disorder involving lipid synthesis, metabolism, and transport that functionally determines hepatic fibrosis procession.

Keywords: Lipidomics, *Rhizoma Paridis*, hepatic Fibrosis, DILI, traditional Chinese medicine

Abbreviations: AA, arachidonic acid; AcOEtE, ethyl acetate extracts of *Rhizoma Paridis;* ALF, acute liver failure; ALT, alanine transaminase; AST, aspartate transaminase; Cer, Ceramide; CL, cardiolipin; DHA, docosahexaenoic acid; DCME, dichloromethane extracts of *Rhizoma Paridis;* DMePE Dimethyl-phosphatidyl ethanolamine; EPA, eicosapentaenoic acid; FC, fold change value; H&E, hematoxylin and eosin; HSC hepatic stellate cells; LC-PUFA, Long-chain polyunsaturated fatty acids; LPI, lysophosphatidylinositol; MTBE methyl-tert-butyl ether; NAFLD, Non-alcoholic fatty liver disease; NASH, Non-alcoholic steatohepatitis; PBS, phosphate-buffered solution; PC, glycerophosphocholine; PCA, principal component analysis; PE, glycerophosphoethanolamine; PEE, petroleum ether extracts of *Rhizoma Paridis;* PG, glycerophosphoglycerol; PLS-DA, partial least squares discriminate analysis; PI glycerophosphoinositol; PS, glycerophosphoserine; PUFA, polyunsaturated fatty acid; QC, quality control; qPCR, quantitative real-time polymerase chain reaction; Sph, sphingosine; TNF, tumor necrosis factor; WSBE, water-saturated n-butanol extracts of *Rhizoma Paridis;* WE, water extracts of *Rhizoma Paridis.*

INTRODUCTION

Drug-induced liver injury (DILI), which can be caused by conventional clinical drugs, herbal medications, and dietary supplements (Kuna et al., 2018; Tillmann et al., 2019), is also the most common cause of acute liver failure in the United States and Europe (Fontana et al., 2014). DILI can be affected by many factors, such as gender, age, ethnicity, pregnancy, alcohol consumption, and their interaction (Kumar et al., 2021). Therefore, early identification of DILI is essential primarily to improve drug safety and reduce the cost of drug development.

In a state of persistent liver injury (metabolic, cholestatic, or toxic), hepatocellular damage triggers a series of events that culminate in the activation of quiescent hepatic stellate cells (HSC) to a myofibroblastic (activated) HSC state (Mederacke et al., 2013). Multiple pathways direct HSC activation and ultimately leads to increased secretion of extracellular matrix proteins such as collagens that eventually accumulate in the liver parenchyma and lead to liver fibrosis (Friedman, 2008). Hepatic fibrosis is a repair response to diffuse over deposition and abnormal distribution of extracellular matrices such as glycoproteins, collagen, and proteoglycans after various injuries to the liver and is a critical step in the progression of various chronic liver diseases to cirrhosis. Although there have been many advances in basic and clinical research on liver fibrosis in recent years, there is still a lack of ideal drugs to treat liver fibrosis.

Rhizoma Paridis, which has significant hemostatic and anti-tumor effects, is the main rhizome of *Paris Polyphylla* var *yunnanensis* (Franch.) Hand. -Mazz, or *Paris Polyphylla* Smith var. *chinensis* (Franch.) Hara (Qin et al., 2018). Relevant studies have shown that *Rhizoma Paridis* is hepatotoxic. Polyphylin I, II, VI, and VII were cytotoxic to both hepatocytes-HL-7702 and HepaRG cells. Furthermore, Polyphylin I, which can induce HepG2 cells' apoptosis through intracellular and extracellular apoptotic pathways, was proved to be the most cytotoxic among them (Zeng et al., 2020).

Zebrafish (*Danio rerio*), also known as a kind of tropical freshwater fish with ornamental value, is an important vertebrate model organism in scientific research, especially in studying the regenerative capacity of organisms (Goldshmit et al., 2012). Zebrafish and humans share up to 87% significant genome sequence similarity. It can overcome the limitations of cell-based *in vitro* assays and perform high-throughput *in vitro* screening (Bauer et al., 2021). Zebrafish are increasingly used in toxicity and targeted drug-related studies and have proved to be an essential vertebrate model for studying biological processes and functions (Barros et al., 2008; Ali et al., 2011; He et al., 2013).

This study aimed to investigate the potential hepatotoxicity of *Rhizoma Paridis* and its possible mechanism. To this end, we extracted *Rhizoma Paridis* by using petroleum ether, dichloromethane, ethyl acetate, n-butanol, and water, respectively. We examined the dose-toxicity curves of these five extracts by using zebrafish larvae. The relevant physicochemical indicators, including ALT/AST, hematoxylin-eosin staining, and acridine orange staining, were conducted to evaluate the liver damage of different extracts to zebrafish larvae.

The chemical composition contained in extracts of *Rhizoma Paridis* was also analyzed by UHPLC-Q-Exactive Orbitrap MS. Modern lipidomics technology based on mass spectrometry has been used in this study to provide significant insights into the metabolism and alterations in lipids through the identification and qualitative analysis of individual lipid species. Meanwhile, lipid uptake, transport, metabolism, and inflammation-related genes were examined separately by quantitative real-time PCR (qPCR) in zebrafish larvae after exposure.

MATERIALS AND METHODS
Chemicals and Materials
The HPLC grade methanol, acetonitrile, and water (Optima™ LC/MS grade) were purchased from Fisher Chemical, United States of America. Formic acid (HPLC grade) was purchased from CNW, Germany. 2-propanol (HPLC grade) was purchased from Merck (Darmstadt, Germany). MTBE (HPLC grade) was purchased from Adamas-beta. Ammonium acetate (HPLC grade) was purchased from Sigma-Aldrich (St. Louis, MO, United States). Petroleum ether, dichloromethane, ethyl acetate, n-butanol (analytical grade) were purchased from Sinopharm Chemical Reagent Co., Ltd (Shanghai, China). Ultrapure water was prepared using a Milli-Q water purification system (Millipore Corp. Billerica, MA, United States). Analytical grade ethanol and methanol were purchased from Beijing Chemical Works (Beijing, China).

Preparation of *Rhizoma Paridis*
The dried roots of *Rhizoma Paridis* were collected from Maoshan town, Luquan country, Yunnan province, in October 2019. Professor Liu Chunsheng, who works at Beijing University of Chinese Medicine and is the head of the department of Chinese Medicine Identification, identified and checked the quality of these roots.

Extraction and Fractionation
Rhizoma Paridis was powdered and successively extracted with five different solvents, petroleum ether, dichloromethane, ethyl acetate, water-saturated n-butanol, and water. The specific extraction method was as follows: The *Rhizoma Paridis* powder was wrapped with filter paper and placed in a Soxhlet extractor with solvent and extracted by heated reflux extraction within 2 h, followed by cooling and filtration. A rotary evaporator was used to recover the solvent, after which the remaining mixture was lyophilized into powder and stored at −4°C for further study. The extraction rates of ethyl acetate extract and dichloromethane extract of *Rhizoma Paridis* were 2.51 and 1.14%. The main components of the ethyl acetate extracts were analyzed using UPLC-Q-Orbitrap MS methods, which were described in detail in **Supplementary Table S1**.

Animals and Experimental Design
Zebrafish Larvae Maintenance
Zebrafish wild-type (AB) were maintained in Farming System (ESEN, Beijing, China) in Beijing Key Lab for Quality Evaluation

of Chinese Materia Medica, with a 14:10-h light/dark cycle and 28.5 °C water temperature. Fish were fed with brine shrimp three times a day. The male and female zebrafish were allowed to mate naturally every morning at 7 a.m. And healthy eggs were collected and cultured in embryo water (5.4 mmol/L KCl, 0.137 mol/L NaCl, 0.25 mmol/L Na$_2$HPO$_4$, 0.44 mmol/L K$_2$HPO$_4$, 1.3 mmol/L CaCl$_2$, 1.0 mmol/L MgSO$_4$, 4.2 mmol/L NAHCO3). Zebrafish embryos can take nutrients from the yolk sac before 7dpf. Healthy 4dpf larvae were screened by microscope (Zeiss, Germany) for further experiments.

Treatment of Zebrafish Larvae

Randomly selected 4dpf zebrafish larvae were placed in 12-well plates with 20 fish per well and exposed to different concentrations of *Rhizoma Paridis* extracts for 24 h, including petroleum ether extracts (PEE), dichloromethane extracts (DCME), ethyl acetate extracts (AcOEtE), water-saturated n-butanol extracts (WSBE) and water extracts (WE) of *Rhizoma Paridis* (dissolved in 0.5% dimethyl sulfoxide (DMSO)). Each extract contained different concentrations (containing both safe and lethal doses), and each concentration was repeated in three wells. Meanwhile, normal zebrafish culture water was used as a negative control group. During the exposure period, the number of dead zebrafish larvae in each experimental group was counted every 6 h, and the dead bodies were promptly removed. The entire experiment was carried out at a constant temperature of 28°C and repeated three times in parallel. At the end of the experiment, the number of surviving zebrafish larvae in the different treatment groups was counted to calculate the mortality rate of each group.

Then, the 4dpf zebrafish larvae were given the maximum non-lethal dose concentration of DCME and AcOEtE. 20 samples per well and six wells in parallel for each group, the blank group was given zebrafish embryo water. 24 h after administration, samples were collected and washed 3 times with embryo culture water and deionized water, respectively. Three wells of each group were fixed in 4% paraformaldehyde, and the remaining samples were stored at -80 °C for further study.

Biochemical and Histological Analysis
Determination of Biochemical Parameters in Zebrafish Larvae

At 24 h postexposure, 80 zebrafish larvae were collected from each group, and a certain amount of phosphate-buffered solution (PBS, pH 7.4) was added. The specimens were homogenized by a homogenizer. Afterward, the specimens were centrifuged for about 20 min (2,000 rpm). The supernatant was carefully collected. Aspartate transaminase (AST) and alanine transaminase (ALT) levels were determined by using diagnostic kits according to the manufacturer's protocols (Jiangsu Yutong Biotechnology Institute, Jiangsu, China). The activity of ALT and AST were determined at 450 nm after adding stop solution.

Histopathology Analysis

After 24 h exposure, zebrafish larvae were fixed with 4% paraformaldehyde for at least 24 h. For hematoxylin and eosin (H&E) staining analysis, zebrafish larvae were dehydrated using

ethanol in ascending order and placed in xylene to make them gradually transparent, followed by paraffin embedding. Then 4 μm thick slides were prepared for H&E staining. For acridine orange staining, the embryos were washed 3 times with water and PBS at the end of exposing, and 1 ml of the acridine orange staining solution was added to each well and stained at 28°C for 20 min. The results were observed under a transmission electron microscope (ZEISS, German).

Sample Preparation for Lipidomics Analysis

Zebrafish larvae samples (50 mg) were placed in 2 ml Eppendorf tubes, and 280 μL of extraction solution (methanol: water, 2:5), 400 μL of methyl-tert-butyl ether (MTBE) along with a 6 mm diameter grinding bead were added to the tube. Then, ground for 6 min (−10°C, 50 Hz) using a frozen tissue grinder. After that, the samples were extracted by low-temperature ultrasound for 30 min (5°C, 40 kHz), followed by 30 min of standing (−20°C). Then, samples were centrifuged at 13,000 g for 15 min at 4°C, and 350 μL of supernatant was added into the EP tube, followed by blow-drying with nitrogen gas. 100 μL of extraction solution (isopropanol: acetonitrile, 1:1) was added and re-solubilized, vortexed for 30 s, and low-temperature ultrasonic extraction for 5min (5 °C, 40 KHz). The extracts were centrifuged at high speed for 10 min (13,000g, 4°C), and the supernatant was pipetted into the injection vial with an internal cannula for analysis. In addition, 20 μL of supernatant was mixed for each sample as the quality control sample.

A Q-Exactive HF-X mass spectrometer (Thermo Scientific high-resolution) was coupled in tandem with a UHPLC system with a DuoSpray ion source operating in positive electrospray (ESI+) and negative electrospray (ESI-) modes (AB Sciex, Foster City, CA). After every 5–15 samples, a QC sample was inserted, and an automatic mass calibration was performed to examine the stability of the entire essay. An Accucore C30 column (100 mm × 2.1 mm i. d. 2.6 μm; Thermo) was used for the separation of lipids. The temperature of the column was maintained at 40 °C. Mobile phase A was 50% acetonitrile in water (containing 0.1% formic acid, 10 mmol/L ammonium acetate), and mobile phase B was acetonitrile: isopropanol: water (10:88:2, v/v/v, containing 0.02% formic acid, 2 mmol/L ammonium acetate). The flow rate was 0.4 ml/min, and the gradient analysis was performed with a gradient starting from 35% mobile phase B, 60% B (4 min), 85% B (12 min), 100% B (15–17 min), and 35% B (18–20 min). After UHPLC separation, samples were analyzed by Q ExactiveTM HF-X for mass spectrometry with the following instrument parameter settings: ion mode, positive and negative; MS1 scan range, 200-2000; Irospray voltage Floating (ESI+, V), 3.0 kV; ionspray Voltage Floating (ESI-, V), −3.0 kV; heater temperature, 370°C; sheath gas flow rate, 60 psi; aux gas flow rate, 20 psi; capillary temperature, 350°C; Normalized collision energy, 20-40-60 (V). Details are described in **Supplementary Table S2**.

Quantitative Real-Time PCR Analysis of Related Gene Expression

Total RNA was extracted from collected samples using TianGen RNA Extraction Kit (Takara, Tokyo, Japan) following

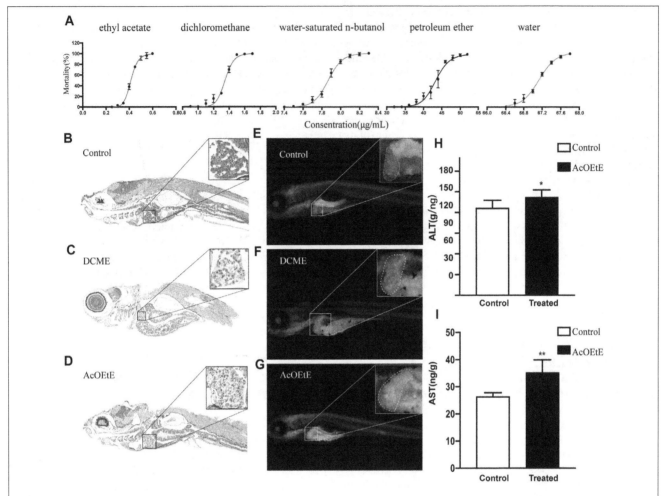

FIGURE 1 | Concentration-mortality curves, tissue sections (×400), and biochemical indicator analysis **(A)** Concentration-mortality curves of five solvent extracts of *Rhizoma Paridis*, including petroleum ether extracts (PEE), dichloromethane extracts (DCME), ethyl acetate extracts (AcOEtE), water-saturated n-butanol extracts (WSBE), and water extracts (WE) **(B-D)** H&E staining of zebrafish larvae sections from the control, DCME, and AcOEtE groups **(E-G)** Acridine orange staining of zebrafish larvae from the control, DCME, and AcOEtE groups **(H-I)** The levels of ALT and AST of control and AcOEtE groups. Data are expressed as mean ± SD. **$p < 0.01$ compared with the control group, *$p < 0.05$ compared with control group.

manufacturer instructions. The isolated total RNA from the different groups was converted into complementary DNA (cDNA) using the FastKing RT Kit (Tiangen Biotech Co., Ltd., Beijing, China). Sequences of primers used in the qPCR were designed with primer-blast (https://ncbi.nlm.nih.gov/tools/primer-blast/) and synthesized by the Biomed gene technology co. LTD. (Beijing, China). (**Supplementary Table S3**). Quantitative real-time PCR was performed using TransStart Top Green qPCR SuperMix (TransGen Biotech, Beijing, China) with the ABI 7500 Real-Time PCR System (Applied Biosystems, Foster City, CA, United States). Relative mRNA expression levels were determined using the following thermal cycling conditions: 95°C for 3 min, followed by 40 cycles of 60°C for 20 s, 60°C, 9°C for 15 s, and 6°C for 10 s, and 9°C for 15 s. The relative quantification was then calculated by the expression $2^{-\Delta\Delta Ct}$. All data were statistically analyzed as the fold-change between the exposed groups and the control. The experiment was conducted in triplicate.

Statistical Analysis

The components of the samples were separated by chromatography and continuously scanned into the mass spectrometer, and the mass spectrometer was continuously scanned for data acquisition. The raw data were imported into LipidsearchTM 4.1 (Thermo Fisher, United States) for baseline filtering, peak identification, integration, retention time correction, and peak alignment to obtain a data matrix containing retention time, mass-to-charge ratio, and peak intensity information. The MS and MS/MS mass spectra were matched with the metabolic database with the MS mass error set to less than 10 ppm, and the metabolites were identified based on the secondary mass spectra matching score. The main parameters are as follows: precursor tolerance: 5 ppm, product tolerance: 5 ppm, product icon threshold: 1%. For the LipidSearch extracted data, the lipid molecules in the missing value 20% group were removed, and the missing values were filled with the minimum value, QC verified with RSD ≤30% and the total peak area of the data was normalized. Subsequently, model construction and discrimination of multivariate statistics were performed using the ropls R package, which included unsupervised principal component analysis (PCA) and orthogonal partial least squares discriminant analysis (OPLS-DA). Among them, PCA analysis uses unite-variance to scale transform the data, and (O) PLSDA uses Pareto to scale transform the data. The values of R^2 and Q^2 were calculated to assess how good the quality of both models was. Volcano plots were plotted using the R package ggplot2. One-way statistical analyses included Student's t-test and mutation multiple analysis. Volcano maps were drawn using r software for hierarchical clustering and correlation analysis. Differences between groups (p-values) were assessed using Graphpad Prism 8.0 software. Differences in data were first determined using normality and chi-square tests, followed by one-way ANOVA analysis and Dunnett's t-test. $*p \leq 0.05$ and $* *p \leq 0.01$ were statistically significant for the AcOEtE group compared to the DMSO group.

RESULTS

Toxicity of Different Solvent Extracts of *Rhizoma Paridis*

Previous studies have shown that the aqueous extracts of *Rhizoma Paridis* exhibited hepatotoxicity to zebrafish and SD rats and cytotoxicity to L02 cells (Zhao et al., 2020). However, there have been no studies on the differences in toxicity of extracts from different solvents on *Rhizoma Paridis*. Our study compared the toxicity of different extracts of *Rhizoma Paridis* on zebrafish larvae. The "dose-toxicity curve" of different extracts is shown in **Figure 1A**. The results showed that the different extracts of *Rhizoma Paridis* exhibited a wide variation in toxicity to zebrafish larvae. As shown in **Figure 1A**, the ethyl acetate extracts of *Rhizoma Paridis* (AcOEtE) were the most toxic fraction, followed by dichloromethane extracts (DCME), petroleum ether extracts (PEE), water-saturated n-butanol extracts (WSBE), and water extracts (WE).

Afterward, AcOEtE and DCME were selected as the more toxic fraction to investigate whether they are hepatotoxic and potentially induce hepatic fibrosis. The administered concentrations are their respective maximum non-lethal concentrations, for AcOEtE was 0.3 μg/ml, and DCME was 1 μg/ml. Randomly selected 4dpf zebrafish larvae were placed in 12-well plates with 20 fish per well and exposed to 0.3 μg/ml AcOEtE and 1 μg/ml DCME for 24 h respectively. Pathological changes were observed in zebrafish larvae 24 h after the administration of AcOEtE and DCME.

Histological and Biochemical Analysis

The results of H&E (**Figures 1B–D**) showed that AcOEtE and DCME had caused varying degrees of liver damage to zebrafish larvae, with inflammatory cell infiltration and mild vacuolated lipid droplets in both groups. In contrast, AcOEtE was significantly more hepatotoxic to zebrafish larvae than DCME, and significant histopathological changes could be observed in the AcOEtE group, including significant hepatic steatosis, partial

nuclear fragmentation, and the appearance of hepatic fibrous nodules. Acridine orange staining showed that both AcOEtE and DCME promoted apoptosis in the hepatocytes of zebrafish larvae to some extent (**Figure 1E–G**). Meanwhile, the results of ALT/AST (**Figure 1H**) after 24 h administration of AcOEtE to zebrafish larvae showed that both ALT/AST significantly increased in the treated group compared to the control group.

Identification of Chemical Compounds in the AcOEtE

Previous studies have been conducted on the chemical composition of *Rhizoma Paridis* and saponins, which are usually considered the main components. In this study, we used UPLC and high-resolution Q-Exactive Orbitrap MS to identify the constituents of AcOEtE. Based on the high-resolution parent ions and their characteristic ions, we have identified 98 relevant components, including Polyphyllin I, Polyphyllin VI, Polyphyllin E, Dioscin, Diosgenin, Protodioscin, Gracillin, etc. The chemical compositions are shown in **Supplementary Table S4**.

Lipid Analysis and Multivariate Analysis of UHPLC-Q Exactive HF-X Mass Spectrometer Data

Lipidomics, derived from metabolomics, emerged in 2003 and has rapidly evolved to focus on the qualitative and quantitative screening of metabolites in biological samples, with two main analytical approaches: 1) the non-targeted and 2) the targeted approach (Lee and Yokomizo, 2018). This study performed lipidomic analysis on zebrafish larvae treated with AcOEtE and control groups based on the UHPLC-Q Exactive HF-X-MS technique, respectively. **Supplementary Figure S1** shows an example of the total ion chromatogram (TIC) of the QC group in positive and negative ion mode, which showed good separation.

Principal Component Analysis (PCA) and Orthogonal Projection of Latent Structure Discriminant Analysis (OPLS-DA) are powerful statistical modeling tools that provide insight into the separation between experimental groups based on the results from the MS analysis instrument and determine whether an experimental sample is anomalous based on its dispersion trend (Worley and Powers, 2016). As can be seen from **Figures 2A–D**, the QC samples were tightly aggregated in ESI+ and ESI- modes, indicating that the instrument was in good operating condition. Both PCA and OPLS-DA results completely distinguish the AcOEtE group from the control group, indicating that endogenous metabolite levels in the treated group have changed significantly compared to the control group.

The results showed that R^2X (cum), R^2Y (cum), and Q^2 of the OPLS-DA model for the cationic model were 0.486, 0.996, and 0.944, respectively, while R^2X (cum), R^2Y (cum), and Q^2 of the anionic model were 0.568, 0.998 and 0.958, respectively (**Figures 2C,D**). $Q^2 > 0.5$ indicated that the model's predictive ability was good, but only using Q^2 is still not enough to prove the model's reliability, and the replacement test-permutation test is also commonly used to judge the model. A 200-time permutation

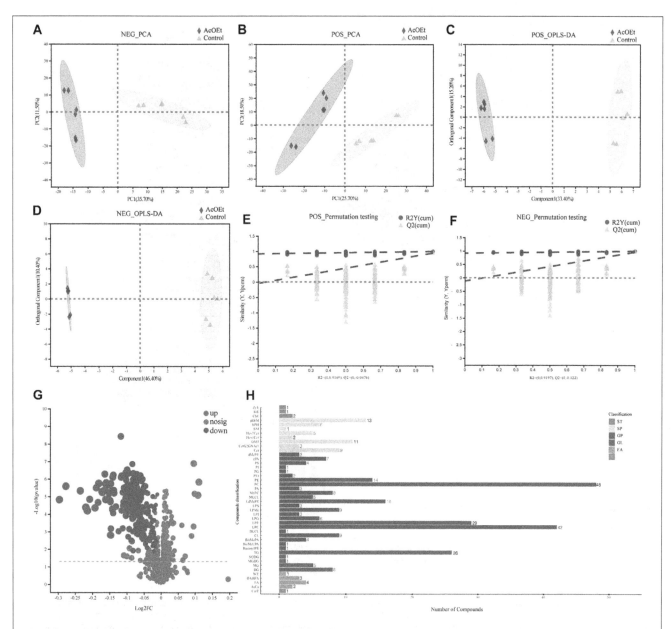

FIGURE 2 | Score plot of PCA and OPLS-DA models of zebrafish larvae **(A, B)** Scores plot of PCA model, obtained from AcOEtE group and control group (NEG and POS) **(C,D)** Scores plot of OPLS-DA model, obtained from AcOEtE group and control group (NEG and POS) **(E,F)** The score of the OPLS-DA model, obtained from the AcOEtE group and control group (NEG and POS). The R^2 factor estimates a good fit, while the Q^2 coefficient determines the predictive value of the created model, referring to the percentage of correctly classified samples using cross-validation. Two hundred permutations were performed, and the resulting R^2 and Q^2 values were plotted (Red circle): R^2 (Pink triangle): Q^2. The two dashed lines represent the regression lines of R^2 and Q^2, respectively **(G)** volcano plot of Model-Control, the blue points represent the down-regulated lipids, red points represent the up-regulated lipids (VIP >1.0, p-value < 0.05) **(H)** The number of detected lipids was based on a non-targeted lipidomics strategy between the AcOEtE and control groups. The horizontal axis represents the number of lipids in the subclass, and the vertical axis represents the subclasses of lipids.

test was performed to validate the OPLS-DA model. Compared to the original points, the Q^2 and R^2 values on the left side are lower, while the intercept of the regression line at the Q2 point with the vertical axis (left side) is less than 0.05 in the envelope test (**Figures 2E,F**). This indicates that the model is valid and can make accurate predictions for the samples in the experiment.

Each high-resolution mass spectrometry peak extracted by compound Discoverer TM was initially screened and classified

into lipid subspecies based on their different cleavage patterns and further confirmed by comparing precise mass determination and the given molecular formula with Lipidsearch (Thermo Fisher, United States) on the lipid database for further confirmation. The International Lipid Classification and Nomenclature Committee classify lipid compounds into eight types, each containing different subclasses, and each subclass can be further divided into different molecular species. We then

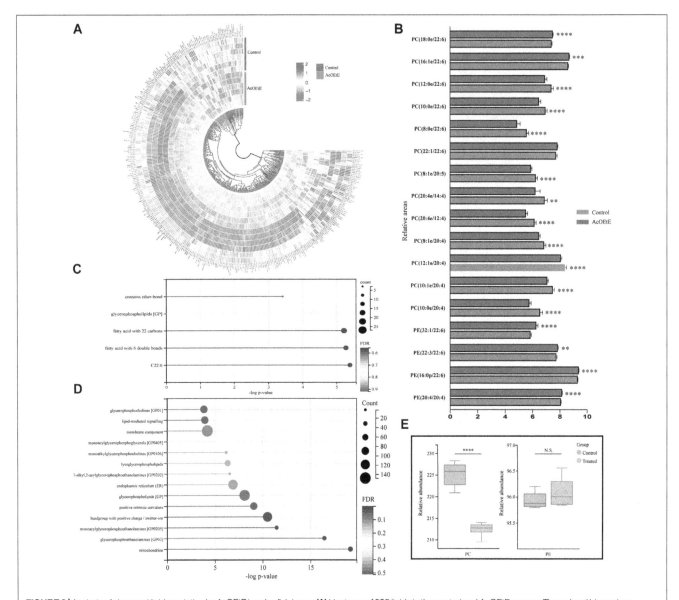

FIGURE 3 | Analysis of abnormal lipid regulation by AcOEtE in zebrafish larvae **(A)** Heatmap of 325 lipids in the control and AcOEtE groups. The red and blue colors indicate the increased and decreased levels, respectively **(B)** Relative intensity analysis of subclasses containing eicosatetraenoic acid or docosahexaenoic acid between the control and AcOEtE groups **(C)** LION-term enrichment analysis of all up-regulated lipids in the AcOEtE group compared to the control group **(D)** LION-term enrichment analysis of all down-regulated lipids in the AcOEtE group **(E)** PCs and PEs in control and AcOEtE groups showed a rise in total concentration. *$p < 0.05$, **$p < 0.01$ compared with the control group.

screened the metabolites for those that were altered in zebrafish larvae after administration. The significance of the variables in the projection (VIP >1) values generated in OPLS-DA was applied in the positive and negative ion model, respectively, resulting in 325 differential metabolites were screened out (**Figure 2G**), covering five lipid categories and 43 lipid subclasses, with phosphatidylcholines (PCs), PEs, and triglycerides (TGs) were the most abundant (**Figure 2H**).

We analyzed the lipid data using clustered heat maps to understand further the differences in lipid metabolism between the AcOEtE and control groups, as shown in **Figure 3A**. The heatmap visualizes the relative increase (red) or decrease (blue) of lipids in each group of samples. 269 lipids were significantly

downregulated, and 56 lipids were significantly upregulated in the AcOEtE group compared to the Control group.

Hierarchical clustering analysis strongly emphasized the enrichment of CL and PE in glycerophospholipid, sphingomyelin (Sph), and Cer in sphingolipids, and sterol lipid. Specifically, among the sphingolipids, six out of nine Cers, three out of five Hex2Cers, and two out of six Sphs showed significant upregulation in the AcOEtE group. Glycerophospholipids were identified in a total of 23 subclasses, and five of these subclasses were significantly upregulated in the AcOEtE group, including CLs, PEs, phosphatidylglycerols (PGs), LPIs, and dimethyl-phosphatidylethanolamines (dMePEs).

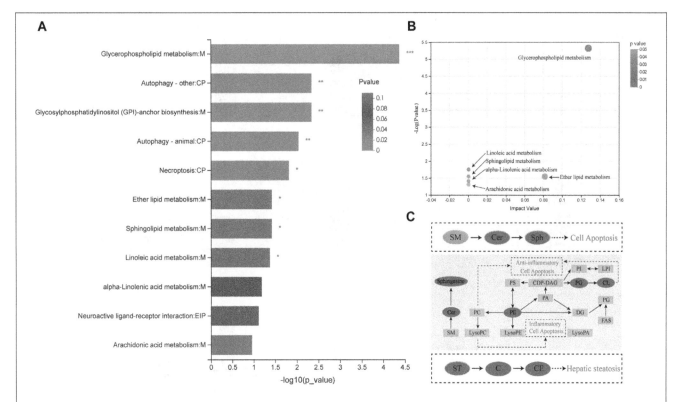

FIGURE 4 | Different lipid species are associated with metabolism **(A)** Pathway enrichment analysis of lipid metabolites by KEGG. Results include α-linolenic and linoleic acid metabolism, arachidonic acid metabolism, glycerolipid metabolism, fatty acid extension in mitochondria, fatty acid biosynthesis, fatty acid metabolism, steroid biosynthesis, and bile acid biosynthesis (*$p < 0.05$, **$p < 0.01$ compared with the control group) **(B)** Pathway topology enrichment analysis of lipid metabolites by KEGG **(C)** Network of changes in potential biomarkers of the AcOEtE group compared to the Control group. Red, upregulated biomarkers; blue, downregulated biomarkers.

Then, we performed a further generalization study with the Lipid Ontology website (http://www.lipidontology.com/) on 269 down-regulated lipids and 59 up-regulated lipids, which were significantly increased by AcOEtE exposure. The results showed that a total of 14 lipids containing docosahexaenoic acid, 15 lipids containing fatty acids with six double bonds, 18 lipids containing fatty acids with 22 carbon atoms, 27 glycerophospholipids, and three lipids containing ether bonds were among the 59 lipids up-regulated after AcOEtE exposure. These five physicochemical properties occupy the top five positions in terms of contribution to lipid upregulation, as shown in **Figure 3C**. Meanwhile, we can see that the 269 lipids down-regulated are mainly related to mitochondria, endoplasmic reticulum, cell membrane components, positive intrinsic curvature of the cell membrane, head group of lipids with positive charge/zwitterion, and lipid-mediated signaling, etc. As shown in **Figure 3D**.

PCs and PEs were the most abundant phospholipids in mammalian cells and showed significant changes in various diseases. Long-chain polyunsaturated fatty acids (LC-PUFA) were defined as polyunsaturated fatty acids with more than 20 carbon atoms and two or more double bindings (Sarwar Inam, 2017). Eicosapentaenoic acid (EPA, C20:5n-3), arachidonic acid (AA, C20:4n-6) and docosahexaenoic Acid (DHA, C22:6 n-3) were considered as the most important LC-PUFA. We

investigated the changes of PCs and PEs between the AcOEtE and control groups and focused on the changed subclasses that contained four or more double bonds. The results of our research suggested that among the 48 significantly altered PC subclasses detected in the AcOEtE group, 16 subclasses are composed of unsaturated fatty acids that contain more than 20 carbon atoms and two or more double bonds. Among the 48 significantly changed PC subclasses, four were significantly upregulated, accounting for 8.3%. It is worth mentioning that all the upregulated subclasses were LC-PUFA, specifically three subclasses were docosahexaenoic acid and one docosatetraenoic acid. Of the 14 significantly altered PE subclasses, five subclasses are composed of unsaturated fatty acids that contain more than 20 carbon atoms and two or more double bonds. Compared with the control group, 11 PE subclasses of the AcOEtE group showed significant upregulation, accounting for 78.6%, of which five contained docosahexaenoic acid and one contained docosahexaenoic acid, as is shown in **Figure 3B**. The PC/PE ratio is often used clinically to detect inflammatory conditions in the organism. Compared to the control group, the PCs mainly were downregulated in the administered group, while PEs were upregulated overall in the AcOEtE group (except for the two short-chain lipids), which led to a substantial downregulation of the ratio (**Figure 3E**).

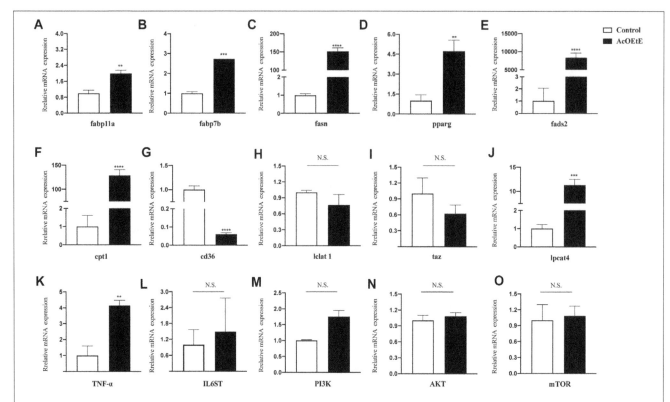

FIGURE 5 | Gene expressions after AcOEtE administration to zebrafish larvae were detected by qPCR. including **(A)** fabp11a **(B)** fabp7b **(C)** fasn **(D)** pparg **(E)** fads2 **(F)** cpt1 **(G)** cd36 **(H)** lclat1 **(I)** taz **(J)** lpcat4 **(K)** TNF-α **(L)** IL6ST **(M)** PI3K **(N)** AKT and **(O)** mTOR. All values are expressed as the mean ± SD of three or more independent experiments. ***p < 0.001; **p < 0.01; *p < 0.05.

In addition, all four sterol lipids subclasses detected in the AcOEtE group, including ChE (24:5), ChE (24:6), StE (24:7), and ZyE (24:5), were all long-chain sterols and upregulated, which may be related to signaling pathway conduction.

To determine the pathways by which AcOEtE affects lipid metabolism in zebrafish larvae, scipy (Python) software was used for analysis. p-value was analyzed and resulted in 39 metabolites mapped to the KEGG metabolic pathway for overexpression and pathway topology analysis. Different metabolite species were analyzed using Scipy. p-value corrected less than 0.05, and finally, 11 lipid metabolic pathways were found to have occurred a game (**Figure 4A**). By the relative positions of the compounds in the pathways, their pathway composite importance scores were calculated with a total score of 1. As shown in **Figure 4A**. The figure shows that glycerophospholipid metabolism, ether lipid metabolism, linoleic acid metabolism, and sphingolipid metabolism had the highest impact factors.

The results of KEGG topology statistics are shown in **Figure 4B**, where each bubble represents a KEGG pathway, and the vertical axis indicates the enrichment significance of metabolite involvement in the pathway-log10 (p-value); the bubble size represents the Impact Value; the more significant the bubble, the greater the importance of the pathway. Five pathways can be found in the figure, including map00564 (Glycerophospholipid metabolism), map00591 (Linoleic acid metabolism), map00590 (Sphingolipid metabolism), map00592

(alpha-Linolenic acid metabolism), and map00565 (Ether lipid metabolism).

Effect of Critical Lipid-Relating Genes by AcOEtE

To determine the underlying mechanism of the abnormal lipid metabolism, the transcription levels of genes that participated in lipid metabolism were further assessed by qPCR (**Figure 5**). Our results indicated that AcOEtE affected genes related to lipid synthesis, metabolism, and transport in zebrafish larvae, such as fabp11a, fabp7b, fasn, pparg, fads2, cpt1, cd36, and enzyme activities related to mitochondrial function were also activated, such as lclat1, Lpcat4, and Taz. Genes related to inflammation were also upregulated, such as TNF-α, IL6ST. As found in our lipidomics results, these genes are involved in the glycerophospholipid metabolic pathway, α-linolenic acid metabolic pathway. Meanwhile, we found a tendency for the PI3K-AKT-mTOR pathway to be upregulated, although it did not show significance, as shown in **Figure 5M–O**.

DISCUSSION

In this study, we investigated the dose-toxicity relationship of different extracts of *Rhizoma Paridis* on zebrafish larvae. We studied the induction of hepatic fibrosis after administration of AcOEtE (ethyl acetate extracts of *Rhizoma Paridis*) and DCME (dichloromethane extracts of *Rhizoma Paridis*) by pathological morphological observation and physicochemical index analysis.

Then, we investigated the effect of AcOEtE on lipid homeostasis in zebrafish larvae by using lipidomics techniques to search for biomarkers that may play a key role in inducing hepatic fibrosis. To the best of our knowledge, this is the first study of hepatotoxicity and hepatic fibrosis in a zebrafish larvae model using lipidomic techniques, which may provide a good reference for future hepatotoxicity studies and clinical applications of *Rhizoma Paridis*.

Compared with the control group, after ingestion of a specific dose of AcOEtE, the lipid homeostasis in zebrafish larvae was disrupted and exhibited pathological fibrosis changes. We examined the mRNA levels of pro-inflammatory factors IL6ST and TNF-α in zebrafish larvae of the AcOEtE group, and both were upregulated. Genes related to fat synthesis and transport, such as the fatty acid-binding protein FABP family, were also detected. FABPs is a single molecular weight intracellular protein family, mainly involved in the transport and metabolism of fatty acids. We examined Fabp7b and Fabp11a, and both showed a significant upregulation trend in the AcOEtE groups. Upregulation of fabp11a and fabp7b genes leads to increased hepatic fatty acid uptake, affecting the subsequent lipid transport process and increasing hepatic lipid deposition and ultimately hepatic steatosis (Ahn et al., 2012; Yan et al., 2015). Fasn is an essential nuclear transcription factor that regulates hepatic lipid metabolism and is a crucial regulator of fatty acid metabolism, and its excessive upregulation leads to hepatic lipid disorders in zebrafish, which in turn causes hepatic lipid accumulation (Chicco and Sparagna, 2007; Knebel et al., 2018; Peng et al., 2018). There was a strong correlation between increased pparg expression and liver fat accumulation. In addition, pparg overexpression was accompanied by increased transcription of several inflammatory marker genes (Westerbacka et al., 2007; Yamazaki et al., 2011). Also upregulated was the fatty acid dehydrogenase 2 (fads2), a key enzyme in synthesizing polyunsaturated fatty acids.

Changes in the Glycerophospholipid Metabolism Pathway

The results of lipidomic studies showed that zebrafish larvae underwent significant changes in the glycerophospholipid metabolic pathway after administration of AcOEtE, with the more significant changes being in PC and PE. There was a total of 48 PCs and 14 PEs were detected to be significantly altered in the AcOEtE group, of which 4 PC subclasses were upregulated (8.33%), and 11 PEs were upregulated (78.57%), suggesting that the homeostasis of PEs and PCs is disturbed in the glycerophospholipid metabolic pathway, and lead to changes in membrane lipid composition, which could affect the physical properties and functional integrity of membranes, leading to apoptosis, inflammation and hepatic fibrosis (Li et al., 2006; Wu et al., 2019). Puneet Puri et al. showed that total PCs were reduced in the livers of humans with Non-alcoholic fatty liver

disease (NAFLD) and Non-alcoholic steatohepatitis (NASH) (Puri et al., 2007). Arendt et al. found that NAFLD and NASH patients had significantly lower PC/PE ratios in liver and erythrocyte membranes than healthy people (Owen and McIntyre, 1978). Charalampos et al. also found that the PC/PE ratio showed a negative correlation with ALT and AST and thus hypothesized that the PC/PE ratio correlated with the pathology of liver tissue (Papadopoulos et al., 2020).

Dimethyl-phosphatidyl ethanolamine (DMePE) is an intermediate in the sequential methylation of PE, and this metabolic pathway is one of the main metabolic pathways for the *de novo* synthesis of PC (Cole et al., 2012). In this study, the amount of PC was reduced in the AcOEtE group compared to the control group, while the amount of DMPE was significantly increased, possibly due to an impairment in this biosynthetic pathway.

Our experimental results also revealed that the Lysophosphatidylcholine (LPC) of the AcOEtE group showed a tendency to be down-regulated to some extent compared to the control group. A total of 42 isoforms were detected in LPC, which were all down-regulated in the AcOEtE group compared to the control group. LPCs are essential signaling molecules with multiple biological functions. LPC affects lipid metabolism throughout the liver and has been found to down-regulate genes involved in fatty acid oxidation and upregulate genes involved in cholesterol biosynthesis (Hollie et al., 2014). Tanaka et al. found that downregulation of serum LPC was significantly correlated with hepatic upregulation of LPcat1-4 and the pro-inflammatory cytokines TNF-α upregulated the expression of Lpcat2/4 mRNA levels in primary hepatocytes (Tanaka et al., 2012). Our experiment showed that the AcOEtE group had a higher level of Lpcat4 compared to the control group. Furthermore, it was also found that TNF-α was significantly upregulated, and IL6ST showed an upregulation trend in the AcOEtE group, indicating that the upregulated expression of Lpcat4 was associated with inflammatory cytokines.

Another possible reason for the overall downregulation of PCs in the AcOEtE group is the involvement of the alpha-linolenic acid metabolic pathway. PCs could be converted to alpha-linolenic acids, which could be further converted to stearidonic acids in the alpha-linolenic acid metabolic pathway. The KEGG pathway analysis of lipidomic results supports this hypothesis, as does the upregulation of activity of fads2 enzyme (an enzyme required for the conversion of PCs to α-linolenic acid) in the AcOEtE group.

CL plays an essential role in mitochondrial bioenergetic processes and is localized and synthesized in the inner mitochondrial membrane, where biosynthesis occurs (Paradies et al., 2019). Also, excess CL has been shown to have a detrimental effect on mitochondria. CL is closely associated with respiratory chain proteins and is therefore very sensitive to peroxidation, which may lead to the induction of an apoptotic cascade response, ultimately leading to programmed cell death (Petrosillo et al., 2001; Paradies et al., 2002; Paradies et al., 2014). To our Experimentally, CL species containing longer fatty acyl chains were found to be significantly increased in the AcOEtE group. We also examined the level of genes involved in mitochondrial activities inside the AMPK pathway. Carnitine palmitoyltransferase-1 (cpt1) is an enzyme responsible for transporting long-chain fatty acids for β-oxidation, regulating cellular differentiation and lipid metabolism (Zhang et al., 2014). Cpt1 is a rate-controlling enzyme for fatty acid β-oxidation, catalyzing the condensation of acyl-coenzyme A with levulinic acid to form acylcarnitine esters, which are subsequently transported to mitochondria for further catabolism (McGarry and Brown, 1997). In our experiments, we found that the activity of cpt1 was significantly upregulated in the AcOEtE group, which could explain the overactive mitochondrial function in the CL supersaturation state and the translocation and processing of long-chain fatty acids involved in the glycerophospholipid metabolic pathway.

Phosphatidylglycerol (PG) is a glycerophospholipid that is an intermediate product of the CDP-DG (CDP 1,2-diacyl-sn-glycerol) synthetic pathway and a precursor for the synthesis of CL (Kiyasu et al., 1963; Hostetler et al., 1971). The upregulation of PGs in the experimental results may be related to the over-activation of the synthetic pathway of CLs. Our results revealed that PG (18:1/20:5) content was upregulated in the AcOEtE group, and all nine subclasses detected in CL were upregulated. The upregulation did not occur in the five isoforms of MLCL. The activities of the Lclat1 gene and Taz gene were examined, and both were downregulated, indicating that the MLCL to CL conversion pathway was inhibited, possibly as an antiphase protective mechanism of the organism. Compared to the control group, LPG was not upregulated in the administered group, but the enzyme activity of LPG to PG was upregulated, which explained why the PG content was upregulated. Meanwhile, we examined the activity of the cd36 enzyme and found that cd36 underwent significant downregulation. Cd36 is a scavenger receptor that functions in the high-affinity tissue uptake of long-chain fatty acids (FA) and is involved in cellular fatty acids FA uptake. In the AMPK pathway, cd36 could directly promote the further conversion of fatty acids to Fatty Acyl-Coa, while there was a significant upregulation of the mitochondria-related enzyme cpt1, indicating that mitochondria-related functions were activated.

Changes in the Sphingolipid Metabolism Pathway

Our results identified upregulation of Cer and sphingomyelin (Sph) in the AcOEtE group (**Figure 3A**), both of which are included in the sphingolipid metabolic pathway. Cers and ceramide-derived sphingolipids are structural components of cell membranes associated with oxidative stress and inflammation and may play a role in developing Hepatic fibrosis. Inflammation and an oversupply of saturated fatty acids stimulate the continuous synthesis of new Cers (Kasumov et al., 2015). Our results showed that significant upregulation of nine Cer subclasses occurred in the AcOEtE group compared to the control group, while qPCR results also indicated that AKT was suppressed in the AcOEtE group compared to the control group. The level of Cer was increased after the administration of AcOEtE, which may lead to apoptosis of hepatocytes.

As for Sph, present in animal cell membranes, it is usually composed of choline phosphate and Cer or PE head groups. In our study, some of the Sphs in the AcOEtE group were also upregulated. Despite its very low abundance, it is an essential structural component of the cell membrane (Quehenberger et al., 2010; Rodriguez-Cuenca et al., 2017). It was found that after 16 weeks of high fat and high cholesterol administration to mice, the Sph content in their liver increased significantly (Sanyal and Pacana, 2015). Cer, Sph, and sphingosine 1-phosphate (S1P) can be interconverted, a delicate balance known as the "sphingosine rheostat" (Musso et al., 2018). If Cer and Sph are increased, then apoptosis, senescence, and growth arrest are induced.

In addition, three of the five Hex2Cer isoforms were found to be upregulated. Kang-Yu Peng has reported a positive correlation between Hex2Cer and NASH, and increased Hex2Cer levels were detected in human liver cancer tissues. Also, animal studies showed that pharmacological inhibition of Hex2Cer synthase improved steatosis. These observations provide a strong rationale for further investigation of the role of Hex2Cer in the transition from NAFLD to NASH and possibly hepatocellular carcinoma.

Other Lipid Changes

Compared to the control group, the AcOEtE group showed a significant increase in sterol esters, including cholesterol ester (ChE), Zymosterol ester (ZyE), and Stigmasteryl ester (StE). Excessive ChE can lead to fat accumulation in the liver, which can cause abnormal liver function in the long term. It was shown that C57BL/6J mice fed a high-fat, high-cholesterol diet developed severe hepatic steatosis, massive inflammation, and perisinusoidal fibrosis, which was associated with adipose tissue inflammation and reduced plasma lipocalin levels. In contrast, mice fed a high-fat diet without cholesterol developed only simple steatosis (El Kasmi et al., 2013).

CONCLUSION

In this study, the histological assessment was combined with physicochemical index analysis to demonstrate that ethyl acetate extracts of *Rhizoma Paridis* (AcOEtE) induced liver injury and hepatic fibrosis in zebrafish larvae. Lipidomic analysis based on Q-Exactive HF-X mass spectrometer combined with pathway analysis strategies revealed that AcOEtE induced changes in the lipid profile of zebrafish larvae, mainly significant changes in glycerophospholipid metabolites containing long-chain polyunsaturated fatty acids (LCPUFA), accompanied by changes in the sphingolipid pathway. The significant changes in glycerophospholipids were not only in their subclasses such as PE, PC, and CL but also in the composition of lipids containing long-chain polyunsaturated fatty acids (ω-3 fatty acids and ω-6 fatty acids). By analyzing different metabolites, we found that the mechanism of AcOEtE induced hepatic fibrosis was closely related to the glycerophospholipid-mediated inflammatory response as well as the mitochondrial metabolism involved in CL. Based on the reproducibility of the quality control results, the method was considered reliable. In conclusion, this study revealed the mechanism of AcOEtE leading to liver injury and hepatic fibrosis from the lipid molecular level, which provides new ideas for further research on the safe clinical use of *Rhizoma Paridis*.

AUTHOR CONTRIBUTIONS

CL and MW contributed to the study design, study conduct, and drafting of the manuscript. TF, ZL, YC, and TH contributed to the data collection, data interpretation. DF, ZW, QF, and MC contributed to data analysis. HZ, CZ, and RL revised the manuscript.

REFERENCES

Ahn, J., Lee, H., Jung, C. H., and Ha, T. (2012). Lycopene Inhibits Hepatic Steatosis via microRNA-21-Induced Downregulation of Fatty Acid-Binding Protein 7 in Mice Fed a High-Fat Diet. *Mol. Nutr. Food Res.* 56 (11), 1665–1674. doi:10.1002/mnfr.201200182

Ali, S., Champagne, D. L., Spaink, H. P., and Richardson, M. K. (2011). Zebrafish Embryos and Larvae: a New Generation of Disease Models and Drug Screens. *Birth Defects Res. C Embryo Today* 93 (2), 115–133. doi:10.1002/bdrc.20206

Barros, T. P., Alderton, W. K., Reynolds, H. M., Roach, A. G., and Berghmans, S. (2008). Zebrafish: an Emerging Technology for *In Vivo* Pharmacological Assessment to Identify Potential Safety Liabilities in Early Drug Discovery. *Br. J. Pharmacol.* 154 (7), 1400–1413. doi:10.1038/bjp.2008.249

Bauer, B., Liedtke, D., Jarzina, S., Stammler, E., Kreisel, K., Lalomia, V., et al. (2021). Exploration of Zebrafish Larvae as an Alternative Whole-Animal Model for Nephrotoxicity Testing. *Toxicol. Lett.* 344, 69–81. doi:10.1016/j.toxlet.2021.03.005

Chicco, A. J., and Sparagna, G. C. (2007). Role of Cardiolipin Alterations in Mitochondrial Dysfunction and Disease. *Am. J. Physiol. Cell Physiol* 292 (1), C33–C44. doi:10.1152/ajpcell.00243.2006

Cole, L. K., Vance, J. E., and Vance, D. E. (2012). Phosphatidylcholine Biosynthesis and Lipoprotein Metabolism. *Biochim. Biophys. Acta* 1821 (5), 754–761. doi:10.1016/j.bbalip.2011.09.009

El Kasmi, K. C., Anderson, A. L., Devereaux, M. W., Vue, P. M., Zhang, W., Setchell, K. D., et al. (2013). Phytosterols Promote Liver Injury and Kupffer Cell Activation in Parenteral Nutrition-Associated Liver Disease. *Sci. Transl Med.* 5 (206), 206ra137. doi:10.1126/scitranslmed.3006898

Fontana, R. J., Hayashi, P. H., Gu, J., Reddy, K. R., Barnhart, H., Watkins, P. B., et al. (2014). Idiosyncratic Drug-Induced Liver Injury Is Associated with Substantial Morbidity and Mortality within 6 Months from Onset. *Gastroenterology* 147 (1), 96–108.e4. doi:10.1053/j.gastro.2014.03.045

Friedman, S. L. (2008). Hepatic Stellate Cells: Protean, Multifunctional, and Enigmatic Cells of the Liver. *Physiol. Rev.* 88 (1), 125–172. doi:10.1152/physrev.00013.2007

Goldshmit, Y., Sztal, T. E., Jusuf, P. R., Hall, T. E., Nguyen-Chi, M., and Currie, P. D. (2012). Fgf-dependent Glial Cell Bridges Facilitate Spinal Cord Regeneration in Zebrafish. *J. Neurosci.* 32 (22), 7477–7492. doi:10.1523/JNEUROSCI.0758-12.2012

He, J. H., Guo, S. Y., Zhu, F., Zhu, J. J., Chen, Y. X., Huang, C. J., et al. (2013). A Zebrafish Phenotypic Assay for Assessing Drug-Induced Hepatotoxicity. *J. Pharmacol. Toxicol. Methods* 67 (1), 25–32. doi:10.1016/j.vascn.2012.10.003

Hollie, N. I., Cash, J. G., Matlib, M. A., Wortman, M., Basford, J. E., Abplanalp, W., et al. (2014). Micromolar Changes in Lysophosphatidylcholine Concentration Cause Minor Effects on Mitochondrial Permeability but Major Alterations in Function. *Biochim. Biophys. Acta* 1841 (6), 888–895. doi:10.1016/j.bbalip.2013.11.013

Hostetler, K. Y., Van den Bosch, H., and Van Deenen, L. L. (1971). Biosynthesis of Cardiolipin in Liver Mitochondria. *Biochim. Biophys. Acta* 239 (1), 113–119. doi:10.1016/0005-2760(71)90201-3

Kasumov, T., Li, L., Li, M., Gulshan, K., Kirwan, J. P., Liu, X., et al. (2015). Ceramide as a Mediator of Non-alcoholic Fatty Liver Disease and Associated Atherosclerosis. *PLoS one* 10 (5), e0126910. doi:10.1371/journal.pone.0126910

Kiyasu, J. Y., Pieringer, R. A., Paulus, H., and Kennedy, E. P. (1963). The Biosynthesis of Phosphatidylglycerol. *J. Biol. Chem.* 238, 2293–2298. doi:10.1016/s0021-9258(19)67968-8

Knebel, B., Hartwig, S., Jacob, S., Kettel, U., Schiller, M., Passlack, W., et al. (2018). Inactivation of SREBP-1a Phosphorylation Prevents Fatty Liver Disease in Mice: Identification of Related Signaling Pathways by Gene Expression Profiles in Liver and Proteomes of Peroxisomes. *Int. J. Mol. Sci.* 19 (4), 980. doi:10.3390/ijms19040980

Kumar, N., Surani, S., Udeani, G., Mathew, S., John, S., Sajan, S., et al. (2021). Drug-induced Liver Injury and prospect of Cytokine Based Therapy; A Focus on IL-2 Based Therapies. *Life Sci.* 278, 119544. doi:10.1016/j.lfs.2021.119544

Kuna, L., Bozic, I., Kizivat, T., Bojanic, K., Mrso, M., Kralj, E., et al. (2018). Models of Drug Induced Liver Injury (DILI) - Current Issues and Future Perspectives. *Curr. Drug Metab.* 19 (10), 830–838. doi:10.2174/1389200219666180523095355

Lee, H. C., and Yokomizo, T. (2018). Applications of Mass Spectrometry-Based Targeted and Non-targeted Lipidomics. *Biochem. Biophys. Res. Commun.* 504 (3), 576–581. doi:10.1016/j.bbrc.2018.03.081

Li, Z., Agellon, L. B., Allen, T. M., Umeda, M., Jewell, L., Mason, A., et al. (2006). The Ratio of Phosphatidylcholine to Phosphatidylethanolamine Influences Membrane Integrity and Steatohepatitis. *Cell Metab* 3 (5), 321–331. doi:10.1016/j.cmet.2006.03.007

McGarry, J. D., and Brown, N. F. (1997). The Mitochondrial Carnitine Palmitoyltransferase System. From Concept to Molecular Analysis. *Eur. J. Biochem.* 244 (1), 1–14. doi:10.1111/j.1432-1033.1997.00001.x

Mederacke, I., Hsu, C. C., Troeger, J. S., Huebener, P., Mu, X., Dapito, D. H., et al. (2013). Fate Tracing Reveals Hepatic Stellate Cells as Dominant Contributors to Liver Fibrosis Independent of its Aetiology. *Nat. Commun.* 4, 2823. doi:10.1038/ncomms3823

Musso, G., Cassader, M., Paschetta, E., and Gambino, R. (2018). Bioactive Lipid Species and Metabolic Pathways in Progression and Resolution of Nonalcoholic Steatohepatitis. *Gastroenterology* 155 (2), 282–e8.e288. doi:10.1053/j.gastro.2018.06.031

Owen, J. S., and McIntyre, N. (1978). Erythrocyte Lipid Composition and Sodium Transport in Human Liver Disease. *Biochim. Biophys. Acta* 510 (1), 168–176. doi:10.1016/0005-2736(78)90138-4

Papadopoulos, C., Panopoulou, M., Mylopoulou, T., Mimidis, K., Tentes, I., and Anagnostopoulos, K. (2020). Cholesterol and Phospholipid Distribution Pattern in the Erythrocyte Membrane of Patients with Hepatitis C and Severe Fibrosis, before and after Treatment with Direct Antiviral Agents: A Pilot Study. *Maedica (Bucur)* 15 (2), 162–168. doi:10.26574/maedica.2020.15.2.162

Paradies, G., Paradies, V., Ruggiero, F. M., and Petrosillo, G. (2014). Oxidative Stress, Cardiolipin and Mitochondrial Dysfunction in Nonalcoholic Fatty Liver Disease. *World J. Gastroenterol.* 20 (39), 14205–14218. doi:10.3748/wjg.v20.i39.14205

Paradies, G., Paradies, V., Ruggiero, F. M., and Petrosillo, G. (2019). Role of Cardiolipin in Mitochondrial Function and Dynamics in Health and Disease: Molecular and Pharmacological Aspects. *Cells* 8 (7), 728. doi:10.3390/cells8070728

Paradies, G., Petrosillo, G., Pistolese, M., and Ruggiero, F. M. (2002). Reactive Oxygen Species Affect Mitochondrial Electron Transport Complex I Activity through Oxidative Cardiolipin Damage. *Gene* 286 (1), 135–141. doi:10.1016/s0378-1119(01)00814-9

Peng, J., Yu, J., Xu, H., Kang, C., Shaul, P. W., Guan, Y., et al. (2018). Enhanced Liver Regeneration after Partial Hepatectomy in Sterol Regulatory Element-Binding Protein (SREBP)-1c-Null Mice Is Associated with Increased Hepatocellular Cholesterol Availability. *Cell Physiol Biochem* 47 (2), 784–799. doi:10.1159/000490030

Petrosillo, G., Ruggiero, F. M., Pistolese, M., and Paradies, G. (2001). Reactive Oxygen Species Generated from the Mitochondrial Electron Transport Chain Induce Cytochrome C Dissociation from Beef-Heart Submitochondrial Particles via Cardiolipin Peroxidation. Possible Role in the Apoptosis. *FEBS Lett.* 509 (3), 435–438. doi:10.1016/s0014-5793(01)03206-9

Puri, P., Baillie, R. A., Wiest, M. M., Mirshahi, F., Choudhury, J., Cheung, O., et al. (2007). A Lipidomic Analysis of Nonalcoholic Fatty Liver Disease. *Hepatology* 46 (4), 1081–1090. doi:10.1002/hep.21763

Qin, X. J., Ni, W., Chen, C. X., and Liu, H. Y. (2018). Untiring Researches for Alternative Resources of Rhizoma Paridis. *Nat. Prod. Bioprospect* 8 (4), 265–278. doi:10.1007/s13659-018-0179-5

Quehenberger, O., Armando, A. M., Brown, A. H., Milne, S. B., Myers, D. S., Merrill, A. H., et al. (2010). Lipidomics Reveals a Remarkable Diversity of Lipids in Human Plasma. *J. Lipid Res.* 51 (11), 3299–3305. doi:10.1194/jlr.M009449

Rodriguez-Cuenca, S., Pellegrinelli, V., Campbell, M., Oresic, M., and Vidal-Puig, A. (2017). Sphingolipids and Glycerophospholipids - the "ying and Yang" of Lipotoxicity in Metabolic Diseases. *Prog. Lipid Res.* 66, 14–29. doi:10.1016/j.plipres.2017.01.002

Sanyal, A. J., and Pacana, T. (2015). A Lipidomic Readout of Disease Progression in A Diet-Induced Mouse Model of Nonalcoholic Fatty Liver Disease. *Trans. Am. Clin. Climatol Assoc.* 126, 271–288.

Sarwar Inam, A. (2017). Effects of LC-PUFA (Long Chain Poly Unsaturated Fatty Acids) in Infancy. *Adv. Obes. Weight Manage. Control.* 7, 325–327. doi:10.15406/aowmc.2017.07.00207

Tanaka, N., Matsubara, T., Krausz, K. W., Patterson, A. D., and Gonzalez, F. J. (2012). Disruption of Phospholipid and Bile Acid Homeostasis in Mice with Nonalcoholic Steatohepatitis. *Hepatology* 56 (1), 118–129. doi:10.1002/hep.25630

Tillmann, H. L., Suzuki, A., Barnhart, H. X., Serrano, J., and Rockey, D. C. (2019). Tools for Causality Assessment in Drug-Induced Liver Disease. *Curr. Opin. Gastroenterol.* 35 (3), 183–190. doi:10.1097/MOG.0000000000000526

Westerbacka, J., Kolak, M., Kiviluoto, T., Arkkila, P., Sirén, J., Hamsten, A., et al. (2007). Genes Involved in Fatty Acid Partitioning and Binding, Lipolysis, Monocyte/macrophage Recruitment, and Inflammation Are Overexpressed in the Human Fatty Liver of Insulin-Resistant Subjects. *Diabetes* 56 (11), 2759–2765. doi:10.2337/db07-0156

Worley, B., and Powers, R. (2016). PCA as a Practical Indicator of OPLS-DA Model Reliability. *Curr. Metabolomics* 4 (2), 97–103. doi:10.2174/2213235X04666160613122429

Wu, Y., Chen, Z., Darwish, W. S., Terada, K., Chiba, H., and Hui, S. P. (2019). Choline and Ethanolamine Plasmalogens Prevent Lead-Induced Cytotoxicity and Lipid Oxidation in HepG2 Cells. *J. Agric. Food Chem.* 67 (27), 7716–7725. doi:10.1021/acs.jafc.9b02485

Yamazaki, T., Shiraishi, S., Kishimoto, K., Miura, S., and Ezaki, O. (2011). An Increase in Liver PPARγ2 Is an Initial Event to Induce Fatty Liver in Response to a Diet High in Butter: PPARγ2 Knockdown Improves Fatty Liver Induced by High-Saturated Fat. *J. Nutr. Biochem.* 22 (6), 543–553. doi:10.1016/j.jnutbio.2010.04.009

Yan, J., Liao, K., Wang, T., Mai, K., Xu, W., and Ai, Q. (2015). Dietary Lipid Levels Influence Lipid Deposition in the Liver of Large Yellow Croaker (Larimichthys Crocea) by Regulating Lipoprotein Receptors, Fatty Acid Uptake and Triacylglycerol Synthesis and Catabolism at the Transcriptional Level. *PLoS One* 10 (6), e0129937. doi:10.1371/journal.pone.0129937

Zeng, Y., Zhang, Z., Wang, W., You, L., Dong, X., Yin, X., et al. (2020). Underlying Mechanisms of Apoptosis in HepG2 Cells Induced by Polyphyllin I through Fas Death and Mitochondrial Pathways. *Toxicol. Mech. Methods* 30 (6), 397–406. doi:10.1080/15376516.2020.1747125

Zhang, Y. F., Yuan, Z. Q., Song, D. G., Zhou, X. H., and Wang, Y. Z. (2014). Effects of Cannabinoid Receptor 1 (Brain) on Lipid Accumulation by Transcriptional Control of CPT1A and CPT1B. *Anim. Genet.* 45 (1), 38–47. doi:10.1111/age.12078

Zhao, C., Wang, M., Jia, Z., Li, E., Zhao, X., Li, F., et al. (2020). Similar Hepatotoxicity Response Induced by Rhizoma Paridis in Zebrafish Larvae, Cell and Rat. *J. Ethnopharmacol* 250, 112440. doi:10.1016/j.jep.2019.112440

18

Allium victorialis L. Extracts Promote Activity of FXR to Ameliorate Alcoholic Liver Disease: Targeting Liver Lipid Deposition and Inflammation

Zhen-Yu Cui [1†], Xin Han [2†], Yu-Chen Jiang [1], Jia-Yi Dou [1], Kun-Chen Yao [1], Zhong-He Hu [1], Ming-Hui Yuan [1], Xiao-Xue Bao [1], Mei-Jie Zhou [1], Yue Liu [1], Li-Hua Lian [1], Xian Zhang [3], Ji-Xing Nan [1,4*] and Yan-Ling Wu [1*]*

[1]Key Laboratory for Traditional Chinese Korean Medicine of Jilin Province, College of Pharmacy, Yanbian University, Yanji, China, [2]Chinese Medicine Processing Centre, College of Pharmacy, Zhejiang Chinese Medical University, Hangzhou, China, [3]Agricultural College, Yanbian University, Yanji, China, [4]Clinical Research Center, Affiliated Hospital of Yanbian University, Yanji, China

*Correspondence:
Yan-Ling Wu
ylwu@ybu.edu.cn
Ji-Xing Nan
jxnan@ybu.edu.cn
Xian Zhang
zhangxian@ybu.edu.cn

[†]These authors have contributed equally to this work

Allium victorialis L. (AVL) is a traditional medicinal plant recorded in the Compendium of Materia Medica (the Ming Dynasty). In general, it is used for hemostasis, analgesia, anti-inflammation, antioxidation, and to especially facilitate hepatoprotective effect. In recent years, it has received more and more attention due to its special nutritional and medicinal value. The present study investigates the effect and potential mechanism of AVL against alcoholic liver disease (ALD). C57BL/6 mice were fed Lieber–DeCarli liquid diet containing 5% ethanol plus a single ethanol gavage (5 g/kg), and followed up with the administration of AVL or silymarin. AML12 cells were stimulated with ethanol and incubated with AVL. AVL significantly reduced serum transaminase and triglycerides in the liver and attenuated histopathological changes caused by ethanol. AVL significantly inhibited SREBP1 and its target genes, regulated lipin 1/2, increased PPARα and its target genes, and decreased PPARγ expression caused by ethanol. In addition, AVL significantly enhanced FXR, LXRs, Sirt1, and AMPK expressions compared with the EtOH group. AVL also inhibited inflammatory factors, NLRP3, and F4/80 and MPO, macrophage and neutrophil markers. *In vitro*, AVL significantly reduced lipid droplets, lipid metabolism enzymes, and inflammatory factors depending on FXR activation. AVL could ameliorate alcoholic steatohepatitis, lipid deposition and inflammation in ALD by targeting FXR activation.

Keywords: *Allium victorialis* L, alcoholic liver disease, lipid deposition, inflammation, farnesoid X receptor

---

Abbreviations: ALD, alcoholic liver disease; AMPK, adenosine 5'-monophosphate (AMP)-activated protein kinase; CYP2E1, cytochrome P4502E1; FAS, fatty acid synthase; FXR, farnesoid X receptor; LXRs, liver X receptors; NLRP3, NLR family pyrin domain containing 3; NRs, nuclear hormone receptors; PPARα, peroxisome proliferators-activated receptor α; RXRα, retinoid X receptor α; SCD-1, stearoyl-coenzyme A desaturase 1; SIRT1, NAD-dependent deacetylase Sirtuis; SREBP1, sterol-regulatory element binding protein 1.

INTRODUCTION

Alcohol consumption is highly addictive and associated with social, economic, and multifarious health problems (Galicia-Moreno and Gutiérrez-Reyes, 2014). Although moderate drinking is beneficial to physical and mental health, such as prevention of heart disease, hypertension, and diabetes, excessive and prolonged drinking leads to alcoholic liver disease (ALD) (Berger et al., 1999; Sacco et al., 1999). ALD is the main pathogenic factor contributing to morbidity of liver diseases worldwide. Generally, alcohol is first metabolized to acetaldehyde by alcohol dehydrogenase and partly metabolized by cytochrome P4502E1 (CYP2E1), catalase in hepatocyte microsomes and peroxisomes (Liu, 2014). This process would synthesize fatty acids, accumulate triglycerides (TGs) and further lead to fatty liver disease. Simple fatty liver is the early stage in ALD progression and would subsequently lead to steatosis, alcoholic hepatitis, fibrosis, and even cirrhosis with continuous consumption of excessive amounts of alcohol (Shearn et al., 2013; Addolorato et al., 2016). So far, there has been no specific drug to prevent or treat fatty liver. And it is still critical to develop an effective therapeutic drug for ALD, which not only prevents progression and reduces fat deposition but also accelerates regeneration and stability of hepatocytes and promotes liver activity.

Hepatic steatosis is part of the early adaptive response of the liver against some chronic stimulus. Inflammation might occur before hepatic steatosis and subsequently lead to steatosis. During the progression of steatosis, nutrients and their metabolites can also induce the secretion of adipokines and inflammatory factors by adipocytes, macrophages, and other cells, which is called metabolically triggered inflammation (Hotamisligil, 2006). ALD in patients is often accompanied by dyslipidemia, elevation of free fatty acids, and related lipotoxicity, insulin resistance and intestinal endotoxin, which contribute to stimulate and maintain the production and release of proinflammatory cytokines. Thus, inflammation is involved in the development of ALD.

Current researches have indicated that alcohol and its metabolites play critical roles in ALD development through hepatotoxicity, oxidative stress, lipid peroxidation, and ethanol metabolic enzyme system. Hepatosteatosis is the early abnormality in the pathogenesis of ALD due to chronic alcohol abuse and metabolic syndrome. Chronic alcoholism can effect fat synthesis and inhibit fatty acid oxidation, including upregulating SREBP1 and PPARγ by targeting key transcriptional genes associated with metabolic processes (Esfandiari et al., 2005; Esfandiari et al., 2007). Chronic alcohol consumption increased expressions of SREBP1 and PPARγ that is related to the activation of NAD-dependent deacetylase Sirtuis (Sirt) and adenosine 5'-monophosphate (AMP)–activated protein kinase (AMPK) (Lieber et al., 2008). Moreover, chronic alcohol intake could break the mutual effect between farnesoid X receptor (FXR; NR1H4) and retinoid X receptor α (RXRα; NR2B1) via acetylation and inactivation of FXR (Wu et al., 2014). FXR is a nuclear hormone receptor (NR), which is involved in the regulation of bile acid homeostasis and

further in liver disease via the gut–liver axis (Forman et al., 1995; Seol et al., 1995). A previous study had shown that chronic alcohol consumption impaired FXR activity, and activated FXR attenuates hepatic liver injury, steatosis, and cholestasis induced by ETOH (Wu et al., 2014). FXR activation decreases TG levels to regulate lipogenesis through the downregulation of SREBP1 or upregulation of PPARα, mediating fatty acid oxidation (Pineda Torra et al., 2003; Watanabe et al., 2004; Ding et al., 2014). Thus, the present study focuses on the important role FXR plays in the development of ALD caused by Lieber–DeCarli ethanol liquid diet and contributes to alterations of lipid deposition and inflammation through a newly discovered potential mechanism.

Allium victorialis L. (AVL) is a species of the genus Allium (family Alliaceae) and widely spread in most parts of the world. AVL is a kind of medicinal and edible plant, and its stems and leaves are edible. AVL is also used as pickles in soy sauce, wrapped pork, or kimchi, which are loved by many people for their delicious tastes. "Qianjin Yaofang·Shi Zhi Juan," the earliest dietotherapy book in Chinese history written by Sun Si-Miao (the Tang Dynasty, 618–907A.D.), also recorded that AVL could be used to treat liver disease according to the traditional Chinese medicine theory. The ancient traditional Chinese medical books recorded AVL as pungent, slightly warm, and nontoxic and that it could be used to treat body warmth and heat accumulation, clear damp heat, and eliminate miasma, especially in the abdominal digestive system. According to ancient traditional medicine, liver disease is considered to present symptoms of damp heat, toxins, and miasma; therefore, clearing away the heat and removing the dampness is the first choice of treatment. In recent years, AVL has received much attention due to its diverse pharmacological properties, such as anti-obesity, anticancer, antioxidant, hepatoprotective, and so on (Shirataki et al., 2001; Tang et al., 2017). Some studies have found that the extract of AVL could significantly inhibit the formation of tumor nodules in lung tissue and act as a rewarding supplement for cancer prevention and therapy (Kim et al., 2014). Up to now, more than 200 components have been isolated from AVL. The main active components of AVL include volatile oils, flavonoids, steroids, steroidal saponins, carbohydrates, etc. Besides these, plentiful flavonoids isolated from AVL presented functions on regulating neurotransmitters (Woo et al., 2012). In a previous study, the contents of flavonoids in AVL were roughly determined by HPLC analysis by taking rutin, kaempferol, and quercetin as standard references. The authors aimed to explore the improvement effect of AVL on ETOH-induced adipose degeneration in mice, and this study was designed to investigate the effect of AVL on hepatic steatosis and inflammation and reveal the potential role of FXR-mediated by AVL against ALD.

MATERIALS AND METHODS

Plant Material

The samples of *Allium victorialis* L. (AVL) (**Figure 1A**) were wild and grown in Hunchun City of Jilin province and were authenticated by Professor Xian Zhang, Agricultural College,

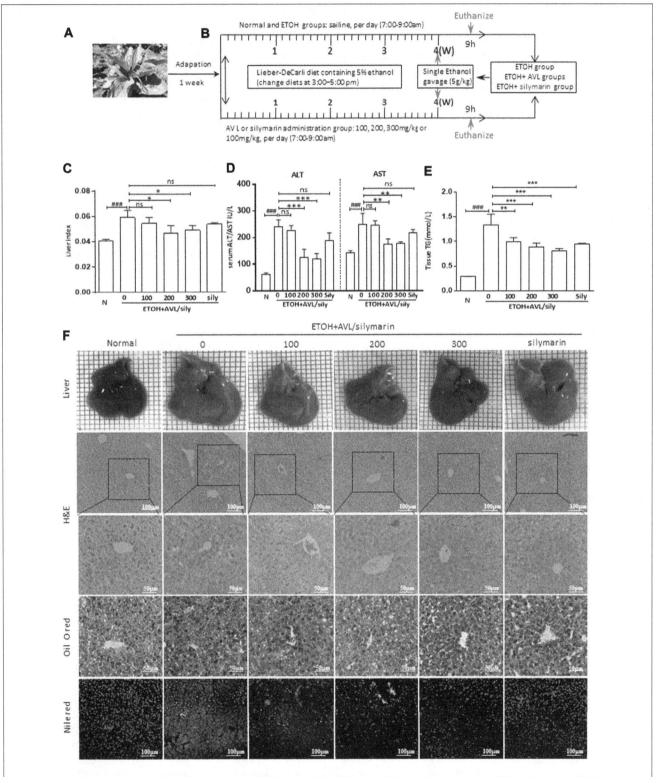

FIGURE 1 | AVL effectively attenuated alcohol-induced fatty liver. **(A)** Picture of AVL. **(B)** Procedures for the animal experiments. **(C)** Liver index levels. **(D)** Serum ALT and AST activities. **(E)** Tissue TG levels. **(F)** Liver appearance picture, H&E stain (×200 and ×400 magnifications), Oil red O stain (×400 magnification), Nile red staining (×200 magnification). $^{###}p < 0.001$ compared with normal group; $^*p < 0.05$, $^{**}p < 0.01$, $^{***}p < 0.001$ compared with EtOH group; ns, not significant.

Yanbian University, China. A voucher specimen (YBUCP20171212) was deposited in the Herbarium of the Agricultural College, Yanbian University, China.

Fresh AVL (1000 g) was soaked in ethanol for 24 h, followed by reflux extraction for 2 h. After filtration, the filter residue was collected and reflux extraction carried out 3 times. The powder of AVL was obtained by vacuum distillation and drying at 80°C. AVL extracts were analyzed by HPLC in supplement data.

Reagents

The reagent strips for ALT/AST and TG were purchased from Changchun Huili Biotech Co., Ltd. (Changchun, China). Primary antibodies against GAPDH (ab8245), MPO (ab45977), lipin 1 (ab70138), LXRα (ab41902), lipin 2 (ab176347), CYP2E1 (ab28146), NLRP3 (ab4207), Sirt1 (ab110304), PPARγ (ab19481), SREBP1 (ab3259), F4/80 (ab6640), and Opti-MEM® were obtained from Abcam (Cambridge, MA, United States). Primary antibodies against ASC (sc514414), PPARα (sc9000), LXRβ (sc34341), IL6 (sc28343), IL1R1 (sc393998), and caspase 1 (sc622) were purchased from Santa Cruz Biotechnology Inc. (Santa Cruz, CA, United States). Primary antibodies against FXR (cs4173), p-AMPKα (cs2531), AMPKα (cs2532), p-AMPKβ1/2 (cs4181), AMPKβ1/2 (cs4150), LKB1 (cs3047), p-LKB1 (cs3482), p-ACC (cs11818), and ACC (cs3676) were purchased from Cell Signaling Technology (Beverly, MA, United States). Lipofectamine® 2000 Transfection Reagent was purchased from Thermo Fisher Scientific (Carlsbad, CA, United States). The BCA Protein Assay Kit was obtained from Beyotime (Jiangsu, China). All other chemicals and reagents were obtained from Sigma-Aldrich (Shanghai, China).

Protocols for the Animal Experiments

Male C57BL/6 mice (body weight, 22–24 g) (SPF, SCXK [J] 2016-0003) purchased from Changchun Yisi Laboratory Animal Technology Co., Ltd. (Jilin, China) were housed under conditions of constant temperature (22 ± 2°C), relative humidity (50–60%), and light (12-h light–dark cycles) for 1 week. The animal experiment was handled in accordance with the Guide for the Care and Use of Laboratory Animals of Yanbian University (Resolution number, 201801022). After a week of acclimatization, all mice were randomly divided into six groups (six mice per group): normal group, EtOH group, EtOH plus AVL (100-, 200-, and 300-mg/kg) groups, and EtOH plus silymarin (100-mg/kg) group. The mice in the normal group were fed control Lieber–DeCarli liquid diet (TP 4030C, Trophic Animal Feed High-Tech Co., Ltd., China), and the mice in the other groups were fed Lieber–DeCarli liquid diet containing ethanol (TP 4030D, Trophic Animal Feed High-Tech Co., Ltd., China). The concentrations of ethanol were from 1 to 4% (v/v) for first 5 days, and then followed by 5% ethanol for 4 weeks. All mice were allowed free access to distilled water during the experiment. EtOH plus AVL or silymarin groups were daily gavaged with AVL (100, 200, and 300 mg/kg) or silymarin (100 mg/kg), and the normal and EtOH groups were daily administrated equal volumes of saline. Except for the normal group, the mice in the other groups were single gavaged with

ethanol (5 g/kg) at the end of the fourth week. After the final administration, the mice were sacrificed under anesthesia. Finally, the serum and livers were collected for subsequent experiments. The detailed modeling procedures are described in **Figure 1B**.

Cell Culture and Treatment

AML12 and HepG2 cells were generous gifts from Professor Dr. Jung Joon Lee of Korea Research Institute of Bioscience and Biotechnology (Daejeon, Korea). The AML12 cells were incubated in DMEM/F-12 with a mixture of insulin–transferrin–selenium (1%), dexamethasone (40 ng/ml), GlutaMAX (1%), and nonessential amino acids, while HepG2 cells were incubated in DMEM. DMEM contains penicillin (100 U/ml), streptomycin (100 mg/ml), and 10% fetal bovine serum (FBS) under the conditions of 5% CO_2 at 37°C. For MTT assay, AML12 cells were cultured in 96-well plates at a density of 1×10^4 cells per well and treated with AVL (0–100 μg/ml) or EtOH (0–200 mM). The cells were cultured in 35-mm dishes at a density of 5×10^6 cells per dish and were treated with EtOH (50 mM) with or without AVL.

Transfection of HepG2 Cells With Plasmid

The transfections of FXR and control plasmid were conducted using the Lipofectamine® 2000 Transfection Reagent according to the manufacturer's protocols. The cells were cultured in a 24-well plate at a density of 6×10^4 cells per dish, then transfected with Opti-MEM® containing 0.2 μg of FXR plasmid or a negative control and 1.5 μL Lipofectamine® 2000 Transfection Reagent at the confluence of 90–95%. The cells were incubated under the condition of 5% CO_2 at 37°C for 48 h and then Opti-MEM® substituted with DMEM containing 10% FBS and EtOH (50 mM) with or without AVL (12.5 μg/ml).

Serum Transaminase and Tissue TG Assay

The serum samples were collected by centrifugation at 3000 rpm and 4°C for 30 min. The liver was homogenized with saline and the homogenate obtained. Serum AST/ALT and tissue TG were measured using Assay kit according to the manufacturer's instructions, which was provided by Changchun Meeting of Biological Co., Ltd. (Changchun, China).

Immunostaining

Parts of the liver tissues were fixed with 10% formalin solution and embedded in paraffin. Frozen sections were prepared with Tissue-Tek® O.C.T. Compound. After dewaxing hydration, the sections were treated with hematoxylin and eosin (H&E) solution following the manufacturer's instructions. The frozen sections were fixed with the mixture of acetone and methanol or paraformaldehyde, and stained with Oil red O and Nile red stains, also following the manufacturer's instructions. For immunofluorescence (Han et al., 2019), the frozen sections were fixed with the mixture of methanol and acetone, dried at room temperature, washed with PBS, and then blocked with 5% goat serum. The slides were incubated with the primary antibody at 4°C overnight and incubated with Alexa Fluor Goat pAb with

TABLE 1 | Primer sequences used in real-time PCR.

Genes	Sense (5' to 3')	Antisense (3' to 5')
SREBP1	CTTGTGCAGTGCCAGCC	GCCCAATACGGCCAAATCC
FASN	AAAGTCCTTGTCCAGGTACG	AGGTCTTGGAGATGGCAGAA
SCD1	TGAGGCGAGCAACTGACTAT	GGCACCGTCTTCACCTTCT
ACLY	TTGTGGACATGCTCAGGAAC	AAGGTAGTGCCCAATGAAGC
Cpt2	AGTATCTGCAGCACAGCATC	ACTTCTGTCTTCCTGAACTGG
PPARα	AGGCTGTAAGGGCTTCTTTC	ATTGTGTACATCCCGACAG
ACOX1	CGTGCAGCCAGATTGGTAG	CGCCACTTCCTTGCTCTTC
fabp	AAGTGTCCGCAATGAGTTC	CTTGACGACTGCCTTGACTT
IL18	TGACTGTAGAGATAATGCAC	ATCATGTCCTGGGACACTTC
IL1α	CAGTGAAATTTGACATGGGTG	CAGGCATCTCCTTCAGCAG
TNF-α	GAGCACTGAAAGCATGATCC	GAGGGTTTGCTACAACATGG
NLRP3	GCCTACAGTTGGGTGAAATG	GTCAGCTCAGGCTTTTCTTC
IL1β	TCTTTGAAGAAGAGCCCATCC	CTAATGGGAACGTCACACAC
GAPDH	ACCACAGTCCATGCCATCAC	TCCACCACCCTGTTGCTGTA

rat IgG at room temperature. The nuclei were stained with DAPI and observed under fluorescence microscope.

Western Blot Analysis

Protein was extracted from liver tissue or cells with RIPA lysis buffer. Equal amounts of protein were separated using 6–15% sodium dodecyl sulfate–polyacrylamide-gel electrophoresis and transferred onto a polyvinylidene fluoride membrane (GE, Freiburg, Germany). The membranes were blocked with skim milk and then incubated with indicated primary antibodies overnight at 4°C, followed with a horseradish peroxidase–conjugated secondary antibody. Finally, the protein bands were visualized with BeyoECL Plus detection reagent (Beyotime, Nanjing, Jiangsu, China) and exposed to an X-ray film. Each band's densitometry was quantified using Bio-Rad Quantity One software.

Real-Time PCR

Total RNA was isolated from liver tissue or cells using the Eastep Super total RNA Extraction Kit (Promega Biological Products Ltd., Shanghai, China) according to the manufacturer's instructions. Samples of RNA were reverse transcribed into complementary DNA (cDNA). Relative gene expression was assessed by real-time PCR, which was performed on an Agilent Mx3000P QPCR System in a mixture containing Power SYBR® Green PCR Master Mix (Life Technologies, Carlsbad, CA), and specific primers are listed in **Table 1**. GAPDH was used as a housekeeping gene to quantify relative fold difference, and the relative fold difference was quantified using the comparative threshold cycle ($\Delta\Delta Ct$) method.

Statistical Analysis

All data in experiments were expressed as mean ± SD. The comparison between groups was evaluated by GraphPad Prism (GraphPad Software, San Diego, CA, United States). One-way analysis of variance and Tukey's multiple comparison tests were used to perform statistical analyses. Statistically significant differences between groups were defined as p-values no more than 0.05.

RESULTS

Allium victorialis L. Effectively Attenuated Alcohol-Induced Fatty Liver

With the Lieber–DeCarli liquid diet containing 5% (vol/vol) ethanol and single ethanol gavage (5 g/kg), the liver index, serum ALT/AST levels, and hepatic TG levels were significantly increased compared to the normal group, while AVL treatments markedly decreased these alternations compared to the EtOH group (**Figures 1C–E**).

As shown in **Figure 1F**, the liver images of the normal mice show a smooth surface, soft texture, and sharp edges. In the EtOH group, the liver tissue of the mice appeared swollen, rough, and tarnished. With AVL or silymarin administration, the liver surface was smoothened and the swelling reduced; however, silymarin administration showed less change than AVL (300 mg/kg).

The H&E analysis showed that the liver in the EtOH group showed massive steatosis compared with that in the normal group, and more fibrous connective tissue in the central region of the hepatic lobules had caused irregular deformation and increased liver injury. All these obvious pathological changes were significantly improved with AVL treatment (**Figure 1F**). In addition, Oil red O and Nile red staining showed that EtOH could induce the formation of lipid droplets in the liver compared to the normal group; however, lipid droplets in the AVL or silymarin groups were less abundant and much smaller than those in the EtOH group (**Figure 1F**). These results indicate that AVL showed hepatoprotective effect against liver injury and steatosis induced by EtOH.

Allium victorialis L. Administrations Regulated Lipid-Related Proteins Induced by EtOH

SREBP1 plays a critical role in alcoholic liver disease, and it could regulate the transcription of downstream signaling, such as FASN, SCD, and ACLY. CYP2E1 is a key pathway in the regulation of lipid peroxidation and oxidative stress induced by ethanol. EtOH elevated protein and mRNA levels of SREBP1, the protein level of CYP2E1, and the mRNA levels of FASN, SCD, and ACLY compared to the normal group. AVL treatment could significantly inhibit protein or mRNA expressions of SREBP1, CYP2E1, FASN, SCD, and ACLY compared to the EtOH group (**Figures 2A,D**), and silymarin showed no obvious regulating in CYP2E1 (**Figure 2A**). In immunohistochemical staining, AVL or silymarin obviously decreased the positive expressions of SREBP1 (in brown) compared to the ETOH group (**Figure 2C**).

Both lipin 1 and lipin 2 are the first central regulatory enzymes in the regulation of lipid metabolism in the liver (Song et al., 2018). As is shown in **Figure 2B**, alcohol intake increased the protein expression of lipin 1 and decreased the protein expression of lipin 2 compared to the normal group, whereas these changes were reversed by AVL treatment compared to the EtOH group (**Figure 2B**). In **Figure 2E**, EtOH stimulation obviously inhibited

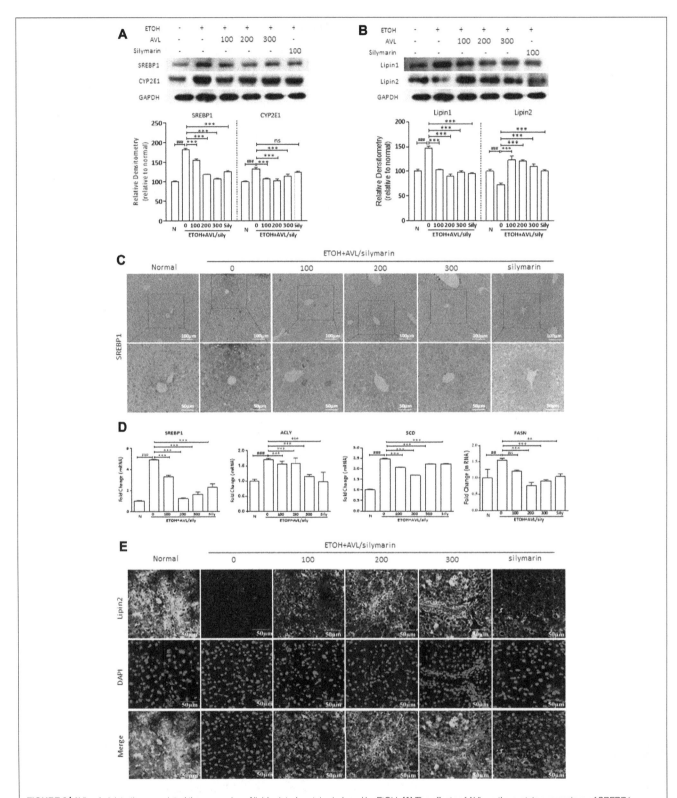

FIGURE 2 | AVL administrations regulated the expression of lipid-related proteins induced by EtOH. (A) The effects of AVL on the protein expressions of SREBP1 and CYP2E1. (B) The effects of AVL on the protein expressions of lipin 1 and lipin 2. Densitometric values were normalized against GAPDH. The same GAPDH was used in Panels 2A,B and in **Figure 3D** and **Figure 4A**. (C) Immunohistochemical staining analysis of SREBP1 (×200 and ×400 magnification). (D) Representative QPCR analysis for SREBP1, ACLY, SCD, and FASN. (E) Immunofluorescence staining analysis of lipin 2 (×600 magnification). Data are presented as mean ± SD (n = 3). ##p < 0.01, ###p < 0.001 compared with normal group; **p < 0.01, ***p < 0.001 compared with EtOH group.

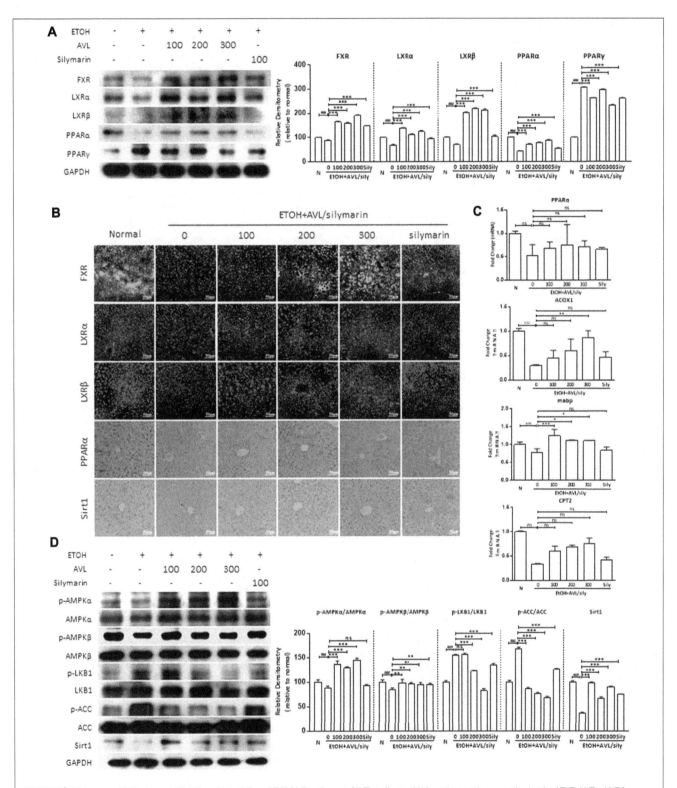

FIGURE 3 | AVL improved lipid accumulation through regulation of FXR/LXR pathways. **(A)** The effects of AVL on the protein expression levels of FXR, LXRα, LXRβ, PPARα, and PPARγ. Densitometric values were normalized against GAPDH. **(B)** Immunofluorescence staining analysis of FXR, LXRα, and LXRβ (×200 magnification), and immunohistochemical staining analysis of PPARα and SIRT1 (×400 magnification). **(C)** Representative QPCR analysis for expressions of mRNA expression of PPARα, ACOX1, mabp, and CPT2. **(D)** The effects of AVL on the protein expression levels of p/t-AMPKα, p/t-AMPKβ, p/t-LKB1, p/t-ACC, and Sirt1. Densitometric values were normalized against GAPDH. The same GAPDH was used in **Figures 2A,B**, Panel 3D, and **Figure 4A**. Data are presented as mean ± SD (n = 3). $^{###}p < 0.001$ compared with normal group; $^{*}p < 0.05$, $^{**}p < 0.01$, $^{***}p < 0.001$ compared with EtOH group; ns, not significant.

the immunofluorescence expression of lipin 2 (in green) compared to the normal group (**Figure 2E**), while AVL or silymarin treatment significantly increased the expressions of lipin 2 compared to the EtOH group (**Figure 2E**). These results suggest that AVL downregulates lipid synthesis and upregulates fatty acid oxidation, and eventually ameliorates hepatic steatosis.

Allium victorialis L. Improved Lipid Accumulation Through Regulation of Farnesoid X Receptor/Liver X Receptor Pathways

FXR and liver X receptors (LXRs), which belong to the NRs supergene family, can regulate the lipid metabolism gene in metabolic diseases. As shown in **Figure 3A**, ethanol significantly decreased the protein expressions of FXR, LXRα, and LXRβ compared to the normal group, whereas AVL or silymarin treatments significantly increased the expressions of FXR, LXRα, and LXRβ compared to the EtOH group. Consistent with these changes, the results of the immunofluorescence staining showed that positive expressions of LXRα, LXRβ (in red), and FXR (in green) were significantly decreased in the EtOH group than in the normal group, AVL treatments significantly enhanced these expressions compared to the EtOH group, and silymarin had little effect on the expressions of these proteins (**Figure 3B**). These results indicate that AVL regulated lipid metabolism by FXR and LXRs activation.

PPARα and PPARγ, members of the ligand-activated NRs transcription factor superfamily, are involved in lipogenesis, and in energy and glucose homeostasis. In the EtOH group, the protein expression of PPARα was deceased and that of PPARγ increased compared to the normal group, whereas AVL treatments significantly increased the expression of PPARα and decreased the expression of PPARγ compared to the EtOH group (**Figure 3A**). The regulation of AVL on PPARα expression was also supported by immunohistochemistry staining, which showed positive expression (in brown) (**Figure 3B**). Moreover, alcohol intake decreased mRNA expressions of the PPARα-regulated genes—ACOX1, mabp, and CPT2, while AVL administrations obviously ameliorated these changes caused by EtOH. These results demonstrate that AVL regulated PPARα-mediated fatty acid oxidation (**Figure 3C**). In addition, AVL significantly regulated AMPKα/β, LKB1, and ACC phosphorylation and Sirt1 compared to the ETOH group (**Figure 3D**). The effect of AVL on Sirt1 was also verified by the immunohistochemistry staining (**Figure 3B**). Thus, AVL regulated AMPK/LKB1/ACC and Sirt1 signaling pathway against ALD.

Allium victorialis L. Ameliorated Ethanol-Induced Hepatic Inflammation

Inflammation plays a key role in the development of hepatic fibrosis. Inflammasomes are large intracellular multiprotein complexes involved in the development of inflammatory disorders, and NLRP3 is a danger-signal sensor to a regulatory

node of inflammatory diseases. The protein expression of NLRP3 significantly increased in the EtOH group than in the normal group (**Figure 4A**). EtOH resulted in a marked inflammatory response in the liver as evidenced by increased expression levels of NLRP3 and ASC, which promoted the inflammatory response with releases of inflammatory cytokines, including IL6, caspase1-p10, IL1R1, and IL1β. Caspase-1 is a protease associated with inflammatory reaction and produces mature IL1β and IL18. Thus, we found AVL and silymarin administrations significantly decreased the expressions of NLRP3, ASC, IL6, caspase1, IL1R1, and IL1β. However, silymarin showed no significant decrease of ASC compared to the EtOH group (**Figure 4A**). The mRNA expressions of NLRP3, IL1β, IL18, IL1α, and TNF-α were significantly decreased by AVL (**Figure 4B**). Immunofluorescence staining also indicated that AVL significantly decreased the expressions of MPO, NLRP3, and F4/80 compared to the EtOH group (**Figure 4C**). These results demonstrated that AVL inhibits the release of inflammatory factors and the related inflammatory response, and further ameliorated ethanol-induced hepatic inflammation.

Allium victorialis L. Improved Lipid Accumulation and Inflammation *in vitro*

EtOH (50, 100, and 200 mM) did not significantly reduce the cell viability of AML12 compared with the negative control (**Figures 5A,B**). AVL (6.25–100 μM) significantly reduced the cell viability of AML12 compared with the negative control without AVL (**Figure 5B**). Consequently, ETOH (50 mM) and AVL (3.125, 6.25, and 12.5 μM) were chosen in the subsequent experiments.

AVL could significantly regulate protein expressions of SREBP1 and lipin 1/2 compared to the EtOH group (**Figure 5C**), which was supported by the immunofluorescence staining of lipin 1/2 (**Figures 5F,G**). In Oil red O staining, AVL obviously decreased the lipid droplets induced by EtOH (**Figure 5E**). AVL treatments could inhibit NLRP3, IL1α, TNF-α, and IL18 at the gene level (**Figure 5D**). These results demonstrate that AVL could inhibit lipid droplets by regulating the expression of SREBP1, lipin 1/2, and inflammation *in vitro*.

Farnesoid X Receptor Is Necessary for *Allium victorialis* L. to Ameliorated EtOH-Induced Liver Lipid Deposition

The LXRs and FXR could regulate the lipid metabolism gene in metabolic and digestive diseases. As we expected, AVL treatments could reverse the reductions of FXR, LXRα, and LXRβ in AML12 cells stimulated with EtOH (**Figure 6A**), which were further verified by immunofluorescent staining of FXR and LXRα (**Figures 6B,C**).

To further confirm that AVL ameliorates alcoholic fatty liver by activating FXR mediation on lipid accumulation, HepG-2 cells were transfected with FXR (NR1H4) shRNA and then treated with EtOH, and with or without AVL. The FXR deficiency was appropriately achieved by FXR shRNA (**Figure 6D,E**). EtOH-mediated decrease of LXRα and LXRβ was strengthened by FXR shRNA, which was also attenuated by AVL interference

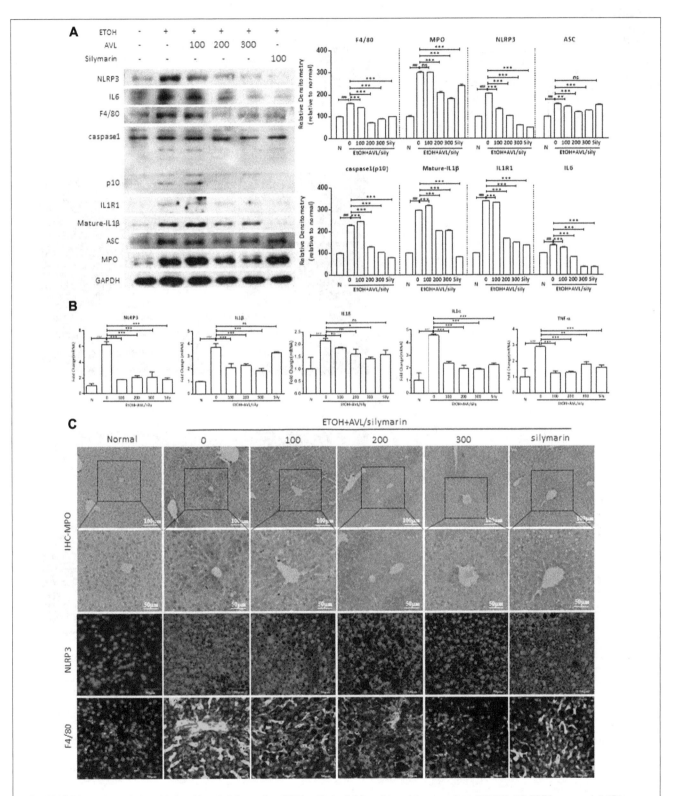

FIGURE 4 | AVL ameliorated ethanol-induced hepatic inflammation. **(A)** The effects of AVL on the protein expressions of NLRP3, IL6, F4/80, caspase1, IL1R1, IL1β, ASC, and MPO. Densitometric values were normalized against GAPDH. The same GAPDH was used in **Figure 2A,B**, **Figure 3D**, and Panel 4A. **(B)** Representative QPCR analysis for NLRP3, ASC, IL6, caspase1-p10, IL1R1, and mature-IL1β. **(C)** Immunohistochemical staining analysis of MPO (×200 and ×400 magnification), and immunofluorescence staining analysis of NLRP3 and F4/80 (×600 magnification). Data are presented as mean ± SD (*n* = 3). ###*p* < 0.001 compared with normal group; *p* < 0.05, **p* < 0.01, ***p* < 0.001 compared with EtOH group; ns, not significant.

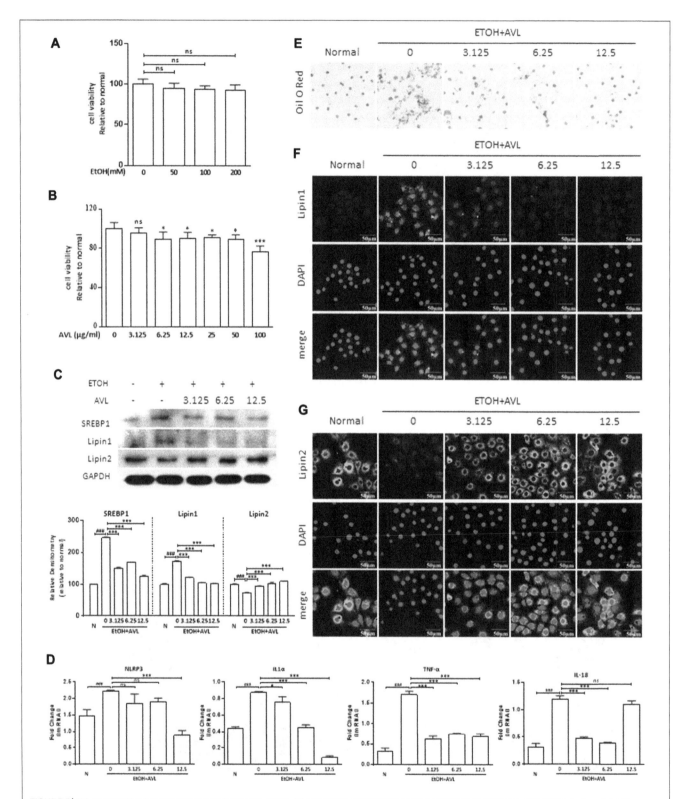

FIGURE 5 | AVL improved lipid accumulation and inflammation *in vitro*. **(A)** MTT assay on cell viability of AML12 with EtOH treatment. **(B)** MTT assay on cell viability of AML12 with AVL treatment. **(C)** The effects of AVL on the protein expressions of SREBP1, lipin 1, and lipin 2. Densitometric values were normalized against GAPDH. The same GAPDH was used in Panel 5C and **Figure 6A**. **(D)** Representative QPCR analysis for NLRP3, IL1α, TNF-α, and IL18. **(E)** Oil red O staining. **(F)** Immunofluorescence staining analysis for lipin 1. **(G)** Immunofluorescence staining analysis for lipin 2. Data are presented as mean ± SD ($n = 3$). ###$p < 0.001$ compared with normal group; *$p < 0.05$, **$p < 0.01$, ***$p < 0.001$ compared with EtOH group; ns, not significant.

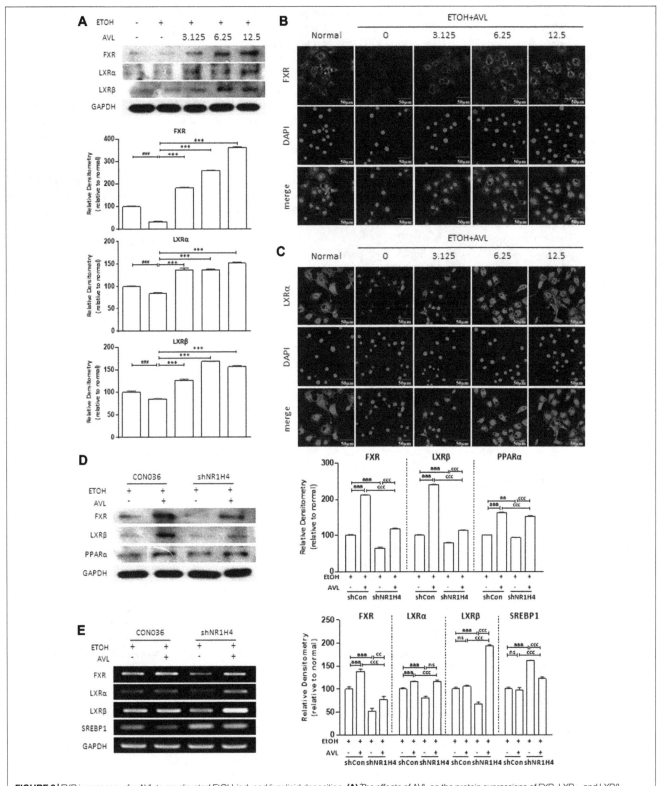

FIGURE 6 | FXR is necessary for AVL to ameliorated EtOH-induced liver lipid deposition. **(A)** The effects of AVL on the protein expressions of FXR, LXRα, and LXRβ in AML12 cells. Densitometric values were normalized against GAPDH. The same GAPDH was used in **Figure 5C** and Panel 6A. **(B)** Immunofluorescence staining analysis for FXR in AML12 cells. **(C)** Immunofluorescence staining analysis for LXRα in AML12 cells. Densitometric values were normalized against GAPDH. Data are presented as mean ± SD (n = 3). $^{##}p < 0.001$, $^{###}p < 0.001$ compared with the normal group; $^{***}p < 0.001$ compared with the ETOH group. **(D)** The effects of AVL on the protein expressions of FXR, LXRα, LXRβ, and PPARα undergoing shFXR. **(E)** Representative real-time PCR analysis for expressions of FXR, LXRα, LXRβ, and SREBP1 undergoing shFXR. Densitometric values were normalized against GAPDH. $^{aaa}p < 0.001$ CON036 treatment vs CON036-AVL group, $^{cc}p < 0.01$, $^{ccc}p < 0.001$ CON036-AVL vs shRNA (FXR)-AVL group, shRNA (FXR) vs shRNA (FXR)-AVL group; ns, not significant.

(**Figures 6D,E**). FXR deficiency also resulted in the decreasing of PPARα (**Figure 6D**), and the increase of SREBP1 (**Figure 6E**). These results suggest that FXR is necessary for AVL to ameliorated EtOH-induced liver lipid deposition, and FXR activation might be the potential therapeutic target for AVL against ALD.

DISCUSSION

Excessive alcohol consumption is responsible for the development of ALD, with a spectrum comprising alcoholic fatty liver, alcoholic steatohepatitis, and so on. The present study found that AVL could attenuate ALD induced by Lieber–DeCarli liquid diet containing ethanol. The mouse model induced by Lieber–DeCarli ethanol liquid diet plus single-binge ethanol feeding synergistically induces liver injury, inflammation, and fatty liver, which mimics acute-on-chronic alcoholic liver injury in patients (Bertola et al., 2013). AVL is a medical and edible plant, which is the guarantee for the safety of AVL usage. Our previous study also showed that AVL is safe for use alone in treatment and caused no liver histopathological changes. AVL could decrease liver index, serum transaminase, and TG accumulation, which has been further verified by histopathological examination. AVL also could ameliorate metabolic disorders and inflammation by inhibiting liver lipid deposition and inflammation factors caused by alcohol. In EtOH-induced metabolic dysregulation, it was found that FXR played an important role during AVL mediation against ALD, and FXR was necessary for AVL to regulate alcoholic steatosis and meta-inflammation.

Studies have found that FXR is a key bile acid–activated receptor that plays a critical role in the regulation of lipid and glucose metabolisms, anti-inflammation, cholestasis, and so on (Tung and Carithers, 1999; Ferrell et al., 2019). The action of activated FXR on the regulation of lipogenesis can be attributed to the downregulation of TG levels. Activated FXR can downregulate the expressions of SREBP1C and its downstream target genes, such as FAS, SCD-1, and ACC, which are related to fatty acid synthesis and TGs by inducing the expression of SHP (Watanabe et al., 2004; Song et al., 2020). Consistent with previous studies, the current results indicate that AVL can activate FXR to regulate lipid deposition, which has been verified by the decrease of SREBP1 and its target genes, and of PPARα and its target genes. The silencing of the FXR gene *in vitro* further indicates that FXR is necessary for AVL in regulating alcohol-induced lipid accumulation and inflammation. Our study provides new insights into the mechanism by which FXR controls metabolic disorders and inflammation in ALD.

Moreover, the increase of SREBP1 may relate to AMPK phosphorylation. AMPK plays a critical role in regulating fatty acid oxidation pathways and inhibiting lipid synthesis. Alcohol can inhibit AMPK phosphorylation, and increase the

expression of SREBP1 and suppressed adenylyl cyclase activity, finally contributing to hepatic steatosis (Subauste and Burant, 2007; Yao et al., 2017a; Yao et al., 2017b). Studies have shown that both Sirt1 and AMPK are two key factors in controlling lipid metabolism (Zhu et al., 2016). Activated Sirt1 could promote AMPK phosphorylation, and it also can be regulated by phosphorylation AMPK on the contrary, while loss of Sirt1 could increase hepatic steatosis and inflammation in mice (Choi et al., 2015; Li et al., 2015). In addition, AMPK phosphorylation can be activated by FXR and mediate oxidative stress (Zhang et al., 2017). These results may suggest that AVL can activate the Sirt1–AMPK signaling pathway via activation of FXR to further inhibit lipid accumulation.

Besides FXR, NRs also include PPARs, LXRs, and PXP, which are associated with various pathologies, such as cholestasis, inflammation, hepatic steatosis, fibrosis, and cancer (Tardelli et al., 2018). Among these NRs, LXRs play an important role in the metabolism of lipids, bile acids, and carbohydrates, and PPARγ with LXR could modulate macrophage activation by regulating several anti-inflammatory responses (Han et al., 2021). In the present study, the silencing of the FXR gene could decrease expressions of PPARα and LXRβ, which might lead to the release of inflammatory cytokines and the increase of SREBP1 expression, which further prove that AVL ameliorates ALD by targeting FXR activation.

Ethanol can regulate the expression of lipin 1/2 by regulating AMPK and SREBP1 signaling pathways (Bi et al., 2015). Lipin 1 can promote the synthesis of TGs and the oxidation of fatty acids during lipid metabolism (You et al., 2017). Like lipin 1, lipin 2 also plays a critical role in lipid metabolism, and it can regulate NLRP3 inflammasome by activating the P2X7 receptor, which in turn regulates inflammatory responses (Lordén et al., 2017). As expected, alcohol can upregulate the expression of lipin 1 and downregulate lipin 2, which were related to lipid metabolism and inflammatory, while AVL can reverse the changes of lipin 1 and lipin 2 induced by alcohol and further decrease lipid accumulation and the release of inflammatory cytokines. All these results demonstrate that AVL can ameliorate ethanol-induced liver injury by regulating energy metabolism and inflammation.

In conclusion, the findings of this study suggest that AVL would ameliorate alcoholic steatohepatitis, lipid deposition, and inflammation in ALD by targeting FXR activation, and further present that AVL targeting FXR might be an attractive candidate or strategy for ALD treatment. As a medicinal food homologous plant, AVL is worth including in product development for potent anti-alcohol related diseases and can be widely applied in the health industry. However, further studies may need to focus on the effective parts or chemical components isolated from AVL to improve its efficacy and targeted regulation accuracy.

AUTHOR CONTRIBUTIONS

Y-LW and J-XN contributed to the design of the study, acquisition of data, and analysis and interpretation of the data. XZ prepared AVL extract. Z-YC, XH, and other authors contributed to the acquisition of data and analysis and interpretation of data. Y-LW, Z-YC, and XH participated in drafting or revising the manuscript. All authors approved the final version of the manuscript for submission.

REFERENCES

Addolorato, G., Mirijello, A., Barrio, P., and Gual, A. (2016). Treatment of Alcohol Use Disorders in Patients with Alcoholic Liver Disease. *J. Hepatol.* 65, 618–630. doi:10.1016/j.jhep.2016.04.029

Berger, K., Ajani, U. A., Kase, C. S., Gaziano, J. M., Buring, J. E., Glynn, R. J., et al. (1999). Light-to-Moderate Alcohol Consumption and the Risk of Stroke Among U.S. Male Physicians. *N. Engl. J. Med.* 341, 1557–1564. doi:10.1056/NEJM199911183412101

Bertola, A., Mathews, S., Ki, S. H., Wang, H., and Gao, B. (2013). Mouse Model of Chronic and Binge Ethanol Feeding (The NIAAA Model). *Nat. Protoc.* 8, 627–637. doi:10.1038/nprot.2013.032

Bi, L., Jiang, Z., and Zhou, J. (2015). The Role of Lipin-1 in the Pathogenesis of Alcoholic Fatty Liver. *Alcohol Alcohol* 50, 146–151. doi:10.1093/alcalc/agu102

Choi, Y. H., Bae, J. K., Chae, H. S., Kim, Y. M., Sreymom, Y., Han, L., et al. (2015). α-Mangostin Regulates Hepatic Steatosis and Obesity through SirT1-AMPK and PPARγ Pathways in High-Fat Diet-Induced Obese Mice. *J. Agric. Food Chem.* 63, 8399–8406. doi:10.1021/acs.jafc.5b01637

Ding, L., Pang, S., Sun, Y., Tian, Y., Yu, L., and Dang, N. (2014). Coordinated Actions of FXR and LXR in Metabolism: From Pathogenesis to Pharmacological Targets for Type 2 Diabetes. *Int. J. Endocrinol.* 2014, 751859. doi:10.1155/2014/751859

Esfandiari, F., Villanueva, J. A., Wong, D. H., French, S. W., and Halsted, C. H. (2005). Chronic Ethanol Feeding and Folate Deficiency Activate Hepatic Endoplasmic Reticulum Stress Pathway in Micropigs. *Am. J. Physiol. Gastrointest. Liver Physiol.* 289, G54–G63. doi:10.1152/ajpgi.00542.2004

Esfandiari, F., You, M., Villanueva, J. A., Wong, D. H., French, S. W., and Halsted, C. H. (2007). S-Adenosylmethionine Attenuates Hepatic Lipid Synthesis in Micropigs Fed Ethanol with a Folate-Deficient Diet. *Alcohol. Clin. Exp. Res.* 31, 1231–1239. doi:10.1111/j.1530-0277.2007.00407.x

Ferrell, J. M., Pathak, P., Boehme, S., Gilliland, T., and Chiang, J. Y. L. (2019). Deficiency of Both Farnesoid X Receptor and Takeda G Protein-Coupled Receptor 5 Exacerbated Liver Fibrosis in Mice. *Hepatology* 70, 955–970. doi:10.1002/hep.30513

Forman, B. M., Goode, E., Chen, J., Oro, A. E., Bradley, D. J., Perlmann, T., et al. (1995). Identification of a Nuclear Receptor that Is Activated by Farnesol Metabolites. *Cell* 81, 687–693. doi:10.1016/0092-8674(95)90530-8

Galicia-Moreno, M., and Gutiérrez-Reyes, G. (2014). The Role of Oxidative Stress in the Development of Alcoholic Liver Disease. *Rev. Gastroenterol. Mex* 79, 135–144. doi:10.1016/j.rgmx.2014.03.001

Han, X., Cui, Z. Y., Song, J., Piao, H. Q., Lian, L. H., Hou, L. S., et al. (2019). Acanthoic Acid Modulates Lipogenesis in Nonalcoholic Fatty Liver Disease via FXR/LXRs-Dependent Manner. *Chem. Biol. Interact* 311, 108794. doi:10.1016/j.cbi.2019.108794

Han, X., Wu, Y., Yang, Q., and Cao, G. (2021). Peroxisome Proliferator-Activated Receptors in the Pathogenesis and Therapies of Liver Fibrosis. *Pharmacol. Ther.* 222, 107791. doi:10.1016/j.pharmthera.2020.107791

Hotamisligil, G. S. (2006). Inflammation and Metabolic Disorders. *Nature* 444, 860–867. doi:10.1038/nature05485

Kim, H. J., Park, M. J., Park, H. J., Chung, W. Y., Kim, K. R., and Park, K. K. (2014). Chemopreventive and Anticancer Activities of Allium Victorialis Var. Platyphyllum Extracts. *J. Cancer Prev.* 19, 179–186. doi:10.15430/JCP.2014.19.3.179

Li, X., Lian, F., Liu, C., Hu, K. Q., and Wang, X. D. (2015). Isocaloric Pair-Fed High-Carbohydrate Diet Induced More Hepatic Steatosis and Inflammation Than High-Fat Diet Mediated by miR-34a/SIRT1 Axis in Miceflammation Than

High-Fat Diet Mediated by miR-34a/SIRT1 axis in Mice. *Sci. Rep.* 5, 16774. doi:10.1038/srep16774

Lieber, C. S., Leo, M. A., Wang, X., and Decarli, L. M. (2008). Alcohol Alters Hepatic FoxO1, P53, and Mitochondrial SIRT5 Deacetylation Function. *Biochem. Biophys. Res. Commun.* 373, 246–252. doi:10.1016/j.bbrc.2008.06.006

Liu, J. (2014). Ethanol and Liver: Recent Insights into the Mechanisms of Ethanol-Induced Fatty Liver. *World J. Gastroenterol.* 20, 14672–14685. doi:10.3748/wjg.v20.i40.14672

Lordén, G., Sanjuán-García, I., de Pablo, N., Meana, C., Alvarez-Miguel, I., Pérez-García, M. T., et al. (2017). Lipin-2 Regulates NLRP3 Inflammasome by Affecting P2X7 Receptor Activation. *J. Exp. Med.* 214, 511–528. doi:10.1084/jem.20161452

Pineda Torra, I., Claudel, T., Duval, C., Kosykh, V., Fruchart, J. C., and Staels, B. (2003). Bile Acids Induce the Expression of the Human Peroxisome Proliferator-Activated Receptor Alpha Gene via Activation of the Farnesoid X Receptor. *Mol. Endocrinol.* 17, 259–272. doi:10.1210/me.2002-0120

Sacco, R. L., Elkind, M., Boden-Albala, B., Lin, I. F., Kargman, D. E., Hauser, W. A., et al. (1999). The Protective Effect of Moderate Alcohol Consumption on Ischemic Stroke. *JAMA* 281, 53–60. doi:10.1001/jama.281.1.53

Seol, W., Choi, H. S., and Moore, D. D. (1995). Isolation of Proteins that Interact Specifically with the Retinoid X Receptor: Two Novel Orphan Receptors. *Mol. Endocrinol.* 9, 72–85. doi:10.1210/mend.9.1.7760852

Shearn, C. T., Smathers, R. L., Jiang, H., Orlicky, D. J., Maclean, K. N., and Petersen, D. R. (2013). Increased Dietary Fat Contributes to Dysregulation of the LKB1/AMPK Pathway and Increased Damage in a Mouse Model of Early-Stage Ethanol-Mediated Steatosis. *J. Nutr. Biochem.* 24, 1436–1445. doi:10.1016/j.jnutbio.2012.12.002

Shirataki, Y., Motohashi, N., Tani, S., Sunaga, K., Sakagami, H., Satoh, K., et al. (2001). Antioxidative Activity of Allium Victorialis L. Extracts. *Anticancer Res.* 21, 3331–3339. doi:10.1097/00001813-200109000-00010

Song, J., Cui, Z. Y., Lian, L. H., Han, X., Hou, L. S., Wang, G., et al. (2020). 20S-Protopanaxatriol Ameliorates Hepatic Fibrosis, Potentially Involving FXR-Mediated Inflammatory Signaling Cascades. *J. Agric. Food Chem.* 68, 8195–8204. doi:10.1021/acs.jafc.0c01978

Song, J., Han, X., Yao, Y. L., Li, Y. M., Zhang, J., Shao, D. Y., et al. (2018). Acanthoic Acid Suppresses Lipin1/2 via TLR4 and IRAK4 Signalling Pathways in EtOH- and Lipopolysaccharide-Induced Hepatic Lipogenesis. *J. Pharm. Pharmacol.* 70, 393–403. doi:10.1111/jphp.12877

Subauste, A. R., and Burant, C. F. (2007). Role of FoxO1 in FFA-Induced Oxidative Stress in Adipocytes. *Am. J. Physiol. Endocrinol. Metab.* 293, E159–E164. doi:10.1152/ajpendo.00629.2006

Tang, X., Olatunji, O. J., Zhou, Y., and Hou, X. (2017). Allium Tuberosum: Antidiabetic and Hepatoprotective Activities. *Food Res. Int.* 102, 681–689. doi:10.1016/j.foodres.2017.08.034

Tardelli, M., Claudel, T., Bruschi, F. V., and Trauner, M. (2018). Nuclear Receptor Regulation of Aquaglyceroporins in Metabolic Organs. *Int. J. Mol. Sci.* 19, E1777. doi:10.3390/ijms19061777

Tung, B. Y., Jr, and Carithers, R. L. (1999). Cholestasis and Alcoholic Liver Disease. *Clin. Liver Dis.* 3, 585–601. doi:10.1016/s1089-3261(05)70086-6

Watanabe, M., Houten, S. M., Wang, L., Moschetta, A., Mangelsdorf, D. J., Heyman, R. A., et al. (2004). Bile Acids Lower Triglyceride Levels via a Pathway Involving FXR, SHP, and SREBP-1c. *J. Clin. Invest.* 113, 1408–1418. doi:10.1172/JCI21025

Woo, K. W., Moon, E., Park, S. Y., Kim, S. Y., and Lee, K. R. (2012). Flavonoid Glycosides from the Leaves of Allium Victorialis Var. Platyphyllum and Their Anti-Neuroinflammatory Effects. *Bioorg. Med. Chem. Lett.* 22, 7465–7470. doi:10.1016/j.bmcl.2012.10.043

Wu, W., Zhu, B., Peng, X., Zhou, M., Jia, D., and Gu, J. (2014). Activation of Farnesoid X Receptor Attenuates Hepatic Injury in a Murine Model of

Alcoholic Liver Disease. *Biochem. Biophys. Res. Commun.* 443, 68–73. doi:10.1016/j.bbrc.2013.11.057

Yao, Y. L., Han, X., Li, Z. M., Lian, L. H., Nan, J. X., and Wu, Y. L. (2017). Acanthoic Acid Can Partially Prevent Alcohol Exposure-Induced Liver Lipid Deposition and Inflammation. *Front. Pharmacol.* 8, 134. doi:10.3389/fphar.2017.00134

Yao, Y. L., Han, X., Song, J., Zhang, J., Li, Y. M., Lian, L. H., et al. (2017). Acanthoic Acid Protectsagainst Ethanol-Induced Liver Injury: Possible Role of AMPK Activation and IRAK4 Inhibition. *Toxicol. Lett.* 281, 127–138. doi:10.1016/j.toxlet.2017.09.020

You, M., Jogasuria, A., Lee, K., Wu, J., Zhang, Y., Lee, Y. K., et al. (2017). Signal Transduction Mechanisms of Alcoholic Fatty Liver Disease: Emer Ging Role of Lipin-1. *Curr. Mol. Pharmacol.* 10, 226–236. doi:10.2174/1874467208666150817112109

Zhang, Y., Xu, Y., Qi, Y., Xu, L., Song, S., Yin, L., et al. (2017). Protective Effects of Dioscin against Doxorubicin-Induced Nephrotoxicity via Adjusting FXR-Mediated Oxidative Stress and Inflammation. *Toxicology* 378, 53–64. doi:10.1016/j.tox.2017.01.007

Zhu, J., Ren, T., Zhou, M., and Cheng, M. (2016). The Combination of Blueberry Juice and Probiotics Reduces Apoptosis of Alcoholic Fatty Liver of Mice by Affecting SIRT1 Pathway. *Drug Des. Devel Ther.* 10, 1649–1661. doi:10.2147/DDDT.S102883

19

Animal and Organoid Models of Liver Fibrosis

Yu-long Bao[1†], Li Wang[1†], Hai-ting Pan[1], Tai-ran Zhang[1], Ya-hong Chen[2], Shan-jing Xu[3], Xin-li Mao[3,4,5] and Shao-wei Li[4,5*]*

[1] College of Basic Medicine, Inner Mongolia Medical University, Hohhot, China, [2] Health Management Center, Taizhou Hospital of Zhejiang Province Affiliated to Wenzhou Medical University, Linhai, China, [3] School of Medicine, Shaoxing University, Shaoxing, Chian, [4] Key Laboratory of Minimally Invasive Techniques & Rapid Rehabilitation of Digestive System Tumor, Taizhou Hospital of Zhejiang Province Affiliated to Wenzhou Medical University, Linhai, China, [5] Department of Gastroenterology, Taizhou Hospital of Zhejiang Province Affiliated to Wenzhou Medical University, Linhai, China

Correspondence:
Shao-wei Li
li_shaowei81@hotmail.com
Xin-li Mao
maoxl@enzemed.com

[†] *These authors have contributed equally to this work*

Liver fibrosis refers to the process underlying the development of chronic liver diseases, wherein liver cells are repeatedly destroyed and regenerated, which leads to an excessive deposition and abnormal distribution of the extracellular matrix such as collagen, glycoprotein and proteoglycan in the liver. Liver fibrosis thus constitutes the pathological repair response of the liver to chronic injury. Hepatic fibrosis is a key step in the progression of chronic liver disease to cirrhosis and an important factor affecting the prognosis of chronic liver disease. Further development of liver fibrosis may lead to structural disorders of the liver, nodular regeneration of hepatocytes and the formation of cirrhosis. Hepatic fibrosis is histologically reversible if treated aggressively during this period, but when fibrosis progresses to the stage of cirrhosis, reversal is very difficult, resulting in a poor prognosis. There are many causes of liver fibrosis, including liver injury caused by drugs, viral hepatitis, alcoholic liver, fatty liver and autoimmune disease. The mechanism underlying hepatic fibrosis differs among etiologies. The establishment of an appropriate animal model of liver fibrosis is not only an important basis for the in-depth study of the pathogenesis of liver fibrosis but also an important means for clinical experts to select drugs for the prevention and treatment of liver fibrosis. The present study focused on the modeling methods and fibrosis characteristics of different animal models of liver fibrosis, such as a chemical-induced liver fibrosis model, autoimmune liver fibrosis model, cholestatic liver fibrosis model, alcoholic liver fibrosis model and non-alcoholic liver fibrosis model. In addition, we also summarize the research and application prospects concerning new organoids in liver fibrosis models proposed in recent years. A suitable animal model of liver fibrosis and organoid fibrosis model that closely resemble the physiological state of the human body will provide bases for the in-depth study of the pathogenesis of liver fibrosis and the development of therapeutic drugs.

Keywords: liver, fibrosis, animal, organoid, model

INTRODUCTION

Liver fibrosis is a pathophysiological process caused by a variety of pathogenic factors that induce the abnormal proliferation of connective tissue in the liver. The repair and healing processes of liver injury can be accompanied by the development of liver fibrosis, and if the factors underlying such injury are not addressed, the process of fibrosis continues, eventually leading to cirrhosis (Hernandez-Gea and Friedman, 2011; Parola and Pinzani, 2019). Viruses, toxins, drugs, alcohol, hereditary factors, metabolism, cholestasis and parasites, among other factors, can damage liver cells, destroying the dynamic balance between collagen fiber synthesis, deposition, degradation and absorption, thus leading to the development of liver fibrosis. Therefore, liver fibrosis is not a unique disease; instead, different factors can lead to it, and regardless of the factors causing the relevant liver injury, the fibrosis process is similar (Mehal et al., 2011; Sebastiani et al., 2014; Kamdem et al., 2018; Testino et al., 2018).

The stimulation of different factors can lead to liver cell damage, which in turn causes inflammation. A continuous inflammatory response often leads to the formation of fibrosis. This is because inflammation causes cell damage, which further enhances the release of inflammatory mediators, such as cytokines and chemokines. These mediators recruit a large number of inflammatory cells to the site of inflammation, such as lymphocytes, neutrophils, eosinophils, basophils, mast cells and macrophages. The collected inflammatory cells further activate effector cells, which promote fibrosis (Hernandez-Gea and Friedman, 2011; Koyama and Brenner, 2017; Parola and Pinzani, 2019). The activation of hepatic stellate cells (HSCs) is the core event of liver fibrosis. HSCs are activated and differentiated into myofibroblasts (MFBs), which secrete and deposit a large amount of extracellular matrix (ECM). When liver injury persists for a long time, chronic inflammatory stimulation and the continuous deposition of ECM together lead to the gradual replacement of normal liver tissue by fibrous tissue (Higashi et al., 2017; Zhangdi et al., 2019; **Figure 1**). As a common pathological stage of chronic liver disease, liver fibrosis is necessary for the development of liver cirrhosis and even liver cancer. Indeed, persistent liver inflammation and fibrosis are known to eventually induce cirrhosis and liver cancer (Uehara et al., 2013).

Studies in rodent models and humans have shown that liver fibrosis is reversible if the damage is ameliorated in a timely manner (Campana and Iredale, 2017). Matrix Metallopeptidase 13 (MMP13) is involved in the degradation of newly formed matrix during the recovery of liver fibrosis in rats. Although not all HSCs express MMP13, the production of MMP13 by HSCs plays a critical role in the process of fibrosis recovery (Watanabe et al., 2000). MMP9 secreted by Kupffer plays a key role in reversing hepatic fibrosis induced by thioacetamide (TAA) in mice (Feng et al., 2018). Dendritic cells can promote fibrosis regression by producing MMP9 (Jiao et al., 2012).

At present, the mechanism underlying liver fibrosis is unclear, and recent research has mostly focused on the etiology and mechanism of the disease. Although there has been some progress in the diagnosis and treatment of fibrosis, effective drugs and treatment are still lacking. The prevention, treatment and

even reversal of liver fibrosis have always been the key to the successful treatment of chronic liver injury. The pathogenesis of liver fibrosis is of great clinical significance for the development of therapeutic drugs and overall improvement of therapeutic approaches. It is therefore important to study the pathogenesis of liver fibrosis and develop therapeutic drugs to construct the animal model of liver fibrosis with similar pathogeneses.

We herein report various liver fibrosis models, which are classified according to the modeling method used, to facilitate their utility as a reference for liver fibrosis researchers.

CHEMICAL DRUG-INDUCED LIVER FIBROSIS MODEL

Chemical liver fibrosis is induced by chemicals that can cause hepatotoxicity. The liver cells are damaged and consequently repaired, resulting in the abnormal growth of connective tissue in the liver. Models of chemical-induced liver injury are usually injected intraperitoneally, which is relatively easy to perform and results in stable development for use in studies concerning clinical liver fibrosis.

Carbon Tetrachloride (CCl$_4$)

Carbon tetrachloride is a colorless non-polar organic compound, highly toxic, that can dissolve many substances such as fat and paint. It is a typical liver poison, but the concentration and frequency of exposure can affect its action site and toxicity. CCl$_4$ directly damages liver cells (mainly endothelial cells and hepatic parenchyma cells in the hepatic portal vein region) by altering the permeability of lysosomes and mitochondrial membranes (Weber et al., 2003). The oxidase system in liver cells can also form highly active free radical metabolites through CYP2E1, leading to severe central lobular necrosis (Zangar et al., 2000). The damage mechanism of CCl4 is mainly oxidative damage caused by lipid peroxidation. Cytochrome P450 enzyme, especially CYP2E1, converts CCl4 into highly toxic trichloromethyl radical ($\cdot$CCl$_3$) and trichloromethyl peroxide ($\cdot$CCl$_3$O$_2$) (Slater et al., 1985; Unsal et al., 2020). This model has been widely used to study the pathogenesis of liver fibrosis and cirrhosis.

More standardized procedures are needed for experimental liver fibrosis studies due to dramatic changes in animal welfare regulations in Europe. Scholten proposed standard operating procedure (SOPs) for the CCl$_4$ mouse model and summarized the widely accepted experimental model for inducing liver injury leading to liver fibrosis (Scholten et al., 2015). The toxicological mechanism of liver fibrosis induced by CCl$_4$ may be related to multiple biological processes, pathways and targets (Dong et al., 2016). After 15 weeks of CCl$_4$ induction, multiple well-differentiated hepatocellular carcinoma (HCC) cells were found in the livers of all mice. CD133 was significantly up-regulated after CCl$_4$ treatment, and the levels of desmin and glial fibrillary acidic protein, the representative markers of HSC, were also significantly increased. The EGF expression was significantly reduced, contrary to what has been observed in humans. In A/J mice, chronic liver injury induced by CCl$_4$ differs from HCC

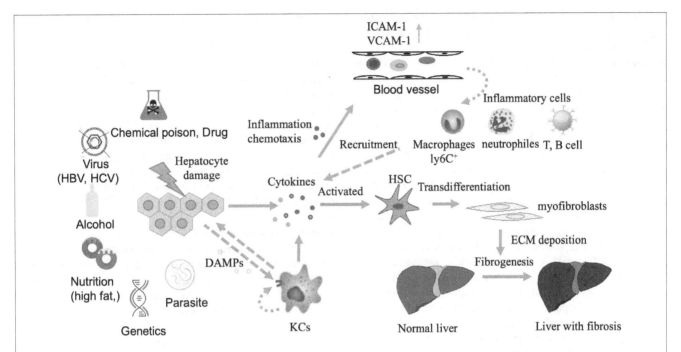

FIGURE 1 | The mechanism of liver fibrosis. Liver damage can be caused by a variety of factors (e.g., chemical poisons, viruses, alcohol, nutrition, genetics, parasites, etc.). Injuries of liver cells release a variety of cytokines, among which damage-associated molecular patterns(DAMPs) (such as S100 family, high mobility group protein, etc.) can activate Kuffers (KCs) cells to produce inflammatory cytokines. Inflammatory cytokines can play a role through autocrine and paracrine. At this point, vascular permeability at the injured site increases, vascular endothelium simultaneously expresses high adhesion molecules, and inflammatory cells in the blood chemotaxis to the injured site under the action of chemokines, leading to the occurrence of inflammation. Multiple cytokines produced at the site of liver injury activate resting HSCs, causing HSCs to differentiate into myofibroblasts and produce ECM deposition. If the injury and inflammation are persistent or recurring, the deposition of ECM cannot be reversed, leading to liver fibrosis.

induced by human cirrhosis (Fujii et al., 2010). The collagen expression was found to be significantly increased after CCl$_4$ injury, and the number of cells expressing cytoglobin was also increased. Cytoglobin may be an early biomarker of liver fibrosis (Man et al., 2008). In addition to intraperitoneal injection, CCl4 can also be inhaled to establish a liver fibrosis model. Rats were exposed to CCl4 vapor twice a week for 30 s each time, while phenobarbital (0.3 g/L) was added to drinking water. The duration of inhalation was increased by 30 s after the first three sessions and by 1 min after every three sessions until a steady state was reached for 5 min. After 9 weeks, it can lead to liver fibrosis (Leeming et al., 2013; Marfà et al., 2016). Compared with intraperitoneal injection, inhalation route is a complex process, with great individual differences, and can cause multiple organ damage. An intraperitoneal injection can reach the liver directly from the hepatic portal vein. The animal model of liver fibrosis induced by CCl$_4$ is relatively low-cost to develop, and the implementation method is relatively simple. Furthermore, it is a classic model and one of the earliest, most widely used and most frequently selected by researchers.

TAA

Thioacetamide is an organic compound with the molecular formula CH$_3$CSNH$_2$, found as a colorless or white crystal. TAA is widely used as a model for inducing experimental liver fibrosis, and can also be used to induce acute liver failure and liver tumors by controlling the dose and duration of administration.

The TAA model is suitable for the study of connective tissue metabolism in fibrotic and cirrhotic models (Müller et al., 1988). TAA itself is not hepatotoxic, and its active metabolites covalently bind to proteins and lipids, causing oxidative stress leading to central lobular necrosis of the liver. Compared with CCl$_4$, TAA resulted in more periportal inflammatory cell infiltration and more pronounced ductal hyperplasia. The intraperitoneal administration of 150 mg/kg of TAA 3 times per week for 11 weeks in rats and TAA administration in drinking water at 300 mg/L for 2-4 months in mice can successfully and repetitively cause chronic liver injury and fibrosis (Wallace et al., 2015). The continued administration of TAA (after the continuous TAA injection for more than 11 weeks) induced sustained liver fibrosis in common marmosets, and this primate-like model of liver fibrosis was thus able to be used to evaluate the therapeutic effect of liver fibrosis (Inoue et al., 2018). In *Macaca fascicularis* fibrosis models induced by TAA and CCl$_4$, TAA induced significant fibrosis, but CCl$_4$ did not. Both TAA and CCl$_4$ increased the Child-Pugh score, but only the TAA model showed an increased retention of indocyanine green. TAA-induced *M. fascicularis* fibrosis was similar to Child-Pugh grade B fibrosis in humans. This model is evaluable by clinical indicators and can be used in preclinical studies (Matsuo et al., 2020). Although both CCl$_4$ and TAA-induced liver injury and fibrosis are dependent on CYP2E1, in some cases, CYP2A5 may have a protective effect against TAA-induced liver injury and fibrosis but has no effect on the hepatotoxicity of CCl$_4$ (Hong et al., 2016). The serum amino acid pattern in the TAA-induced chronic cirrhosis model is partially similar to the corresponding human disease (Fontana et al., 1996). The hepatic fibrosis model of rats was established by injecting TAA solution for 7 weeks. Serum and urine samples were collected weekly for a nuclear magnetic resonance metabolomics analysis to search for differential metabolites associated with TAA-induced injury. That study helped clarify the role of metabolic dynamics in the course of hepatic fibrosis disease (Wei et al., 2014). The levels of fibrogenic cytokines, such as transforming growth factor-β(TGF-β), platelet derived growth factor (PDGF) and connective tissue growth factor (CTGF), also increased in the liver tissue of all three models, but the levels of CTGF in the liver tissue and serum were the highest in the CCl4 group (Park et al., 2016). After 12-week oral administration of TAA in rats, bile duct fibrosis was induced, characterized by tubular hyperplasia surrounded by fibrous tissue (Hata et al., 2013). Both CCl4 and TAA can cause lipid oxidative damage in liver cells. The model of liver fibrosis induced by CCl4 is more suitable for studying the mechanism of spontaneous reversal of liver fibrosis. The hepatic fibrosis model induced by TAA is more suitable for the study of the mechanism of hepatic fibrosis, the screening of therapeutic drugs and the reliability evaluation of hepatic fibrosis serological markers.

DMN and Diethylnitrosamine (DEN)

The toxicity of various nitrosamines in animals and humans is well established, and trace amounts of DEN or DMN can cause severe liver injury in either the enteric or oral form. The most prominent manifestations are extensive neutrophilic infiltration, extensive central lobular hemorrhaging and necrosis, bile duct hyperplasia, fibrosis, bridging necrosis and ultimately HCC. Due to the stability of DMN- and DEN-induced liver changes, the administration of these agents to rodents has become a commonly used experimental model (Tolba et al., 2015).

Iron deposition and fat accumulation were shown to play an important role in the pathological changes of DMN-induced liver fibrosis in rats (He et al., 2007). Rats were intraperitoneally injected with DMN 3 days a week for 3 weeks. Severe central lobular congestion and hemorrhaging and necrosis were observed on day 7. On day 14, central lobular necrosis and numerous neutrophils infiltration were observed. Collagenous fibrous deposition was seen on day 21, along with severe central lobular necrosis, focal fatty changes, bile duct hyperplasia and bridging necrosis and fibrosis around the central vein. DMN-induced liver injury in rats seems to be an animal model similar to early human cirrhosis (George et al., 2001). The model shows significantly increased liver collagen fibraldehyde content due to DMN administration, and the cross-linking of liver fibrosis collagen induced by DMN is greater than that in normal liver. Furthermore, the deposition of type III collagen is more obvious than that of type I collagen in early fibrosis (George and Chandrakasan, 1996). The percentage of collagen fibrosis in rat liver fibrosis induced by DMN has been shown to be closely correlated with the serum levels of hyaluronic acid (HA), laminin (LN) and type IV collagen (Li et al., 2005). After 4 weeks of DEN treatment, 30% of zebrafish showed hyperplasia of reticular fibers. After 6 weeks, reticular and collagen fibers showed active

hyperplasia, and the proliferation rate of reticular fibers increased to 80%, successfully generating a stable liver fibrosis model in zebrafish (Wang et al., 2014).

In the comparative study of dimethylnitrosamine (DMN), CCl4 and TAA rat liver fibrosis models, lipid peroxidation was highest in the CCl4 model, and the serum liver enzyme levels increased with severity. The DMN and TAA models showed significant changes in liver fibrosis. The Alpha-SAM levels significantly increased in the DMN model. In summary, while the modeling time with this method is short, its development is simple, and the fibrosis degree is stable. However, because of the toxicity of nitrosamines, researchers should ensure proper safety measures are taken.

Acetaminophen (APAP)

Acetaminophen overdose is a major cause of drug-induced acute liver failure in many developed countries. Mitochondrial oxidative stress is considered the core event of APAP-induced liver injury (Yoon et al., 2016; Yan et al., 2018). N-acetyl-p-phenylquinone imine (NAPQI), a metabolite of APAP, is hepatotoxic and can increase the mRNA expression of α-SMA, COL1A1, COL3A1 and TGF-β, inducing the phosphorylation of ERK1/2 and SMAD2/3 and nuclear translocation of EGR-1 in hepatic stellate LX2 cells. The long-term administration of APAP can induce liver fibrosis in mice (Bai et al., 2017). When the liver is first exposed to APAP, a necrotizing inflammatory process is kicked off, followed by liver regeneration. However, the liver begins to form fibrosis after the second exposure to APAP (AlWahsh et al., 2019). Of note, a new model of cirrhosis in which rats were gavaged with corn oil daily and APAP 500 mg/day for 3 weeks resulted in the development of focal biliary cirrhosis (Tropskaya et al., 2020).

IMMUNE DAMAGE-INDUCED LIVER FIBROSIS MODEL

Immune liver injury liver fibrosis mainly refers to liver fibrosis caused by clinical autoimmune hepatitis (AIH) and virus infection, but such animal models of immune liver injury lack the sustained replication stage of human virus infection and the pathological process of sustained damage of human liver immunity.

Concanavalin A (ConA), a lectin purified from Brazilian kidney bean (Soares et al., 2011), is widely used in the mouse model of immune-mediated hepatitis. Unlike other models of liver injury, ConA-induced injury is mainly caused by the activation and recruitment of T cells to the liver (Heymann et al., 2015). Therefore, the pathogenesis of the ConA model has something in common with human immune-mediated hepatitis, such as AIH (Wang et al., 2012) and viral hepatitis. The mouse hepatitis model induced by ConA (20 mg/kg, 12 h) reflects most of the pathogenicity of human type I AIH. This provides a reliable animal model for the study of the immune pathogenesis of AIH and the rapid evaluation of new therapeutic methods (Ye et al., 2018). In acute autoimmune liver injury induced by ConA, HSCs are activated early, and the expression of TGF-β1 and TGF-β3 is unbalanced, which may be related to liver dysfunction and fibrosis development (Wang et al., 2017). Repeated injections of Con A resulted in liver fibrosis in mice (Louis et al., 2000). The model of immune fibrosis in mice was established by injecting saffra protein A (0.3 mg/body) once a week for 4 weeks. IFN-β can inhibit liver cell damage caused by repeated injections of ConA but has no effect on the development of fibrosis (Tanabe et al., 2007).

ALCOHOL-INDUCED LIVER FIBROSIS MODEL

Alcoholic liver disease (ALD) is a chronic liver disease caused by long-term heavy drinking. Fatty liver is usually present in the initial stage, which can develop into alcoholic hepatitis, alcoholic liver fibrosis and alcoholic cirrhosis. Almost all heavy drinkers develop fatty liver, but only 20-40% develop more severe ALD, and the underlying mechanism leading to disease progression is still unclear (Tsukamoto and Lu, 2001; Seitz et al., 2018). Although rodents differ from humans with regard to their alcohol metabolism (Holmes et al., 1986) and immune system, experimental animal models of ALD, especially rodent models, have been widely used in the study of human ALD (Mathews et al., 2014; Lamas-Paz et al., 2018).

After the daily administration of alcohol to rats for 16 weeks, the rates of liver steatosis, necrosis, inflammation and fibrosis were increased (Zhou et al., 2013). Chronic ethanol feeding (10 days free oral Lieber-decarli ethanol liquid diet) plus single alcoholic ethanol feeding induced liver injury, inflammation and fatty liver, simulating acute and chronic alcoholic liver injury in humans. This simple model is very useful for the study of ALD and other organs damaged by alcohol consumption (Bertola et al., 2013). Mice treated with CCl_4 combined with ethanol (up to 16%) showed extremely high rates of fibrotic alcoholic fatty liver disease 7 weeks later. The pattern of steatosis, inflammation and fibrosis involved in ALD in this mouse model is similar to that in humans and is suitable as a preclinical model for drug development (Brol et al., 2019). The same CCl_4 vapor exposure combined with chronic alcohol feeding resulted in extensive liver fibrosis in rats at week 5 and micronodular cirrhosis at week 10. This animal model simulates how some chronic liver damage in humans may be due to the presence of other hepatotoxins in the environment that play a role in enhancing the effects of alcohol (Hall et al., 1991). A new experimental model of porcine hepatosclerosis was established by CCl_4 and ethanol. Cirrhosis was induced by the intraperitoneal injection of CCl_4 twice a week for 9 weeks. Corn flour was the only food consumed during the period, and a 5% alcohol-water mixture was consumed. After 9 weeks, 83.3% of the pigs had cirrhosis, and 33.3% had died (Zhang et al., 2009). In combination with chronic alcohol administration and a non-alcoholic steatohepatitis (NASH)-induced high-fat diet, this new model enables the study of the combined effects of alcohol and a high-fat diet on liver injury, which may contribute to the development of liver fibrosis by enhancing TLR_4 signaling (Gäbele et al., 2011). To cause progressive alcoholic liver injury, the animal must be given too

much alcohol and maintain a persistently high blood alcohol level. Because of the rats' natural aversion to alcohol, the method of feeding them alcoholic liquid food was greatly restricted. In addition, the experiment cycle is long, the cost is high and the success rate is low, so it has been rarely used. At present, the more commonly used method is alcohol combined with chemical poison gavage, during the control of diet to replicate the model of alcoholic liver fibrosis. The model has the advantages of simple operation, short cycle and high molding rate.

DIET METABOLISM-INDUCED LIVER FIBROSIS MODEL

Non-alcoholic fatty liver disease (NAFLD) is a clinicopathological syndrome characterized by excessive fat deposition in hepatocytes except for alcohol and other clear liver damage factors, which is closely related to insulin resistance and genetic susceptibility of acquired metabolic stress liver injury (Cobbina and Akhlaghi, 2017). NAFLD is becoming a common chronic liver injury due to lifestyle changes. NAFLD can cause inflammation, ballooning degeneration of hepatocytes, and varying degrees of fibrosis, known as non-alcoholic steatohepatitis (NASH). Patients with advanced liver fibrosis or cirrhosis are at risk of developing complications, such as HCC and esophageal varices (Stål, 2015).

A choline-deficient high-fat (CDHF) diet induces NASH in mice. Hepatic histopathology has shown that a CDHF diet causes severe steatosis, inflammation and pericellular fibrosis (Honda et al., 2017). A modified choline-deficient, L-amino acid-defined, high-fat diet (CDAHFD) rapidly induces liver fibrosis in mice. This model will contribute to a better understanding of human NASH disease and may be useful for the development of effective treatments (Matsumoto et al., 2013). $AIM^{-/-}$ mice fed the D09100301 diet showed similar phenotypes to non-obese patients with NAFLD, indicating their utility as a pathophysiological model for studying obesity-induced HCC (Komatsu et al., 2019). Dietary control combined with chemical toxicants may be an effective means of reducing the modeling time of diet-induced NAFLD models. A fast food diet (FFD) combined with a trace dose of CCL_4 (0.5 mL/kg body weight) for 8 weeks resulted in histological features of NAFLD, including steatosis, inflammation and fibrosis, in Wistar rat models within 8 weeks, suggesting that the model has potential utility in developing NAFLD and anti-fibrosis therapy (Chheda et al., 2014). Furthermore, using a high-fat, high-fructose and high-cholesterol diet combined with a weekly low dose of CCL_4 as an accelerant shortened the cycle of a mouse NASH model of fibrosis and HCC (Tsuchida et al., 2018). The mechanism of fatty liver fibrosis is still unclear, among which oxidative stress/lipid peroxidation is an important cause of fatty liver fibrosis. Unlike alcoholic fatty liver, which leads directly to liver fibrosis, non-alcoholic fatty liver must pass through an intermediate stage of steatohepatitis before it can develop into liver fibrosis. In other words, inflammation itself is a prerequisite for fatty liver fibrosis. The diet-induced NASH mouse model is characterized by good simulation of obesity, type

2 diabetes mellitus, dyslipidemia, and metabolic syndrome, but with less liver fibrosis.

SURGERY-INDUCED LIVER FIBROSIS MODEL

Cholestasis is an obstruction of both bile flow formation and excretion. Continuous cholestasis leads to chronic inflammation, which damages bile duct cells and liver cells, activates MFBs through a number of regulatory factors and causes the excessive deposition of ECM, leading to liver fibrosis (Li and Apte, 2015).

Surgical bile duct ligation (BDL) is one of the most widely used experimental models of cholestatic liver injury in mice and rats. The BDL model is a classic model of liver fibrosis. BDL was first achieved by the double ligation of bile ducts in rats. In brief, at 7-10 days after surgery, bile duct stenosis, increased bile duct pressure, upstream dilatation of bile ducts, increased liver volume composed of portal vein and bile duct hyperplasia are observed (Rodríguez-Garay et al., 1996). BDL protocols have been improved over time, but basically, animals are anesthetized and then undergo laparotomy. The bile duct is exposed from the abdominal cavity and ligated twice using a surgical cord. Mice and rats that undergo the procedure develop a strong fibrotic response (Kirkland et al., 2010). During the procedure, the animal can be placed on a heated plate at 37°C and permanently connected to the anesthesia system. At the time of the operation, the bile ducts are double-ligated but not dissected. This procedure induces highly repeatable morphological phenotypic changes in the liver and allows for the study of fiber formation at specific points in time (Tag et al., 2015). The standard model for cholestasis studies is total BDL (tBDL), but this model can cause severe liver damage in mice, so a new cholestasis model using partial BDL (pBDL) has been established (Heinrich et al., 2011). A mouse model of recanalization of biliary tract obstruction was previous established by performing anastomosis between the gallbladder and jejunum (G-J anastomosis), which has some value for studying the recovery from cholestasis liver fibrosis (Yoshino et al., 2021).

TRANSGENIC ANIMAL LIVER FIBROSIS MODEL

A chronic hepatitis C virus infection leads to liver fibrosis and cirrhosis. For a long time, chimpanzees were the only available non-human model of HCV infection (Pellicoro et al., 2014). Since the host range of HBV is relatively narrow and it only infects humans, it is very difficult to establish an animal model of HBV infection. Only chimpanzees and tupaia have previously been used for infection experiments (Walter et al., 1996; Dandri et al., 2005). The construction of humanized liver chimeric transgenic mice enables the stable regrowth of human liver cells in mice, and even the normal function and morphology of human liver, which has become an important bridge between mouse and

human preclinical studies (Katoh et al., 2008). Hepatitis virus infects human TK-NOG mice and UPA-SCID mice with severe combined immunodeficiency (UPA-SCID). All human TK-NOG and UPA-SCID mice injected with hepatitis B virus infected serum developed viremia. The occurrence of HCV viremia in TK-NOG mice was significantly higher than that in UPA-SCID mice. TK-NOG mice are more beneficial for the study of hepatitis virus virology and the evaluation of antiviral drugs (Kosaka et al., 2013).

In addition to humanized mice, many transgenic mice were constructed for the study of liver fibrosis according to the different pathogenesis of liver fibrosis and the key functional genes of liver fibrosis regulation (Hayashi and Sakai, 2011). Immunodeficiency NOD induced natural killer T cell (NKT) transgenic population mediated spontaneous multi-organ chronic inflammation and fibrosis, non-obese diabetic inflammation and fibrosis (N-IF) mice. Due to fibrosis components, early onset, spontaneity, and reproducibility, this novel mouse model provides further insight into the underlying mechanisms that mediate the transformation of chronic inflammation into fibrosis (Fransén-Pettersson et al., 2016). Although the pathology of BDL is similar to chronic cholestasis in humans, the severity of surgical stress and cholestasis injury limits the application of the BDL model. MDR2 (ABCB4) is a mouse homologous gene MDR3 (ABCB4) that encodes a tubule phospholipid transporter. MDR2-/- mice, also known as ABCB4-/- mice, are another mature model of chronic cholestatic liver injury (Ikenaga et al., 2015). MDR2 knockout (MDR2 -/-) mice are a genetic model similar to patients with primary sclerosing cholangitis (Nishio et al., 2019). Transgenic mice that overexpress the transforming growth factor-β1 (TGF-β1) fusion gene [C-reactive protein (CRP)/TGF-β1] are able to control the expression level of TGF-β1. This model can be used to study the regulation of collagen synthesis, fibrinolysis and the degree of reversibility of liver fibrosis. CRP/TGF-β1 transgenic mouse model can be used as an anti-fibrofactor test model (Kanzler et al., 1999). Similarly, TGF-β1 overexpression transgenic mice were established based on the tetracycline regulation gene expression system. This model will help to analyze the role of TGF-β1 in fibrogenesis (Ueberham et al., 2003). The role of platelet-derived growth factor A (PDGF-A) in the formation of liver fibrosis in vivo can be evaluated in transgenic mice with hepatocellular specific overexpression of PDGF-A by the C-reactive protein (CRP) gene promoter (Thieringer et al., 2008). Metalloproteinase-1 tissue inhibitor (TIMP-1) is upregulated during liver fibrogenesis, but its role in liver fibrosis and carcinogenesis in mice is not necessarily direct (Thiele et al., 2017). Transgenic mice overexpressing human TIMP-1 (HTIMP-1) in the liver under the control of albumin promoter/enhancer can be used to investigate the role of TIMP-1 in promoting liver fibrosis (Yoshiji et al., 2000). Mouse models carrying human apolipoprotein E* 3-leiden and cholesterol ester transfer protein, fed a "Western" diet, lead to liver inflammation and fibrosis that are highly dependent on genetic background and have a large overlap of pathways between human diseases (Hui et al., 2018).

TABLE 1 | Advantages and disadvantages of different methods in hepatic fibrosis models.

Model type	Model	species	Method	Advantages	Disadvantages	References
Chemical drug-induced liver fibrosis model	Carbon tetrachloride	Mouse/Rat	Intraperitoneal injection/inhalation	Simplicity of operator, commonly used, high reproducibility	Highly toxic and volatile, different from human liver fibrosis	Slater et al., 1985; Weber et al., 2003; Leeming et al., 2013; Scholten et al., 2015; Marfà et al., 2016; Unsal et al., 2020
	Thioacetamide	Mouse/Rat/ Monkey	Intraperitoneal injection	Simplicity of operator, commonly used, high reproducibility	Highly toxic	Müller et al., 1988; Fontana et al., 1996; Wei et al., 2014; Wallace et al., 2015; Inoue et al., 2018
	Dimethylnitrosamine or diethylnitrosamine	Mouse/Rat/ Zebra fish	Intraperitoneal injection	Simplicity of operator, commonly used, high reproducibility	Highly toxic and volatile	George et al., 2001; Wang et al., 2014; Tolba et al. 2015
	Acetaminophen	Mouse/Rat	Intraperitoneal injection, gavage	Simplicity of operator, similar to the drug liver fibrosis	—	Yoon et al., 2016; Yan et al., 2018; Tropskaya et al., 2020
Immune damage-induced liver fibrosis model	Concanavalin A	Mouse/Rat	tail vein injection	High success rate, low animal mortality and simple operation	Similar to liver fibrosis caused by chronic virus or autoimmunity in humans	Tanabe et al., 2007; Wang et al., 2012; Heymann et al., 2015; Ye et al., 2018
Alcohol-induced liver fibrosis model	Alcohol	Mouse/Rat	Gavage	Suitable for the study of alcoholic liver disease	Alcohol tolerance in rodents	Bertola et al., 2013; Zhou et al., 2013
	Alcohol combined with chemical poisons	Mouse/Rat/Pig	Gavage	Suitable for the study of alcoholic liver disease, short model cycle	Alcohol tolerance in rodents	Hall et al., 1991; Zhang et al., 2009; Brol et al., 2019
Diet metabolism-induced liver fibrosis model	Dietary deficiencies	Mouse/Rat	Feeding	Close to human NASH	Long time t develop mild fibrosis	Matsumoto et al., 2013; Honda et al., 2017
	Dietary deficiencies combined with chemical poisons	Mouse/Rat	Feeding	Close to human NASH	—	Chheda et al., 2014; Tsuchida et al., 2018
Surgery-induced liver fibrosis model	Surgical bile duct ligation	Mouse/Rat	Surgery	Fast molding and high repeatability Close to human cholestatic injury	Surgical operation required, high mortality rate	Rodríguez-Garay et al., 1996; Kirkland et al., 2010; Heinrich et al., 2011; Tag et al., 2015
Transgenic animal liver fibrosis model	Humanized liver chimeric transgenic mice	Mouse	Transgenic mice combined with human hepatocyte transplantation	Simulate the process of human infection with hepatitis virus	Transplant surgery is complicated. The source of primary human hepatocytes was deficient	Katoh et al. 2008; Kosaka et al., 2013
	Transgenic/knockout mice	Mouse	Transgenic mice	Identify the role of a gene in liver fibrosis	Long time to develop Expensive price	Kanzler et al., 1999; Ueberham et al., 2003; Thieringer et al., 2008; Fransén-Pettersson et al., 2016; Nishio et al., 2019; Yoshiji et al., 2000
Organoid liver fibrosis modes	Liver organoids	Human/Mouse	3D in vitro culture technology	Homology with target organs Functionally similar with target organs	High model cost Difficulty of model Uncontrollable factors	Leite et al., 2016; Artegiani and Clevers, 2018; Coll et al., 2018; Ouchi et al., 2019; Pingitore et al., 2019; Prior et al., 2019; Brovold et al., 2020; Chusilp et al., 2020; Elbadawy et al., 2020

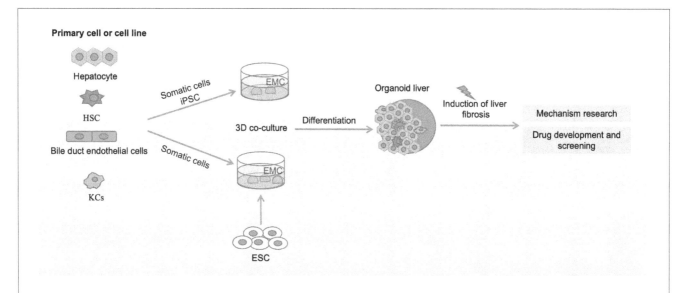

FIGURE 2 | Organoid models of liver fibrosis. The generation of liver organoids and liver fibrosis models. liver organoid can be constructed by 3D co-culture of embryonic stem cells (ESC) and somatic hepatocytes, 3D coculture of induced pluripotent stem cells, and then through induction and differentiation of different developmental stages, and finally can be developed into liver organoids in the reactor. The establishment of liver fibrosis model using liver organoids can be used to study the mechanism of liver fibrosis and drug development and screening.

ORGANOID LIVER FIBROSIS MODES

Studying tissue and organ biology in mammals is challenging, and progress may be hampered by the availability of samples and ethical issues, especially in humans (Rossi et al., 2018). Although traditional 2D cell culture systems have many advantages, these models lack the ability to maintain *in situ* cellular characteristics and reflect cell-to-cell and cell-to-matrix interactions. The primary cells obtained by purification and isolation will also lose their original functions and characteristics after 2D culture *in vitro*. Organoids are 3D organ-like cells that are derived from embryonic or adult stem cells that are cultured *in vitro* and have a definite structure and function. Although these cellular structures are not human organs in the true sense, they can mimic real organs in structure and function, so they are playing an increasingly important role in scientific research. Organoids *in vitro* culture systems are characterized by self-renewing stem cell populations that include cells capable of differentiating into organs with similar spatial tissue functions (Artegiani and Clevers, 2018). Organoids can be used to simulate organ development and disease, and have a wide range of applications in basic research, drug development, and regenerative medicine (Lancaster and Knoblich, 2014; Huch et al., 2017; Xia et al., 2019). While mouse models and cell lines have advanced our understanding of liver biology and related diseases, they have significant drawbacks in simulating human liver tissue, particularly its complex structure and metabolic function. Currently, a variety of liver organoids have been established from induced pluripotent stem cells, embryonic stem cells, hepatoblasts and adult tissue-derived cells (Prior et al., 2019).

HepaRG (Hep) and primary human HSCs were cultured into 3D spheres in 96-well plates. The metabolic capacity of the organoid exceeds 21 days. This novel liver organ culture model

is the first capable of detecting hepatocellular dependence and compound-induced HSC activation and represents an important advance in the *in vitro* compound assessment of drug-induced liver fibrosis (Leite et al., 2016). Induced pluripotent stem cell-hepatic stellate cells (iPSC-HSCs) are very similar to primary human HSCs at the transcriptional, cellular, and functional levels. iPSC-HSCs exhibit a static phenotype when they remain 3D spherical with HepaRG hepatocytes, but are activated in response to wound-healing mediator stimulation and hepatocytotoxicity, resulting in fibrotic responses and secretion of procollagen, and accumulation of retinol in lipid droplets, similar to their *in vivo* counterparts. Thus, this protocol provides a powerful *in vitro* system for studying stellate cell development, modeling liver fibrosis, and screening for drug toxicity (Coll et al., 2018). Activated hepatic stellate cells (aHSCs) produced by 2D culture were coated in a 3D collagen gel to form a spherical structure, which created a stiffer environment and expressed higher levels of TIMP1 and LOXL2 compared to LX-2 cells cultured in 2D culture. This model proposes a fibrosis model that can be combined with the multicellular model to more accurately reflect the impact of severe fibrosis on liver function (Brovold et al., 2020). Using organoids from intrahepatic bile ducts, APAP was used to induce organoid injury in culture medium. The injury model suggested that bile duct cell apoptosis and its fibrotic response played a role in the initiation of the fibrotic process of bile duct diseases, such as biliary atresia (BA) (Chusilp et al., 2020). Genetically susceptible NAFLD organoid systems composed of hepatocytes (HepG2) and HSCs (LX-2) can be used to clarify the molecular mechanisms underlying the accumulation of lipids that induces the early stage of fibrogenesis. In addition, these systems can be used to identify new compounds for treating NASH through high-throughput drug screening (Pingitore et al., 2019). It is difficult to select

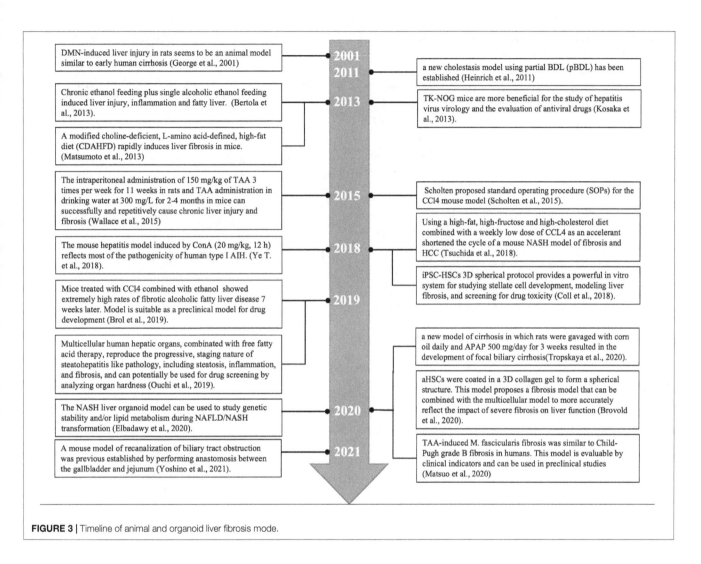

DMN-induced liver injury in rats seems to be an animal model similar to early human cirrhosis (George et al., 2001)

Chronic ethanol feeding plus single alcoholic ethanol feeding induced liver injury, inflammation and fatty liver. (Bertola et al., 2013).

A modified choline-deficient, L-amino acid-defined, high-fat diet (CDAHFD) rapidly induces liver fibrosis in mice. (Matsumoto et al., 2013)

The intraperitoneal administration of 150 mg/kg of TAA 3 times per week for 11 weeks in rats and TAA administration in drinking water at 300 mg/L for 2-4 months in mice can successfully and repetitively cause chronic liver injury and fibrosis (Wallace et al., 2015)

The mouse hepatitis model induced by ConA (20 mg/kg, 12 h) reflects most of the pathogenicity of human type I AIH. (Ye T. et al., 2018).

Mice treated with CCl4 combined with ethanol showed extremely high rates of fibrotic alcoholic fatty liver disease 7 weeks later. Model is suitable as a preclinical model for drug development (Brol et al., 2019).

Multicellular human hepatic organs, combined with free fatty acid therapy, reproduce the progressive, staging nature of steatohepatitis like pathology, including steatosis, inflammation, and fibrosis, and can potentially be used for drug screening by analyzing organ hardness (Ouchi et al., 2019).

The NASH liver organoid model can be used to study genetic stability and/or lipid metabolism during NAFLD/NASH transformation (Elbadawy et al., 2020).

A mouse model of recanalization of biliary tract obstruction was previous established by performing anastomosis between the gallbladder and jejunum (Yoshino et al., 2021).

2001
2011
2013
2015
2018
2019
2020
2021

a new cholestasis model using partial BDL (pBDL) has been established (Heinrich et al., 2011)

TK-NOG mice are more beneficial for the study of hepatitis virus virology and the evaluation of antiviral drugs (Kosaka et al., 2013).

Scholten proposed standard operating procedure (SOPs) for the CCl4 mouse model (Scholten et al., 2015).

Using a high-fat, high-fructose and high-cholesterol diet combined with a weekly low dose of CCL4 as an accelerant shortened the cycle of a mouse NASH model of fibrosis and HCC (Tsuchida et al., 2018).

iPSC-HSCs 3D spherical protocol provides a powerful in vitro system for studying stellate cell development, modeling liver fibrosis, and screening for drug toxicity (Coll et al., 2018).

a new model of cirrhosis in which rats were gavaged with corn oil daily and APAP 500 mg/day for 3 weeks resulted in the development of focal biliary cirrhosis(Tropskaya et al., 2020).

aHSCs were coated in a 3D collagen gel to form a spherical structure. This model proposes a fibrosis model that can be combined with the multicellular model to more accurately reflect the impact of severe fibrosis on liver function (Brovold et al., 2020).

TAA-induced M. fascicularis fibrosis was similar to Child-Pugh grade B fibrosis in humans. This model is evaluable by clinical indicators and can be used in preclinical studies (Matsuo et al., 2020)

FIGURE 3 | Timeline of animal and organoid liver fibrosis mode.

media and extracellular matrix that can co-maintain multiple cell lineages. A novel organ-like culture method was developed for co-differentiation of epithelial and mesenchymal lineages from PSCs. Using 11 different health and disease pluripotent cell lines, a repeatable method was developed to obtain multicellular human liver-like organs composed of hepatocytes, stellate cells, and Kupffer like cells that exhibit transcriptome similarity to tissue of *in vivo* origin. These multicellular human hepatic organs (HLOs), in combination with free fatty acid therapy, reproduce the progressive, staging nature of steatohepatitis like pathology, including steatosis, inflammation, and fibrosis, and can potentially be used for drug screening by analyzing organ hardness (Ouchi et al., 2019). Liver organoids were generated from mice with mild (NASH A), moderate (NASH B), and severe (NASH C) methionine and choline deficiency diets-induced NASH models that reproduce the characteristics of NASH disease liver tissue. The NASH liver organoid model can be used to study genetic stability and/or lipid metabolism during NAFLD/NASH transformation (Elbadawy et al., 2020).

In conclusion, organoid technology is one of the most important advances in stem cell research. Organoids are three-dimensional cell cultures that reproduce some of the key cell types and structural characteristics of the organs they represent. Organoids remove the confounding variables that might be introduced by animal models and are more complex than homogenized cell cultures. Organoid culture has a high degree of gene stability, maintaining the genotype and phenotype of the source tissue. Thus, organoids can be used to model diseases, to study the mechanisms and progression of diseases, and to predict patients' individual responses to drug therapy (**Figure 2**).

CONCLUSION AND PERSPECTIVES

A reasonable model of liver fibrosis should resemble the characteristics and pathogenesis of human disease. It is universally recognized that "animal welfare" includes five freedoms: freedom from hunger and thirst; comfort; freedom from pain, injury and disease; freedom from fear and sadness and expression of nature. In laboratory animals, it is difficult to achieve all five freedoms at the same time. In particular, damage to these creatures' health is often a byproduct of the natural course of research. Due to such factors as animal suffering and scientific exploration, the three R principles are widely recognized: including replacement, reduction and refinement (Lindsjö et al., 2016). This requires animal experiments to have stable experimental methods, a high mold-forming rate and good reproducibility. Thus far, researchers have successfully developed a number of hepatic fibrosis models using different experimental animals and different methods. However, due to the complexity of the pathogenesis of human liver fibrosis and differences in the genetic background between human and other animal species, there is no modeling method that can perfectly replicate the process of human liver fibrosis. Researchers can only use different models of liver fibrosis to mimic, as much as possible, the different pathologies that cause liver fibrosis in humans. **Table 1** briefly compares the advantages and disadvantages of different liver fibrosis models (**Table 1**). Although the liver fibrosis model induced by chemical poisons is different from the pathogenesis of human liver fibrosis, it is often used to study the mechanism of liver fibrosis due to its simple operation and good reproducibility. The immune-induced liver injury fibrosis model most closely replicates the clinical situation, which is similar to the liver fibrosis caused by human AIH and virus infection. Due to the complex pathogenesis of ALD and NAFLD, and the great differences between animal genetics, metabolism and immunity and human beings, it is relatively difficult to construct a model similar to human diseases through liver fibrosis induced by alcohol and the diet metabolism. BDL can simulate liver fibrosis induced by cholestasis, requiring only a short time with good reproducibility for model construction. However, it has drawbacks of substantial operational requirements, the need for an aseptic surgical setting and high animal mortality. Humanized transgenic chimeric mice and transgenic/knockout mice are emerging modeling methods that have been established in recent decades. Humanized liver chimeric transgenic mice constitute a good animal model of hepatitis virus infection, and transgenic/knockout mice are a good animal model for studying

the role of the functional genes involved in liver fibrosis. The latest organoid model makes up for the great difference between the traditional *in vitro* cell culture and human organs. Liver organoids are expected to be a useful new model for *in vitro* experiments that closely resembles the actual situation in human liver diseases. Although the techniques are becoming more advanced, liver fibrosis models are becoming more complex. Researchers continue to make various models of liver fibrosis in order to bring them closer to the true pathogenesis of human liver fibrosis (**Figure 3**). Each model has its advantages and disadvantages, and it remains a challenge to identify the most reasonable and stable hepatic fibrosis model.

AUTHOR CONTRIBUTIONS

All authors contributed to the writing and editing of the manuscript and contributed to the article and approved the submitted version.

FUNDING

This work was supported in part by the Program of Inner Mongolia Autonomous Region Tumor Biotherapy Collaborative Innovation Center, Medical Science and Technology Project of Zhejiang Province (2021PY083), Program of Taizhou Science and Technology Grant (20ywb29), Major Research Program of Taizhou Enze Medical Center Grant (19EZZDA2), Key Technology Research and Development Program of Zhejiang Province (2019C03040), and Open Fund of Key Laboratory of Minimally Invasive Techniques & Rapid Rehabilitation of Digestive System Tumor of Zhejiang Provinces (21SZDSYS01 and 21SZDSYS09).

REFERENCES

AlWahsh, M., Othman, A., Hamadneh, L., Telfah, A., Lambert, J., Hikmat, S., et al. (2019). Second exposure to acetaminophen overdose is associated with liver fibrosis in mice. *EXCLI J.* 18, 51–62.

Artegiani, B., and Clevers, H. (2018). Use and application of 3D-organoid technology. *Hum. Mol. Genet.* 27:ddy187. doi: 10.1093/hmg/ddy187

Bai, Q., Yan, H., Sheng, Y., Jin, Y., Shi, L., Ji, L., et al. (2017). Long-term acetaminophen treatment induced liver fibrosis in mice and the involvement of Egr-1. *Toxicology* 382, 47–58. doi: 10.1016/j.tox.2017.03.008

Bertola, A., Mathews, S., Ki, S. H., Wang, H., and Gao, B. (2013). Mouse model of chronic and binge ethanol feeding (the NIAAA model). *Nat. Protoc.* 8, 627–637. doi: 10.1038/nprot.2013.032

Brol, M. J., Rösch, F., Schierwagen, R., Magdaleno, F., Uschner, F. E., Manekeller, S., et al. (2019). Combination of CCl with alcoholic and metabolic injuries mimics human liver fibrosis. *Am. J. Physiol. Gastroint. Liver Physiol.* 317, G182–G194. doi: 10.1152/ajpgi.00361.2018

Brovold, M., Keller, D., and Soker, S. (2020). Differential fibrotic phenotypes of hepatic stellate cells within 3D liver organoids. *Biotechnol. Bioeng.* 117, 2516–2526. doi: 10.1002/bit.27379

Campana, L., and Iredale, J. P. (2017). Regression of Liver Fibrosis. *Semin. Liver Dis.* 37:1597816. doi: 10.1055/s-0036-1597816

Chheda, T. K., Shivakumar, P., Sadasivan, S. K., Chanderasekharan, H., Moolemath, Y., Oommen, A. M., et al. (2014). Fast food diet with CCl4 microdose induced hepatic-fibrosis–a novel animal model. *BMC Gastroenterol.* 14:89. doi: 10.1186/1471-230X-14-89

Chusilp, S., Lee, C., Li, B., Lee, D., Yamoto, M., Ganji, N., et al. (2020). A novel model of injured liver ductal organoids to investigate cholangiocyte apoptosis with relevance to biliary atresia. *Pediatr. Surg. Int.* 36, 1471–1479. doi: 10.1007/s00383-020-04765-2

Cobbina, E., and Akhlaghi, F. (2017). Non-alcoholic fatty liver disease (NAFLD) - pathogenesis, classification, and effect on drug metabolizing enzymes and transporters. *Drug Metab. Rev.* 49, 197–211. doi: 10.1080/03602532.2017.1293683

Coll, M., Perea, L., Boon, R., Leite, S. B., Vallverdú, J., Mannaerts, I., et al. (2018). Generation of Hepatic Stellate Cells from Human Pluripotent Stem Cells Enables In Vitro Modeling of Liver Fibrosis. *Cell Stem Cell* 23, 101.e–113.e. doi: 10.1016/j.stem.2018.05.027

Dandri, M., Volz, T. K., Lütgehetmann, M., and Petersen, J. (2005). Animal models for the study of HBV replication and its variants. *J. Clin. Virol.* 34(Suppl. 1), S54–S62.

Dong, S., Chen, Q.-L., Song, Y.-N., Sun, Y., Wei, B., Li, X.-Y., et al. (2016). Mechanisms of CCl4-induced liver fibrosis with combined transcriptomic and proteomic analysis. *J. Toxicol. Sci.* 41, 561–572. doi: 10.2131/jts.41.561

Elbadawy, M., Yamanaka, M., Goto, Y., Hayashi, K., Tsunedomi, R., Hazama, S., et al. (2020). Efficacy of primary liver organoid culture from different stages of non-alcoholic steatohepatitis (NASH) mouse model. *Biomaterials* 237:119823. doi: 10.1016/j.biomaterials.2020.119823

Feng, M., Ding, J., Wang, M., Zhang, J., Zhu, X., and Guan, W. (2018). Kupffer-derived matrix metalloproteinase-9 contributes to liver fibrosis resolution. *Int. J. Biol. Sci.* 14, 1033–1040. doi: 10.7150/ijbs.25589

Fontana, L., Moreira, E., Torres, M. I., Fernández, M. I., Ríos, A., Sánchez de Medina, F., et al. (1996). Serum amino acid changes in rats with thioacetamide-induced liver cirrhosis. *Toxicology* 106, 197–206. doi: 10.1016/0300-483x(95)03177-h

Fransén-Pettersson, N., Duarte, N., Nilsson, J., Lundholm, M., Mayans, S., Larefalk, Å, et al. (2016). A New Mouse Model That Spontaneously Develops Chronic Liver Inflammation and Fibrosis. *PLoS One* 11:e0159850. doi: 10.1371/journal.pone.0159850

Fujii, T., Fuchs, B. C., Yamada, S., Lauwers, G. Y., Kulu, Y., Goodwin, J. M., et al. (2010). Mouse model of carbon tetrachloride induced liver fibrosis: Histopathological changes and expression of CD133 and epidermal growth factor. *BMC Gastroenterol.* 10:79. doi: 10.1186/1471-230X-10-79

Gäbele, E., Dostert, K., Dorn, C., Patsenker, E., Stickel, F., and Hellerbrand, C. (2011). A new model of interactive effects of alcohol and high-fat diet on hepatic fibrosis. *Alcohol Clin. Exp. Res.* 35, 1361–1367. doi: 10.1111/j.1530-0277.2011.01472.x

George, J., and Chandrakasan, G. (1996). Molecular characteristics of dimethylnitrosamine induced fibrotic liver collagen. *Biochim. Biophys. Acta* 1292, 215–222. doi: 10.1016/0167-4838(95)00202-2

George, J., Rao, K. R., Stern, R., and Chandrakasan, G. (2001). Dimethylnitrosamine-induced liver injury in rats: the early deposition of collagen. *Toxicology* 156, 129–138. doi: 10.1016/s0300-483x(00)00352-8

Hall, P. D., Plummer, J. L., Ilsley, A. H., and Cousins, M. J. (1991). Hepatic fibrosis and cirrhosis after chronic administration of alcohol and "low-dose" carbon tetrachloride vapor in the rat. *Hepatology* 13, 815–819. doi: 10.1016/0270-9139(91)90246-r

Hata, M., Iida, H., Yamanegi, K., Yamada, N., Ohyama, H., Hirano, H., et al. (2013). Phenotypic characteristics and proliferative activity of hyperplastic ductule cells in cholangiofibrosis induced by thioacetamide in rats. *Exp. Toxicol. Pathol.* 65, 351–356. doi: 10.1016/j.etp.2011.11.004

Hayashi, H., and Sakai, T. (2011). Animal models for the study of liver fibrosis: new insights from knockout mouse models. *Am. J. Physiol. Gastrointest Liver Physiol.* 300, G729–G738. doi: 10.1152/ajpgi.00013.2011

He, J.-Y., Ge, W.-H., and Chen, Y. (2007). Iron deposition and fat accumulation in dimethylnitrosamine-induced liver fibrosis in rat. *World J. Gastroenterol.* 13, 2061–2065. doi: 10.3748/wjg.v13.i14.2061

Heinrich, S., Georgiev, P., Weber, A., Vergopoulos, A., Graf, R., and Clavien, P.-A. (2011). Partial bile duct ligation in mice: a novel model of acute cholestasis. *Surgery* 149, 445–451. doi: 10.1016/j.surg.2010.07.046

Hernandez-Gea, V., and Friedman, S. L. (2011). Pathogenesis of liver fibrosis. *Annu. Rev. Pathol.* 6, 425–456. doi: 10.1146/annurev-pathol-011110-130246

Heymann, F., Hamesch, K., Weiskirchen, R., and Tacke, F. (2015). The concanavalin A model of acute hepatitis in mice. *Lab. Anim.* 49(1 Suppl.), 12–20. doi: 10.1177/0023677215572841

Higashi, T., Friedman, S. L., and Hoshida, Y. (2017). Hepatic stellate cells as key target in liver fibrosis. *Adv. Drug Deliv. Rev.* 121, 27–42. doi: 10.1016/j.addr.2017.05.007

Holmes, R. S., Duley, J. A., Algar, E. M., Mather, P. B., and Rout, U. K. (1986). Biochemical and genetic studies on enzymes of alcohol metabolism: the mouse as a model organism for human studies. *Alcohol Alcohol.* 21, 41–56.

Honda, T., Ishigami, M., Luo, F., Lingyun, M., Ishizu, Y., Kuzuya, T., et al. (2017). Branched-chain amino acids alleviate hepatic steatosis and liver injury in choline-deficient high-fat diet induced NASH mice. *Metabolism* 69, 177–187. doi: 10.1016/j.metabol.2016.12.013

Hong, F., Si, C., Gao, P., Cederbaum, A. I., Xiong, H., and Lu, Y. (2016). The role of CYP2A5 in liver injury and fibrosis: chemical-specific difference. *Naunyn Schmiedebergs Arch. Pharmacol.* 389, 33–43. doi: 10.1007/s00210-015-1172-8

Huch, M., Knoblich, J. A., Lutolf, M. P., and Martinez-Arias, A. (2017). The hope and the hype of organoid research. *Development* 144, 938–941. doi: 10.1242/dev.150201

Hui, S. T., Kurt, Z., Tuominen, I., Norheim, F., Davis, R. C., Pan, C., et al. (2018). The Genetic Architecture of Diet-Induced Hepatic Fibrosis in Mice. *Hepatology* 68, 2182–2196. doi: 10.1002/hep.30113

Ikenaga, N., Liu, S. B., Sverdlov, D. Y., Yoshida, S., Nasser, I., Ke, Q., et al. (2015). A new Mdr2(-/-) mouse model of sclerosing cholangitis with rapid fibrosis progression, early-onset portal hypertension, and liver cancer. *Am. J. Pathol.* 185, 325–334. doi: 10.1016/j.ajpath.2014.10.013

Inoue, T., Ishizaka, Y., Sasaki, E., Lu, J., Mineshige, T., Yanase, M., et al. (2018). Thioacetamide-induced hepatic fibrosis in the common marmoset. *Exp. Anim.* 67, 321–327. doi: 10.1538/expanim.17-0156

Jiao, J., Sastre, D., Fiel, M. I., Lee, U. E., Ghiassi-Nejad, Z., Ginhoux, F., et al. (2012). Dendritic cell regulation of carbon tetrachloride-induced murine liver fibrosis regression. *Hepatology* 55, 244–255. doi: 10.1002/hep.24621

Kamdem, S. D., Moyou-Somo, R., Brombacher, F., and Nono, J. K. (2018). Host Regulators of Liver Fibrosis During Human Schistosomiasis. *Front. Immunol.* 9:2781. doi: 10.3389/fimmu.2018.02781

Kanzler, S., Lohse, A. W., Keil, A., Henninger, J., Dienes, H. P., Schirmacher, P., et al. (1999). TGF-beta1 in liver fibrosis: an inducible transgenic mouse model to study liver fibrogenesis. *Am. J. Physiol.* 276, G1059–G1068. doi: 10.1152/ajpgi.1999.276.4.G1059

Katoh, M., Tateno, C., Yoshizato, K., and Yokoi, T. (2008). Chimeric mice with humanized liver. *Toxicology* 246:12. doi: 10.1016/j.tox.2007.11.012

Kirkland, J. G., Godfrey, C. B., Garrett, R., Kakar, S., Yeh, B. M., and Corvera, C. U. (2010). Reversible surgical model of biliary inflammation and obstructive jaundice in mice. *J. Surg. Res.* 164, 221–227. doi: 10.1016/j.jss.2009.08.010

Komatsu, G., Nonomura, T., Sasaki, M., Ishida, Y., Arai, S., and Miyazaki, T. (2019). AIM-deficient mouse fed a high-trans fat, high-cholesterol diet: a new animal model for nonalcoholic fatty liver disease. *Exp. Anim.* 68, 147–158. doi: 10.1538/expanim.18-0108

Kosaka, K., Hiraga, N., Imamura, M., Yoshimi, S., Murakami, E., Nakahara, T., et al. (2013). A novel TK-NOG based humanized mouse model for the study of HBV and HCV infections. *Biochem. Biophys. Res. Commun.* 441, 230–235. doi: 10.1016/j.bbrc.2013.10.040

Koyama, Y., and Brenner, D. A. (2017). Liver inflammation and fibrosis. *J. Clin. Invest.* 127, 55–64. doi: 10.1172/JCI88881

Lamas-Paz, A., Hao, F., Nelson, L. J., Vázquez, M. T., Canals, S., Gómez Del Moral, M., et al. (2018). Alcoholic liver disease: Utility of animal models. *World J. Gastroenterol.* 24, 5063–5075. doi: 10.3748/wjg.v24.i45.5063

Lancaster, M. A., and Knoblich, J. A. (2014). Organogenesis in a dish: modeling development and disease using organoid technologies. *Science* 345:1247125. doi: 10.1126/science.1247125

Leeming, D. J., Byrjalsen, I., Jiménez, W., Christiansen, C., and Karsdal, M. A. (2013). Protein fingerprinting of the extracellular matrix remodelling in a rat model of liver fibrosis–a serological evaluation. *Liver Int.* 33, 439–447. doi: 10.1111/liv.12044

Leite, S. B., Roosens, T., El Taghdouini, A., Mannaerts, I., Smout, A. J., Najimi, M., et al. (2016). Novel human hepatic organoid model enables testing of drug-induced liver fibrosis in vitro. *Biomaterials* 78:026. doi: 10.1016/j.biomaterials.2015.11.026

Li, C.-H., Piao, D.-M., Xu, W.-X., Yin, Z.-R., Jin, J.-S., and Shen, Z.-S. (2005). Morphological and serum hyaluronic acid, laminin and type IV collagen changes in dimethylnitrosamine-induced hepatic fibrosis of rats. *World J. Gastroenterol.* 11, 7620–7624. doi: 10.3748/wjg.v11.i48.7620

Li, T., and Apte, U. (2015). Bile Acid Metabolism and Signaling in Cholestasis, Inflammation, and Cancer. *Adv. Pharmacol.* 74, 263–302. doi: 10.1016/bs.apha.2015.04.003

Lindsjö, J., Fahlman, Å, and Törnqvist, E. (2016). ANIMAL WELFARE FROM MOUSE TO MOOSE–IMPLEMENTING THE PRINCIPLES OF THE 3RS IN WILDLIFE RESEARCH. *J. Wildl. Dis.* 52(2 Suppl.), S65–S77. doi: 10.7589/52.2S.S65

Louis, H., Le Moine, A., Quertinmont, E., Peny, M. O., Geerts, A., Goldman, M., et al. (2000). Repeated concanavalin A challenge in mice induces an interleukin 10-producing phenotype and liver fibrosis. *Hepatology* 31, 381–390. doi: 10.1002/hep.510310218

Man, K.-N. M., Philipsen, S., and Tan-Un, K. C. (2008). Localization and expression pattern of cytoglobin in carbon tetrachloride-induced liver fibrosis. *Toxicol. Lett.* 183, 36–44. doi: 10.1016/j.toxlet.2008.09.015

Marfà, S., Morales-Ruiz, M., Oró, D., Ribera, J., Fernández-Varo, G., and Jiménez, W. (2016). Sipa1l1 is an early biomarker of liver fibrosis in CCl4-treated rats. *Biol. Open* 5, 858–865. doi: 10.1242/bio.018887

Mathews, S., Xu, M., Wang, H., Bertola, A., and Gao, B. (2014). Animals models of gastrointestinal and liver diseases. Animal models of alcohol-induced liver disease: pathophysiology, translational relevance, and challenges. *Am. J. Physiol. Gastrointest Liver Physiol.* 306, G819–G823. doi: 10.1152/ajpgi.00041.2014

Matsumoto, M., Hada, N., Sakamaki, Y., Uno, A., Shiga, T., Tanaka, C., et al. (2013). An improved mouse model that rapidly develops fibrosis in non-alcoholic steatohepatitis. *Int. J. Exp. Pathol.* 94:12008. doi: 10.1111/iep.12008

Matsuo, M., Murata, S., Hasegawa, S., Hatada, Y., Ohtsuka, M., and Taniguchi, H. (2020). Novel liver fibrosis model in Macaca fascicularis induced by thioacetamide. *Sci. Rep.* 10:2450. doi: 10.1038/s41598-020-58739-4

Mehal, W. Z., Iredale, J., and Friedman, S. L. (2011). Scraping fibrosis: expressway to the core of fibrosis. *Nat. Med.* 17, 552–553. doi: 10.1038/nm0511-552

Müller, A., Machnik, F., Zimmermann, T., and Schubert, H. (1988). Thioacetamide-induced cirrhosis-like liver lesions in rats–usefulness and reliability of this animal model. *Exp. Pathol.* 34, 229–236. doi: 10.1016/s0232-1513(88)80155-5

Nishio, T., Hu, R., Koyama, Y., Liang, S., Rosenthal, S. B., Yamamoto, G., et al. (2019). Activated hepatic stellate cells and portal fibroblasts contribute to cholestatic liver fibrosis in MDR2 knockout mice. *J. Hepatol.* 71, 573–585. doi: 10.1016/j.jhep.2019.04.012

Ouchi, R., Togo, S., Kimura, M., Shinozawa, T., Koido, M., and Koike, H. (2019). Modeling Steatohepatitis in Humans with Pluripotent Stem Cell-Derived Organoids. *Cell Metab.* 30, 374.e–384.e. doi: 10.1016/j.cmet.2019.05.007

Park, H.-J., Kim, H.-G., Wang, J.-H., Choi, M.-K., Han, J.-M., Lee, J.-S., et al. (2016). Comparison of TGF-β, PDGF, and CTGF in hepatic fibrosis models using DMN, CCl4, and TAA. *Drug Chem. Toxicol.* 39, 111–118. doi: 10.3109/01480545.2015.1052143

Parola, M., and Pinzani, M. (2019). Liver fibrosis: Pathophysiology, pathogenetic targets and clinical issues. *Mol. Aspects Med.* 65, 37–55. doi: 10.1016/j.mam.2018.09.002

Pellicoro, A., Ramachandran, P., Iredale, J. P., and Fallowfield, J. A. (2014). Liver fibrosis and repair: immune regulation of wound healing in a solid organ. *Nat. Rev. Immunol.* 14, 181–194. doi: 10.1038/nri3623

Pingitore, P., Sasidharan, K., Ekstrand, M., Prill, S., Lindén, D., and Romeo, S. (2019). Human Multilineage 3D Spheroids as a Model of Liver Steatosis and Fibrosis. *Int. J. Mol. Sci.* 20:20071629. doi: 10.3390/ijms20071629

Prior, N., Inacio, P., and Huch, M. (2019). Liver organoids: from basic research to therapeutic applications. *Gut* 68, 2228–2237. doi: 10.1136/gutjnl-2019-319256

Rodríguez-Garay, E. A., Agüero, R. M., Pisani, G., Trbojevich, R. A., Farroni, A., and Viglianco, R. A. (1996). Rat model of mild stenosis of the common bile duct. *Res. Exp. Med.* 196, 105–116. doi: 10.1007/s004330050017

Rossi, G., Manfrin, A., and Lutolf, M. P. (2018). Progress and potential in organoid research. *Nat. Rev. Genet.* 19, 671–687. doi: 10.1038/s41576-018-0051-9

Scholten, D., Trebicka, J., Liedtke, C., and Weiskirchen, R. (2015). The carbon tetrachloride model in mice. *Lab. Anim.* 49(1 Suppl.):23677215571192. doi: 10.1177/0023677215571192

Sebastiani, G., Gkouvatsos, K., and Pantopoulos, K. (2014). Chronic hepatitis C and liver fibrosis. *World J. Gastroenterol.* 20, 11033–11053. doi: 10.3748/wjg.v20.i32.11033

Seitz, H. K., Bataller, R., Cortez-Pinto, H., Gao, B., Gual, A., Lackner, C., et al. (2018). Alcoholic liver disease. *Nat. Rev. Dis. Primers* 4:16. doi: 10.1038/s41572-018-0014-7

Slater, T. F., Cheeseman, K. H., and Ingold, K. U. (1985). Carbon tetrachloride toxicity as a model for studying free-radical mediated liver injury. *Philos. Trans. R. Soc. Lond. B Biol. Sci.* 311, 633–645. doi: 10.1098/rstb.1985.0169

Soares, P. A. G., Nascimento, C. O., Porto, T. S., Correia, M. T. S., Porto, A. L. F., and Carneiro-da-Cunha, M. G. (2011). Purification of a lectin from Canavalia ensiformis using PEG-citrate aqueous two-phase system. *J. Chromatogr. B Analyt. Technol. Biomed. Life Sci.* 879, 457–460. doi: 10.1016/j.jchromb.2010.12.030

Stål, P. (2015). Liver fibrosis in non-alcoholic fatty liver disease - diagnostic challenge with prognostic significance. *World J. Gastroenterol.* 21, 11077–11087. doi: 10.3748/wjg.v21.i39.11077

Tag, C. G., Sauer-Lehnen, S., Weiskirchen, S., Borkham-Kamphorst, E., Tolba, R. H., Tacke, F., et al. (2015). Bile duct ligation in mice: induction of inflammatory liver injury and fibrosis by obstructive cholestasis. *J. Vis. Exp.* 2015:52438. doi: 10.3791/52438

Tanabe, J., Izawa, A., Takemi, N., Miyauchi, Y., Torii, Y., Tsuchiyama, H., et al. (2007). Interferon-beta reduces the mouse liver fibrosis induced by repeated administration of concanavalin A via the direct and indirect effects. *Immunology* 122, 562–570. doi: 10.1111/j.1365-2567.2007.02672.x

Testino, G., Leone, S., Fagoonee, S., and Pellicano, R. (2018). Alcoholic liver fibrosis: detection and treatment. *Minerva Med.* 109, 457–471. doi: 10.23736/S0026-4806.18.05844-5

Thiele, N. D., Wirth, J. W., Steins, D., Koop, A. C., Ittrich, H., Lohse, A. W., et al. (2017). TIMP-1 is upregulated, but not essential in hepatic fibrogenesis and carcinogenesis in mice. *Sci. Rep.* 7:714. doi: 10.1038/s41598-017-00671-1

Thieringer, F., Maass, T., Czochra, P., Klopcic, B., Conrad, I., Friebe, D., et al. (2008). Spontaneous hepatic fibrosis in transgenic mice overexpressing PDGF-A. *Gene* 423, 23–28. doi: 10.1016/j.gene.2008.05.022

Tolba, R., Kraus, T., Liedtke, C., Schwarz, M., and Weiskirchen, R. (2015). Diethylnitrosamine (DEN)-induced carcinogenic liver injury in mice. *Lab. Anim.* 49(1 Suppl.), 59–69. doi: 10.1177/0023677215570086

Tropskaya, N. S., Kislyakova, E. A., Vilkova, I. G., Kislitsyna, O. S., Gurman, Y. V., Popova, T. S., et al. (2020). Experimental Model of Cirrhosis of the Liver. *Bull. Exp. Biol. Med.* 169, 416–420. doi: 10.1007/s10517-020-04899-2

Tsuchida, T., Lee, Y. A., Fujiwara, N., Ybanez, M., Allen, B., Martins, S., et al. (2018). A simple diet- and chemical-induced murine NASH model with rapid progression of steatohepatitis, fibrosis and liver cancer. *J. Hepatol.* 69, 385–395. doi: 10.1016/j.jhep.2018.03.011

Tsukamoto, H., and Lu, S. C. (2001). Current concepts in the pathogenesis of alcoholic liver injury. *FASEB J.* 15, 1335–1349. doi: 10.1096/fj.00-0650rev

Ueberham, E., Löw, R., Ueberham, U., Schönig, K., Bujard, H., and Gebhardt, R. (2003). Conditional tetracycline-regulated expression of TGF-beta1 in liver of transgenic mice leads to reversible intermediary fibrosis. *Hepatology* 37, 1067–1078. doi: 10.1053/jhep.2003.50196

Uehara, T., Ainslie, G. R., Kutanzi, K., Pogribny, I. P., Muskhelishvili, L., Izawa, T., et al. (2013). Molecular mechanisms of fibrosis-associated promotion of liver carcinogenesis. *Toxicol. Sci.* 132, 53–63. doi: 10.1093/toxsci/kfs342

Unsal, V., Cicek, M., and Sabancilar, I. (2020). Toxicity of carbon tetrachloride, free radicals and role of antioxidants. *Rev. Environ. Health* 2020:48. doi: 10.1515/reveh-2020-0048

Wallace, M. C., Hamesch, K., Lunova, M., Kim, Y., Weiskirchen, R., Strnad, P., et al. (2015). Standard operating procedures in experimental liver research: thioacetamide model in mice and rats. *Lab. Anim.* 49(1 Suppl.), 21–29. doi: 10.1177/0023677215573040

Walter, E., Keist, R., Niederöst, B., Pult, I., and Blum, H. E. (1996). Hepatitis B virus infection of tupaia hepatocytes in vitro and in vivo. *Hepatology* 24, 1–5. doi: 10.1053/jhep.1996.v24.pm0008707245

Wang, H.-X., Liu, M., Weng, S.-Y., Li, J.-J., Xie, C., He, H.-L., et al. (2012). Immune mechanisms of Concanavalin A model of autoimmune hepatitis. *World J. Gastroenterol.* 18, 119–125. doi: 10.3748/wjg.v18.i2.119

Wang, K., Liu, L., Dai, W., Chen, X., Zheng, X., and Hou, J. (2014). Establishment of a hepatic fibrosis model induced by diethylnitrosamine in zebrafish. *Nan Fang Yi Ke Da Xue Xue Bao* 34, 777–782.

Wang, L., Tu, L., Zhang, J., Xu, K., and Qian, W. (2017). Stellate Cell Activation and Imbalanced Expression of TGF-1/TGF-3 in Acute Autoimmune Liver Lesions Induced by ConA in Mice. *Biomed. Res. Int.* 2017:2540540. doi: 10.1155/2017/2540540

Watanabe, T., Niioka, M., Hozawa, S., Kameyama, K., Hayashi, T., Arai, M., et al. (2000). Gene expression of interstitial collagenase in both progressive and recovery phase of rat liver fibrosis induced by carbon tetrachloride. *J. Hepatol.* 33, 224–235. doi: 10.1016/s0168-8278(00)80363-3

Weber, L. W. D., Boll, M., and Stampfl, A. (2003). Hepatotoxicity and mechanism of action of haloalkanes: carbon tetrachloride as a toxicological model. *Crit. Rev. Toxicol.* 33, 105–136. doi: 10.1080/713611034

Wei, D.-D., Wang, J.-S., Wang, P.-R., Li, M.-H., Yang, M.-H., and Kong, L.-Y. (2014). Toxic effects of chronic low-dose exposure of thioacetamide on rats based on NMR metabolic profiling. *J. Pharm. Biomed. Anal.* 98, 334–338. doi: 10.1016/j.jpba.2014.05.035

Xia, X., Li, F., He, J., Aji, R., and Gao, D. (2019). Organoid technology in cancer precision medicine. *Cancer Lett.* 457, 20–27. doi: 10.1016/j.canlet.2019.04.039

Yan, M., Huo, Y., Yin, S., and Hu, H. (2018). Mechanisms of acetaminophen-induced liver injury and its implications for therapeutic interventions. *Redox Biol.* 17, 274–283. doi: 10.1016/j.redox.2018.04.019

Ye, T., Wang, T., Yang, X., Fan, X., Wen, M., Shen, Y., et al. (2018). Comparison of Concanavalin a-Induced Murine Autoimmune Hepatitis Models. *Cell Physiol. Biochem.* 46, 1241–1251. doi: 10.1159/000489074

Yoon, E., Babar, A., Choudhary, M., Kutner, M., and Pyrsopoulos, N. (2016). Acetaminophen-Induced Hepatotoxicity: a Comprehensive Update. *J. Clin. Transl. Hepatol.* 4, 131–142. doi: 10.14218/JCTH.2015.00052

Yoshiji, H., Kuriyama, S., Miyamoto, Y., Thorgeirsson, U. P., Gomez, D. E., Kawata, M., et al. (2000). Tissue inhibitor of metalloproteinases-1 promotes liver fibrosis development in a transgenic mouse model. *Hepatology* 32, 1248–1254. doi: 10.1053/jhep.2000.20521

Yoshino, K., Taura, K., Iwaisako, K., Masano, Y., Uemoto, Y., Kimura, Y., et al. (2021). Novel mouse model for cholestasis-induced liver fibrosis resolution by cholecystojejunostomy. *J. Gastroenterol. Hepatol.* 2021:15406. doi: 10.1111/jgh.15406

Zangar, R. C., Benson, J. M., Burnett, V. L., and Springer, D. L. (2000). Cytochrome P450 2E1 is the primary enzyme responsible for low-dose carbon tetrachloride metabolism in human liver microsomes. *Chem. Biol. Interact.* 125, 233–243. doi: 10.1016/s0009-2797(00)00149-6

Zhang, J. J., Meng, X. K., Dong, C., Qiao, J. L., Zhang, R. F., Yue, G. Q., et al. (2009). Development of a new animal model of liver cirrhosis in swine. *Eur. Surg. Res.* 42, 35–39. doi: 10.1159/000167855

Zhangdi, H.-J., Su, S.-B., Wang, F., Liang, Z.-Y., Yan, Y.-D., Qin, S.-Y., et al. (2019). Crosstalk network among multiple inflammatory mediators in liver fibrosis. *World J. Gastroenterol.* 25, 4835–4849. doi: 10.3748/wjg.v25.i33.4835

Zhou, J.-Y., Jiang, Z.-A., Zhao, C.-Y., Zhen, Z., Wang, W., and Nanji, A. A. (2013). Long-term binge and escalating ethanol exposure causes necroinflammation and fibrosis in rat liver. *Alcohol Clin. Exp. Res.* 37, 213–222. doi: 10.1111/j.1530-0277.2012.01936.x

Permissions

The contributors of this book come from diverse backgrounds, making this book a truly international effort. This book will bring forth new frontiers with its revolutionizing research information and detailed analysis of the nascent developments around the world.

We would like to thank all the contributing authors for lending their expertise to make the book truly unique. They have played a crucial role in the development of this book. Without their invaluable contributions this book wouldn't have been possible. They have made vital efforts to compile up to date information on the varied aspects of this subject to make this book a valuable addition to the collection of many professionals and students.

This book was conceptualized with the vision of imparting up-to-date information and advanced data in this field. To ensure the same, a matchless editorial board was set up. Every individual on the board went through rigorous rounds of assessment to prove their worth. After which they invested a large part of their time researching and compiling the most relevant data for our readers.

The editorial board has been involved in producing this book since its inception. They have spent rigorous hours researching and exploring the diverse topics which have resulted in the successful publishing of this book. They have passed on their knowledge of decades through this book. To expedite this challenging task, the publisher supported the team at every step. A small team of assistant editors was also appointed to further simplify the editing procedure and attain best results for the readers.

Apart from the editorial board, the designing team has also invested a significant amount of their time in understanding the subject and creating the most relevant covers. They scrutinized every image to scout for the most suitable representation of the subject and create an appropriate cover for the book.

The publishing team has been an ardent support to the editorial, designing and production team. Their endless efforts to recruit the best for this project, has resulted in the accomplishment of this book. They are a veteran in the field of academics and their pool of knowledge is as vast as their experience in printing. Their expertise and guidance has proved useful at every step. Their uncompromising quality standards have made this book an exceptional effort. Their encouragement from time to time has been an inspiration for everyone.

The publisher and the editorial board hope that this book will prove to be a valuable piece of knowledge for researchers, students, practitioners and scholars across the globe.

List of Contributors

Liang Shan
Department of Pharmacy, The Second People's Hospital of Hefei, Hefei Hospital Affiliated to Anhui Medical University, Hefei, China
Anhui Province Key Laboratory of Major Autoimmune Diseases, Anhui Medical University, Hefei, China
Inflammation and Immune Mediated Diseases Laboratory of Anhui Province, Hefei, China
The Key Laboratory of Major Autoimmune Diseases, Hefei, China

Fengling Wang, Dandan Zhai, Xiangyun Meng and Jianjun Liu
Department of Pharmacy, The Second People's Hospital of Hefei, Hefei Hospital Affiliated to Anhui Medical University, Hefei, China

Xiongwen Lv
Anhui Province Key Laboratory of Major Autoimmune Diseases, Anhui Medical University, Hefei, China
Inflammation and Immune Mediated Diseases Laboratory of Anhui Province, Hefei, China
The Key Laboratory of Major Autoimmune Diseases, Hefei, China

Wenzhang Dai
Senior Department of Hepatology, The Fifth Medical Center of Chinese PLA General Hospital, Beijing, China
School of Pharmacy, Hunan University of Chinese Medicine, Changsha, China

Qin Qin, Zhie Fang and Yanzhong Han
Senior Department of Hepatology, The Fifth Medical Center of Chinese PLA General Hospital, Beijing, China

Xiaohe Xiao
Senior Department of Hepatology, The Fifth Medical Center of Chinese PLA General Hospital, Beijing, China
School of Pharmacy, Hunan University of Chinese Medicine, Changsha, China
China Military Institute of Chinese Materia, The Fifth Medical Centre, Chinese PLA General Hospital, Beijing, China

Qing Liang, Meina Zhang, Yudi Hu, Yujie Chen, Pengxin Xue, Qiyuan Li and Kejia Wang
National Institute for Data Science in Health and Medicine, School of Medicine, Xiamen University, Xiamen, China

Wei Zhang
Department of Pathology, The 971 Hospital of People's Liberation Army Navy, Qingdao, China

Ping Zhu
Department of Gynecology and Obstetrics, The 971 Hospital of People's Liberation Army Navy, Qingdao, China

Yongqiang Ai, Wei Shi, Xiaobin Zuo, Xiaoming Sun, Yuanyuan Chen, Wenqing Mu, Kaixin Ding, Qiang Li, Jing Zhao, Zhi-e Fang, Lutong Ren, Tingting Liu, Ziying Wei, Wenqing Mou, Li Lin and Yan Yang
Department of Hepatology, The Fifth Medical Centre, Chinese PLA General Hospital, Beijing, China

Ruisheng Li
Research Center for Clinical and Translational Medicine, The Fifth Medical Center of Chinese PLA General Hospital, Beijing, China
Senior Department of Hepatology, The Fifth Medical Center of Chinese PLA General Hospital, Beijing, China

Xueai Song
China Military Institute of Chinese Materia, The Fifth Medical Centre, Chinese PLA General Hospital, Beijing, China

Xiaoyan Zhan and Zhaofang Bai
Department of Hepatology, The Fifth Medical Centre, Chinese PLA General Hospital, Beijing, China
China Military Institute of Chinese Materia, The Fifth Medical Centre, Chinese PLA General Hospital, Beijing, China

Florian Hamberger, Young Seon Mederacke, Richard Taubert and Ingmar Mederacke
Department of Gastroenterology, Hepatology and Endocrinology, Hannover Medical School, Hannover, Germany

Georg Hansmann, Ekaterina Legchenko and Philippe Chouvarine
Department of Pediatric Cardiology and Critical Care, Hannover Medical School, Hannover, Germany

Martin Meier
Laboratory Animal Science, Small Animal Imaging Center, Hannover Medical School, Hannover, Germany

Danny Jonigk
Institute of Pathology, Hannover Medical School, Hannover, Germany
Member of the German Center for Lung Research (DZL), Biomedical Research in Endstage and Obstructive Lung Disease Hannover (BREATH), Hannover, Germany

Tatiana Kisseleva
Department of Surgery, University of California, San Diego, La Jolla, CA, USA

David A. Brenner
Department of Medicine, University of California, San Diego, La Jolla, CA, USA

Shuang Liang
Department of Surgery, University of California, San Diego, La Jolla, CA, USA
Department of Medicine, University of California, San Diego, La Jolla, CA, USA

Joeri Lambrecht, Inge Mannaerts and Leo A. van Grunsven
Liver Cell Biology Lab, Department of Biomedical Sciences, Vrije Universiteit Brussel, Brussels, Belgium

Ya-Ru Yang
Department of Clinical Pharmacology, Second Hospital of Anhui Medical University, Hefei, China

Shuang Hu, Fang-Tian Bu, Hao Li, Cheng Huang, Xiao-Ming Meng, Lei Zhang, Xiong-Wen Lv and Jun Li
Inflammation and Immune Mediated Diseases Laboratory of Anhui Province, School of Pharmacy, Anhui Institute of Innovative Drugs, Anhui Medical University, Hefei, China
Institute for Liver Diseases of Anhui Medical University, Anhui Medical University, Hefei, China

Fa-Da Wang, Jing Zhou and En-Qiang Chen
Center of Infectious Diseases, West China Hospital, Sichuan University, Chengdu, China

Xiaoqi Nie
Department of Oncology, Tongji Hospital, Huazhong University of Science and Technology, Wuhan, China
Department of Dermatology, Tongji Hospital, Huazhong University of Science and Technology, Wuhan, China

Qianqian Yu, Long Li, Minxiao Yi, Bili Wu, Yongbiao Huang, Hu Han and Xianglin Yuan
Department of Oncology, Tongji Hospital, Huazhong University of Science and Technology, Wuhan, China

Yonghui Zhang
School of Pharmacy, Tongji Medical College, Huazhong University of Science and Technology, Wuhan, China

Chen Chen, Lingbiao Wang, Sen Yang, Wenjing Ye, Minrui Liang and Hejian Zou
Department of Rheumatology, Huashan Hospital, Fudan University, Shanghai, China
Institute of Rheumatology, Immunology and Allergy, Fudan University, Shanghai, China

Jinfeng Wu
Department of Dermatology, Huashan Hospital, Fudan University, Shanghai, China

Meijuan Lu and Ming Guan
Department of Laboratory Medicine, Huashan Hospital, Fudan University, Shanghai, China

Jing Xie, Yuzhou Ding, Bingyan Liu, Zhonghuan Shao, Yuanyuan Liu and Yunqiu Xie
National Drug Clinical Trial Center, The First Affiliated Hospital of Bengbu Medical College, Bengbu, China

Huan Zhou
National Drug Clinical Trial Center, The First Affiliated Hospital of Bengbu Medical College, Bengbu, China
School of Pharmacy, Bengbu Medical College, Bengbu, China
School of Public Foundation, Bengbu Medical University, Bengbu, China

Xingyu Zhu, Minhui Zhu, Cuixia He, Yuanyuan Xu, Rongfang Shan, Ying Wang and Xiangdi Zhao
National Drug Clinical Trial Center, The First Affiliated Hospital of Bengbu Medical College, Bengbu, China
School of Pharmacy, Bengbu Medical College, Bengbu, China

Yue Su and Jiaxiang Ding
National Drug Clinical Trial Center, The First Affiliated Hospital of Bengbu Medical College, Bengbu, China
School of Public Foundation, Bengbu Medical University, Bengbu, China

Yan Yao and Tao Xu
Inflammation and Immune Mediated Diseases Laboratory of Anhui Province, Anhui Institute of Innovative Drugs, School of Pharmacy, Anhui Medical University, Hefei, China

Yifan Ren
National Local Joint Engineering Research Center for Precision Surgery and Regenerative Medicine, Shaanxi Provincial Center for Regenerative Medicine and Surgical Engineering, First Affiliated Hospital of

Xi'an Jiaotong University, Xi'an, China
Department of General Surgery, The Second Affiliated Hospital of Xi'an Jiaotong University, Xi'an, China

Rongqian Wu
National Local Joint Engineering Research Center for Precision Surgery and Regenerative Medicine, Shaanxi Provincial Center for Regenerative Medicine and Surgical Engineering, First Affiliated Hospital of Xi'an Jiaotong University, Xi'an, China

Meng Xu
Department of General Surgery, The Second Affiliated Hospital of Xi'an Jiaotong University, Xi'an, China

Qing Cui
Department of Cardiology, Xi'an Central Hospital, Xi'an, China

Jia Zhang, Wuming Liu and Yi Lv
National Local Joint Engineering Research Center for Precision Surgery and Regenerative Medicine, Shaanxi Provincial Center for Regenerative Medicine and Surgical Engineering, First Affiliated Hospital of Xi'an Jiaotong University, Xi'an, China
Department of Hepatobiliary Surgery, First Affiliated Hospital of Xi'an Jiaotong University, Xi'an, China

Zheng Wu
Department of Hepatobiliary Surgery, First Affiliated Hospital of Xi'an Jiaotong University, Xi'an, China

Yuanyuan Zhang
Department of Department of Pediatrics, First Affiliated Hospital of Xi'an Jiaotong University, Xi'an, China

Zhiyong Li
School of Pharmacy, Chengdu University of Traditional Chinese Medicine, Chengdu, China
Department of Hepatology, Fifth Medical Center of Chinese PLA General Hospital, Beijing, China

Zhilei Wang
TCM Regulating Metabolic Diseases Key Laboratory of Sichuan Province, Hospital of Chengdu University of Traditional Chinese Medicine, Chengdu, China
Department of Hepatology, The Fifth Medical Centre, Chinese PLA General Hospital, Beijing, China

Fang Dong
School of Public Health and Health Management, Shandong First Medical University and Shandong Academy of Medical Sciences, Shandong, China

Li Ma
School of Traditional Chinese Medicine, Capital Medical University, Beijing, China

Tian-Yu Zhao, Qing-Wei Cong, Fang Liu, Li-Ying Yao and Ying Zhu
Liver Disease Center of Integrated Traditional Chinese and Western Medicine, The First Affiliated Hospital of Dalian Medical University, Dalian, China

Zhifa Wang
Department of Rehabilitation Medicine, Chaohu Hospital of Anhui Medical University, Hefei Anhui, China

Xiaoke Yang
Department of Rheumatology and Immunology, The First Affiliated Hospital of Anhui Medical University, Hefei, China

Siyu Gui
Department of Ophthalmology, The Second Affiliated Hospital of Anhui Medical University, Hefei, China

Fan Yang and Zhuo Cao
The First Clinical Medical College, Anhui Medical University, Hefei, China

Rong Cheng, Xiaowei Xia and Chuanying Li
Department of Gastroenterology, Anhui Provincial Children's Hospital, Hefei, China

Chaofeng Li, Mingshuang Wang, Zhiqi Li, Yang Chen, Dan Feng, Zhaoyi Wang, Qiqi Fan, Meilin Chen, Ruichao Lin and Chongjun Zhao
Beijing Key Lab for Quality Evaluation of Chinese Materia Medica, School of Chinese Materia Medica, Beijing University of Chinese Medicine, Beijing, China

Tao He, Tingting Fu and Honggui Zhang
School of Chinese Materia Medica, Beijing University of Chinese Medicine, Beijing, China

Zhen-Yu Cui, Yu-Chen Jiang, Jia-Yi Dou, Kun-Chen Yao, Zhong-He Hu, Ming-Hui Yuan, Xiao-Xue Bao, Mei-Jie Zhou, Yue Liu, Li-Hua Lian and Yan-Ling Wu
Key Laboratory for Traditional Chinese Korean Medicine of Jilin Province, College of Pharmacy, Yanbian University, Yanji, China

Xin Han
Chinese Medicine Processing Centre, College of Pharmacy, Zhejiang Chinese Medical University, Hangzhou, China

Xian Zhang
Agricultural College, Yanbian University, Yanji, China

Ji-Xing Nan
Key Laboratory for Traditional Chinese Korean Medicine of Jilin Province, College of Pharmacy, Yanbian University, Yanji, China
Clinical Research Center, Affiliated Hospital of Yanbian University, Yanji, China

Yu-long Bao, Li Wang, Hai-ting Pan and Tai-ran Zhang
College of Basic Medicine, Inner Mongolia Medical University, Hohhot, China

Ya-hong Chen
Health Management Center, Taizhou Hospital of Zhejiang Province Affiliated to Wenzhou Medical University, Linhai, China

Shan-jing Xu
School of Medicine, Shaoxing University, Shaoxing, Chian

Xin-li Mao
School of Medicine, Shaoxing University, Shaoxing, Chian
Key Laboratory of Minimally Invasive Techniques & Rapid Rehabilitation of Digestive System Tumor, Taizhou Hospital of Zhejiang Province Affiliated to Wenzhou Medical University, Linhai, China
Department of Gastroenterology, Taizhou Hospital of Zhejiang Province Affiliated to Wenzhou Medical University, Linhai, China

Shao-wei Li
Key Laboratory of Minimally Invasive Techniques & Rapid Rehabilitation of Digestive System Tumor, Taizhou Hospital of Zhejiang Province Affiliated to Wenzhou Medical University, Linhai, China
Department of Gastroenterology, Taizhou Hospital of Zhejiang Province Affiliated to Wenzhou Medical University, Linhai, China

Index

Printed in the USA
CPSIA information can be obtained
at www.ICGtesting.com
JSHW062236071123
51533JS00031B/77